# Evidence-Based Procedural Dermatology

Murad Alam

Editor

# Evidence-Based
# Procedural Dermatology

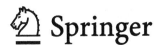 Springer

*Editor*
Murad Alam, MD, MSCI
Chief, Section of Cutaneous and Aesthetic Surgery
Professor, Departments of Dermatology, Otolaryngology, and Surgery
Feinberg School of Med, Northwestern University
Chicago, IL, USA

ISBN 978-0-387-09423-6    e-ISBN 978-0-387-09424-3
DOI 10.1007/978-0-387-09424-3
Springer New York Dordrecht Heidelberg London

Library of Congress Control Number: 2011938458

Printed on acid-free paper

Springer is part of Springer Science+Business Media (www.springer.com)

# Preface

Procedural dermatology is an old profession. Documented, well-described skin modification methods date from the ancient Egyptian, Indian, and Greek periods. Early practitioners no doubt carefully observed their outcomes and honed their techniques to improve results. Modern dermatologists use a similar approach. What has changed is the formalization of the steps for evaluating safety and efficacy of operative procedures. Experience and good technical skills remain important, but self-confidence is no longer enough to convince others of the validity of a particular approach.

Evidence-based medicine, a term coined by Sackett et al. as recently as the 1980s, was initially defined as "the conscientious, explicit, and judicious use of the best evidence in making decisions about the care of individual patients [1]." Evidence-based dermatology already has textbooks, including a fine eponymous second edition crafted by Williams, Bigby, Diepgen, Herxheimer, Naldi, and Rzany, and another similarly entitled volume by Maibach, Bashir, and McKibbon. In addition, there is the user-friendly ebderm.org web site, created and maintained by Barzilai.

This is the first evidence-based textbook for procedural dermatology. Unlike prior evidence-based dermatology texts, which have included excellent chapters on procedural dermatology, the purpose of the present volume is not to focus on procedural topics of special importance, or those for which there is abundant evidence. Rather, we cover the spectrum of procedural dermatology, from skin cancer surgery to laser techniques, from minor cosmetic injections to major cosmetic surgery, and all the way to emergent procedures of as yet uncertain utility. The evidence for some of these may be limited, murky, or even absent. However, it is our conviction that more and better evidence cannot be accumulated unless the starting point in every area is well-characterized.

So, the purpose of this volume is twofold. First, it should be of practical value to dermatologists who are treating or counseling patients. Second, it may help those proceduralists who are designing new studies to collect further evidence.

Finally, some notes on nomenclature. Since 2003, the Accreditation Council of Graduate Medical Education (ACGME) in the United States has recognized "procedural dermatology" as the subspecialty concerned with surgical treatment of diseases of the skin and subcutaneous tissues, with the three principal areas being cutaneous oncologic surgery, cutaneous reconstructive surgery, and cutaneous cosmetic surgery. Beyond dermatology residency, 12-month fellowship training in procedural dermatology is overseen by the ACGME. Hence the title of this book. To preclude inaccurate value judgments, we have avoided the qualifiers "aesthetic" or "cosmetic" in the chapter titles. For instance, reconstruction after cancer can be as cosmetically important as repair of photoaging; similarly, so-called cosmetic procedures can be used to treat medical disease and traumatic scarring.

Chicago, IL                                          Murad Alam, MD, MSCI

## Reference

1. McLeod RS. Evidence-based surgery. In: Norton JA, et al., editors. Surgery: basic science and clinical evidence. 2nd ed. New York: Springer; 2008. p. 21–35.

# Acknowledgments

Many thanks to the staff at Springer for making this book possible. Brian Belval first approached us with the idea, and Catherine Paduani and Shelley Reinhardt have been kind in seeing this project to its completion. We also thank Natalie Kim and Natalie Pace for the careful administrative work to see this through to completion. Finally, we are indebted to the chapter authors, expert surgeons all, who took the time to write and review the very stylized and technical articles required for this volume.

# Contents

# Levels of Evidence

There are many different methods for grading level of evidence. The chapter contributors in this volume have been encouraged to use the following two classification schemes [1]

| Level | Type of evidence |
|-------|------------------|
| I | Evidence from systematic review or meta-analysis of randomized controlled trials |
| II | Evidence from at least one randomized controlled trial |
| III | Evidence from at least one well-designed controlled study without randomization (e.g., cohort study) |
| IV | Evidence from at least one other type of well-designed quasi-experimental study (e.g., case-control study) |
| V | Evidence from well-designed nonexperimental descriptive studies (comparative, correlation, or case studies) |
| VI | Evidence from expert committee reports or opinions, and/or clinical experience of respected authorities |

| Level | Grade of evidence |
|-------|-------------------|
| A | At least one randomized controlled trial as part of a body of literature of overall good quality and consistency addressing the specific recommendation (evidence levels I, II) |
| B | Well-conducted clinical studies but no randomized clinical trials on the topic of recommendation (evidence III, IV, and V) |
| C | Indicates that directly applicable clinical studies of good quality are absent (evidence level VI) |

Please note that the two grading systems are similar, but slightly different and overlapping.

In the text, tables, and summary boxes, study citations are followed by a pair of grades, one from each system above, in bold and in parentheses.

For example:
The study discussed in Smith et al. [2] (II/A).

For example:

| Findings | Evidence level |
|---|---|
| Patients should be… | II/A |
| Patients with ethnic skin should… | VI/C |
| Etc. | |

# Reference

1. Stone C, editor. The evidence for plastic surgery. Shrewsbury: TFM Publishing; 2008.

# Contributors

**Murad Alam, MD, MSCI** Department of Dermatology, Northwestern University, Chicago, IL, USA

Section of Cutaneous and Aesthetic Surgery, Feinberg School of Medicine, Northwestern University, Chicago, IL, USA

**Kenneth A. Arndt, MD** SkinCare Physicians, Chestnut Hill, MA, USA

Section of Dermatologic Surgery and Cutaneous Oncology, Yale University School of Medicine, New Haven, CT, USA

Dartmouth Medical School, Hanover, NH, USA

**Nidhi Avashia, MD** Department of Dermatology and Cutaneous Surgery, University of Miami Miller School of Medicine, Miami, FL, USA

**Marc R. Avram, MD** Department of Dermatology, New York Presbyterian Hospital, Weill Cornell Medical College, New York, NY, USA

**Ashish C. Bhatia, MD, FAAD** Department of Dermatology, Feinberg School of Medicine, Northwestern University, Chicago, IL, USA

The Dermatology Institute of DuPage Medical Group, Naperville, IL, USA

**Christopher K. Bichakjian, MD** Department of Dermatology, Cutaneous Surgery and Oncology, University of Michigan, Alfred Taubman Center, Ann Arbor, MI, USA

**Kenneth Beer, MD, PA** Esthetic Surgical and General Dermatology, West Palm Beach, FL, USA

**Anjali Butani, MD** Butani Dermatology, Orange, CA, USA

**Rawat Charoensawad, MD** Department of Dermatology, Suphannahong Dermatology Institute, Prathmuwan, Lumpinee, Thailand

**David H. Ciocon, MD** Division of Dermatology, Albert Einstein College of Medicine, Yeshiva University, Bronx, NY, USA

**Murray A. Cotter, MD, PhD** Dermatologic Surgery and Laser Center, University of California, San Francisco, CA, USA

Dermatology Associates of Northern Michigan, Petoskey, MI, USA

**Shraddha Desai, MD** Division of Dermatology, Loyola University - Stritch School of Medicine, Maywood, IL, USA

**Jeffrey S. Dover, MD, FRCPC** SkinCare Physicians, Chestnut Hill, MA, USA

Section of Dermatologic Surgery and Cutaneous Oncology, Yale University School of Medicine, New Haven, CT, USA

Dartmouth Medical School, Hanover, NH, USA

**Zoe Diana Draelos, MD** Department of Dermatology, Duke University School of Medicine, High Point, NC, USA

**Mohamed L. ElSaie, MD, MBA** Department of Dermatology and Cutaneous Surgery, University of Miami Miller School of Medicine, Miami, FL, USA

**Douglas Fife, MD, FAAD, FACMS** Surgical Dermatology & Laser Center, Las Vegas, NV, USA

**Bahar Firoz, MD, MPH** Department of Dermatology, University of Texas Health Science Center, San Antonio, TX, USA

**Hayes Gladstone, MD** Division of Dermatologic Surgery, Department of Dermatology, Stanford University, Redwood City, CA, USA

**Elizabeth Grossman, MD** Department of Dermatology, Northwestern University, Chicago, IL, USA

**Monica L. Halem, MD** Department of Dermatology, Columbia University Medical Center/New York Presbyterian Hospital, Dermatologic Surgery Unit, New York, NY, USA

**Conway C. Huang, MD** Department of Dermatology, University of Alabama at Birmingham, Birmingham, AL, USA

**Ali Jabbari, MD** Ronald O. Perelman Department of Dermatology, NYU Medical Center, New York, NY, USA

**Misbah H. Khan, MD, FAAD** Department of Dermatology, Weill Cornell Medical Center, New York, NY, USA

**Darius J. Karimipour, MD** Department of Dermatology, University of Michigan Hospitals, Ann Arbor, MI, USA

**Arash Kimyai-Asadi, MD** Dermsurgery Associates, Houston, TX, USA

**Joy H. Kunishige, MD** Zitelli & Brodland Skin Cancer Center, Pittsburgh, PA, USA

Northwest Dermatology, Hoffman Estates, IL, USA

**Brenda LaTowsky, MD, PLC** Skin Care Physicians, Chestnut Hill, MA, USA

Paradise Valley Dermatology, Phoenix, AZ, USA

**Naomi Lawrence, MD** Division of Dermatologic Surgery,
Cooper University Hospital, Marlton, NJ, USA

**Erica H. Lee, MD** Department of Dermatology Service,
Memorial Sloan-Kettering Cancer Center, New York, NY, USA

Department of Dermatology, New York University Medical Center,
New York, NY, USA

**Vicki J. Levine, MD, FAAD** Department of Dermatology,
New York University Medical Center, New York, NY, USA

**Alan L. Levy, MD** Division of Dermatology, Department of Medicine,
Vanderbilt University, One Hundred Oaks, Nashville, TN, USA

**Su Luo, MD** Department of Dermatology and Cutaneous Surgery,
University of Miami Miller School of Medicine, Miami, FL, USA

**Jennifer L. MacGregor, MD** SkinCare Physicians, Chestnut Hill, MA, USA

Division of Dermatology, Georgetown University Hospital,
Washington, DC, USA

**Gabriel J. Martinez-Diaz, MD** Department of Dermatology,
University of Pittsburgh, Pittsburgh, PA, USA

**Shivani Nanda, MD** Feinberg School of Medicine,
Northwestern University, Chicago, IL, USA

**Alexander Nast, MD** Division of Evidence Based Medicine (dEBM),
Klinik für Dermatologie, Charité – Universitätsmedizin, Berlin, Germany

**Kishwer S. Nehal, MD** Department of Dermatology Service,
Memorial Sloan-Kettering Cancer Center, New York, NY, USA

**Shari A. Nemeth, MD, MS** Department of Dermatology,
Mayo Clinic Arizona, Scottsdale, AZ, USA

Division of Dermatologic Surgery, Cooper University Hospital,
Marlton, NJ, USA

**Isaac M. Neuhaus, MD** Dermatologic Surgery and Laser Center,
University of California, San Francisco, CA, USA

**Keyvan Nouri, MD** Department of Dermatology and Cutaneous Surgery,
University of Miami Miller School of Medicine, Miami, FL, USA

**Asha Patel** Department of Dermatology, Columbia University Medical
Center/New York Presbyterian Hospital, Dermatologic Surgery Unit,
New York, NY, USA

**Désirée Ratner, MD** Department of Dermatology, Columbia University
Medical Center/New York Presbyterian Hospital, Dermatologic Surgery Unit,
New York, NY, USA

**Babar K. Rao, MD** Department of Dermatology, Robert-Wood
Johnson University Hospital, University of Medicine and Dentistry
New Jersey, New Brunswick, NJ, USA

**Nicole E. Rogers, MD, FAAD** Department of Dermatology,
Tulane University School of Medicine, Old Metairie Dermatology,
Metairie, LA, USA

**Berthold Rzany, MD** Division of Evidence Based Medicine (dEBM),
Klinik für Dermatologie, Charité – Universitätsmedizin Berlin, Germany

**Neil S. Sadick, MD** Weil Medical College, Cornell University, New York,
NY, USA

**Roberta D. Sengelmann, MD, FAAD** Santa Barbara, CA, USA

Department of Dermatology, University of California, Irvine, CA, USA

**John Starling III, MD** Department of Dermatology, University
of Michigan Hospitals, Ann Arbor, MI, USA

Dermatology Associates of Wisconsin, S.C., Oshkosh, WI, USA

**Thomas Stasko, MD, FAAD, FACMS** Division of Dermatology,
Department of Medicine, Vanderbilt University, One Hundred Oaks,
Nashville, TN, USA

**Jane Unaeze, MD** Division of Dermatology, Albert Einstein College
of Medicine, Yeshiva University, Bronx, NY, USA

**Voraphol Vejjabhinanta, MD** Department of Dermatology,
Siriraj Hospital, Bangkoknoi, Bangkok, Thailand

**Yue (Emily) Yu, MD, PhD** Department of Dermatology, Boston University
School of Medicine, Boston, MA, USA

**Siegrid S. Yu, MD** Dermatologic Surgery and Laser Center,
University of California, San Francisco, CA, USA

**John A. Zitelli, MD** Department of Dermatology, University of Pittsburgh
Medical Center, Pittsburgh, PA, USA

# Mohs Surgery

### Alan L. Levy and Thomas Stasko

## Introduction

In the early 1940s, Dr. Frederic Mohs first published a technique for the removal of skin cancers utilizing in vivo tissue fixation by the application of a zinc chloride paste directly to the skin, followed by excision and specimen mounting for histologic evaluation the next day. The procedure was based on the principles that cutaneous malignancies grow in a contiguous manner from a central origin and complete removal is necessary and sufficient for tumor local tumor control. Since that time the practice of Mohs micrographic surgery (MMS) has evolved into the fresh tissue technique with frozen sections. This procedure omits fixation of the tissue in situ prior to excision and rapidly processes the tissue after excision using an embedding medium and a cryostat to freeze and section the specimen prior to histologic staining. MMS is divided into two phases: surgery and pathology. There are great variations in technique among Mohs surgeons regarding tumor debulking, the removal of layers and the marking of specimens. The common elements for all Mohs procedures include a clinical delineation of tumor margins, removal of the clinical tumor with 1–3 mm margins with a disc or saucer shape, marking of the tumor bed to allow correlation of the surgical site with the excised specimen, and mapping of the specimen. During mapping, the tissue is cut into appropriate pieces and the edges are dyed with different colored inks to identify individual margins. The colors are coded to the corresponding edges on the tissue map. In the pathology phase of the procedure, the tissue is embedded in an appropriate medium in a manner that places the skin edge and the deep/central portion of the specimen in the same plane. The embedded tissue is frozen and sectioned on a cryostat in 2–6 μm sections. Once sections are mounted they are stained with either hematoxylin and eosin or toluidine blue based on the tumor type and the preference of the surgeon. The sectioning and staining process takes 15–45 min depending on variables such as tissue size, lab volume, and histotechnician technique. After slide preparation, the surgeon becomes the pathologist and examines the slides for the presence of tumor. With the Mohs procedure, the physician can examine the complete deep and peripheral margins of the tissue for the presence of residual tumor. Positive tumor is marked in the appropriate area on the map that is taken back to the bedside where the surgery phase resumes. Using the shape of the defect and the markings made in the wound edges, the area of residual tumor is outlined along with an appropriate margin. The process is repeated until histologically clear deep and peripheral margins are verified. Reconstruction of the surgical defect may follow clearance of the tumor with the Mohs procedure or the wound may be allowed to heal by second intention (Fig. 1.1).

A.L. Levy • T. Stasko (✉)
Division of Dermatology, Department of Medicine,
Vanderbilt University, One Hundred Oaks, 719 Thompson
Lane, Suite 26300, Nashville, TN 37204, USA
e-mail: tom.stasko@vanderbilt.edu

M. Alam (ed.), *Evidence-Based Procedural Dermatology*,
DOI 10.1007/978-0-387-09424-3_1, © Springer Science+Business Media, LLC 2012

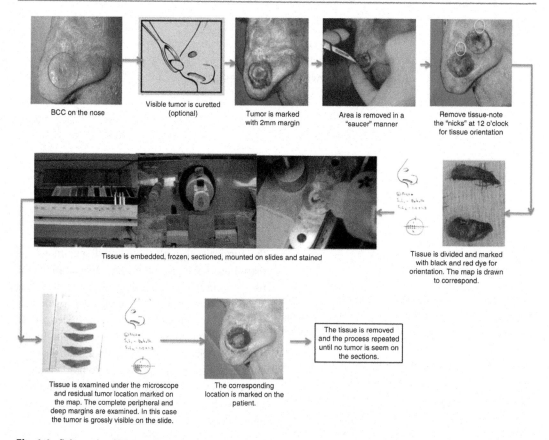

BCC on the nose

Visible tumor is curetted (optional)

Tumor is marked with 2mm margin

Area is removed in a "saucer" manner

Remove tissue-note the "nicks" at 12 o'clock for tissue orientation

Tissue is embedded, frozen, sectioned, mounted on slides and stained

Tissue is divided and marked with black and red dye for orientation. The map is drawn to correspond.

Tissue is examined under the microscope and residual tumor location marked on the map. The complete peripheral and deep margins are examined. In this case the tumor is grossly visible on the slide.

The corresponding location is marked on the patient.

The tissue is removed and the process repeated until no tumor is seem on the sections.

**Fig. 1.1** Schematic of Mohs micrographic surgery

## Mohs Micrographic Surgery for Basal Cell Carcinoma and Squamous Cell Carcinoma

### Consensus Documents

#### American Academy of Dermatology

The American Academy of Dermatology (AAD) officially calls the procedure MMS instead of its many synonyms such as chemosurgery, fixed tissue technique, fresh tissue technique, microscopically controlled surgery, Mohs histographic surgery, or Mohs technique. According to the organization's website (www.aad.org), MMS offers a very high cure rate and is used for large or aggressive tumors and tumors in areas at high risk for recurrence. "Guidelines of care for Mohs micrographic surgery" produced by the Guidelines/Outcomes Committee of the AAD in 1995 [1] defines Mohs surgery as a "surgical method for the removal of tissue including certain neoplasms [that] have high potential for cure with maximal preservation of normal tissue." The goal of MMS is complete tumor removal with maximal preservation of normal tissue. The AAD recognizes the number of well-accepted surgical and nonsurgical modalities for the treatment of skin cancer, and advises consideration for the type of lesion, lesion history, and patient's general medical history and risk factors and that MMS is "not indicated for the treatment of all skin tumors." Table 1.1 lists indications for cutaneous malignancies.

**Table 1.1** Indications for MMS as set forth by the AAD Guidelines in 1995 [1]

| Basal cell carcinoma | Squamous cell carcinoma | Melanoma | Other neoplasms |
|---|---|---|---|
| High risk for recurrence | High risk for recurrence | Data are accumulating | Ill-defined |
| Ill-defined or field-fire type | Ill-defined | supporting efficacy of | Subclinic extension |
| Anatomic location | Anatomic location | narrow surgical margins | Examples |
| History of incomplete | History of incomplete | using MMS for certain | Verrucous carcinoma |
| excision | excision | types/locations | Keratocanthomas |
| Prior radiation therapy | Prior radiation therapy | | (aggressive, recurrent, |
| History of recurrence | Large size | | or mutilating) |
| Large size | Perineural or | | Dermatofibrosarcoma |
| Histologic pattern | perivascular involvement | | protuberans |
| | Anaplastic histology | | Atypical fibroxanthoma |
| | Deep tissue or bone | | Malignant fibrous |
| | involvement' | | histiocytoma |
| | | | Leiomyosarcoma |
| Need for tissue preservation | Need for tissue | | Adenocystic carcinoma of |
| | preservation | | the skin |
| Rapid growth/aggressive | Rapid growth/aggressive | | Sebaceous carcinoma |
| behavior | behavior | | Extramammary Paget's disease |
| Immunosuppression | Immunosuppression | | Erythroplasia of Queyrat |
| | High risk for metastasis | | Oral and central facial |
| | Long-standing duration | | paranasal sinus neoplasms |
| | Certain genodermatoses | | Microcystic adnexal |
| | | | carcinoma |
| | | | Merkel cell carcinoma |
| | | | Apocrine carcinoma of the skin |
| | | | Aggressive or locally |
| | | | recurrent benign tumors |

## British Association of Dermatologists

In 1999, Telfer et al. [2] (III/B) established guidelines for the treatment of BCC by MMS. Five criteria based on level of evidence A/IIi (defined as "good evidence to support the use of the procedure obtained from well-designed controlled trials without randomization") were established as indications for MMS: high-risk site (eyes, ears, lips, nose, and nasolabial folds), aggressive histological subtype (morpheaform, infiltrative, and micronodular), recurrent BCCs, size >2 cm especially in high-risk sites, and tumors with perineural involvement.

## National Comprehensive Cancer Network (VI/B)

Within the 2011 Clinical Practice Guidelines in Oncology [3], the National Comprehensive Cancer Network (NCCN), a global alliance of cancer specialists at 21 centers, maintains that the goal of primary treatment of skin cancer is cure along

**Table 1.2** NCCN categories of evidence and consensus

| |
|---|
| Category 1: Uniform NCCN consensus, based on high-level evidence |
| Category 2A: Uniform NCCN consensus, based on lower-level evidence including clinical experience |
| Category 2B: Nonuniform NCCN consensus (but no major disagreement), based on lower-level evidence including clinical experience |
| Category 3: Major NCCN disagreement over the appropriateness of the recommendation |

From 2011 Clinical Practice Guidelines in Oncology, The National Comprehensive Cancer Network (NCCN) [3]

with maximal maintenance of function and cosmetic outcome. NCCN guideline evidence levels are shown in Table 1.2. All recommendations are category 2A, except as noted. Surgical modalities "offer the most effective and efficient means for accomplishing cure," but optimal results include considerations of function, cosmesis, and patient preference. For nonmelanoma skin cancer, the NCCN distinguishes between low- and high-risk

**Table 1.3** Low- and high-risk features for BCC and SCC

|  | Low risk | High risk[a] |
| --- | --- | --- |
| **Basal cell carcinoma** |  |  |
| Location and size | Trunk, extremities < 20 mm | Trunk, extremities ≥ 20 mm |
|  | Cheeks, forehead, scalp, and neck < 10 mm | Cheeks, forehead, scalp, and neck ≥ 10 mm |
|  | Mask area of face, chin, mandible, preauricular/postauricular areas, genitalia, hands, and feet < 6 mm | Mask area of face, chin, mandible, preauricular/postauricular areas, genitalia, hands, and feet ≥ 6 mm |
| Borders | Well-defined | Poorly defined |
| Primary vs. recurrent | Primary | Recurrent |
| Immunosuppression | No | Yes |
| Site of prior radiation | No | Yes |
| Histologic subtype | Nodular, superficial | Morpheaform, sclerosing, mixed infiltrative, or micronodular features in any portion |
| **Squamous cell carcinoma** |  |  |
| Location and size | Trunk, extremities < 20 mm | Trunk, extremities ≥ 20 mm |
|  | Cheeks, forehead, scalp, and neck < 10 mm | Cheeks, forehead, scalp, and neck ≥ 10 mm |
|  | Mask area of face, chin, mandible, preauricular/postauricular areas, genitalia, hands, and feet < 6 mm | Mask area of face, chin, mandible, preauricular/postauricular areas, genitalia, hands, and feet ≥ 6 mm |
| Borders | Well-defined | Poorly defined |
| Primary vs. recurrent | Primary | Recurrent |
| Immunosuppression | No | Yes |
| Site of prior radiation | No | Yes |
| Site of chronic inflammation | No | Yes |
| Rapid growth | No | Yes |
| Neurologic symptoms | No | Yes |
| Histologic maturity | Well-differentiated | Moderately or poorly differentiated |
| Histologic subtype | Nonaggressive (e.g., keratoacanthoma type, verrucous carcinoma) | Acantholytic, adenosquamous, or desmoplastic |
| Modified Breslow depth[b] | <4 mm | ≥4 mm |
| Perineural or vascular involvement | No | Yes |

Adapted from the 2011 NCCN Clinical Practice Guidelines in Oncology™ [3]
[a]Any high-risk factor places the patient in the high-risk category
[b]Exclude parakeratosis or scale/crust or from base of ulcer if present

tumors based on several parameters outlined in Table 1.3. In low-risk BCC, MMS is indicated after positive margins are found on excision with postoperative margin assessment. Equally acceptable treatment, however, is re-excision for tumors on the trunk or extremities or radiation therapy. MMS is indicated for all high-risk BCC in surgical candidates. Local excision is acceptable for large (≥20 mm) lesions on the trunk or extremities if no other high-risk factors are present and if 10 mm surgical margins are functionally and cosmetically feasible.

Recommendations for low-risk squamous cell carcinoma are similar to low-risk BCC provided 4–6 mm clinical margins can be taken around the lesion during excision. If margins are positive after excision, MMS is indicated for all lesions. Another option is excision with complete circumferential peripheral and deep margin assessment (CCPDMA) with permanent or frozen section. Repeat excision with routine margin assessment is only advisable for low-risk lesions on the trunk or extremities. For high-risk SCC, MMS is the treatment of choice for surgical candidates. As in the case of high-risk BCC, local excision is appropriate for large (≥20 mm) lesions on the trunk or extremities if excision with 10 mm clinical margins is possible. In both BCC and SCC, if margins are persistently positive, MMS is indicated. For very aggressive or extensive malignancies, MMS may fail to clear the tumor due to bone involvement or danger to a vital structure. Other cases may be cleared with MMS, yet extensive perineural or large-nerve involvement is revealed on examination. In these cases, adjuvant radiation therapy is recommended. Radiation therapy can be used as primary therapy for all BCCs and SCCs in nonsurgical candidates over 60 years old (category 2B evidence).

High-risk patients who include organ transplant recipients, immunosuppressed patients (HIV, drug-induced, lymphoma/leukemia), those with xeroderma pigmentosa, and long-term PUVA exposure should be treated as having high-risk nonmelanoma skin cancer and MMS is a treatment options for tumors in these patients. Since these patients frequently have multiple tumors, many of which are low-risk, other destructive modalities (cryosurgery, electrodessication and curretage, or photodynamic therapy) may be appropriately employed (category 2A evidence). Surgery in immunosuppressed patients with multiple adjacent tumors and carcinoma, in situ, may be limited to removal of invasive malignancies and topical or destructive modalities utilized for in situ disease. In cases where this "field effect" is significant, the surgeon should limit tissue rearrangement as much as possible.

According to the NCCN guidelines, excision of cutaneous malignancy accompanied by complete deep and peripheral margin assessment is recommended for all high-risk tumors. Tumor resection can be accomplished by either MMS or standard surgical excision. According to the NCCN, however, "…intra-operative frozen section assessment is not acceptable as an alternative to MMS unless it includes a complete assessment of all deep and peripheral margins. The descriptive term complete CCPDMA underscores the panel's belief that intraoperative assessment of all tissue margins is the key to complete tumor removal. MMS is preferred because of its documented efficacy."

## American College of Mohs Surgeons (ACMS)

Consensus documentation from the American College of Mohs Surgery (http://www.mohscollege.org) reports, MMS offers the highest success rate of all treatments for skin cancer and is the treatment of choice for cancers of the face and other sensitive areas as it offers complete removal of the malignancy with maximal sparing of the normal tissue. The report cites clinical studies conducted at the Mayo Clinic [4], the University of Miami School of Medicine [5], and Royal Perth Hospital in Australia [6] which demonstrate that MMS provides 5 year cure rates exceeding 99% for new cancers, and 95% for recurrent cancers. The American College of Mohs Surgeons (ACMS) describes their members as physicians who have undergone 1–2 years of fellowship training after dermatology residency in a Mohs College approved program. The procedure is referred to as "the most advanced and effective treatment procedure for skin cancer available today."

Specifically, MMS is recommended when the tumor involves cosmetically and functionally sensitive areas such as the eyelids, nose, ears, lips, fingers, toes, and genitalia. It is also appropriate for recurrent tumors, tumors occurring in or around scar tissue, and neoplasms that are large, ill-defined, of a histologically aggressive subtype, or rapidly and uncontrollably growing. The ACMS addresses cost as one of the major criticisms of the procedure and the resultant expense to the healthcare system with the rising incidence of skin cancers. Two studies are cited, both from Archives of Dermatology [7, 8], that show MMS is not more expensive than standard excision and actually less costly than radiation therapy or excision in ambulatory surgery centers (IV/B). Because MMS maximizes margin control and minimizes the risk of recurrence, an argument is made for long-term healthcare savings by elimination of larger, more complex surgery for recurrent skin cancers.

## Reviews

Lang and Osguthorpe [9] (V/B) reviewed the indications and limitations of MMS and its role in a multidisciplinary approach to skin cancer treatment. The general indications are based on previous retrospective systematic reviews, literature reviews, and case series and are categorized by location, clinical features, and histologic features. Indications based on location include tumors in embryonic fusion planes, in anatomic areas associated with a high risk for recurrence, and in anatomic areas where maximal preservation of tissue is mandatory (e.g., H-zone of the face, digits, and anogenital area). Clinical indications are large tumors, recurrent tumors, ill-defined tumors, and "field-fire" basal cell carcinomas. Histological indications include morpheaform and metatypical basal cell carcinoma, deeply penetrating tumors, incompletely excised tumors, tumors with an aggressive growth pattern (infiltrating, micronodular, and macronodular with "spikey" projections), and tumors with perineural involvement. All of these indications have in common the potential for extensive subclinical spread and therefore can benefit from the complete margin analysis afforded by MMS. The authors discuss the multiple advantages (maximal cure rate and preservation of tissue and the ability to extend surgical extirpation to patients at high risk for complications after general anesthesia) and the disadvantages (increased cost if used to treat inappropriate cases, patient exhaustion if prolonged, and requires special training for physician and ancillary staff) of MMS. Specific limitations and implied contraindications are discussed as well. It may not be advisable to use MMS as primary therapy or monotherapy for tumors at high risk for metastatic disease, those with disconnected tumor foci or multicentricity, cases where there are difficulties distinguishing malignant findings from normal anatomy on pathology, and excessively large tumors that may result in mutilation. In these cases, other treatment modalities and/or adjunctive therapy with radiotherapy or retinoids are advocated for optimal outcome. The authors conclude that, in considering the employment of MMS to treat a cutaneous malignancy, the physician must consider its location, histology, size, and history of and tendency for recurrence. The authors emphasize the crucial need for high quality histologic preparations for MMS to be effective.

Lambert and Siegle [10] (V/B) performed a review of MMS in 1990 for NMSC and proposed that MMS is the "preferred treatment for high-risk primary basal and squamous cell carinomas." High-risk tumors are further defined as those located in anatomic areas at greater risk for recurrence (nose, lateral forehead, nasolabial folds, periorbital area, periauricular area, and over embryonic fusion planes), histologically aggressive basal cell carcinomas, tumors >1.5 cm in diameter, clinically ill-defined tumors, and recurrent tumors. The authors claim that due to its precision and high success rate in an office-based surgery setting, MMS is "highly cost-effective"; however, no specific cost-analysis was discussed to support this assertion.

In 1991, Leslie and Greenway [11] (VI/B) composed a review of MMS for the Australasian Journal of Dermatology. The authors cite the often-referenced data from Rowe et al. [12] of cure rates of 99% for primary BCC, 94.4% for recurrent BCC, and 94% for SCC (see below). Indications for MMS are reported and are assumed to be based on referenced retrospective reviews and case studies. The authors state that MMS is indicated for all recurrent and some primary basal cell carcinomas (aggressive histologic subtypes, multicentric tumors, rapid growth/ aggressive clinical behavior, of large size (not quantified), located in the central face, nasolabial folds, periorbital area, periauricular area, on the hands, feet, or genitalia, exhibiting perineural or perivascular spread), incompletely removed BCCs, and collision tumors (not defined) and BCCs with involvement of deep tissue or bone are also asserted indications. For squamous cell carcinoma, indications are the same for BCC, plus those in areas of previous radiation, mucocutaneous tumors, and Bowen's disease in high-risk anatomic areas. The evidence for these indications is not delineated in this review, and although several directly applicable clinical studies are referenced, it is unclear exactly on which of these the indications are based.

Shriner et al. [13] offered a review of MMS in July 1998 (IV/B). A description of the technique as well as its indications, training, and limitations is presented. The indications are based on

**Table 1.4** Criteria for MMS

| |
| --- |
| Recurrent tumors |
| Tumors located in anatomic areas associated with a high risk of local recurrence[a] |
| Tumors overlying the embryonic fusion planes |
| Tumors located in areas in which tissue preservation is mandatory |
| Tumors located in areas in which the highest cure rate is mandatory |
| Aggressive tumors |
| Large tumors |
| Tumors with poorly defined clinical margins |
| Incompletely excised tumors |
| Tumors arising in irradiated skin |
| Tumors with perineural involvement |
| Tumors with increased risk of metastasis |
| Tumors arising in immunosuppressed patients |

Adapted from Shriner et al. [13]
[a]Nasolabial fold, pinna, medial and lateral canthi, and periauricular area

retrospective reviews and case series by several other authors and are listed in Table 1.4. Limitations of MMS are also cited in this review. The authors assert MMS is labor intensive. The procedure utilizes specialized laboratory personnel, trained nursing staff, histologic diagnosis by the surgeon, and may require multiple surgeries in a single day. The increases in labor are not quantified in comparison to other treatment modalities, nor are they qualified by any potential increase in effectiveness of MMS. Another cited disadvantage is time spent by the patient. The time can be extensive from 2 h to over 8 h in complex cases. Comparing this disadvantage of MMS to standard surgical excision while including the benefit of lower risk for recurrence with MMS, is difficult. Positive margins are reported to occur in approximately 5–30% of primary excisions depending on surgical margins and tumor type [14–18]. Another limitation is maintaining the precise orientation so crucial for mapping when excising on deeply or contoured structures such as cartilage or bone. In addition, fat and muscle are challenging to process in horizontal sections, especially when taken without epidermis. A fourth limitation of MMS discussed in this review is the increase in histopathology technical errors due to processing artifacts in frozen specimen processing and the increased difficulty in interpreting slides of frozen tissue compared to paraffin-embedded tissue. Technical or slide/mapping interpretation errors have been reported as responsible for over three-fourths of recurrences after MMS [19]. Cost of therapy was also addressed. The authors note MMS is usually less costly than alternative options such as radiation therapy and wide local excision for indicated malignancies, but discouraged using MMS for nonindicated tumors such as small nodular basal cell carcinomas of the trunk where simple excision or alternative destructive techniques offer an acceptable cure rate and are frequently more cost-effective.

## Cohort Studies/Case Series

There is a vast amount of literature regarding the treatment of skin cancer, both medical and surgical. The most widely used outcome measure when comparing cancer treatment modalities is recurrence. However, there is a paucity of high quality randomized comparisons of outcomes of the treatment modalities employed for skin cancer treatment. The bulk of the literature addressing the use of MMS for skin cancer consists of case studies, systematic reviews, and meta-analyses. Case studies are frequently limited by inadequate power, short follow-up periods, and single institution investigators. The latter two study types combine heterogeneous data from individual studies and perpetuate inherent biases in each. Most of the literature is retrospective, nonrandomized, and suffers from selection bias. For example, the level of risk for a type of skin cancer often drives the decision of which treatment is used and influences the likelihood of recurrence after therapy. Retrospective studies examining the effectiveness of MMS for nonmelanoma skin cancer therefore may be biased, as those tumors treated with MMS are frequently at higher risk and thus at greater inherent risk for recurrence. The only way to avoid selection bias is randomization. In addition, there is a notable lack of uniformity between studies in reporting methods for and classification of a "recurrence," which obviously affects outcomes analysis. In the next section, we look at the evidence for the use of MMS from both prospective and retrospective case series, systematic chart reviews, and cohort studies.

## Prospective Studies

The existing prospective outcomes-based data for MMS for the treatment of nonmelanoma skin cancer is quite limited. The rest of the prospective studies for MMS concern BCC and SCC. The following prospective studies provide evidence for the use of MMS for BCC and SCC.

### Australian Mohs Database: Intro
The Australian Mohs Database is a large prospective, multicenter, investigational case series of all patients treated with MMS in Australia between 1993 and 2002. It was started after the creation of the Mohs subdivision of the Australasian College of Dermatologists with the purpose of conducting collaborative outcomes analysis for MMS by fellowship-trained Australian Mohs surgeons and has produced many publications (Table 1.5). Strict recurrence rates for 5 years of follow-up are reported for basal cell carcinoma overall, squamous cell carcinoma overall, squamous cell carcinoma in situ, basosquamous carcinoma, periocular tumors, tumors with perineural invasion (PNI), tumors of the lip, and other malignancies treated with MMS between 1993 and 1999. An advantage of this project is the large numbers of tumors prospectively included. The lack of follow-up with modified life-table data, considered the most useful in reporting recurrence rates, is a limitation to the information found from this study. Follow-up was obtained by questionnaires sent to the treating Mohs surgeon at the end of the 5 year period. Thus, there was no weighted credit for tumor-free follow-up of less than 5 years.

### Australian Mohs Database: BCC
In the study by Leibovitch et al. [20] (V/B), recurrence rates were reported for BCC treated with MMS in Australia over a 5-year follow-up. Inclusion criteria were all BCCs referred for MMS, most were on the head and neck (98%). Of the 3,370 cases treated, 44% were recurrent BCC. Subclinical extension was measured as the difference in the clinical size of the tumor and the final defect size and was found to be double the tumor size in 22.1% of cases. The authors found an overall recurrence rate of 2.6% (86 in 3,370), primary BCC recurrence rate of 1.4% (26 in 1,886), and recurrent BCC recurrence rate of 4.0% (60 in 1,484). Interestingly, the size of the tumor was less than 2 cm in over three-fourths of patients both with and those without recurrences at 5 years. Thus, in this series, no association between tumor size and recurrence could be determined, nor were there significant relationships between postexcision defect size or subclinical extension and recurrence. Significance was found, however, between the mean number of Mohs layers required for tumor clearance and recurrence, as those without recurrence averaged 1.72 layers and those with recurrence 2.11 layers. In addition, the longer duration of tumor before MMS was significantly associated with risk for recurrence in these cases.

### Australian Mohs Database: SCC
In a related study by Leibovitch et al. [21] (V/B), recurrence rates were determined for SCC for the same population of patients from the Australian Mohs Database over the same follow-up period noted above. Again, the majority (96%) of cases treated with MMS were located on the head and neck. There were 381 SCCs treated for which 5-year follow-up data was available. Of these, 15 recurred (overall recurrence rate of 3.9%). The recurrence rates for primary and recurrent SCC after treatment were 2.6% (9 in 229) and 5.9% (9 in 152), respectively. The most common sites of recurrence were the nose, ears, and forehead (these three locations accounted for 73% of all recurrences). There were no cases of metastasis over the 5-year follow-up after treatment with MMS. These rates correlate with previous numbers by Rowe et al. who found a recurrence rate on 3.1% for primary SCC treated by MMS compared with recurrence rates of 8.1% found with standard surgical excision and 10.9% for all other non-Mohs treatment modalities [22].

**Table 1.5** Studies from the Australian Mohs database

| References | Tumor | Cases | % Recurrent | Subclinical extension | RR (%) | Mean stages |
|---|---|---|---|---|---|---|
| Australian Mohs database | | | | | | |
| Leibovitch et al. [20] | BCC | 3,370 | 44 | 22.1 | 2.6 | 1.72 primary, 2.11 recurrent follow-up 5 years |
| Leibovitch et al. [21] | SCC | 381 | 40 | 18.6 | 3.9 | 1.6±0.8 |
| Leibovitch et al. [23] | SCCIS | 95 | 0 | 18.7 | 6.3 | 2.0±0.9 |
| Leibovitch et al. [35] | BCC with PNI | 78 | 60 | 40.8 | 7.7 | 2.5 |
| Leibovitch et al. [38] | SCC with PNI | 70 | 49 | 47.7 | 8.0 | 2 |
| Malhotra et al. [42] | Periocular BCC | 347 | 26 | N/A | 2.0 | N/A |
| Malhotra et al. [43] | Periocular SCC | 78 | 27 | N/A | 3.6 | 1.8 primary, 2.0 recurrent follow-up 5 years |
| Malhotra et al. [43] | Periocular SCCIS | 36 | 47 | N/A | 8.3 | 2.1 primary, 2.6 recurrent follow-up to date |

A separate report was published the same year by the same institution in Australia for SCCIS [23]. As in invasive SCC, the majority of the 95 cases of SCCIS (93%) treated with MMS were located on the head and neck. The overall recurrence rate was 6.3%; for primary lesions, 2.5% and for recurrent lesions, 9.1%. Although 83% of recurrences occurred in recurrent lesions, these data were not statistically significant.

The lack of randomization with other treatment modalities lowers the quality of evidence provided by these papers. Nonetheless, this long term, highly powered series highlights the efficacy of this treatment, and lends support to MMS as the standard of care for high-risk BCC, SCC, and SCCIS (IV/B). Data from the Australian Mohs Database regarding outcomes of MMS for periocular tumors and tumors with PNI will be discussed in their respective sections below.

### Other Prospective Studies: BCC

The study by Julian and Bowers [24] (V/B) analyzed recurrences in 73 primary BCCs and 155 recurrent BCCs treated with MMS and followed for 5 years. The authors investigated the need, practicality, and efficacy of the procedure for selected tumors with a small prospective, non-comparative study. Their criteria for inclusion were large tumors in a cosmetically sensitive area, morpheaform BCC, tumors in embryonic folds, and persistently recurrent tumors. One-hundred and thirty-one patients were followed for at least 5 years for recurrence. The authors demonstrated a raw recurrence rate of 1.3% (1 in 73) for primary BCC and 2.5% (4 in 155) for recurrent BCC. The overall strict recurrence rate was 3.8% (5 in 131). This study gives further support to the use of MMS for high-risk BCC. Given the small number of cases, the evidence is limited. In addition, nonreproducible calculation of the total number of recurrent and primary BCC cases that completed 5 years of follow-up confuses the data and makes the strict recurrence rates unreliable.

### Retrospective Studies

Most of the English literature for outcomes analysis of the use of MMS for BCC and SCC is retrospective and consist primarily of systematic chart reviews and case series. We limited inclusion in this chapter to those relevant studies with at least 3 years of follow-up data, unless limited clinical data precluded this exclusion or studies provided important clinical evidence despite limited follow-up.

Two consecutive retrospective case series were published by Mohs [25, 26] (V/B), and in total comprise the largest published series of patients with BCC treated with MMS with 5-year follow-up. The data included 9,351 cases treated with the fixed tissue technique for extensive tumors and 196 cases with the fresh tissue technique. Mohs found an overall recurrence rate of 1.0%, 0.7% for primary BCC and 3.2% for recurrent BCC.

Mohs also published a 6% recurrence rate for SCC [27]. These rates must be interpreted with caution as locally recurrent lesions were not considered recurrent if another MMS cleared the residual tumor.

Robins performed a retrospective study of 2,966 BCCs of the face and scalp in patients from 1965 to 1980 who were treated with MMS [28] (V/B) and followed for at least 5 years. Nearly three-fourths (72.5%) of all tumors he treated were processed by fresh tissue technique and 27.5% by fixed tissue technique. Half were primary and half were recurrent. He found an overall recurrence rate of 2.6%, primary BCC recurrence rate of 1.8%, and recurrent BCC recurrence rate of 3.4%. The author compares these data to recurrence rate of 5–10% for primary and 40% for recurrent BCCs treated by "standard procedures."

Robins et al. [29] reported a retrospective analysis of 414 cases of SCC treated with MMS between 1966 and 1980 and found a recurrence rate of 3.4%. Higher rates of recurrence were found for men, age younger than 40, greater than 4 stages, and tumors larger than 5 cm. The authors suggest taking an additional layer past the tumor-free plane to decrease the increased recurrence in high risk cases.

MMS in its ideal form should be able to provide 100% cure rates for histologically distinctive tumors such as BCC. To better elucidate the reasons for recurrence after MMS, Dzubow [30] (V/B) published a case series in 1987 that illustrated technical and interpretive errors that contributed to tumor recurrence after MMS. In his review of three cases, Dzubow found that incomplete skin edge on histologic preparation, tumor-masking inflammatory reaction, and incomplete deep edge were likely culprits in these cases. In addition, he noted that perineural or lymphatic involvement, true tumor multifocality, poor host immunity, and difficulty in distinguishing normal anatomical structures from tumor may contribute to MMS failure. In 1994, Hruza [19] (V/B) performed a large retrospective review of 2,414 tumors treated by MMS and reviewed the cause for error in each recurrence. The author found a recurrence rate of 1.4% for MMS over at least 5 years follow-up. After review of each recurrence, Hruza concluded

that technical or interpretive errors accounted for over three-fourths of the recurrences in MMS. Similar to Rowe et al. [12], Hruza found that although most studies cite 5-year follow-up data, 20% of recurrences developed more than 5 years after MMS. Errors occurred in histologic examination in 35% of recurrent cases, slide preparation in 52%, and mapping in 13%. Seven recurrences could not be explained. This influential study provides evidence for the efficacy of MMS for NMSC, and it highlights the necessary attention to detail, high quality of histologic tissue preparation, and procedural thoroughness required to maintain the superior rates of cure that MMS provides for NMSC.

A retrospective analysis by Campbell et al. [31] (V/B) was performed on 296 MMS cases performed between 1991 and 2004 and sent to a plastic surgeon who removed an additional margin of unspecified size for permanent sectioning. This study allowed a unique opportunity for an immediate evaluation of the accuracy of MMS. Out of 296 tumors (99% basal cell and squamous cell carcinomas), only 1 (0.3%) had persistence of tumor after "clear" margins were obtained by MMS. Although limited by one Mohs surgeon, this study underscores the accuracy of MMS and supports the conclusions of Hruza.

In 2004, Smeets et al. [32] (V/B) from the Netherlands performed an analysis of a retrospective cohort 720 BCC located on the face and neck treated between 1992 and 1999 with MMS. The authors defined a recurrence as a histologically confirmed BCCC within 5 mm of a scar and recorded overall recurrence rates of 4.5% with 3.2% for primary BCC and 6.7% for recurrent BCC. They concluded that MMS is the treatment of choice for a subset of BCCs that are histologically aggressive, leave a large postoperative defect, are recurrent, or require more than four Mohs stages. Several limitations of the study should be taken into consideration. First, because only 292 tumors were available for 5-year follow-up (37% of cases had less than 3 years of follow-up), the authors used raw recurrence rates and estimated the 5-year cumulative probability of recurrence using Kaplan–Meier survival analysis. This yielded rates which differ from the strict

5-year recurrence rate of 10%. Second, the authors note that most recurrences were found in tumors treated within the first 2 years reviewed in the study and suggest that the surgeons improved with time leading to fewer errors in later years. This implies a lack of consistency of the surgeons' skills in performing this technical procedure over the study period. Third, there is no information regarding the training or accreditation of the physicians performing the Mohs surgeries. No information regarding the number of cases treated per year or the breakdown of primary vs. recurrent BCC per year was provided, but in both 1993 and 1994, 12% of tumors recurred. The reason for such high recurrence rates is unclear, and these rates are outliers compared with studies noted above. One reason may be the high number of multiply recurrent BCCs (12%) and histologically aggressive BCC (55%).

## Tumors with Perineural Invasion

PNI is defined by the presence of tumor in or around a nerve. It is known to be associated with large (2 cm) tumors, tumors of the head and neck, recurrent, aggressive, and poorly differentiated tumors. It is reported to occur in 2.5–14% of SCCs and 1–3% of histologically aggressive BCCs [33, 34]. Extensive subclinical spread is frequently found in tumors with perineural involvement and they carry a higher risk of recurrence and metastasis. Randomized controlled trials comparing different treatment modalities for tumors with PNI are lacking. The studies below support the use of MMS for the treatment of cutaneous neoplasms with PNI, given MMS's ability to track the tumor until clearance.

### BCC with PNI
Data from the aforementioned Australian Mohs Database was used by Leibovitch et al. [35] (V/B) to determine recurrence rates for BCC with PNI for the same population of patients over a 5-year follow-up period. Of 78 patients diagnosed with BCC with PNI on initial histopathology, six recurred (7.7%). All six were recurrent BCC and 5 of the 6 were from males. This study also showed

a statistically significant increase in risk for recurrence in BCCs with perineural spread as only 2.4% of BCCs without perineural spread recurred after MMS. These data correlate with an earlier prospective study by Ratner et al. [36] (V/B) of 78 patients with BCC which that required two or more stages of MMS to clear. Eight of these (10%) were found to have PNI. The author also presented data at the American College of MMS and Cutaneous Oncology Meeting, Portland, Oregon, May 1998 detailing a retrospective review of 320 BCCs. Forty-five percent of those requiring two or more stages of MMS had PNI, suggestive of tumors with extensive subclinical spread and at higher risk for recurrence.

Hanke et al. [37] reviewed ten cases of BCC with PNI, nine of which were treated with MMS. The authors reported an 11% recurrence rate over a mean follow-up of 18 months.

### SCC with PNI
Leibovitch et al. [38] reported recurrence rates for SCC with PNI. Of 70 patients diagnosed with SCC with PNI on initial histopathology, 25 had 5-year follow-up data and two of these recurred (8%). It should be noted that 37 of 70 patients in this review received adjuvant radiotherapy. Initial clinical tumor size, postoperative defect size, subclinical extension, and mean number of MMS levels were significantly increased in cases with PNI vs. those without. The authors found the increase in recurrence rate for SCC with perineural spread to be statistically significant as only 3.7% of patients with SCC without PNI recurred after MMS. The authors conclude that MMS offers the highest cure rate in these tumors. The authors state that "…the high sensitivity of MMS in detecting PNI and the low 5-year recurrence rate compared with standard excision make it the preferred mode of treatment for BCC with PNI" and "…although MMS offers the highest cure rate, it still results in a significant recurrence rate, emphasizing the long-term monitoring of these patients." To explain the higher rate of recurrence in SCC with PNI, the authors suggest that apparent skip areas of perineural involvement due to folding and tortuosity of nerves in tissue may cause focal apparent discontinuity and thus a false

negative reading on pathologic examination. These skip areas may provide the appearance of uninvolved regions with an otherwise proximally or distally invaded nerve. Because of the potential for multifocality of nerve involvement by such tumors, some investigators recommend taking an additional layer of normal tissue beyond the tumor-free plane to insure clearance of lesions with perineural involvement [9, 36, 37, 39].

Standard surgical excision of SCC with PNI is reported to have recurrence and regional metastatic rates of 47 and 35%, respectively [40]. By contrast, in the study by Cottel [39] (V/B) no recurrences and one metastasis was reported in 16 SCCs with PNI treated by MMS over an average follow-up of 16 months. It is notable that eight of these patients received adjunctive radiotherapy. Lawrence and Cottel analyzed survival rates for 44 patients with SCC with PNI treated with MMS between 1978 and 1991. The authors defined recurrence as "the reappearance of SCC at the site of MMS or as metastatic disease" and reported three recurrences (6.8%). Only 33 cases were followed for 3 years or more, and three cases were followed for less than 1 year. Using life-table analysis, the authors concluded that patients with perineural SCC an 88.7% survival rate after MMS which compares favorably with prior studies of surgical excision of SCC with PNI which show survival rates less than 30% [40, 41]. This study demonstrates improved cure rates and supports the use of MMS for these high-risk tumors. There use of radiation in cases of perineural involvement remains controversial as no randomized controlled clinical trials have been performed for its use in SCC treated with MMS.

### Other Tumors: PNI

Feasel et al. [33] performed a literature review of PNI in multiple cutaneous neoplasms in addition to BCC and SCC that display PNI and are amenable to MMS including keratoacanthoma, eccrine carcinoma, and microcystic adnexal carcinoma (MAC). The authors support MMS as the treatment of choice for BCC with PNI and review case reports and reviews supporting its role in the treatment of the other cutaneous neoplasms as listed. The authors assert that the "…increased sensitivity in the detection of PNI and lower rates

of recurrence when compared to traditional surgical techniques suggest MMS as the preferred therapy for several cutaneous malignancies with PNI."

### Periocular BCC

Malhotra et al. [42, 43] (V/B) reported 5-year follow-up data from the Australian Mohs Database for periocular basal cell carcinoma (347 cases) and squamous cell carcinoma (78 cases). Recurrence rates were 2.0 and 3.6%, respectively. For primary periocular basal cell carcinoma there were no recurrences out of 256 primary tumors and seven recurrences out of 90 previously treated tumors for strict 5-year recurrence rates of 0 and 7.8%, respectively. Of the seven recurrences, five were located in the medial canthus. Although interesting in light of studies corroborating the high recurrence rates for tumors in this location, this was not a statistically significant predictor of recurrence in this study. These data are similar to others noted below.

Other retrospective analyses investigating the use of MMS for periocular basal cell and squamous cell carcinoma have been performed. Robins et al. [44] retrospectively reviewed cure rates for 631 periocular basal cell carcinomas treated by MMS. The recurrence rates were found to be 1.9% for primary BCC and 6.4% for recurrent BCC. This study found that 100% of the periocular BCCs recurrent after initial treatment with MMS were located in the medial canthus. In addition, overall recurrence rate for medial canthus BCC treated with MMS was 9.5%, over 2× higher than for BCCs in other periocular locations. Recurrence in the medial canthus was 3× higher if previously treated by radiotherapy. The authors conclude that the high rate of recurrence in this area reflects more common use of radiation to treat primary tumors in this area. Therefore, the authors claim MMS is indicated for the treatment of periocular BCCs and especially those in the medial canthus.

In 1986, Mohs [45] reported a retrospective analysis of 1,124 primary and 290 recurrent eyelid BCCs. The study demonstrated 5-year strict recurrence rates of 0.6% for primary and 7.6% for recurrent. This study confirmed recurrence rates found in previous studies. For example, in the review by Ceilley and Anderson [46], the investigators reported a 0% recurrence rate one year after treatment with MMS. Others have reported recurrence rates of 0–2% over a mean follow-up of 3 years for periorbital BCC treated with MMS [4, 47].

The potential consequences of recurrence in periorbital BCC with PNI are highlighted in a noncomparative case series by Wong et al. [48] in which 22% (4/18) of cases with PNI led to enucleation. The authors reported a 2.2% recurrence rate for 97 primary BCCs treated with excision followed by en face frozen section processing over a 5 year follow-up period. Six periocular BCCs were treated with MMS with no recurrences over 1.7 years of follow-up.

Case reports [49–51] and case series [52–54] (V/B) support the use of MMS for ocular sebaceous carcinoma with a local recurrence rate of 12%. Extraocular sebaceous carcinoma has been successfully treated with MMS [55, 56].

## Lip and External Ear

Existing evidence supports MMS for the treatment of cancers located in other high-risk anatomical sites such as the lip and ear and outcomes data compares favorably to conventional methods of treatment. The 5-year determinate survival rate for treatment with conventional methods (standard excision, radiation, or combination therapy) was found to be around 80% in one large series [57]. Mohs and Snow published the largest series of patients (V/B) with 1,448 cases of squamous cell carcinoma of the lip treated with MMS. They reported a 5-year recurrence rate of 5.8%. Size was a useful prognostic factor in this study as tumors smaller than 2 cm had a recurrence rate of 3.4% as opposed to 40.3% for tumors greater than 2 cm. In addition, excluding advanced cases with advanced disease including local lymph node involvement, the recurrence rate decreases to 3–4%. In the retrospective review of 50 early (T1 or T2N0M0) SCC located on the lip treated with MMS by Holmkvist and Roenigk [58] (V/B), 8% of patients had local recurrence over a 5-year follow-up period. The authors support the use of MMS for SCC of the lip. However, they warn that

the potential for tumor multifocality may reveal a limitation for any method of treatment and propose that the recurrences may actually have been new primary cancers. All recurrences occurred in the setting of severe actinic cheilitis, and no patients who underwent adjuvant carbon dioxide laser ablation had recurrences, suggesting adjunctive treatment of adjacent actinic damage may prevent recurrence or the development of new primary squamous cell carcinoma.

Mohs et al. [59] (V/B) reported on the efficacy of MMS for the treatment of primary BCC located on the external ear. In this study of 1,032 patients treated with MMS, Mohs demonstrated a raw recurrence rate of 1.3% (13 in 1,032) and a strict recurrence rate of 1.7% (13 in 748).

## Conclusions

Multiple retrospective studies and several prospective studies exist supporting the use of MMS for the ablation of BCC and SCC. In general it is well-established that MMS is the most precise treatment modality for nonmelanoma skin cancer and provides the lowest rates of recurrence in all situations. Given the high and increasing incidence of these tumors, however, costs of the procedure must be balanced with the improved cure rates. The higher costs are offset in cases where recurrence is likely from standard treatment methods, such as tumors with significant subclinical extension. Therefore, the overall impression is that MMS is indicated for tumors in high-risk anatomic sites, large tumors, basal cell carcinomas with aggressive histologic growth patterns, incompletely excised tumors, tumors in precarious functional or cosmetic areas, and tumors in immunocompromised hosts.

## Mohs Surgery for Tumors Other Than BCC and SCC

### Melanoma

#### Introduction

MMS for definitive treatment of melanoma in situ (MIS) and superficially invasive and invasive melanoma was first examined by Mohs [60] and since then has been widely studied. The existing body of evidence for the treatment of melanoma and MIS consists of retrospective chart reviews and case reports/series from single institutions, with small power and relatively short-term follow-up. Melanoma and especially MIS may have extensive subclinical spread similar to basal cell and squamous cell carcinoma and thus are potentially reasonable candidates for MMS and its ability to detect underlying branching tumor strands.

## Accuracy of Frozen Sections

Since the ability to detect tumor on histologic preparations is critical to the success of MMS, high quality, clear slides are needed to employ MMS for melanoma. Due to the freezing of tissue during Mohs processing, artifactual cytoplasmic retraction may be produced in normal keratinocytes leading to diagnostic confusion with proliferating melanocytes in MIS. Thus, there is argument over the accuracy of frozen sections in histopathologic rendering of melanoma. Some authors warn of decreased sensitivity of frozen sectioning for detecting atypical melanocytes. Barlow et al. [61] (V/C) reported that frozen sections were 59% sensitive and 81% specific for LM based on reinterpretation of 50 slides with permanent sections read by a dermatopathologist (V/C). These data might be biased as all 50 were considered the more difficult cases to interpret and the cases considered straightforward on frozen section analysis were omitted. Studies by Nield et al. [62] and Shafir et al. [63] found differences in melanoma thickness when frozen sections were compared with permanent sections, suggesting limitations of frozen sectioning in melanoma. On the other hand, 30 of 31 melanomas were correctly diagnosed on frozen section in the latter study. Zitelli et al. [64, 65] (V/B) reported 100% sensitivity and 90% specificity for detecting melanoma and atypical melanocytes at the margins of melanoma with Mohs frozen sectioning compared with permanent sections. In a retrospective study by Zitelli et al. [66] discussed below, the investigators found an overall recurrence rate of 0.5%. The authors compared their results with the average of those reported by

Pitman et al. [67] at a mean of 6% recurrence rate for traditional surgical excision of MIS. The authors conclude that these low recurrence rates are evidence that frozen sections are accurate for the rendering of melanoma but caution that experience and histotechnical expertise are requisite for the lowest recurrence rates.

Bienert et al. [68] (V/B) reported 92 patients with biopsy proven facial MIS or melanoma treated by MMS and followed for a mean follow-up period of 33 months. The authors found a local recurrence rate of 0%, although one patient died of metastatic melanoma. No in situ or invasive melanoma was identified on 117 tissue margins on permanent sections that were interpreted as negative on frozen section. The authors concluded that the 100% correlation between frozen section margins and permanent controls supports the accuracy of MMS in the treatment of facial melanoma. Likewise, in a recent prospective study, Bene et al. [69] (V/B) measured the accuracy of Mohs frozen sectioning for MIS by confirming margin clearance with paraffin-embedded sections. The study included 167 cases of MIS that were cleared using MMS with frozen sections. After the surgeons cleared the tumor on frozen sections, a 1 mm rim of skin was taken for permanent sections for evaluation by a dermatopathologist. Eight of 167 cases had positive margins on permanent sections (95.1% clearance rate). All of these were successfully treated with one re-excision of 3 mm margins. For a mean follow-up of 63 months, only two recurrences were reported for a recurrence rate of 1.8%.

## Modifications of MMS

Because of the difficulty of interpreting melanoma and MIS from frozen sections reported in the literature, modifications of MMS such as the use of immunohistochemical stains and "slow Mohs" have been described and put into clinical practice. The latter describes a technique in which horizontal permanent sections following each MMS stage are analyzed in attempt to take advantage of both complete margin control and improved visualization of melanocytes with permanent tissue fixation. The variation in technique makes comparison among studies of "Mohs micrographic surgery" for melanoma difficult. Recurrence rates including these modified MMS range from 0.5 to 3% over 2–9 years of follow up [70, 71] (VI/C).

In the retrospective study by Cohen et al. [72] (V/B) and the extended follow-up report in 1998 [73], 45 patients with LM or LMM were analyzed for recurrence after treatment with MMS. The authors debulked the clinically apparent lesion or scar with an unspecified margin and then excised a 2–3 mm margin as the first Mohs layer. Another 2–3 mm margin around this defect was taken for paraffin-embedded permanent sections to be examined by a dermatopathologist. If the permanent margins were positive, surgery was resumed the next day using sequential excisions with permanent sectioning. This was repeated until negative or equivocal margins were found. The authors found a recurrence rate over nearly 5 years of 2.2% (1 in 45). Firm conclusions regarding the evidence of the efficacy of MMS for the treatment of LM or LMM cannot be drawn from this study as pure MMS was not employed; however, the study does support the use of Mohs technique until margins are deemed clear followed by permanent sectioning as a "check" on the frozen interpretation as well as for analysis of initial debulking layer for the presence of invasive disease.

The lack of consensus as to the histologic definition of MIS makes comparison between studies less useful. Some authors define MIS as nests and contiguous atypical melanocytes along the basal layer. Others believe the lateral margins of MIS include scattered single atypical melanocytes. These cells may be hard to distinguish from normal melanocytes on frozen or permanent sectioning. Immunohistochemical staining has been increasingly employed to help clarify this distinction by highlighting melanocytes. Several stains have been reported in MMS including HMB-45, S-100, Mel-5, and MART-1/melan-A. Although many studies support the use of HMB-45, evidence is increasing that MART-1/melan-A is the more accurate stain for MIS and MM. Albertini et al. [74] (V/B) studied 42 cases of MIS treated by MMS with MART-1/melan-A staining and reviewed 18 studies to compare its sensitivity to HMB-45 in melanoma. Based on their and others findings, the authors suggest that MART-1/melan-A "…may be the best marker currently available for MMS." Zalla et al. [75] in an earlier review in 2000 (V/B) claimed that MART-1/melan-A staining was more crisp and accurate and stained 6 of 7 HMB-45-negative tumors. The authors conclude that MART-1/melan-A provides the most reliable staining and "…is the stain of choice" for melanoma based on their findings.

Kelley and Starkus [76] (V/B) found 100% concordance in seven cases of LM using frozen sectioning with paraffin-embedded permanent staining after staining with MART-1. The authors note, "there was a striking difference in the ability to detect melanocytes in the MART-1-stained slides as compared with frozen sections stained with H&E." More recently, Mallipeddi et al. [77] reported the processing of MMS sections using microwave technology with paraffin-embedded tissue and staining with H&E. The described protocol takes 2 h to complete. The authors claim no difference in visualization of normal vs. abnormal melanocyte as well as in the rendering of other epidermal and dermal anatomy compared to standard paraffin processing and significant improvement in these parameters over frozen H&E sectioning, commonly used in MMS.

## MMS for Melanoma In Situ

Guidelines set forth by the NIH [78] in 1992 and agreed upon by the NCCN [79] and the AAD [80] recommend excision with a 5 mm margin for MIS. Multiple retrospective chart reviews and case series discuss the use of microscopic margin control for MIS. There are currently no prospective randomized, controlled clinical trials that offer a high quality comparison of MMS to other surgical modalities. A potentially important confounding factor is the possibility of a focus of invasive melanoma within a biopsy proven MIS. A case series by Megahed et al. [81] of 104 cases originally diagnosed as MIS, found 29% to be invasive upon reevaluation. Thus, inaccurate staging may lead to improper management if standard surgical excision with predetermined margins based on the original diagnosis is undertaken.

In the prospective case review by Bricca et al. [82] (V/B), 331 MIS were treated with MMS with a cure rate of 99.7% at nearly 5 years of follow-up. The authors excised the clinically apparent tumor with 3 mm margins and sent this initial specimen for permanent sections. The first layer was taken with another 3 mm around the debulking defect and processed by Mohs technique. One-third of cases were stained with HMB-45. Similar cure rates for lentigo maligna, a subtype of MIS occurring of sites of chronic sun-exposure of the head and neck, were noted by the retrospective case review by Bhardwaj et al. [83]. In this report, initial clinical margins were outlined with a Wood's light, and the lesion was excised with a 1–2 mm margin and sent for permanent analysis. Another 2–3 mm were taken around the defect and processed by the Mohs technique. The authors reported a recurrence rate of 0.6% (1 in 158) over an average of 38 months follow-up. 38% of these lesions (including the one that recurred after MMS) were either recurrent or incompletely excised prior to inclusion. All of the tissue in this study was stained with Mel-5.

Temple and Arlette [84] (V/B) reported a case series of 119 lentigo malignas and 8 MIS as well as 69 invasive melanomas treated by MMS. From 1993 to 1997, rather than sending a debulking layer for permanent sectioning, the authors outlined the extent of the clinical lesion with the help of a Wood's lamp and excised the first Mohs layer using 5 mm margins. After 1997, the authors sent this layer for permanent sectioning. Subsequent layers were taken with 2–3 mm margins. Mean follow-up was 30 months with 0% local recurrence rate noted. Four regional recurrences were reported as well as two patients who died of metastatic melanoma.

## MMS for Melanoma

Mohs surgery for 20 cases of melanoma was first described by Mohs [60]. In 1956 [85] and 1977 [86], 31 and 103 more cases, respectively, were described. The technique described in these studies differs from the way MMS is currently practiced. First, chemical fixation prior to surgical excision of the melanoma was exclusively performed. Second, once a tumor-free plane was established, an additional 1–3 cm margin around the wound was removed to capture perilymphatic malignant cells. An overall cure rate of 50% was reported in the 1977 study, however, 69 of 86 (80%) of cases were Clark level 4 or greater. The cure rate was favorable compared with traditional surgical excision for each Clark level. A report by Zitelli et al. [87] provided further evidence for MMS in the treatment of melanoma. The authors reported an overall cure rate of 65% for 200 cases of melanoma, although they included several level V cases. Few of these cases would be expected to achieve cure, regardless of the choice of modality for local surgical control. The authors note that the contiguous growth pattern of early, localized melanoma and its potential for underlying ramifying spread makes it amenable to MMS for treatment. In addition, the advantage of conservation of normal tissue is explored, as wound defect diameters were at least 1.8 cm smaller when treated with MMS compared to standard surgical excision while allowing for resection of subclinical contiguous foci potentially missed on WLE followed by standard vertical sectioning. A key study by Zitelli et al. [66] (V/B) using fresh tissue MMS technique for 553 melanomas revealed 5-year Kaplan–Meier survival rates comparable to or exceeding those reported for standard wide local excision and overall local recurrence rates of 0.05% over 5 years of follow-up. The authors contend that these data confirm the ability to detect melanoma on frozen sections and the efficacy of MMS for definitive treatment of melanoma.

In the same series described above for MIS, Bricca et al. [82] also treated 294 invasive melanomas. The authors reported a 1.6% local recurrence rate (which included satellite and in-transit metastases) for 64 melanomas 1.50–3.99 mm in thickness and a 0% local recurrence rate for the remaining 230 invasive melanomas. MMS compared favorably to conventional surgical excision for all levels of thickness including MIS, although 88.5% of invasive melanomas treated by the conventional excision were thicker than 0.75 mm compared to only 43.5% of those treated by MMS. The authors suggest that the low rates of recurrence validate the ability to detect melanoma on frozen sectioning, particularly with the addition of special histologic stains, and that these rates are dependent upon complete margin analysis rather than clinical margin widths. It is concluded that due to its ability to achieve low recurrence rates with smaller wound size, MMS has advantages over conventional wide local excision in the treatment of MIS and melanoma.

## Conclusions

Complete surgical excision is the "gold standard" for the treatment of localized melanoma. Although reports have shown improved local recurrence rates for MMS over wide local excision [82], no randomized, controlled studies exist to directly compare local recurrence or disease-free survival rates between MMS vs. traditional wide local excision. When scrupulous surgical and histopathologic technique is applied, MMS may be successful in excising localized melanoma with clear margins while sparing normal tissue. In addition, the continued improvement in special stains may provide increased accuracy in detecting melanoma on frozen sections thereby improving the overall sensitivity and specificity of MMS for melanoma.

## Merkel Cell

Merkel cell carcinoma (MCC) is a rare, biologically aggressive cutaneous neuroendocrine tumor most often occurring on the head and neck. Wide surgical excision with or without adjuvant radiotherapy is generally regarded as the treatment of choice for the treatment of localized MCC. Most early sources recommended wide surgical excision with 2.5–3.0 cm margins for localized Stage I disease followed by radiation. A systematic review by Haag et al. [88] (VI/C) suggested wide local excision followed by lymph node dissection if palpable nodes were present and radiation as appropriate therapy for MCC. Lymph node dissection in the absence of palpable disease is controversial. Even with seemingly adequate surgical margins, local recurrence rates range from

12 to 44% and overall survival rates of 39–68% [89, 90]. Tumor size appears to be the most important prognostic parameter for the risk of local recurrence and metastasis and may dictate the need for adjuvant therapy following surgical extirpation. In the retrospective study by Boyer et al. [91] (V/B), the mean surgical margin needed to achieve clearance was 16.7 mm. If margins of 2.0 or 3.0 cm were taken for standard excision, 25 and 12%, respectively, of untreated MCC would have had positive margins. In contradistinction, nearly half of all tumors treated needed 1 cm or smaller margins to achieve tumor-free specimens. Compared with standard surgical excision, recurrence rates for MMS range from 0 to 22% [90–94] (see Table 1.6). The success of MMS for MCC underscores its twofold benefit of identification of subclinical tumor extension and simultaneous tissue conservation.

In the retrospective review by O'Connor et al. [92] (V/B), MMS fared better than surgical excision in terms of local recurrence and regional metastasis over at least 3 years of follow-up. In addition, the authors studied the role of postoperative radiation therapy in the treatment of MCC. Of the 12 cases treated with MMS, 4 received postoperative radiation and 8 did not receive radiation. They found no regional metastasis in those that underwent radiation as opposed to four cases that were not treated with radiation. The role of radiotherapy in the treatment of MCC after MMS was further investigated by Boyer et al. [91] (V/B). Compared with a 16% total recurrence rate without postoperative radiation, there were no recurrences in 20 patients treated with MMS followed by postoperative radiation over an average of 27 months follow-up. The difference, however, was not statistically significant. The authors conclude that MMS is an effective therapy for primary MCC, but, despite the trend towards showing a benefit for radiation, suggest there is insufficient evidence from this study or their review of the current literature to recommend adjuvant radiotherapy. This study was limited by small power, short follow-up, and a small average tumor size of 1.6 cm. A discussion of the evidence for radiotherapy following surgical excision of MCC is beyond the scope of this chapter.

**Table 1.6** Selected studies of MMS for MCC

| References | Treatment | Cases | Local recurrence rate (%) | Regional metastasis rate (%) | Postop XRT # (of cases) | Follow-up |
|---|---|---|---|---|---|---|
| Allen et al. [90] | TSE | 102 | 12 | 39 | 14 | 35 months |
| O'Connor et al. [92] | TSE | 41 | 13 | 49 | N/A | 5 years |
| O'Connor et al. [92] | MMS | 12 | 8 | 33 | 4 | 3 years |
| Snow et al. [93] | MMS | 9 | 22 | 22 | 6 | 30 months |
| Boyer et al. [91] | MMS-XRT | 25 | 4 | 28 | 0 | 28 months |
| Boyer et al. [91] | MMS+XRT | 20 | 0 | 15 | 20 | 27 months |
| Dancey et al. [94] | TSE 1–3 cm margins | 31 | 27 | 50 | 7 | 3 years |

*Allen PJ, Zhang ZF, Coit DG. Surgical management of Merkel cell carcinoma. Ann Surg. 1999 Jan;229(1):97–105

In conclusion, MCC is a rare and aggressive cutaneous malignancy of neuroendocrine origin with a tendency for metastasis. Adequate treatment may require multimodality therapy, including surgery, radiation therapy, and possibly adjuvant chemotherapy. Evidence for the role of MMS in the treatment of this aggressive tumor is mounting, and it may prove to be more effective than standard surgical excision. Randomized controlled trials, however, do not exist, and data is currently limited to retrospective case reviews. MMS is advocated for its tissue-sparing attribute, especially for periorbital, perioral, and perinasal MCCs where 2.5–3.0 cm margins are functionally impossible. Therefore, MMS may be an appropriate treatment for MCC in areas not amenable to very wide surgical excision such as the face and ears. The evidence needed to establish a treatment of choice is lacking and large, prospective clinical trials are needed to optimize therapy of this malignancy.

## Dermatofibrosarcoma Protuberans (DFSP)

DFSP is a locally invasive, slow growing fibrohistiocytic tumor that rarely metastasizes but frequently recurs after surgical excision due to its tendency for extensive deep and peripheral penetration. Taylor and Helwig [95] reported a 49% recurrence rate following standard surgical excision of DFSP, and the recurrence rates for standard surgical excision of DFSP generally range from 10 to 60%. Dawes and Hanke [96] reported a surgical excision width of 1 cm around the primary

tumor would have left residual tumor in 65%; a width of 1.5 cm, 50%; a width of 2 cm, 31%; and 2.5 cm, 15%. Similar results were found in a chart review by Ratner et al. [97] (V/B) which demonstrated that wide local excision with a width of 1 cm around the primary tumor would have left microscopic residual tumor in 70.7%; a width of 2 cm, 39.7%; 3 cm, 15.5%; and 5 cm, 5.2%. Two tumors would have been inadequately excised if standard 3 cm had been used, and two tumors were still positive at a width of 10 cm, emphasizing the importance of deep and peripheral margin microscopic analysis in order to track the direction of subclinical extension while preventing unnecessary normal tissue resection.

Although wide surgical excision using a 3-cm margin reduces the risk of recurrence, evidence continues to accumulate supporting MMS as treatment of choice for this slowly growing but frequently recurrent neoplasm given a cumulative recurrence rate ranging from 0 to 8%. One prospective study [98] complements case series [99–101] and retrospective case reviews [96, 97, 100–108] that offer collective evidence for the use of MMS for the treatment of DFSP (see Table 1.7).

In conclusion, randomized, controlled clinical trials comparing MMS to other surgical or nonsurgical modalities for the treatment of DFSP are lacking. Given the rarity of this tumor, multiinstitutional collaboration is needed for such evidence. However, numerous systematic reviews and case series authored by recognized experts in the field of dermatologic surgery at large tertiary referral centers offer evidence to support the use of MMS as the emerging treatment of choice for DFSP. More recently, several case reports [109] (VI/C)

**Table 1.7**  Selected studies of MMS for DFSP

| References | Cases | Recurrence rate | Follow-up | LOE |
|---|---|---|---|---|
| Robinson [98] | 4 | 0 | 5 years | V/B |
| Hobbs et al. [108] | 10 | 0 | 3.5 years | V/B |
| Parker and Zitelli [139]* | 20 | 0 | 40.4 months | V/B |
| Gloster et al. [104] | 15 | 6.6 | 40 months | V/B |
| Dawes and Hanke [96] | 24 | 8 | 61.25 months | V/B |
| Garcia and Clark [101] | 16 | 0 | 4.4 years | V/B |
| Ratner et al. [97] | 58 | 2 | 4.8 years | V/B |
| Haycox et al. [105] | 10 | 0 | 3.4 years | V/B |
| Haycox et al. [105] meta-analysis | 169 | 2.4 | 3.3 years | V/B |
| Nouri et al. [103] | 20 | 0 | 56.4 months | V/B |
| Nouri et al. [103] meta-analysis | 221 | 2.3 | N/A | V/B |
| Snow et al. [102] | 29 | | 5 years | V/B |
| Snow et al. [102] meta-analysis | 136 | 6.6 | 5 years | V/B |
| Thomas et al. [100] | 35 | 0 | 39 months | V/B |
| Paradisi et al. [106] | 41 | 0 | 5.4 years | V/B |
| Nelson and Arlette [107] | 44 | 0 | 3.3 years | V/B |

*Parker TL, Zitelli JA. Surgical margins for excision of dermatofibrosarcoma protuberans. J Am Acad Dermatol. 1995 Feb;32(2 Pt 1):233–6

and a clinical trial [110] (VI/C) of neoadjuvant imatinib mesylate, a platelet-derived growth factor β (PDGFβ) inhibitor, with MMS have resulted in presurgical tumor shrinkage for tumors positive for the $t(17;22)$ or $r(17;22)$ gene rearrangement and might be considered in locally aggressive, large, or multiply recurrent tumors. Others [111] (VI/C) caution that neoadjuvant treatment might create multifocality resulting in increased recurrence rates after MMS and suggest reserving this protocol for unresectable disease, while employing adjuvant imatinib for all translocation positive DFSPs.

## Atypical Fibroxanthoma

AFX is an uncommon spindle cell tumor with invasive potential occurring most frequently on the head and neck of older white males with chronic actinic damage. There is no evidence-based consensus regarding the treatment of choice for AFX. Treatment data are limited to retrospective comparisons and case series, but most show favorable recurrence rates for MMS.

Retrospective analyses provide support of MMS for the treatment of AFX/MFH. A retrospective cohort study from the Mayo Clinic in 1997 by Davis et al. [112] (V/B), found that compared to wide local excision, treatment of AFX with MMS resulted in a lower recurrence rate (0 vs. 12%) after a mean follow-up period of approximately 30 months for MMS and 74 months for wide local excision [112]. It is noted that the comparison is limited by the difference of 5.5 years more follow-up for WLE. However, as most recurrences are within 2 years of treatment, the difference in recurrence rates cannot be entirely explained by disproportionate follow-up.

A case series by Seavolt and McCall [113] (V/B) reported no recurrences in 13 patients with AFX treated with MMS. Three of these patients had 5-years of follow-up, and six had at least 3 years of follow-up. An average of 2 stages was needed to clear the tumors and the average postoperative defect was 2.9 cm. The authors suggest that based on their results and prior reports, MMS is the preferable treatment modality for this tumor. In the largest retrospective chart review and literature review by Huether et al. [114] (V/B), a strict recurrent rate of 6.9% was reported for 29 AFXs treated by MMS and followed for a mean of 3.3 years.

In a retrospective study of MMS for 20 malignant fibrohistiocytomas (considered by some to be a deeper, more aggressive relative of AFX) and five AFXs, Brown and Swanson [115] (V/B), report a recurrence rate of 0.4% (1 in 25) over an average of 3-years follow-up. The authors report their study lends support for MMS "…as a desired surgical approach for these difficult-to-cure neoplasms." Smaller case studies (VI/C) by Limmer and Clark [116] (6 cases), Leibovitch et al. [117] (4 cases), and Dzubow [118] (4 cases) and case reports (VI/C) by Chilukuri et al. [119] and Hakim [120] report 0% recurrence rates and favor the use of MMS for AFX, especially in cosmetically or functionally sensitive areas such as the ear.

Outcomes for MMS compare favorably with those for standard surgical excision for the treatment of AFX. Fretzin and Helwig [121] reported a recurrence rate of 9% (9/101) over a mean 4 years of follow-up after the treatment of AFX by wide local excision. They noted that the average recurrence rate for wide excision is around 10%, although follow-up data, margin width, and tumor characteristics are often omitted. Others have reported recurrence rates as high as 21% with 1 cm surgical margins [112, 122–124].

## Conclusions

Data appear to indicate a much lower recurrence rate with MMS for the treatment of AFX, although no high quality clinical trials exist. Although evidence is limited to retrospective reports, case studies, and clinical experience of recognized experts in the field, MMS may offer improved cure rates with its concurrent advantage of maximal tissue conservation.

## Microcystic Adnexal Carcinoma

MAC is an uncommon indolent, locally aggressive but rarely metastatic adnexal tumor of the head and neck, most often found on the upper lip of middle-aged adults.

Recurrence rates for standard wide local excision of MAC are notoriously high, with multiple series reporting rates as high as 60% [125–128]. The evidence for MMS for the treatment of MAC is limited to case series and chart reviews, but overall lends support for MMS as the treatment of choice for this tumor. The prospective case

series by Leibovitch et al. [129] (V/B) included a thorough literature review revealing consistently lower recurrence rates for MMS (0–12%). The authors treated 44 MACs by MMS and followed these cases for recurrence. Of the 20 patients available for 5 year follow-up, only 5% (1 in 20) had a recurrence. In a small retrospective case series by Abbate et al. [130], a recurrence rate of 0% was found for four cases of MAC treated by MMS compared to 16.7% (1 in 6) by surgical excision over a mean 30 months of follow-up. No information regarding surgical margins taken was provided. Two of the six cases (33%) treated by surgical excision had positive margins requiring a second procedure.

## Conclusions

Since actual cutaneous involvement of the tumor is often significantly greater than clinical appearance, MMS would intuitively seem to be an ideal surgical treatment modality. Despite the lack of high quality evidence, the general impression available from the literature favors the use of MMS as the treatment of choice for MAC.

## Other Tumors (Angiosarcoma, Adnexal Tumors)

Rare case reports of angiosarcoma treated by MMS favor the technique for local control of tumors of smaller size, usually less than 10 cm in diameter [131, 132]. Employing MMS as a surgical option for angiosarcoma was first suggested in a case report by Goldberg and Kim [131] (VI/C). The authors noted that surgical excision is the treatment of choice for early, localized angiosarcoma less than 10 cm in diameter, and MMS offers a viable treatment option as a tissue-sparing technique. However, this patient was several years later reported to have metastases of angiosarcoma to the brain. A second case of angiosarcoma was reported by Muscarella [132] as well with no recurrence for 20 months. No treatment implications can be made from these cases. Thus, the evidence for MMS as a primary therapeutic modality for angiosarcoma is absent.

Hundreds of case reports exist for both benign and rare cutaneous adnexal neoplasms such as adenoid cystic carcinoma, verrucous carcinoma, neurothekeoma, tubular apocrine adenoma, malignant eccrine spiradenoma, eccrine ductal carcinoma, proliferating tricholemmoma, pilomatrical carcinoma, desmoplastic trichoepithelioma, syringocystadenoma papilliferum, hidradenoma, and papillary eccrine adenoma supporting the use of MMS as a first-line treatment. Multiple case reports and series exist for mucinous carcinoma, eccrine porocarcinoma, and tricholemmal carcinoma. In addition, several case reports exist for the treatment of nonmelanoma skin cancer in unusual sites such as peristomal, periungual, genital, nipple/areaola complex, nasal cavity, within port wine stains, within a nevus, within lichen sclerosus, and associated with EB.

## Randomized Clinical Trials/ Meta-Analyses

A systematic review by Thissen et al. [133] (IV/B) studied the recurrence rates after 5 years for seven different treatment modalities for nonrecurrent BCCs. They limited their study to prospective analyses completed after 1970 that included at least 50 lesions. In this meta-analysis, 18 of the 298 studies that evaluated the efficacy of treatment for BCC met the authors' inclusion criteria resulting in 9,930 primary BCCs to be studied. Tumors treated with MMS had the lowest recurrence rates followed by surgical excision, cryosurgery, and electrodessication and curettage. As is adequately noted in the manuscript, the recurrence rates could not be compared due to lack of uniformity in methods of reporting among the different articles reviewed. In addition, none of the studies reviewed were randomized due to ethical and practical constraints. Therefore, the results must be interpreted cautiously and no consensus guidelines can be drawn from this paper, although the authors' general recommendation of MMS for larger BCCs, those in the H-zone of the face, and those with aggressive histopathology are congruent with previously published guidelines for primary BCC.

There has been one randomized clinical trial of MMS vs. surgical excision for BCC. In 2004, Smeets et al. [134] (II/A) investigated which modality was more effective at reducing recurrence for both primary and recurrent BCC. In this study, 397 primary and 201 recurrent BCCs were treated by either MMS or surgical excision using 3 mm margins. Recurrence rates were analyzed by intent to treat. The authors found that of the primary carcinomas, five (3%) recurred after SE compared with three (2%) after MMS during 30 months of follow-up. Of the recurrent carcinomas, three (3%) recurred after SE and none after MMS during 18 months of follow-up. These differences in recurrence rates between the two tiers were deemed not statistically significant and no definitive conclusion for treatment of choice could be made based on recurrence rates.

Limitations of this study include less than 5 years of follow-up. This may underestimate the true recurrence rate, as it has been reported that only 50% of recurrences occur within the first 2 years and 66% occur within the first 3 years, and 18% of recurrences occur between the fifth and tenth year following treatment [12]. Thus, the reported recurrence rates may be artificially low. This drawback is addressed in the follow-up to this study by Mosterd et al. [135] (II/A) which included 5-year recurrence rate data. In the primary BCC group, there were seven recurrences after surgical excision and four after MMS. In the recurrent BCC group, there were ten recurrences after surgical excision and two after MMS. The differences were statistically significant for recurrent BCC but not for primary BCC, and the authors conclude that MMS "…is preferred over surgical excision for the treatment of facial recurrent BCC." However, because a significant difference in recurrence exists in primary BCC between treatment groups, "…treatment with surgical excision is probably sufficient in most cases of primary BCC." A Cox-regression analysis found an aggressive histological subtype to be a significant risk factor for recurrence in recurrent, but not primary, BCC.

In the meta-analyses performed by Rowe et al. [12, 136] of all studies since 1947 that reported recurrence rates for primary and recurrent BCC treated with various modalities including surgical excision and MMS. The authors found the 5-year recurrence rate for primary (untreated) BCC treated with MMS to be 1% (based on 7,670 tumors) and 8.7% for all non-Mohs modalities (10.1% for surgical excision). For recurrent BCC, the 5 year recurrence rate for MMS was 5.6% and for non-Mohs modalities was 19.9% (17.4% for surgical excision). The authors conclude that MMS is the treatment of choice for recurrent BCC. A second meta-analysis by Rowe et al. [22] reviewed all studies on recurrence of SCC of the skin and lip since 1940. The authors reported the local recurrence rate for primary SCC on the skin and lip was 3.1% for MMS compared with 10.9% for non-Mohs modalities. For recurrent SCC, the recurrence rate was 10% for MMS compared with 23.3% for non-MMS modalities. In addition, recurrence rates for auricular SCC were 5.3% for MMS and 18.7% for non-Mohs modalities, and for SCC with perineural involvement 0% for MMS and 47% for non-Mohs. SCC of size greater than 2 cm recurrence rates and poorly differentiated SCC were 25.2 and 32.6% for MMS and 41.7 and 53.6% for non-Mohs.

## Cost Comparisons

Debate exists as to the overall cost-effectiveness of MMS. To effectively perform MMS extra time, additional resources, and specialized training are requisite. Many authors have attempted to answer the question of whether the increased cost of MMS outweighs the repeatedly reported long-term recurrence free benefit.

The prospective cohort study by Cook and Zitelli [137] (V/B) compared the cost of MMS with office-based surgical excision with permanent sections, office-based surgical excision with frozen sections, and ambulatory surgical facility excision with frozen sections each with same day repair for multiple types of NMSC and for multiple anatomic locations. The authors first planned a non-Mohs surgical excision and proposed likely repairs. Based on these assumptions a cost value was generated for all non-Mohs excisions and compared with the costs incurred by MMS. They found that MMS was marginally (6%) higher in cost than office-based surgical excision with permanent sections for all tumors on the head, neck, and trunk but actually less expensive for office surgical excision with frozen sections and excision in an ambulatory surgery facility for the same locations. For the extremities and the genitalia, MMS was found to be the least expensive surgical option. An obvious limitation of this study is the assumption of reconstructive practices following surgical ablation. There were more flaps (30 vs. 10%) and more grafts (32 vs. 12.8%) for excision vs. MMS, both more expensive procedures than primary closure. Moreover, there were fewer wounds proposed to be left to heal by second intention in the excision group (0 vs. 39.3%), a much cheaper repair option. The authors claim these assumptions "…are based on current surgical standards across the United States," and, although the increase in flaps and grafts may be somewhat arbitrary, the lack of repair by secondary intent is likely to be fairly accurate given the limited number of acceptable anatomic locations for healing by granulation and the generally accepted notion the primary intent repair follows tumor extirpation in most cases. Thus the authors conclude that "….Mohs micrographic surgery is not a costly procedure, nor should its use be limited to high-risk tumors on the central portion of the face. It should be considered a cost-effective treatment with high intrinsic value that compares favorably with traditional surgical excision."

The prospective cohort study by Bialy et al. [8] (IV/B) compared the cost of MMS with surgical excision performed by otolaryngologic surgeons for NMSC of the face and ears. They also reported on the frequency of positive margins after surgical excision, allowing for more accurate representation of the true cost of obtaining negative margins. The authors determined the mean cost per patient for facial and auricular NMSC was $937 for MMS vs. $831 for traditional surgical excision with permanent sections. This figure is comparable to a report from Lear et al. [138] where the mean cost of MMS for complex facial BCCs was $871 (range $630–1,159). The positive margin rate was found to be 32% for surgical excision with permanent sections and 39% for surgical excision with frozen sections. Although this seems a bit on the high side, there are data to support the presence of positive margins after surgical excision of NMSC on the head and neck at a rate ranging from 5 to 30% [14–18]. Taking a subsequent margin clearing procedure into consideration, MMS compared favorably cost-wise with excision followed by MMS or a repeat excision, although these data were not statically significant. Moreover, subgroup analysis of 31 cases where frozen sections were requested by the ENT surgeon found that MMS was significantly less expensive ($956 vs. $1,399) per patient [138]. The data in this study were affected by type of repair and limited by design. As noted by the authors, deep margin control after traditional surgical excision could not be obtained and were assumed to be negative. This may arbitrarily lower the positive margin rate and lower the total cost incurred by surgical excision due to subsequent procedures for margin clearance. Another potential bias reported by the authors was that of the physicians performing either surgical excision or MMS given their knowledge of studied outcomes such as defect size and cost. Overall, however, this was a well-designed study that accurately reflects the common practices of US surgeons performing excisions or MMS followed by their choice of repair and gives some insight into cost comparison analysis of the two treatment modalities.

A detailed cost-analysis was published by Essers et al. [7] (II/A) as an adjunct to the Smeets study in 2004 using the same patient set to determine the cost-effectiveness of MMS vs. surgical excision. The incremental cost-effectiveness ratio (ICER), which is defined as the difference in cost divided by the difference in effectiveness between MMS and surgical excision, was used to determine the cost of using MMS to prevent a single recurrence and found to be $31,236 and $8,649 for primary and recurrent BCC (2001 USD). The authors found that for facial BCCs the total costs were significantly higher than those for surgical excision and conclude that the cost of MMS is too high for widespread implementation. With the exceptions of primary BCC of the ears and recurrent BCC of the cheeks and chin, MMS is "not likely to be considered a cost-effective treatment."

The authors from the Mosterd paper in 2008 again studied the ICER which was found to be approximately $25,063 for primary BCC and $3,389 for recurrent BCC, lower than previous estimates likely because of longer follow-up time (5 years vs. less than 3 years). The researchers argue that for primary BCC of the face, MMS is not cost-effective if you compare the cost of 2 MMS (initial surgery and again for recurrence around $2,744) with the ICER. However, it may well be cost effective for recurrent BCC with an ICER of $3,389. Defect size was found to be significantly larger for recurrent large and histologically aggressive facial BCC with surgical excision than with MMS, thereby leading to poorer cosmesis in the former modality. In patients with aggressive BCC of the face, the authors recommend MMS over surgical excision.

## Conclusions

The Mohs process involves meticulous examination of the tumor margins offering a high cure rate for many cutaneous malignancies while sparing normal tissue. It is widely accepted that this technique is appropriate for high-risk tumors (recurrent or incompletely excised tumors, location in functionally or cosmetically sensitive areas such as the ears and H-zone of the face, size >2 cm, aggressive histopathology, deep extension, and tumors with PNI).

MMS is widely employed as the treatment of choice for skin cancers with high risk of recurrence. Evidence is growing for the utility of MMS for MIS, superficially invasive and invasive melanoma. At present, the body of evidence is mostly limited to retrospective systematic review, case series, and a few prospective noncomparative analyses. Certainly, multicentered, randomized controlled trials are needed to support the use of MMS in less common and aggressive tumors such as melanoma and MCC. In an age of exploding health costs, high quality trials are needed to evaluate relative current and future costs of the procedure compared with other modalities.

In summary, MMS is a highly effective treatment modality for treatment of various types of nonmelanoma skin cancer and superficial melanoma. Consistently high cure rates combined with maximum normal tissue preservation validate MMS as the profound benefit of the procedure. As such, the NCCN has recognized the benefit of MMS for nonmelanoma skin cancer, and it remains a primary therapy for high-risk skin cancer. It is equally important that the high standards of quality of those performing the Mohs technique are maintained as data surfaces that continue to support its use for cutaneous cancer, as this is the principle factor in its success. The high success rate of MMS for any cutaneous malignancy requires that all parts of the procedure function at the highest possible level of accuracy. Rigorous training, experience, and a superior frozen section preparation are paramount in achieving the highest possible cure rates with MMS.

**Evidence-Based Summary**

| Findings | Evidence level |
| --- | --- |
| MMS has several specific indications for the treatment of NMSC | III/B |
| MMS is cost-effective for primary BCC of the ears | II/A |
| MMS has the lowest recurrence rate for primary basal cell carcinoma | IV/B |
| MMS is preferred over surgical excision for facial recurrent BCC | II/A |
| Standard surgical excision is probably sufficient in most primary BCCs | II/A |
| Aggressive histological subtypes of BCC is a significant risk factor for recurrence in recurrent but not primary BCC | II/A |
| MMS is cost-effective for recurrent BCC of the face | II/A |
| MMS is indicated for BCC of the eyes, ears, lips, and nose | III/B |
| MMS is indicated for BCCs > 2 cm in diameter | III/B |
| MMS is indicated for morpheaform, infiltrative, and micronodular BCC | III/B |
| MMS is indicated for BCC with perineural involvement | III/B |
| Surgery offers the most effective and efficient means for a cure of skin cancer | VI/B |
| MMS is indicated for low-risk BCC after positive margins are found on primary excision, but re-excision if on the trunk or radiation | VI/B |
| Local excision is acceptable for BCC > 2 cm on the trunk or extremities if 10 mm margins are functionally and cosmetically feasible | VI/B |
| MMS is indicated for all types of SCC if positive margins are found on primary excision | VI/B |
| According to the NCCN guidelines, MMS is the treatment of choice for high-risk BCC and SCC in surgical candidates | VI/B |
| According to the NCCN guidelines, adjuvant radiation therapy is recommended for perineural involvement of BCC or SCC | VI/B |
| Radiation can be used to treat all NMSC in nonsurgical candidates over 60 | VI/B |
| Intraoperative frozen section is not acceptable as an alternative to MMS unless it includes complete deep and peripheral margin assessment | VI/B |
| MMS is not more expensive than standard excision for treatment of NMSC | IV/B |
| MMS is discouraged for noncontiguous tumors | VI/B |
| MMS is the treatment of choice for tumors in cosmetically and functionally critical areas | VI/B |
| Limitations of MMS include increased time, use of specialized personnel, precision needed during mapping, and frozen section artifacts | VI/B |
| MMS offers lower recurrence rates over standard excision for BCC and SCC | VI/B |
| Debate exists over the cost-effectiveness of MMS vs. standard excision | VI/B |
| MMS is the preferred treatment modality for BCC with PNI | VI/B |
| There is high concordance rates for melanoma on frozen and permanent sections | V/B |
| MMS has been shown to have 5-year survival rates comparable to or exceeding those of wide local excision | V/B |
| MMS is emerging as the treatment of choice for DFSP | V/B |
| Outcomes for MMS compares favorably with WLE for MCC | V/B |

# References

1. Drake LA, Dinehart SM, Goltz RW, Graham GF, Hordinsky MK, Lewis CW, et al. Guidelines of care for Mohs micrographic surgery. American Academy of Dermatology. J Am Acad Dermatol. 1995;33:271–8.
2. Telfer NR, Colver GB, Bowers PW. Guidelines for the management of basal cell carcinoma. British Association of Dermatologists. Br J Dermatol. 1999; 141:415–23.
3. http://www.nccn.org/professionals/physician_gls/ default.asp. Accessed August 30, 2011.
4. Miller PK, Roenigk RK, Brodland DG, Randle HW. Cutaneous micrographic surgery: Mohs procedure. Mayo Clin Proc. 1992;67:971–80.
5. Iriondo M. Mohs micrographic surgery. Compr Ther. 1994;20:369–74.
6. Kumar B, Roden D, Vinciullo C, Elliott T. A review of 24 cases of Mohs surgery and ophthalmic plastic reconstruction. Aust N Z J Ophthalmol. 1997;25: 289–93.
7. Essers BA, Dirksen CD, Nieman FH, Smeets NW, Krekels GA, Prins MH, et al. Cost-effectiveness of Mohs micrographic surgery vs surgical excision for basal cell carcinoma of the face. Arch Dermatol. 2006;142:187–94.
8. Bialy TL, Whalen J, Veledar E, Lafreniere D, Spiro J, Chartier T, et al. Mohs micrographic surgery vs traditional surgical excision: a cost comparison analysis. Arch Dermatol. 2004;140:736–42.
9. Lang Jr PG, Osguthorpe JD. Indications and limitations of Mohs micrographic surgery. Dermatol Clin. 1989;7:627–44.
10. Lambert DR, Siegle RJ. Skin cancer: a review with consideration of treatment options including Mohs micrographic surgery. Ohio Med. 1990;86:745–7.
11. Leslie DF, Greenway HT. Mohs micrographic surgery for skin cancer. Australas J Dermatol. 1991;32:159–64.
12. Rowe DE, Carroll RJ, Day Jr CL. Long-term recurrence rates in previously untreated (primary) basal cell carcinoma: implications for patient follow-up. J Dermatol Surg Oncol. 1989;15:315–28.
13. Shriner DL, McCoy DK, Goldberg DJ, Wagner Jr RF. Mohs micrographic surgery. J Am Acad Dermatol. 1998;39:79–97.
14. Rippey JJ, Rippey E. Characteristics of incompletely excised basal cell carcinomas of the skin. Med J Aust. 1997;166:581–3.
15. Pascal RR, Hobby LW, Lattes R, Crikelair GF. Prognosis of "incompletely excised" versus "completely excised" basal cell carcinoma. Plast Reconstr Surg. 1968;41:328–32.
16. Cataldo PA, Stoddard PB, Reed WP. Use of frozen section analysis in the treatment of basal cell carcinoma. Am J Surg. 1990;159:561–3.
17. Farhi D, Dupin N, Palangie A, Carlotti A, Avril MF. Incomplete excision of basal cell carcinoma: rate and associated factors among 362 consecutive cases. Dermatol Surg. 2007;33:1207–14.
18. Wolf DJ, Zitelli JA. Surgical margins for basal cell carcinoma. Arch Dermatol. 1987;123:340–4.
19. Hruza GJ. Mohs micrographic surgery local recurrences. J Dermatol Surg Oncol. 1994;20:573–7.
20. Leibovitch I, Huilgol SC, Selva D, Richards S, Paver R. Basal cell carcinoma treated with Mohs surgery in Australia II. Outcome at 5-year follow-up. J Am Acad Dermatol. 2005;53:452–7.
21. Leibovitch I, Huilgol SC, Selva D, Hill D, Richards S, Paver R. Cutaneous squamous cell carcinoma treated with Mohs micrographic surgery in Australia I. Experience over 10 years. J Am Acad Dermatol. 2005;53:253–60.
22. Rowe DE, Carroll RJ, Day Jr CL. Prognostic factors for local recurrence, metastasis, and survival rates in squamous cell carcinoma of the skin, ear, and lip. Implications for treatment modality selection. J Am Acad Dermatol. 1992;26:976–90.
23. Leibovitch I, Huilgol SC, Selva D, Richards S, Paver R. Cutaneous squamous carcinoma in situ (Bowen's disease): treatment with Mohs micrographic surgery. J Am Acad Dermatol. 2005;52:997–1002.
24. Julian CG, Bowers PW. A prospective study of Mohs' micrographic surgery in two English centres. Br J Dermatol. 1997;136:515–8.
25. Mohs FE. Chemosurgery: microscopically controlled surgery for skin cancer – past, present and future. J Dermatol Surg Oncol. 1978;4:41–54.
26. Mohs FE. Chemosurgery for the microscopically controlled excision of cutaneous cancer. Head Neck Surg. 1978;1:150–66.
27. Mohs F. Chemosurgery: microscopically controlled surgery for skin cancer. Springfield: Charles C. Thomas; 1978.
28. Robins P. Chemosurgery: my 15 years of experience. J Dermatol Surg Oncol. 1981;7:779–89.
29. Robins P, Dzubow LM, Rigel DS. Squamous-cell carcinoma treated by Mohs' surgery: an experience with 414 cases in a period of 15 years. J Dermatol Surg Oncol. 1981;7:800–1.
30. Dzubow LM. Chemosurgical report: recurrence (persistence) of tumor following excision by Mohs surgery. J Dermatol Surg Oncol. 1987;13:27–30.
31. Campbell RM, Barrall D, Wilkel C, Robinson-Bostom L, Dufresne RG, Jr. Post-Mohs micrographic surgical margin tissue evaluation with permanent histopathologic sections. Dermatol Surg. 2005;31:655–8; discussion 8.
32. Smeets NW, Kuijpers DI, Nelemans P, Ostertag JU, Verhaegh ME, Krekels GA, et al. Mohs' micrographic surgery for treatment of basal cell carcinoma of the face – results of a retrospective study and review of the literature. Br J Dermatol. 2004;151:141–7.
33. Feasel AM, Brown TJ, Bogle MA, Tschen JA, Nelson BR. Perineural invasion of cutaneous malignancies. Dermatol Surg. 2001;27:531–42.
34. Mohs FE, Lathrop TG. Modes of spread of cancer of skin. AMA Arch Derm Syphilol. 1952;66:427–39.
35. Leibovitch I, Huilgol SC, Selva D, Richards S, Paver R. Basal cell carcinoma treated with Mohs surgery in

Australia III. Perineural invasion. J Am Acad Dermatol. 2005;53:458–63.

36. Ratner D, Lowe L, Johnson TM, Fader DJ. Perineural spread of basal cell carcinomas treated with Mohs micrographic surgery. Cancer. 2000;88:1605–13.

37. Hanke CW, Wolf RL, Hochman SA, O'Brian JJ. Chemosurgical reports: perineural spread of basal-cell carcinoma. J Dermatol Surg Oncol. 1983;9: 742–7.

38. Leibovitch I, Huilgol SC, Selva D, Hill D, Richards S, Paver R. Cutaneous squamous cell carcinoma treated with Mohs micrographic surgery in Australia II. Perineural invasion. J Am Acad Dermatol. 2005;53: 261–6.

39. Cottel WI. Perineural invasion by squamous-cell carcinoma. J Dermatol Surg Oncol. 1982;8:589–600.

40. Goepfert H, Dichtel WJ, Medina JE, Lindberg RD, Luna MD. Perineural invasion in squamous cell skin carcinoma of the head and neck. Am J Surg. 1984;148: 542–7.

41. Ballantyne AJ, McCarten AB, Ibanez ML. The extension of cancer of the head and neck through peripheral nerves. Am J Surg. 1963;106:651–67.

42. Malhotra R, Huilgol SC, Huynh NT, Selva D. The Australian Mohs database, part II: periocular basal cell carcinoma outcome at 5-year follow-up. Ophthalmology. 2004;111:631–6.

43. Malhotra R, Huilgol SC, Huynh NT, Selva D. The Australian Mohs database: periocular squamous cell carcinoma. Ophthalmology. 2004;111:617–23.

44. Robins P, Rodriguez-Sains R, Rabinovitz H, Rigel D. Mohs surgery for periocular basal cell carcinomas. J Dermatol Surg Oncol. 1985;11:1203–7.

45. Mohs FE. Micrographic surgery for the microscopically controlled excision of eyelid cancers. Arch Ophthalmol. 1986;104:901–9.

46. Ceilley RI, Anderson RL. Microscopically controlled excision of malignant neoplasms on and around eyelids followed by immediate surgical reconstruction. J Dermatol Surg Oncol. 1978;4:55–62.

47. Arlette JP, Carruthers A, Threlfall WJ, Warshawski LM. Basal cell carcinoma of the periocular region. J Cutan Med Surg. 1998;2:205–8.

48. Wong VA, Marshall JA, Whitehead KJ, Williamson RM, Sullivan TJ. Management of periocular basal cell carcinoma with modified en face frozen section controlled excision. Ophthal Plast Reconstr Surg. 2002; 18:430–5.

49. Dzubow LM. Sebaceous carcinoma of the eyelid: treatment with Mohs surgery. J Dermatol Surg Oncol. 1985;11:40–4.

50. Ratz JL, Luu-Duong S, Kulwin DR. Sebaceous carcinoma of the eyelid treated with Mohs' surgery. J Am Acad Dermatol. 1986;14:668–73.

51. Yount AB, Bylund D, Pratt SG, Greenway HT. Mohs micrographic excision of sebaceous carcinoma of the eyelids. J Dermatol Surg Oncol. 1994;20:523–9.

52. Spencer JM, Nossa R, Tse DT, Sequeira M. Sebaceous carcinoma of the eyelid treated with Mohs micrographic surgery. J Am Acad Dermatol. 2001;44:1004–9.

53. Callahan EF, Appert DL, Roenigk RK, Bartley GB. Sebaceous carcinoma of the eyelid: a review of 14 cases. Dermatol Surg. 2004;30:1164–8.

54. Snow SN, Larson PO, Lucarelli MJ, Lemke BN, Madjar DD. Sebaceous carcinoma of the eyelids treated by mohs micrographic surgery: report of nine cases with review of the literature. Dermatol Surg. 2002;28:623–31.

55. Berlin AL, Amin SP, Goldberg DJ. Extraocular sebaceous carcinoma treated with Mohs micrographic surgery: report of a case and review of literature. Dermatol Surg. 2008;34:254–7.

56. Reina RS, Parry E. Aggressive extraocular sebaceous carcinoma in a 52-year-old man. Dermatol Surg. 2006;32:1283–6.

57. Baker SR, Krause CJ. Carcinoma of the lip. Laryngoscope. 1980;90:19–27.

58. Holmkvist KA, Roenigk RK. Squamous cell carcinoma of the lip treated with Mohs micrographic surgery: outcome at 5 years. J Am Acad Dermatol. 1998;38:960–6.

59. Mohs F, Larson P, Iriondo M. Micrographic surgery for the microscopically controlled excision of carcinoma of the external ear. J Am Acad Dermatol. 1988;19:729–37.

60. Mohs FE. Chemosurgical treatment of melanoma; a microscopically controlled method of excision. Arch Derm Syphilol. 1950;62:269–79.

61. Barlow RJ, White CR, Swanson NA. Mohs' micrographic surgery using frozen sections alone may be unsuitable for detecting single atypical melanocytes at the margins of melanoma in situ. Br J Dermatol. 2002;146:290–4.

62. Nield DV, Saad MN, Khoo CT, Lott M, Ali MH. Tumour thickness in malignant melanoma: the limitations of frozen section. Br J Plast Surg. 1988;41: 403–7.

63. Shafir R, Hiss J, Tsur H, Bubis JJ. Pitfalls in frozen section diagnosis of malignant melanoma. Cancer. 1983;51:1168–70.

64. Zitelli JA, Moy RL, Abell E. The reliability of frozen sections in the evaluation of surgical margins for melanoma. J Am Acad Dermatol. 1991;24:102–6.

65. Zitelli JA, Brown CD, Hanusa BH. Surgical margins for excision of primary cutaneous melanoma. J Am Acad Dermatol. 1997;37:422–9.

66. Zitelli JA, Brown C, Hanusa BH. Mohs micrographic surgery for the treatment of primary cutaneous melanoma. J Am Acad Dermatol. 1997;37: 236–45.

67. Pitman GH, Kopf AW, Bart RS, Casson PR. Treatment of lentigo maligna and lentigo maligna melanoma. J Dermatol Surg Oncol. 1979 Sep;5(9): 727–37.

68. Bienert TN, Trotter MJ, Arlette JP. Treatment of cutaneous melanoma of the face by Mohs micrographic surgery. J Cutan Med Surg. 2003;7:25–30.

69. Bene NI, Healy C, Coldiron BM. Mohs micrographic surgery is accurate 95.1% of the time for melanoma in situ: a prospective study of 167 cases. Dermatol Surg. 2008;34:660–4.

70. Dhawan SS, Wolf DJ, Rabinovitz HS, Poulos E. Lentigo maligna. The use of rush permanent sections in therapy. Arch Dermatol. 1990;126:928–30.
71. Stonecipher MR, Leshin B, Patrick J, White WL. Management of lentigo maligna and lentigo maligna melanoma with paraffin-embedded tangential sections: utility of immunoperoxidase staining and supplemental vertical sections. J Am Acad Dermatol. 1993;29:589–94.
72. Cohen LM, McCall MW, Hodge SJ, Freedman JD, Callen JP, Zax RH. Successful treatment of lentigo maligna and lentigo maligna melanoma with Mohs' micrographic surgery aided by rush permanent sections. Cancer. 1994;73:2964–70.
73. Cohen LM, McCall MW, Zax RH. Mohs micrographic surgery for lentigo maligna and lentigo maligna melanoma. A follow-up study. Dermatol Surg. 1998;24:673–7.
74. Albertini JG, Elston DM, Libow LF, Smith SB, Farley MF. Mohs micrographic surgery for melanoma: a case series, a comparative study of immunostains, an informative case report, and a unique mapping technique. Dermatol Surg. 2002;28:656–65.
75. Zalla MJ, Lim KK, Dicaudo DJ, Gagnot MM. Mohs micrographic excision of melanoma using immunostains. Dermatol Surg. 2000;26:771–84.
76. Kelley LC, Starkus L. Immunohistochemical staining of lentigo maligna during Mohs micrographic surgery using MART-1. J Am Acad Dermatol. 2002;46: 78–84.
77. Mallipeddi R, Stark J, Xie XJ, Matthews M, Taylor RS. A novel 2-hour method for rapid preparation of permanent paraffin sections when treating melanoma in situ with mohs micrographic surgery. Dermatol Surg. 2008;34:1520–6.
78. Diagnosis and Treatment of Early Melanoma. National Institutes of Health Consensus Development Conference Statement on diagnosis and treatment of early melanoma, January 27–29, 1992. Am J Dermatopathol. 1993;15:34–43; discussion 6–51.
79. NCCN clinical practice guidelines in oncology: melanoma [monograph on the Internet]. Jenkintown: National Comprehensive Cancer Network. http://www.nccn.org/professionals/physician_gls/PDF/melanoma.pdf. Accessed 1 March 2006.
80. Sober AJ, Chuang TY, Duvic M, Farmer ER, Grichnik JM, Halpern AC, et al. Guidelines of care for primary cutaneous melanoma. J Am Acad Dermatol. 2001;45: 579–86.
81. Megahed M, Schon M, Selimovic D, Schon MP. Reliability of diagnosis of melanoma in situ. Lancet. 2002;359:1921–2.
82. Bricca GM, Brodland DG, Ren D, Zitelli JA. Cutaneous head and neck melanoma treated with Mohs micrographic surgery. J Am Acad Dermatol. 2005;52:92–100.
83. Bhardwaj SS, Tope WD, Lee PK. Mohs micrographic surgery for lentigo maligna and lentigo maligna melanoma using Mel-5 immunostaining: University of Minnesota experience. Dermatol Surg. 2006;32:690–6; discussion 6–7.
84. Temple CL, Arlette JP. Mohs micrographic surgery in the treatment of lentigo maligna and melanoma. J Surg Oncol. 2006;94:287–92.
85. Mohs F. Chemosurgery in cancer, gangrene, and infections. Springfield: Charles C. Thomas; 1956.
86. Mohs FE. Chemosurgery for melanoma. Arch Dermatol. 1977;113:285–91.
87. Zitelli JA, Mohs FE, Larson P, Snow S. Mohs micrographic surgery for melanoma. Dermatol Clin. 1989;7:833–43.
88. Haag ML, Glass LF, Fenske NA. Merkel cell carcinoma. Diagnosis and treatment. Dermatol Surg. 1995;21:669–83.
89. Suarez C, Rodrigo JP, Ferlito A, Devaney KO, Rinaldo A. Merkel cell carcinoma of the head and neck. Oral Oncol. 2004;40:773–9.
90. Allen PJ, Zhang ZF, Coit DG. Surgical management of Merkel cell carcinoma. Ann Surg. 1999;229:97–105.
91. Boyer JD, Zitelli JA, Brodland DG, D'Angelo G. Local control of primary Merkel cell carcinoma: review of 45 cases treated with Mohs micrographic surgery with and without adjuvant radiation. J Am Acad Dermatol. 2002;47:885–92.
92. O'Connor WJ, Roenigk RK, Brodland DG. Merkel cell carcinoma. Comparison of Mohs micrographic surgery and wide excision in eighty-six patients. Dermatol Surg. 1997;23:929–33.
93. Snow SN, Larson PO, Hardy S, Bentz M, Madjar D, Landeck A, et al. Merkel cell carcinoma of the skin and mucosa: report of 12 cutaneous cases with 2 cases arising from the nasal mucosa. Dermatol Surg. 2001;27:165–70.
94. Dancey AL, Rayatt SS, Soon C, Ilchshyn A, Brown I, Srivastava S. Merkel cell carcinoma: a report of 34 cases and literature review. J Plast Reconstr Aesthet Surg. 2006;59:1294–9.
95. Taylor HB, Helwig EB. Dermatofibrosarcoma protuberans. A study of 115 cases. Cancer. 1962;15: 717–25.
96. Dawes KW, Hanke CW. Dermatofibrosarcoma protuberans treated with Mohs micrographic surgery: cure rates and surgical margins. Dermatol Surg. 1996;22:530–4.
97. Ratner D, Thomas CO, Johnson TM, Sondak VK, Hamilton TA, Nelson BR, et al. Mohs micrographic surgery for the treatment of dermatofibrosarcoma protuberans. Results of a multiinstitutional series with an analysis of the extent of microscopic spread. J Am Acad Dermatol. 1997;37:600–13.
98. Robinson JK. Dermatofibrosarcoma protuberans resected by Mohs' surgery (chemosurgery). A 5-year prospective study. J Am Acad Dermatol. 1985;12: 1093–8.
99. Hafner J, Schutz K, Morgenthaler W, Steiger E, Meyer V, Burg G. Micrographic surgery ("slow Mohs") in cutaneous sarcomas. Dermatology. 1999; 198:37–43.
100. Thomas CJ, Wood GC, Marks VJ. Mohs micrographic surgery in the treatment of rare aggressive cutaneous tumors: the Geisinger experience. Dermatol Surg. 2007;33:333–9.

101. Garcia C, Clark RE, Buchanan M. Dermatofibrosarcoma protuberans. Int J Dermatol. 1996;35: 867–71.
102. Snow SN, Gordon EM, Larson PO, Bagheri MM, Bentz ML, Sable DB. Dermatofibrosarcoma protuberans: a report on 29 patients treated by Mohs micrographic surgery with long-term follow-up and review of the literature. Cancer. 2004;101:28–38.
103. Nouri K, Lodha R, Jimenez G, Robins P. Mohs micrographic surgery for dermatofibrosarcoma protuberans: University of Miami and NYU experience. Dermatol Surg. 2002;28:1060–4; discussion 4.
104. Gloster Jr HM, Harris KR, Roenigk RK. A comparison between Mohs micrographic surgery and wide surgical excision for the treatment of dermatofibrosarcoma protuberans. J Am Acad Dermatol. 1996;35:82–7.
105. Haycox CL, Odland PB, Olbricht SM, Casey B. Dermatofibrosarcoma protuberans (DFSP): growth characteristics based on tumor modeling and a review of cases treated with Mohs micrographic surgery. Ann Plast Surg. 1997;38:246–51.
106. Paradisi A, Abeni D, Rusciani A, Cigna E, Wolter M, Scuderi N, et al. Dermatofibrosarcoma protuberans: wide local excision vs. Mohs micrographic surgery. Cancer Treat Rev. 2008;34:728–36.
107. Nelson RA, Arlette JP. Mohs micrographic surgery and dermatofibrosarcoma protuberans: a multidisciplinary approach in 44 patients. Ann Plast Surg. 2008;60:667–72.
108. Hobbs ER, Wheeland RG, Bailin PL, Ratz JL, Yetman RJ, Zins JE. Treatment of dermatofibrosarcoma protuberans with Mohs micrographic surgery. Ann Surg. 1988;207:102–7.
109. Wright TI, Petersen JE. Treatment of recurrent dermatofibrosarcoma protuberans with imatinib mesylate, followed by Mohs micrographic surgery. Dermatol Surg. 2007;33:741–4.
110. McArthur GA, Demetri GD, van Oosterom A, Heinrich MC, Debiec-Rychter M, Corless CL, et al. Molecular and clinical analysis of locally advanced dermatofibrosarcoma protuberans treated with imatinib: imatinib Target Exploration Consortium Study B2225. J Clin Oncol. 2005;23:866–73.
111. Ortiz AE, Wu JJ, Linden KG. Letter: clear margins after the use of imatinib mesylate prior to resection of extensive dermatofibrosarcoma protuberans. Dermatol Surg. 2008;34:1151.
112. Davis JL, Randle HW, Zalla MJ, Roenigk RK, Brodland DG. A comparison of Mohs micrographic surgery and wide excision for the treatment of atypical fibroxanthoma. Dermatol Surg. 1997;23:105–10.
113. Seavolt M, McCall M. Atypical fibroxanthoma: review of the literature and summary of 13 patients treated with mohs micrographic surgery. Dermatol Surg. 2006;32:435–41; discussion 9–41.
114. Huether MJ, Zitelli JA, Brodland DG. Mohs micrographic surgery for the treatment of spindle cell tumors of the skin. J Am Acad Dermatol. 2001;44: 656–9.
115. Brown MD, Swanson NA. Treatment of malignant fibrous histiocytoma and atypical fibrous xanthomas with micrographic surgery. J Dermatol Surg Oncol. 1989;15:1287–92.
116. Limmer BL, Clark DP. Cutaneous micrographic surgery for atypical fibroxanthoma. Dermatol Surg. 1997;23:553–7; discussion 7–8.
117. Leibovitch I, Huilgol SC, Richards S, Paver R, Selva D. Scalp tumors treated with Mohs micrographic surgery: clinical features and surgical outcome. Dermatol Surg. 2006;32:1369–74.
118. Dzubow LM. Mohs surgery report: spindle cell fibrohistiocytic tumors: classification and pathophysiology. J Dermatol Surg Oncol. 1988;14:490–5.
119. Chilukuri S, Alam M, Goldberg LH. Two atypical fibroxanthomas of the ear. Dermatol Surg. 2003 Apr;29(4):408–10.
120. Hakim I. Atypical fibroxanthoma. Ann Otol Rhinol Laryngol. 2001;110:985–7.
121. Fretzin DF, Helwig EB. Atypical fibroxanthoma of the skin. A clinicopathologic study of 140 cases. Cancer. 1973;31:1541–52.
122. Brown MD. Recognition and management of unusual cutaneous tumors. Dermatol Clin. 2000;18: 543–52.
123. Zalla MJ, Randle HW, Brodland DG, Davis JL, Roenigk RK. Mohs surgery vs wide excision for atypical fibroxanthoma: follow-up. Dermatol Surg. 1997;23:1223–4.
124. Hausner RJ, Vargas-Cortes F, Alexander RW. Dermatofibrosarcoma protuberans with lymph node involvement. A case report of simultaneous occurrence with an atypical fibroxanthoma of the skin. Arch Dermatol. 1978;114:88–91.
125. Burns MK, Chen SP, Goldberg LH. Microcystic adnexal carcinoma. Ten cases treated by Mohs micrographic surgery. J Dermatol Surg Oncol. 1994; 20:429–34.
126. Friedman PM, Friedman RH, Jiang SB, Nouri K, Amonette R, Robins P. Microcystic adnexal carcinoma: collaborative series review and update. J Am Acad Dermatol. 1999;41:225–31.
127. Chiller K, Passaro D, Scheuller M, Singer M, McCalmont T, Grekin RC. Microcystic adnexal carcinoma: forty-eight cases, their treatment, and their outcome. Arch Dermatol. 2000;136:1355–9.
128. Snow S, Madjar DD, Hardy S, Bentz M, Lucarelli MJ, Bechard R, et al. Microcystic adnexal carcinoma: report of 13 cases and review of the literature. Dermatol Surg. 2001;27:401–8.
129. Leibovitch I, Huilgol SC, Selva D, Lun K, Richards S, Paver R. Microcystic adnexal carcinoma: treatment with Mohs micrographic surgery. J Am Acad Dermatol. 2005;52:295–300.
130. Abbate M, Zeitouni NC, Seyler M, Hicks W, Loree T, Cheney RT. Clinical course, risk factors, and treatment of microcystic adnexal carcinoma: a short series report. Dermatol Surg. 2003; 29:1035–8.
131. Goldberg DJ, Kim YA. Angiosarcoma of the scalp treated with Mohs micrographic surgery. J Dermatol Surg Oncol. 1993;19:156–8.

132. Muscarella VA. Angiosarcoma treated by Mohs micrographic surgery. J Dermatol Surg Oncol. 1993;19:1132–3.

133. Thissen MR, Neumann MH, Schouten LJ. A systematic review of treatment modalities for primary basal cell carcinomas. Arch Dermatol. 1999;135: 1177–83.

134. Smeets NW, Krekels GA, Ostertag JU, Essers BA, Dirksen CD, Nieman FH, et al. Surgical excision vs Mohs' micrographic surgery for basal-cell carcinoma of the face: randomised controlled trial. Lancet. 2004;364:1766–72.

135. Mosterd K, Krekels GA, Nieman FH, Ostertag JU, Essers BA, Dirksen CD, et al. Surgical excision versus Mohs' micrographic surgery for primary and recurrent basal-cell carcinoma of the face: a prospective randomised controlled trial with 5-years' follow-up. Lancet Oncol. 2008;9:1149–56.

136. Rowe DE, Carroll RJ, Day Jr CL. Mohs surgery is the treatment of choice for recurrent (previously treated) basal cell carcinoma. J Dermatol Surg Oncol. 1989;15:424–31.

137. Cook J, Zitelli JA. Mohs micrographic surgery: a cost analysis. J Am Acad Dermatol. 1998;39:698–703.

138. Lear W, Mittmann N, Barnes E, Breen D, Murray C. Cost comparisons of managing complex facial basal cell carcinoma: Canadian study. J Cutan Med Surg. 2008;12:82–7.

139. Parker TL, Zitelli JA. Surgical margins for excision of dermatofibrosarcoma protuberans. J Am Acad Dermatol. 1995;32(2 Pt 1):233–6.

## Self-Assessment

1. All of the following statements about Mohs surgery are true except
   (a) Mohs surgery is cost effective for basal cell carcinoma around the eye
   (b) Compared with standard surgical excision, Mohs surgery has a statistically significant lower rate of recurrence for primary BCC on the face
   (c) Mohs surgery is indicated for skin cancer in high-risk anatomic areas, such as the genitalia
   (d) Mohs surgery is encouraged for noncontiguous tumors

2. Evidence supports the use of Mohs surgery for all of the following tumors except
   (a) 0.6 cm infiltrative basal cell carcinoma of the nasal ala
   (b) 1.7 cm nodular basal cell carcinoma of the upper back
   (c) 0.4 cm morpheaform basal cell carcinoma of the chin
   (d) 0.5 cm nodular basal cell carcinoma of the medial canthus

3. The average cited rate of recurrence for dermatofibrosarcoma protuberans treated with Mohs surgery is
   (a) 0–8%
   (b) 10–15%
   (c) 16–25%
   (d) 25–50%

4. Evidence levels for Mohs surgery for the treatment of merkel cell carcinoma is
   (a) III/C
   (b) II/A
   (c) VI/C
   (d) V/B

5. Perineural invasion found on pathology of a squamous cell carcinoma
   (a) Is an indication for Mohs surgery
   (b) Is a contraindication for Mohs surgery
   (c) Portends a lower rate of tumor recurrence or persistence
   (d) Is found in greater than 50% of cases

## Answers

1. d: Mohs surgery is encouraged for noncontiguous tumors
2. b: 1.7 cm nodular basal cell carcinoma of the upper back
3. a: 0–8%
4. d: V/B
5. a: Is an indication for Mohs surgery

# Basal Cell Carcinoma

Monica L. Halem, Désirée Ratner,
and Asha Patel

## Introduction

Cutaneous basal cell carcinoma (BCC) is the most ubiquitous cancer affecting humans worldwide [1]. It is the most common cutaneous malignancy, accounting for approximately 60–75% of all skin cancers [2]. BCC is an indolent, locally invasive, malignant epithelial neoplasm arising from the basilar layer of the epidermis [3]. It slowly progresses, with projections of microtumor spreading in a three-dimensional manner throughout the papillary and reticular dermis [4], and rarely leads to metastasis. BCC is thought to be composed of aberrant follicular germinative cells, also known as trichoblasts, due to its morphological and immunohistochemical similarities to hair follicle structures [5].

## Incidence

The exact incidence of BCC is difficult to measure, since data collection regarding nonmelanoma skin cancer (NMSC) is usually excluded from cancer registries. This problem is further complicated by the variable geographic incidence of NMSC [6]. However, trends indicate that the incidence of BCC is rapidly increasing worldwide, affecting more than one million Americans per year [7]. The estimated average lifetime risk for Caucasians to develop BCC is upwards of 30% [8]. The highest BCC incidence occurs in Australia, and is reported to affect 1–2% of the population each year [9]. In a recent Australian study, the incidence of persons affected multiple times by primary BCC (pBCC) was 705/100,000 person-years; the incidence rate of persons affected once by pBCC was 935/100,000 person-years [10]. Age-standardized yearly rates in the United States have been estimated at up to 407 cases of BCC per 100,000 white men and 212 cases per 100,000 white women [11]. Although the rates remain highest among elderly men, patients with BCC are increasingly likely to be young women as well [12]. Once an individual has developed one BCC, they are more likely to develop another. One meta-analysis estimates that these patients have a 44% risk of developing an additional BCC within 3 years [13].

## Risk Factors

BCC has a predilection for patients with a history of intense ultraviolet (UV) radiation exposure during childhood (0–19 years), Fitzpatrick skin type I–II, blonde/red hair color, light eye color, and with chronic photodamaged skin, which typically occurs over the head and neck region [14]. The most significant risk factor for the development of

M.L. Halem (✉) • D. Ratner • A. Patel
Department of Dermatology, Columbia University
Medical Center/New York Presbyterian Hospital,
Dermatologic Surgery Unit, 161 Fort Washington
Avenue 12th Floor, New York, NY 10032, USA
e-mail: mlh2166@columbia.edu

M. Alam (ed.), *Evidence-Based Procedural Dermatology*,
DOI 10.1007/978-0-387-09424-3_2, © Springer Science+Business Media, LLC 2012

**Table 2.1**  Risk factors for basal cell carcinoma

| |
|---|
| Ultraviolet radiation |
| Arsenic |
| Ionizing radiation |
| Tanning bed use |
| Red or blond hair |
| Light eye color |
| Fitzpatrick skin types I–II |
| Immunosuppression |
| Genodermatoses |

BCC appears to be exposure to UV radiation [15]. However, the timing, pattern, and amount of exposure to UV radiation also seem to be important. The risk of disease is significantly increased by exposure to UV radiation during childhood and adolescence [16], as well as intense intermittent and chronic cumulative sun exposure [17]. Physical factors, including fair complexion, hair and eye color, influence responsiveness to UV radiation and also act as independent risk factors [18]. Other risk factors include a history of diagnostic or therapeutic radiation [19], arsenic exposure [20], immunosuppressive therapy for organ transplant recipients [21], psoralen and UV A radiation [22], and various genodermatoses such as Gorlin's Syndrome and Xeroderma Pigmentosum [23] (Table 2.1). It has been estimated that 16% of renal transplant patients will develop BCC, and their risk increases with the length of their immunosuppression [24]. Several studies have shown that renal transplant recipients have a risk of BCC 10 times that of the general population [25].

## Clinical Presentation

BCCs characteristically arise in body areas exposed to the sun and are most common on the head and neck, followed by the trunk, arms, and legs. In addition, BCCs have been reported in unusual sites, including the axillae, breasts, perianal area, genitalia, palms, and soles. BCCs have been classified into four main types according to clinical and histopathological features: superficial, nodular, micronodular, and infiltrative or morpheaform. In a retrospective study of over 10,000 cases of diagnosed BCCs, 79% were nodular, 15%

were superficial, and 6% were morpheaform [26]. The nodular and morpheaform types were observed on the head and neck 90–95% of the time, whereas 46% of superficial BCCs occurred on the trunk. In another earlier review of 1,039 consecutive cases of BCC, the most common histologic subtypes were mixed 38.6%, nodular 21.0%, superficial 17.4%, and micronodular 14.5% [27]. Nodular BCC is the classic form, which most often presents as a pearly pink to white dome-shaped papule surrounded by a well-demarcated rolled border; prominent telangiectatic vessels may superficially traverse the lesion (Fig. 2.1a, b, and d). Superficial BCC presents as a scaly erythematous patch or plaque (Fig. 2.1c). The morpheaform type, also known as sclerosing, fibrosing, or infiltrative BCC, typically appears as an indurated, whitish, scar-like plaque with indistinct margins (Fig. 2.1e). Uncommon variants, including basosquamous, keratotic, granular-cell, adamantinoid, clear-cell, and BCC with matrical differentiation, have also been described. The value of classifying the histologic appearance of BCC lies in the relationship between histologic subtype and clinical behavior. Aggressive histologic variants include micronodular, infiltrative, basosquamous, morpheaform, and mixed subtypes [28]. Nodular and superficial subtypes generally have a less aggressive clinical course.

## Molecular Pathogenesis

The most recent insight into BCC pathogenesis is the discovery of the hedgehog (HH) signaling pathway (Fig. 2.2). This pathway was originally shown to be necessary for the development of the fruitfly *Drosophila melanogaster*, and was later found to have a crucial role in mammalian development [29]. Sonic HH (SHH) protein binds the tumor-suppressor protein patched homologue 1 (PTCH1), thereby inhibiting PTCH1-mediated suppression of intracellular signaling by another transmembrane protein, the G-protein-coupled receptor smoothened (SMO). The downstream targets of SMO include the GLI family of transcription factors. Currently, it is thought that upregulation of this HH signaling is the pivotal

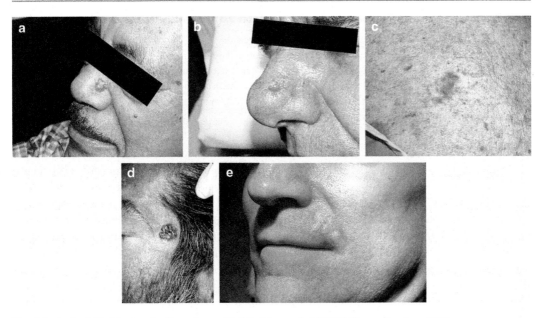

**Fig. 2.1** (**a**, **b**, **e**) Nodular basal cell carcinoma (BCC), (**c**) superficial BCC (**d**) morpheaform BCC

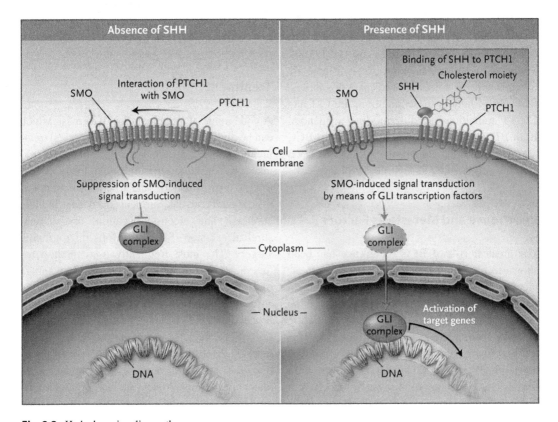

**Fig. 2.2** Hedgehog signaling pathway

**Table 2.2** Low vs. high risk factors of BCC

| Low risk | High risk |
| --- | --- |
| Primary | Recurrence |
| Tumor <2 cm on trunk/Ext | Tumor >2 cm on trunk/Ext |
| Tumor <1 cm on face | Tumor >1 cm on face |
| Complete excision | Incomplete excision |
| Non-aggressive histology | Aggressive histology |
| No perineural invasion | Perineural invasion |
| No perivascular invasion | Perivascular invasion |

**Table 2.3** Treatment options for basal cell carcinoma

| Surgical | Non-Surgical |
| --- | --- |
| Surgical excision | Topical imiquimod |
| Mohs micrographic surgery | Photodynamic therapy |
| Electrodesiccation and curettage | Radiotherapy |
| Cryosurgery | Laser therapy |

abnormality in BCC [30]. Approximately 90% of sporadic BCCs have loss-of-mutations in at least one allele of *PTCH1*, and 10% have activating mutations of downstream SMO protein [31–33]. This loss-of-function mutation of *PTCH1* includes the germ-line mutation found in patients with basal cell nevus syndrome (Gorlin syndrome) [34]. With these mutations and dysregulation of the HH pathway, SMO is active, resulting in continuous activation of target genes [35]. The expression of mRNAs from these target genes is increased in BCCs [32]. Other alterations in the HH pathway that have been implicated in the development of this disease include gain-of-function mutations in SHH and GLI [30]. Mutations in the *p53* tumor-suppressor gene are found in approximately 50% of cases of sporadic BCC [36]. Many of these mutations are C-T and CC-TT transitions at dipyrimidine sequences. Both *PTCH1* and *Tp53* mutations seen in BCC are of the type indicative of exposure to UVB radiation, confirming its significant role.

## Recurrence and Metastasis Factors

The greatest risk of BCC recurrence has been shown to be within the first 5 years after treatment [37]. Risk factors for recurrence include a tumor diameter greater than 2 cm, location on the central part of the face or ears, long-standing duration, incomplete excision, an aggressive histologic growth pattern, and perineural or perivascular involvement (Table 2.2). Tumors with subclinical extension or indistinct borders have a higher recurrence rate than more limited or well-defined tumors [38].

Metastasis of BCC is rare, with metastatic rates ranging from 0.003 to 0.5% [39]. Fewer than 500 cases have been reported in the literature [40]. Risk factors for the development of metastasis are identical to those for recurrence, although they also include a history of persistent, longstanding, untreated BCC, lack of response to conventional methods of treatment, and previous radiation treatment. The median interval between tumor presentation and metastasis is estimated to be 9 years [41]. BCC most often metastasizes via dissemination to regional lymph nodes (40–83%), followed by hematogenous spread to lungs (35–53%), bone, (20–28%), skin (10–17%), and liver (9%) [40]. The prognosis for metastatic disease is poor, with mean survival ranging from 8 months to 4 years [38, 42].

## Treatment

A wide range of treatments for BCC exist, which can be divided into surgical and nonsurgical treatments (Table 2.3). Choice of treatment should take into consideration tumor type, location, histologic growth pattern, and whether the tumor is primary or recurrent. Surgical approaches include curettage and electrodesiccation, cryosurgery, surgical excision (SE), and Mohs micrographic surgery. The most frequently used method for treatment of BCC is SE, which has the advantage of histologic evaluation of the margins of the specimen, although the vertical, or breadloaf, processing that is typically used allows visualization of less than 1% of the entire specimen margin [43]. Mohs micrographic surgery remains as the "gold standard" because of its highest cure rate, complete histological analysis of tumor margins using horizontal sectioning techniques, and preservation of normal tissue [44]. Nonsurgical

**Table 2.4** NCCN risk factors for recurrence

| H&P | Low risk | High risk |
| --- | --- | --- |
| Location/size | "Mask area" of face <6 mm<br>Cheeks/forehead/scalp <10 mm<br>Trunk/extremities <20 mm | "Mask area" of face >6 mm<br>Cheeks/forehead/scalp >10 mm<br>Trunk/extremities >20 mm |
| Borders | Well defined | Poorly defined |
| Primary vs. recurrent | Primary | Recurrent |
| Immunosuppression | (−) | (+) |
| Prior radiation treatment | (−) | (+) |
| Histopathologic subtype | Nodular, superficial | Morpheaform, sclerosing, or mixed |
| Perineural involvement | (−) | (+) |

approaches include radiotherapy, topical and injectable therapies, and photodynamic therapy (PDT). Radiotherapy is an important option for patients who are not surgical candidates, although its use may be limited due to the risk of side effects. Newer topical therapies such as imiquimod and PDT have been shown to be useful for superficial lesions. There are few randomized controlled studies comparing different skin cancer treatments; however, much of the published literature has low patient numbers and short-term follow-up [45]. The remainder of this chapter will highlight consensus documents and analyze the literature comparing the various treatment modalities to gain a more evidence-based approach to the treatment of BCC.

## Consensus Documents

### National Comprehensive Cancer Network (Evidence IIA) [46]

The National Comprehensive Cancer Network (NCCN) Clinical Practice Guidelines in Oncology is one of the most inclusive and updated oncologic references. It is compiled annually into a comprehensive review based on a detailed evaluation of evidence and expert medical opinion. The following key recommendations have been summarized from the NCCN 2009 BCC guidelines.

### Clinical Risk Factors

The NCCN has agreed upon several clinical risk factors that apply to BCC. High risk location and large size are known risk factors for recurrence and metastasis. The panel states that BCCs on the trunk/extremities ≥20 mm, BCCs on the cheeks/forehead/scalp/neck ≥10 mm, or BCCs on the "mask areas" of the face/genitalia/hands/feet ≥6 mm are considered high risk (Table 2.4). "Mask areas" of the face include the following locations: central face, eyelids, eyebrows, periorbital region, nose, cutaneous lip, vermilion lip, chin, mandible, preauricular skin and sulci, postauricular skin and sulci, ear, and temple. The NCCN Panel selected these criteria based on a retrospective review performed at the Skin and Cancer Unit of the NYU School of Medicine [47]. Additional risk factors include poorly defined borders, recurrent tumor, history of prior radiation and perineural involvement. The panel states that if perineural involvement is seen, further workup with MRI should be considered to evaluate the extent of disease further. The panel has also agreed that immunosuppression and long term use of psoralen and UV A light increase the risk of BCC, even though there is little published data confirming that BCCs are more likely to recur or metastasize in immunosuppressed patients [48]. This consensus was mostly based on anecdotal clinical reports and NCCN panel members' own clinical experience. After further evaluating the literature, the NCCN panel decided that young age alone, i.e., age younger than 40-years old, was not an independent clinical risk factor. However, any tumor showing an aggressive histologic growth pattern, regardless of the patient's age, should be considered a high risk tumor.

**Table 2.5** NCCN TNM staging system for non-melanoma skin cancer, adapted from 2008 American Joint Committee on Cancer (AJCC)

| Primary tumor (T) | | Stage grouping | |
|---|---|---|---|
| TX | Primary tumor cannot be assessed | Stage 0 | Tis N0M0 |
| T0 | No evidence of primary tumor | Stage 1 | T1N0M0 |
| Tis | Carcinoma in situ | Stage II | T2N0M0 |
| | | | T3N0M0 |
| T1 | Tumor 2 cm or less in greatest dimension | Stage III | T4N0M0 |
| | | | Any TN1M0 |
| T2 | Tumor more than 2 cm but not more than 5 cm in greatest dimension | Stage IV | Any T |
| | | | Any NM1 |
| T3 | Tumor more than 5 cm in greatest dimension | Histologic Grade (G) | |
| T4 | Tumor invades deep extradermal structures (i.e., cartilage, skeletal muscle, or bone) | GX | Grade cannot be assessed |
| Regional lymph nodes (N) | | G1 | Well differentiated |
| NX | Regional lymph nodes cannot be assessed | G2 | Moderately differentiated |
| N0 | No regional lymph node metastasis | G3 | Poorly differentiated |
| N1 | Regional lymph node metastasis | G4 | Undifferentiated |
| Distant metastasis (M) | | | |
| MX | Distant metastasis cannot be assessed | | |
| M0 | No distant metastasis | | |
| M1 | Distant metastasis | | |

## Histologic Subtypes

The panel concluded that BCCs with an "aggressive growth pattern" on histology were more likely to recur. These histologic subtypes included micronodular, infiltrative, morpheaform, sclerosing, and mixed. Superficial and nodular subtypes were classified as nonaggressive histologic growth patterns.

## Clinical Presentation and Workup

The NCCN has adapted the American Joint Committee on Cancer (AJCC) 2007 tumor staging system for NMSC (Table 2.5). Clinical staging of cutaneous carcinomas, according to the AJCC, is based upon physical inspection and palpation of the lesion and regional lymph nodes. If a lesion appears to be fixed, imaging studies of underlying bony structures are recommended. On pathologic staging, cell differentiation, uniform cell size, infrequent cellular mitoses, nuclear irregularity, and intact intercellular bridges are characteristics of a benign or low-grade tumor [49]. Of note is that these histopathologic features are more relevant to the evaluation of squamous cell carcinoma than BCC, whose cells tend to be monomorphic and basaloid, without mitoses or nuclear irregularity, and with intact intercellular bridges.

The NCCN states that the most important step toward assessing a suspicious lesion is to take a full history and perform a complete skin and regional lymph node examination. An appropriate skin biopsy should be performed on the suspicious lesion including the deep reticular dermis if clinically indicated. If more extensive disease is suspected, appropriate preoperative imaging may be completed to assess the extent of involvement.

## Treatment

Treatment options of BCC are based upon clinical risk factors, consideration of functional and cosmetic outcome, and patient preference. Curettage and electrodesiccation is effective for low-risk tumors. If the lesion is on a hair-bearing site, with a risk of tumor extension into follicular structures, or if high-risk pathological features are present, SE should be strongly considered as an alternative.

Excision with postoperative margin assessment (POMA) is used as a primary treatment for low-risk BCC if the lesion can be excised with 4 mm clinical margins and allowed to heal by secondary intention, or closed with a side-to-side linear repair or skin graft. The lesion qualifies for additional treatment if margins are positive after excision with POMA. These treatments include the following: (1) Mohs micrographic surgery, (2) resection with complete circumferential peripheral and deep-margin assessment (CCPDMA), (3) radiation therapy (reserved for patients ≥60 years), or (4) re-excision with POMA for tumors located on the trunk or extremities.

For high-risk tumors, Mohs surgery or excision with CCPDMA using intraoperative frozen section (IOFS) assessment is recommended. The available evidence suggests that Mohs micrographic surgery is the preferred modality. If negative margins are unachievable with surgery, adjuvant treatment with radiation is recommended.

Radiation therapy, typically using electron beams, is also a first-line treatment option for nonsurgical candidates, particularly patients who are ≥60 years old. Tumors with a size <20 mm typically require treatment margins of 1–1.5 cm, while tumors ≥2 cm require 1.5–2 cm margins. Radiation treatment is contraindicated in patients with genodermatoses predisposing them to skin cancer, as well as patients with connective tissue disease.

Topical therapeutic modalities for BCC are also available, but because of their low cure rates, these are reserved for patients who are not candidates either for surgery or radiation. Treatments for low-risk BCC include topical 5-fluorouracil (5FU), topical imiquimod, PDT, and cryotherapy.

## Monitoring

Appropriate follow-up care to monitor for recurrence is essential, as 30–50% of patients will develop another NMSC during the 5-year follow-up period [50]. Patients with a history of BCC may also be at increased risk for developing melanoma [51]; long-term surveillance and patient education (sun protective measures and self skin examinations) are therefore strongly recommended.

The NCCN states that the primary goal for BCC treatment is to cure the cancer while simultaneously preserving maximum function and cosmesis. Treatment decisions should be customized for each patient to take into account both their medical situation and personal preference (Evidence IIA). A surgical approach is preferred, since it is most efficient and effective with respect to cure rate, but radiation therapy may be considered as primary treatment if function, cosmesis, or patient preference could be affected by a surgical approach (Evidence IIA). In patients at high risk for multiple primary tumors, increased surveillance is recommended, as well as consideration of prophylactic measures for further skin cancer prevention (Evidence IIA). In patients with superficial BCC for whom surgery or radiation treatment is not an option, topical therapies (5-FU, imiquimod, PDT, or cryotherapy) can be considered, despite the fact that cure rates with these agents are lower than with other therapies (Evidence IIA).

## American Cancer Society (Evidence VIC) [52]

The American Cancer Society (ACS) is a nationwide, community-based voluntary health organization headquartered in Atlanta, Georgia, USA. The purpose of the ACS is to disseminate medical information that is accurate and readily available both to the general public and health care providers. The following information has been summarized from the 2008 online ACS skin cancer reference site, which is primarily compiled from the views of physicians and nurses serving on the ACS's Cancer Information Database Editorial Board. This information is based upon the board's interpretation of published medical studies and their own professional experience.

BCC is reported to occur in approximately 8 out of 10 skin cancers, approximately 800,000–900,000 cases per year. BCC is commonly found on sun-exposed areas of the body in middle-aged to older individuals; however, the trend is increasing in younger people. Recurrence may occur after treatment, and as many as half of the population who has had one BCC may develop a new skin cancer within 5 years. Mortality is rare from NMSC, reported to be between 1,000 and 2,000 deaths per year in the US, and typically occurs in older individuals with large untreated lesions or in immunosuppressed patients, such as organ transplant recipients.

Risk factors for acquiring BCC include the following: intense exposure to UV radiation via sunlight and tanning booths, light-colored skin that freckles or burns easily, older age, male gender, exposure to arsenic/industrial tar/coal/paraffin/certain types of oil, medical radiation treatment, prior skin cancer, chronic scars from severe burns or severe skin problems, psoralen and UV-A (PUVA) treated skin for treatment of psoriasis, genetic skin diseases (such as xeroderma pigmentosum or basal cell nevus syndrome), or a weakened immune system.

Preventative measures recommended by the ACS include the following: (1) to protect skin with long-sleeves and long pants with dark, dry fabric preferably with built-in UV protection or laundry rinse-cycle additives; (2) to wear a hat with at least a 2–3 in. brim all around or a shade cap that protects the neck/ears/eyes/forehead/nose/scalp; (3) to wear sunscreen and lip balm with a SPF of 15 or higher, preferably re-applying every 2 h; (4) to wear wrap-around sunglasses that absorb at least 99% of UV rays; (5) to avoid sun exposure between 10 am to 4 pm when UV radiation is the strongest; and (6) to avoid tanning beds and sun lamps.

The ACS recommends routine monthly self-exams performed in front of a full-length mirror and hand-held mirror. Key warning signs for suspicious lesions include a new growth, a growing lesion, or a sore that does not heal within 3 months. A thorough yearly physical examination of any suspicious lesions as well as the entire body is suggested, along with regional lymph node examination as appropriate. Referral to a dermatologist may be advisable and inspection of the suspicious lesion(s) with a dermatoscope may also be indicated. The ACS states that a biopsy is necessary to diagnose a skin cancer. Various biopsy techniques may be performed (shave, punch, incisional, excisional), depending upon the amount of tissue needed to make the diagnosis.

The ACS describes a variety of treatment options, including simple excision, curettage and electrodesiccation, Mohs surgery, cryosurgery, PDT, topical chemotherapy, immune response modifiers, laser surgery, radiation therapy, and systemic chemotherapy. Follow-up care is emphasized and recommended to be every 6 months for the first 5 years after a BCC is diagnosed. Yearly visits to the physician should follow this 5-year period. The ACS also offers an introductory background on clinical trials as another avenue for additional treatment, if patients are interested in future chemoprevention studies or options for treatment of advanced disease.

## National Cancer Institute (Evidence VIC) [53]

The National Cancer Institute (NCI) is a division of the U.S. National Institutes of Health (NIH) located in Bethesda, Maryland, USA. The NCI distributes accurate, up-to-date, comprehensive cancer information from the US government's principal agency for cancer research, which is available to the general public and medical professionals both in print form and online. The following information has been summarized from the online 2005 NCI "What You Need To Know About Skin Cancer" booklet, an NIH publication compiled by NCI health professionals and employees.

BCC is a slow growing skin cancer typically found on areas of the skin that have been exposed to the sun, particularly the face, which rarely spreads to other parts of the body.

Studies have found that risk factors associated with skin cancer include the following: (1) exposure to excessive UV radiation via sun, sunlamps, and tanning beds/booths, (2) physical traits such as fair skin that freckles or burns, red/blonde hair and light-colored eyes, (3) geographic locations such as tropical/warm climates and higher altitudes, (4) chronic scars/burns, (5) chronic skin inflammation or skin ulcers, (6) genodermatoses (xeroderma pigmentosum, basal cell nevus syndrome, albinism), (7) radiation therapy, (8) immunosuppression, (9) personal history of prior skin cancer(s), and (10) family history of skin cancer.

Prevention is emphasized, primarily by protection from excessive sun exposure as well as protecting children from an early age. Staying out of the mid-day sun (mid-morning to late afternoon) and protecting oneself from UV radiation reflection from sand, water, snow, and ice is recommended. Wearing long pants and long-sleeved clothing made with tightly woven fabrics, a wide-brimmed hat, and sunglasses are also suggested. Protection with a broad-spectrum UV-A and UV-B sunscreen with a SPF of at least 15 is essential. Avoidance of sunlamps and tanning booths is also highly recommended.

The NCI recommends that patients be aware of their skin and note skin changes to their physician immediately. A new growth, a sore that does not heal, or change in a pre-existing growth may be warning signs of skin cancer. Specific changes to watch for include the following: (1) a small, smooth, shiny, pale, or waxy lump, (2) a firm, red lump, (3) a sore or lump that bleeds or develops a crust or a scab, (4) a flat red spot that is rough, dry, or scaly and may become itchy or tender, or (5) a red or brown patch that is rough or scaly.

A biopsy is described as a sample taken from skin that does not look normal, which is then evaluated by a pathologist. Types of biopsies include punch, incisional, excisional, and shave. Staging defines the extent of disease. The stage is based on the size of the growth, how deep it is, and whether it has spread to nearby lymph nodes or other structures. The stages of skin cancer are as follows: Stage 0: the cancer involves only the top layer of skin, also known as carcinoma in situ; Stage I, the growth is less than or equal to 2 cm wide; Stage II: the growth is more than 2 cm wide; Stage III: the cancer has spread below the skin to cartilage, muscle, bone, or nearby lymph nodes, but has not spread to other places in the body; Stage IV: the cancer has spread to other places in the body.

The goal of treatment is to effect a cure and depends upon the type and stage of disease, the location, and the general health of the individual. Specialists who treat skin cancer include dermatologists, surgeons, and radiation oncologists. A second opinion for treatment is encouraged if the patient's case can allow for a delay in starting treatment. The NCI offers contact information via telephone and online sources to assist in finding a qualified physician for additional evaluation. Suggested treatment plans include surgery, topical chemotherapy, PDT, or radiation therapy. Surgical options include excisional surgery, Mohs surgery, electrodesiccation and curettage, cryosurgery, laser surgery, and reconstructive surgery. Topical chemotherapy is a modality that may be appropriate if the skin cancer is too large for surgery to be performed without significant functional or cosmetic compromise; 5-FU and imiquimod are two possible options for topical treatment.

Follow-up care after treatment of skin cancer is just as important as the treatment itself. Regular monitoring of the skin by a physician is imperative, as new skin cancers arise more commonly than metastases after skin cancer has been treated. Between physician visits, regular self-skin examinations are highly recommended, and are described in detail with the use of both full-length and hand-held mirrors. Sources of support and basic information on cancer research and clinical trials are available for patients to access if they are interested.

## Randomized Controlled Trials and Meta-Analyses

Evidence-based medicine and clinical trials involving BCC revolve around proving which treatment options are most efficacious in terms of long-term follow-up and which treatments are preferable to patients. The following are brief summaries of randomized controlled trials, organized by treatment modality, that were available via online medical search engines.

### Surgery (Excision, Mohs Micrographic Surgery, Cryosurgery, Radiotherapy)

Smeets et al. [54] (Evidence IIA) compared SE to Mohs surgery (MMS) in a prospective multicenter randomized controlled trial located in the Netherlands. There were 374 participants in the pBCC category and 191 participants in the recurrent BCC (rBCC) category. Inclusion criteria for the pBCC group included at least one untreated histologically confirmed facial BCC of at least 1 cm in diameter, either located in the H zone of the face or of a high/risk aggressive subtype (morpheaform, micronodular, BCC with squamous differentiation, trabecular, infiltrative). Inclusion criteria for the rBCC group were at least one histologically confirmed, facial tumor recurring for the first or second time. Excluded individuals were patients with a life expectancy of less than 3 years. Randomization was done primarily via a computer program (Sampsize 2.0). The primary outcome was recurrence of the carcinoma, and secondary outcomes were incomplete excision, suboptimal esthetic results, and excessive costs of treatment. Follow-up was scheduled at 18 and 30 months post intervention. Three-hundred and ninety-seven primary (198 MMS, 199 SE) and 201 recurrent (99 MMS, 102) tumors were treated. Of patients with primary carcinomas, 21 had both MMS and SE on different tumors. Nine with recurrent carcinomas had both treatments on different skin tumors. Sixty-six primary and 13 recurrent carcinomas were lost to follow-up. Of the primary carcinomas, 3% recurred after SE compared with 2% after MMS after 30 months of follow-up. Of the recurrent carcinomas, 3% recurred after SE and 0% after MMS, after 18 months of follow-up. Four recurrent carcinomas randomly assigned to the SE group were treated with MMS. Although these results slightly favored MMS, they were not found to be significant, and the total operative costs of MMS were in fact higher than those of excision. Treatment with MMS lowered the recurrence rate for both primary and recurrent tumors compared with SE, although not significantly, MMS was recommended for treating aggressive or large facial tumors to avoid larger defects, poor cosmesis, and functional problems. Study limitations included the fact that the study size, although substantial, was inadequate, since enrolling a larger number of patients could have enabled detection of a more significant difference in the recurrence rates of SE vs. MMS. A small number of patients were also lost to follow-up.

Mosterd et al. [55] (Evidence IIA) conducted a prospective multi-center randomized controlled trial in the Netherlands, which compared the effectiveness of SE with Mohs micrographic surgery (MMS) for the treatment of primary and recurrent facial BCCs. This study had a follow-up period of 5 years. Inclusion criteria for the pBCC (pBCC) group included the following: at least one untreated, histologically confirmed facial pBCC, at least 1 cm in diameter, location in the H zone, or aggressive histologic subtype. Inclusion criteria for the rBCC group stated that the lesion must be recurrent for the first or second time. Patients were excluded if they had a life expectancy of less than 3 years. In total, 408 pBCCs and 204 rBCCs in patients from seven hospitals were randomly assigned via a computer to SE or MMS. The primary outcome was recurrence of cancer, diagnosed clinically and histologically. Of the 397 pBCCs that were treated, 127 pBCCs, in 113 patients, were lost to follow-up after 5 years. Of the 11 recurrences that occurred in patients with pBCC, 7 (4.1%) occurred after SE, and 4 (2.5%) occurred in patients after MMS. Out of the 202 rBCCs that were treated, 56 tumors, in 52 patients, were lost to follow-up after 5 years. Two BCCs (2.4%) in two patients treated with MMS recurred, and ten BCCs (12.1%) in ten patients treated with SE recurred. The difference in the number of recurrences between treatments was only significant after MMS in rBCC cases. The authors concluded that MMS is preferable to SE for the treatment of facial rBCC, on the basis of significantly fewer recurrences. However, since there was no significant difference in recurrence of pBCC between interventions, treatment with SE was considered a suitable treatment modality for most cases of pBCC.

Avril et al. [56] (Evidence IIA) compared SE to radiotherapy for facial BCCs less than 4 cm in size in a prospective single-center randomized controlled trial located in France. The primary end point was the failure rate (persistent or recurrent disease) after a follow-up period of 4 years. The secondary end point was the cosmetic result as assessed by the patient, the dermatologist and three persons blinded from the trial. During the clinical trial, 347 patients were treated. Exclusion criteria included BCC on scalp or neck, total removal of BCC at the time of biopsy, patients with five or more BCCs, and a life expectancy of less than 3 years. Of the 174 patients in the surgery group, all of whom underwent resection of entire tumor with a free margin of at least 2 mm from visible borders, 71% had local anesthesia and 91% had frozen section examinations. Of the 173 patients in the radiotherapy group, 55% were treated with interstitial brachytherapy, 33%

with superficial contact therapy, and 12% with conventional radiotherapy. Follow-up was performed at 3, 6, and 12 months after the end of treatment, then yearly until the fourth year. The 4-year failure rate was 0.7% with surgery when compared with 7.5% with radiotherapy. The cosmetic results assessed by four of the five judges were significantly better after surgery compared to radiotherapy. Eighty-seven percent of the surgery-treated patients and 69% of the radiation-treated patients considered the cosmetic result to be good. For treatment of facial BCCs less than 4 cm in diameter, surgery was shown to be the preferred treatment modality.

Thissen et al. [57] (Evidence IIA) compared SE to cryosurgery of primary (nodular/superficial), <2 cm BCCs in the head/neck area, in a prospective single-center randomized controlled trial located in the Netherlands. Exclusion criteria were recurrent lesions, histologic subtypes other than nodular or superficial, tumors larger than 2 cm in diameter, patients with five or more BCCs, contraindications to surgery or cryosurgery, and life expectancy of less than 1 year. The objective was to compare cosmetic outcome 1 year after SE with a safety margin of 3 mm from the visible tumor and cryosurgery using a curette to debulk the tumor and the cone-spray technique. Cosmetic results after both interventions were assessed by five independent professional observers (male dermatologist, female dermatologist, plastic surgeon, dermatologic nurse, and beautician) and by the patients themselves. Ninety-six BCCs were treated either with SE ($n=48$) or cryosurgery ($n=48$). Clinical professionals found the cosmetic results after surgery to be significantly better, as did the patients. Location and size of the tumor did not affect this general preference for SE. From the results of this survey, the authors concluded that cosmetic results after SEs are far better than after cryosurgery.

Hall et al. [58] (Evidence IIA) compared cryotherapy to radiotherapy for BCC in a prospective single-center randomized controlled trial located in the United Kingdom. The tumors included were on the neck, face, eyelids, and trunk. Patients were excluded if they had recurrent tumors, lesions on the nose or pinna, if electrons were the treatment of choice, or if the lesion was near the eye and vision in the other eye was less than 6/18. Patients were evaluated by two physicians at 1, 6, 12, and 24 months after treatment. At each visit, the presence or absence of recurrent tumor was recorded as well as the cosmetic appearance. There were 93 study patients, 49 in the radiotherapy intervention group, and 44 in the cryotherapy intervention group. There was no difference in the age, sex, skin type, or length of history in the two groups. At the end of 1 year, 17 patients had histologically proven recurrence of disease in the cryotherapy group (39%), compared with 2 (4%) treated with radiotherapy. The authors concluded that cryotherapy does not offer a satisfactory alternative to radiotherapy in the treatment of BCC, despite the fact that cryotherapy is reported in the literature as a curative alternative for BCC.

## Photodynamic Therapy

Rhodes et al. [59] (Evidence IIA) compared PDT with topically applied methyl aminolevulinate (MAL PDT) vs. simple excisional surgery for the treatment of primary nodular BCC in a prospective multi-center randomized controlled trial located in Europe. The primary objective was to compare the 5-year lesional recurrence rates between the two treatment modalities. Randomization occurred via a standard computer program. A total of 97 patients, 50 of whom had 53 lesions treated with MAL PDT and 47 of whom had 52 lesions treated by excisional surgery were included in the analysis. Topical MAL was applied for 3 h before illumination (75 $J/cm^2$ of red light at 570–670 nm) for two treatments. Twelve (23%) of the 53 lesions needed four total MAL PDT treatments. Simple excisional surgery with at least 5 mm margins was performed once under local anesthesia for the surgical intervention group. After 5 years, recurrence was noted in 7 (14%) of 49 lesions in the MAL PDT group vs. 2 (4%) of 52 lesions in the surgical intervention group. Estimated sustained lesional complete response rates were 76% for MAL PDT and 96% for excision surgery. However, the cosmetic outcome was more favorable in the MAL PDT intervention group (87 vs. 54%).

After a 5-year follow-up period, surgery was found to have superior efficacy to MAL PDT with respect to recurrence rates. However, MAL PDT could also be considered an effective treatment with a preferable esthetic outcome for primary nodular BCC.

Mosterd et al. [60] (Evidence IIA) compared PDT with topically applied δ-aminolevulinic acid (ALA-PDT) to SE for the treatment of histologically proven nodular BCC in a prospective single-center randomized controlled clinical trial located in the Netherlands. Patients were excluded for the following reasons: pregnancy, life expectancy of less than 5 years, genodermatoses, photosensitivity, recurrent/pigmented BCCs, histologic subtypes other than nodular, or location on concave or hairy skin. One-hundred and seventy-three primary nodular BCCs in 149 patients were analyzed. Primary nodular BCCs were randomly assigned via a computer to either the PDT intervention group (85 lesions) or to the surgical intervention group (88 lesions). Tumors treated with PDT were illuminated twice on the same day, 4 h after application of ALA cream, 3 weeks after debulking. SE was performed with a 3 mm margin, followed by histological examination. In total, 171 primary nodular BCCs in 149 patients were treated. The authors performed a 3-year interim analysis, which showed that the cumulative incidence of failure was significant, 2.3% for surgery and 30.3% for PDT, and therefore concluded that surgery was significantly more effective than ALA-PDT, and preferable to ALA-PDT, in terms of long-term cure rates.

Wang et al. [61] (Evidence IIA) compared PDT with topically applied δ-aminolevulinic acid (ALA-PDT) to cryotherapy for the treatment of histologically proven, nodular, or superficial BCC in a prospective single-center nonblinded randomized controlled phase III clinical trial located in Sweden. The inclusion criteria were histopathologically verified BCCs suitable for PDT or cryosurgery, and age between 20 and 90 years. The exclusion criteria included pregnancy/lactation, severe malignancies, daily intake of vitamins E or C, β-carotene, iron preparations, nonsteroidal anti-inflammatory agents, or strong analgesics in higher than specified doses. Additional exclusion criteria were as follows: BCC on the nose, morphea-like growth pattern, porphyria, abdominal pain of unknown etiology, photosensitivity, and treatment of the BCC with topical steroids type III or IV within the last month. Randomization took place according to a stratified pattern in blocks of ten participants. Eighty-eight patients, 44 women and 44 men, aged 42–88 years, were included in the trial. Forty-seven of the lesions were in the PDT group, and 41 lesions were in the cryosurgery group. Fifty-four percent of lesions were located on the trunk, 28% in the head and neck region, 11% on the legs, and 7% on the arms. The follow-up period was restricted to 1 year with close follow-up for the first 3 months (1, 4, and 8 weeks, then at 3 months). Efficacy (by histopathology at 3 months) was assessed as the recurrence rate, 12 months after the first treatment session. Tolerability was evaluated as the time of healing, pain and discomfort during and after the treatment, as well as the final cosmetic outcome. Histopathologically verified recurrence rates in the two groups were statistically comparable and were 25% for ALA-PDT and 15% for cryosurgery. However, clinical recurrence rates were only 5% for ALA-PDT and 13% for cryosurgery. Additional treatments, usually one, had to be performed in 30% of the lesions in the ALA-PDT group. The healing time was considerably shorter and the cosmetic outcome significantly better with ALA-PDT. Pain and discomfort were equivalent with the two treatment modalities. In terms of efficacy, ALA-PDT was comparable with cryosurgery as a treatment modality for BCC, taking into consideration that retreatments were more often required with ALA-PDT than with cryosurgery.

Basset-Seguin et al. [62] (Evidence IIA) compared PDT with topically applied methyl aminolevulinate (MAL PDT) vs. cryotherapy for the treatment of superficial BCC in a prospective multi-center randomized controlled trial. Sixty patients with 114 lesions were treated with topical MAL applied for 3 h before illumination (570–670 nm, light dose 75 J/cm$^2$) (1 session), and 58 patients with 105 lesions received two freeze-thaw cycles of cryotherapy. Twenty patients with an incomplete response at 3 months received two further MAL PDT sessions and 16 patients received repeat cryotherapy. One hundred lesions treated with MAL PDT and 93 lesions treated with cryotherapy had a complete response 3 months after the last treatment and were evaluable for recurrence after a 5 year follow-up period. There was no difference in 5-year recurrence rates with either treatment (20% with cryotherapy vs. 22% with MAL PDT). However, 60% of patients had an excellent significant cosmetic outcome with MAL PDT vs. 16% with cryotherapy. This study provides support for the use of MAL PDT over cryotherapy as an alternative nonsurgical option for primary superficial BCC.

Soler et al. [63] (Evidence IIA) compared laser light (LL, red-light laser, monochromatic 630 nm) vs. broadband-lamp light (BL, 570–740 nm) with PDT with topically applied δ-aminolevulinic acid (ALA-PDT) for the treatment of superficial BCC in a prospective single-center randomized controlled trial located in Norway. Eighty-three Caucasian patients with 245 previously untreated superficial BCCs (clinical thickness less than 1 mm, diameter less than 3 cm) were included in the study. Patients with fewer than six lesions were included. The patients were randomly allocated on the treatment day to one of the two treatment groups in sets of four patients. None of the patients were treated with both interventions. Group LL comprised 41 patients (27 females and 14 males, mean age 62.4 years) with 111 BCCs. Group BL comprised 42 patients (17 females and 25 males, mean age 62.0 years) with 134 BCCs. Treatment involved topical application of 20% ALA for 3 h before light exposure with either LL or BL. A complete response 6 months after treatment was achieved in 95 lesions (86%) in the LL intervention and 110 lesions (82%) in the BL intervention. Of these, 80 lesions (84%) in the LL intervention and 101 lesions (92%) in the BL intervention were independently evaluated to have an excellent or good cosmetic posttreatment. There was no statistically significant difference in cure rates or cosmetic outcomes between the two groups, but BL in this setting was superior with respect to its lower cost and safety.

Lui et al. [64] (Evidence IIA) designed a study to assess the safety and efficacy of PDT with verteporfin infusion (14 mg/m$^2$) and various levels of red light in the treatment of multiple NMSCs. It was an open-label, randomized, multicenter,

dose ranging phase 2 study conducted in academic dermatology centers in North America. Inclusion criteria included patients with at least two biopsy-proven nonpigmented NMSCs (superficial/nodular BCC or SCC in situ); basal cell nevus syndrome patients were also included in the study. Patients were randomly assigned to receive three different light doses: 60, 120, or 180 J/cm$^2$. To avoid a significant difference in the number of tumors within each treatment group, randomization was stratified by the number of tumors (2–5 tumors, 6–10 tumors, or >10 tumors) and by center. In total, 54 patients with 421 multiple NMSCs were included; 92% of tumors were BCC, 15 patients had basal cell nevus syndrome. Response rates were assessed at 6 months postintervention. Clinical and cosmetic responses were assessed and graded at 6 weeks, 3 months, and 6 months after intervention with optional follow-up visits at 12, 18, and 24 months. The response rate ranged from 69% at 60 J/cm$^2$ to 93% at 180 J/cm$^2$. At the optional 24-month follow-up period (31 patients with 276 tumors), the clinical complete response rate ranged from 51 to 95% (60–180 J/cm$^2$). No significant systemic adverse events were observed, except for pain at the treated tumor sites. The authors concluded that a single course of verteporfin PDT may induce good response rates with favorable esthetic outcomes for patients with multiple NMSCs.

## Imiquimod

Beutner et al. [65] (Evidence IIA) compared imiquimod 5% cream to vehicle cream for the treatment of nodular/superficial BCC in a prospective randomized single-center double-blind pilot trial located in the US. The objective of this pilot study was to evaluate the safety and efficacy of imiquimod 5% cream. Patients were unevenly randomized in a 2:1 ratio to receive imiquimod cream or vehicle cream. There were five treatment schedules: twice daily, once daily, 3 times weekly, twice weekly, and once weekly. Patients continued treatment with study cream until 2 weeks after the target tumor was clinically cleared as determined by the investigator or until 16 weeks of treatment were completed. In total, 35 patients were included, 24 in the imiquimod 5% cream group and 11 in the vehicle cream group in 1 of 5 dosing regimens for up to 16 weeks. At 6 weeks posttreatment, an excisional biopsy of the target site was performed. In terms of histopathologic response, BCC was cleared in all 15 patients (100%) dosed twice daily, once daily, and 3 times weekly; in 3 of 5 (60%) patients dosed twice weekly; 2 of 4 (50%) dosed once weekly; and in 1 of 11 (9%) treated with vehicle. Adverse events largely consisted of local reactions at the target tumor site, with the incidence and severity of local skin reactions associated with escalating dosing regimens. The authors concluded that imiquimod 5% cream showed clinical efficacy in the treatment of BCC compared to vehicle, but that the efficacy needed to be confirmed in larger controlled trials before routine use could be recommended.

Marks et al. [66] (Evidence IIA) conducted a study in Australia and New Zealand to assess the efficacy and safety of different dosing regimens (twice every day, once every day, twice daily 3×/week, once daily 3×/week) of imiquimod 5% cream for the treatment of superficial BCCs in a prospective multi-center randomized open-label dose-response trial. Inclusion criteria were the following: men and women aged 18 years and older, specimen histologically confirming a primary superficial BCC located on the head, neck, trunk, or limbs, lesions with a surface area between 0.5 and 2 cm$^2$; the lesion also had to be free from infection. Exclusion criteria were the following: tumors on areas within 1 cm of the hairline, eyes, nose, mouth, ears, anogenital region, hands, and feet. Ninety-nine patients were randomized to 6 weeks' application of imiquimod 5% cream in 1 of 4 dosing regimens. The treatment site was excised and examined histologically 6 weeks after cessation of intervention. Intention-to-treat analysis revealed 100% (3/3) histologic clearance in the twice-daily regimen, 87.9% (29/33) clearance in the once every day regimen, 73.3% (22/30) clearance in the twice-daily 3×/week regimen, and 69.7% (23/33) clearance in the once-daily 3×/week regimen. Adverse events included a dose-related inflammatory skin reaction at the site of application, which had previously been reported. The authors concluded that imiquimod 5% cream appeared to have potential success as a patient-administered treatment option for treating superficial BCCs.

Shumack et al. [67] (Evidence IIA) designed a study to establish an efficacious and safe dosing regimen of imiquimod 5% cream for the treatment of primary nodular BCC in two phase II clinical trials. One trial was a prospective 6-week randomized open-label dose-response study evaluating four dosing regimens (Australia and New Zealand) and the other was a prospective 12-week randomized vehicle-controlled double-blind dose-response study evaluating four dosing regimens (US based trial). The randomization method was not indicated. Ninety-nine patients were enrolled in the 6-week trial and 92 patients in the 12-week trial. Inclusion criteria were as follows: male or female patients of at least 18-years old, biopsy-confirmed diagnosis of nodular BCC, size between 0.5 and 1.5 cm$^2$, and location greater than 1 cm from the eyes, nose, mouth, ear, and hairline. Morpheaform, infiltrating, and micronodular BCCs were excluded from the study. The 6-week dosing regimen consisted of application of imiquimod once daily for 3 or 7 days/week or twice daily for 3 or 7 days/week. The 12-week dosing regimen consisted of application of imiquimod or vehicle once daily for 3, 5, or 7 days/week, or twice daily for 7 days/week. The tumor was excised in its entirety 6 weeks after treatment and was examined histologically for evidence of residual BCC. The authors reported that dosing once daily for 7 days/week resulted in the highest clearance rate, with 25/35 patients (71%) and 16/21 patients (76%) showing clearance of the tumor histopathologically in the 6- and 12-week studies, respectively. The authors concluded that topical 5% imiquimod cream is well tolerated and most effective in treating nodular BCCs when applied once daily for 7 days/week for either a 6 or 12 week period.

Sterry et al. [68] (Evidence IIA) conducted two studies in Europe to establish the safety and efficacy of occlusion on low dose regimens of imiquimod 5% cream for the treatment of superficial and nodular BCCs. Both trials were prospective 6-week randomized open-label trials in which patients were divided by histologic subtype, superficial (93 patients) vs. nodular (90 patients). Patients were then randomized by computer to one of four treatment groups, applying imiquimod 5% cream 2 or 3 days/week either with or without occlusion. Six weeks following the 6-week intervention period, the tumor was excised in its entirety and histopathologically examined. In both trials, the highest complete response rate was seen in the 3 days/week with occlusion group, with complete response rates of 87% (superficial) and 65% (nodular). Occlusion did not have a statistically significant effect on response rate at either dosing frequency. Response rates for patients treated 3 days/week without occlusion were 76% (superficial) and 50% (nodular). The authors concluded that although there were acceptable safety profiles for both groups, occlusion did not have a statistically significant effect on efficacy for either superficial or nodular BCC tumors.

Geisse et al. [69] (Evidence IIA) compared imiquimod 5% cream vs. vehicle cream, comparing various dosing regimens to find the most effective frequency of dosing with tolerable side effects for the treatment of superficial BCCs in a prospective multi-center randomized double-blind vehicle-controlled phase II 12-week trial, located in the US. Inclusion criteria were as follows: male or female gender, 18 years of age or older, histologically confirmed diagnosis of primary superficial noninfected BCC, and between 0.5 and 2.0 cm$^2$ in size. Exclusion criteria were as follows: tumors within 1 cm of the hairline, eyes, nose, mouth, or ears, the anogenital area or hands and feet, previously treated or rBCC, or target BCC within 5 cm of another BCC. In total, 128 patients were randomized via computer to receive imiquimod (96 patients) or placebo (32 patients) and placed into various dosing schedules: twice daily, once daily, 5 times a week, or 3 times a week. At 6 weeks after the 12-week intervention period, the tumor was clinically evaluated, excised in its entirety, and histopathologically examined for residual BCC. Complete response rates were 100% (10/10), 87.1% (27/31), 80.8% (21/26), and 51.7% (15/29) for patients in the twice daily, once daily, 5 times a week, and 3 times a week imiquimod 5% cream intervention groups, respectively, and only 18.8% (6/32) in the vehicle control group. The authors concluded that imiquimod 5% cream was effective and safe in the treatment

of superficial BCC, and recommended a daily or 5 times a week dosing regimen for a 12-week period.

Geisse et al. [70] (Evidence IIA) conducted two studies in the U.S. to evaluate the efficacy and safety of imiquimod 5% cream vs. vehicle cream for the treatment of superficial BCCs. Two identical prospective multi-center randomized double-blind vehicle-controlled phase III 6-week studies were conducted, in which subjects were computer randomized to 1 of 4 treatment groups: 5×/week (vehicle vs. imiquimod) or 7×/week (vehicle vs. imiquimod). Inclusion criteria were as follows: male or female gender, at least 18 years old, primary histologically-confirmed superficial BCC, at least 0.5 cm$^2$ in area with a maximum diameter of 2 cm, located on the limbs, trunk, neck, or head (excluding the H zone and anogenital area). Exclusion criteria included: aggressive histologic growth pattern, dermatologic disease in the target area that could be exacerbated by imiquimod, or lesions in locations that were not suitable for follow-up excision. The lesions were clinically examined 12 weeks postintervention and then surgically excised in their entirety. The authors reported that composite clearance rates (combined clinical and histological assessments) for the imiquimod intervention were 75% (5×/week) and 73% (7×/week). Histological clearance rates for the imiquimod intervention were 82% (5×/week) and 79% (7×/week). The higher the clearance rate, the more severe the erythema, erosion, and scabbing/crusting that occurred. The authors concluded that the difference in clearance rates between the two imiquimod dosing groups was not significant, but recommended the 5×/week dosing regimen because of its superior safety profile.

Schulze et al. [71] (Evidence IIA) conducted a study in Europe to evaluate the safety and clinical efficacy of imiquimod 5% cream vs. vehicle cream for the treatment of superficial BCC in a prospective multi-center randomized double-blinded vehicle-controlled phase III clinical study. Inclusion criteria were as follows: male or female gender, at least 18 years old, primary histologically-confirmed superficial BCC, at least 0.5 cm$^2$ in area with a maximum diameter of 2 cm, lesion located on the limbs, trunk, neck, or head (excluding the anogenital area and lesions within 1 cm of the hairline, nose, mouth, ears and eyes). Exclusion criteria included: aggressive histologic growth pattern, dermatologic disease in the target area that could be exacerbated by imiquimod, unstable medical conditions, and evidence of metastatic disease. In total, 166 patients were randomized via computer to apply imiquimod (84 patients) or vehicle cream (82 patients) to the tumor once daily, 7×/week for a total of 6 weeks. The treated tumor site was clinically assessed for treatment response at 12 weeks postintervention and was then excised for evaluation; efficacy assessments included composite clearance rates and response rates solely based on histology. Composite clearance was demonstrated in 77% (imiquimod) and 6% (vehicle) of subjects treated. Histological clearance was demonstrated in 80% (imiquimod) and 6% (vehicle) of subjects treated. The authors concluded that imiquimod 5% cream administered 7×/week for 6 weeks is a safe and effective treatment for superficial BCC.

Eigentler et al. [72] (Evidence IIA) conducted a study in Germany to evaluate the efficacy and safety of imiquimod 5% cream in a thrice weekly regimen for 8 vs. 12 weeks for the treatment of nodular BCC in a prospective single-center randomized controlled phase III trial. In total, 102 patients were randomized, but due to drop-out, a total of 90 patients was analyzed (45 in 8 week group, 45 in 12 week group). Of the 90, 70 had a complete clinical clearance (78%) and there was no significant difference between 8 and 12 weeks with respect to efficacy or safety profile. Excisional biopsies were performed at 8 weeks after treatment; complete histopathological clearance was observed in 58 patients (64%). In 12 patients, despite complete clinical clearance, tumor remnants were still detected histopathologically. Adverse events were reported in 92% of the patients and were mainly classified as mild to moderate local inflammation, as is the case in most imiquimod studies. Imiquimod applied in the 3 times weekly for 8 and 12 weeks dosing regimen showed moderate activity against nodular BCCs, with residual cancer seen in more than one third of treated patients. A benign clinical appearance after treatment did not accurately reflect the presence or absence of disease in

nearly 1 out of every 5 patients with nodular BCC. Therefore, the authors recommended excisional biopsy of the treated site because of the concern of residual tumor beneath the surface, even after a complete course of treatment.

## 5-Fluorouracil

Miller et al. [73] (Evidence IIA) conducted a trial in the U.S. to compare the safety, tolerability, and efficacy of six different treatment regimens of 5-FU/epinephrine? gel in patients with BCC in a prospective multi-center open-label randomized controlled trial. Inclusion criteria were the following: 6–15 mm in largest diameter, well-defined margins, and lesions that were at least 50 mm from any other malignancy. Exclusion criteria were the following: pregnant/lactating patients, lesions that had already received treatment, high-risk sites (e.g., eyelids, nose, ears, and the central part of the face), tumors considered to be more appropriately treated with Mohs micrographic surgery, lesions with deep tissue involvement, morpheaform lesions, basal cell nevus syndrome patients, patients with known hypersensitivities or allergies to 5-FU, sulfites, epinephrine, or bovine collagen, patients with a history of autoimmune disease or immunosuppression. The randomization method was not described. A total of 116 patients with biopsy-proven BCCs completed the study and were randomized into the following intervention categories: (1) 1.0 mL 5FU/epi gel once weekly for 6 weeks, (2) 0.5 mL 5FU/epi gel once weekly for 6 weeks, (3) 1.0 mL 5FU/epi gel twice weekly for 3 weeks, (4) 0.5 mL 5FU/epi gel twice weekly for 3 weeks, (5) 0.5 mL 5FU/epi gel twice weekly for 4 weeks, (6) 0.5 mL 5FU/epi gel thrice weekly for 2 weeks. Lesions were observed for 3 months at which time the tumor site was excised for histopathologic examination. The authors found that 91% of the treated tumors (106 of 116) in all regimens had histologically confirmed complete tumor resolution. The best response rate, tolerance, and patient compliance occurred in patients receiving the sixth regimen (0.5 mL of 5FU/epi gel thrice weekly for 2 weeks). The complete response rate based on histologic assessment in this group was 100%.

The authors concluded that treating BCC with 5-FU/epi gel is both safe and effective, and has response rates comparable to surgery, supporting the use of this regimen as a nonsurgical treatment alternative in selected patients.

Romagosa et al. [74] (Evidence IIA) conducted a study in the U.S. to assess the efficacy of phosphatidyl choline (PC) as a vehicle to facilitate the penetration of 5-FU when compared with petrolatum-based 5-FU cream in a prospective single-center double-blind randomized pilot study. In total, 13 patients with 17 biopsy-proven, moderate thickness BCCs were randomized to receive either the intervention, 5% 5-FU in a PC vehicle, or the standard, 5% 5-FU in a petrolatum base, twice daily for a total of 4 weeks. Excisional biopsy of the treated BCC site was performed at week 16. A 90% cure rate (9/10) in those lesions treated with 5% 5-FU in PC vs. a 57% cure rate (4/7) in those treated with 5% 5-FU in a petrolatum-based cream was found. The authors conclude that although the study was unable to detect any statistically significant differences in outcome, these findings may indicate an increase in the short-term eradication of BCC using the novel PC-based vehicle when compared to the standard. However, further larger-scale double-blind therapeutic trials are necessary to establish the efficacy of this treatment modality, including 5-year follow-up studies to fully assess efficacy.

## Interferon Alfa-2b

Edwards et al. [75] (Evidence IIA) conducted a study in the U.S. to assess the efficacy of a novel sustained-release protamine zinc chelated intralesional interferon alfa-2b formulation (ten million IU per injection) in a prospective single-center randomized controlled trial. Sixty-five patients between 35 and 65 years of age were enrolled in this study. Inclusion criteria were the following: one clinically typical, sharply defined BCC with clearly visible margins, size ranging from 0.5 to 1.5 cm for nodular tumors or 2 cm for superficial lesions in the largest diameter, and locations that would be amenable to easy excision. Exclusion criteria included: morphea-like BCC, recurrent cancers, deeply invasive lesions,

periorificial tumors, central facial BCCs, serious or debilitating illness, a history of thromboembolic or cardiovascular disease, radiation therapy to the test site area, history of arsenic ingestion, pregnancy, breast-feeding, immunosuppression, and use of nonsteroidal anti-inflammatory medications. In total, 65 BCCs (33 nodular, 32 superficial) were treated in one of two dosing schedules with the novel intralesional sustained release interferon alfa-2b. Patients in each nodular and superficial group were randomly assigned to receive protamine zinc chelated interferon alfa-2b either in a single dose of ten million IU or in one dose of ten million IU per week for 3 weeks. This randomization thus produced four groups: (1) patients with superficial BCCs treated with one injection (16 subjects); (2) patients with nodular BCCs treated with one injection (17 subjects); (3) patients with superficial BCCs treated with three injections (16 subjects); and (4) patients with nodular BCCs treated with three injections (16 subjects). At week 16, 80% of evaluable tumors treated with three injections and 52% treated with one injection were cured histopathologically. The authors concluded that three injections of sustained-release protamine zinc preparation of interferon alfa-2b showed promise as a practical, effective, and cosmetically suitable treatment for BCCs, but that a larger scale trial would be needed to support wide-scale use.

Cornell et al. [76] (Evidence IIA) conducted a study in the U.S. to compare the efficacy of intralesional interferon alfa-2b ($1.5 \times 10^6$ IU) vs. placebo for treatment of biopsy-proven noduloulcerative or superficial BCCs at a thrice weekly for 3 weeks dosing schedule (cumulative dose of 13.5 million IU) in a prospective multi-center randomized controlled trial. In total, 172 patients were randomized via computer to either the interferon group or placebo group. Exclusion criteria were as follows: previous therapy to the site, immunosuppressive or cytotoxic therapy within prior 4 weeks, exogenous interferon use, lesions in the perioral region or central face, and lesions penetrating deep tissue. Interventions consisted of intralesional injections of either 1.5 million IU of interferon alfa-2b or placebo on 3 alternate days per week for 3 consecutive weeks. Treatment efficacy (by histologic examination) was determined at 16–20 weeks, and demonstrated cure of lesions in 86% of interferon-treated patients and in 29% of placebo-treated patients. Three patients, all in the interferon-treated group, discontinued therapy because of intolerable side effects. At 1 year after initiation of therapy, 81% of interferon recipients and 20% of those given the placebo remained tumor free. Both types of BCC, noduloulcerative and superficial, were equally responsive to treatment with interferon. The authors concluded that in some cases of noduloulcerative or superficial BCCs, intralesional interferon alfa-2b may be an effective nonsurgical alternative treatment.

## Solasodine Glycoalkaloids

Punjabi et al. [77] (Evidence IIA) conducted a study in the U.K. to assess the safety and efficacy of a novel topical therapy, 0.005% mixture of solasodine glycosides (Zycure), vs. vehicle cream for the treatment of histologically-confirmed nodular, cystic, pigmented, and superficial BCC in a prospective multi-center double-blind randomized vehicle-controlled parallel clinical trial. Inclusion criteria were as follows: male or female gender, aged 18 years or older, histologically-confirmed BCC, lesion size of at least 0.5 cm in diameter. Exclusion criteria were as follows: morphea-like BCC, pregnancy, lactation, known sensitivity or allergy to the active medication, immunosuppression, use of 5FU or topical tretinoin within the preceding 2 months, and a history of rBCC after surgery, cryotherapy, or radiotherapy. Subjects included 50 males and 44 females, ranging in age from 32 to 95; 94 patients were randomized on a 2:1 ratio (Zycure=62, Vehicle=32). Treatment consisted of a twice daily regimen, under occlusion with Zycure or vehicle for a total of 8 weeks; follow-up continued at 6 month intervals for 1 year. The primary efficacy endpoint was histologically confirmed clearance of the BCC at the end of the 8-week treatment. Efficacy at 8 weeks was 66% (41/62) in the Zycure group, compared to 25% (8/32) in the vehicle group. Ninety percent (37/41) of the Zycure group completed follow-up at 6-month intervals for 1 year, of whom 78% (29/37) had no recurrence. The authors concluded that the novel solasodine

glycoside cream Zycure was a safe therapy for BCC, with a cure rate of 66% at 8 weeks and 78% at 1 year follow-up, but that larger-scale comparative studies with other topical treatments should be performed to fully assess efficacy.

## Conclusion

Several risk factors are defined by the NCCN as associated with a high risk of recurrence of BCC. Clinical risk factors include a tumor size greater than 2 cm; tumor location on the head and neck, particularly the central portion of the face, eyelids, nose, or ears; tumors with poorly defined borders; recurrent tumors; previous radiotherapy; and immunosuppression. Pathological risk factors include aggressive histologic growth patterns (morpheaform, infiltrative, and basosquamous types) and perineural invasion.

In patients who are candidates for surgery, SE has high cure rates for low risk lesions on the neck, trunk, and arms and legs, as well as selected well-circumscribed tumors on the head and neck. Curettage and electrodesiccation and cryosurgery are cost-effective and appropriate for low-risk lesions but not for morpheaform or recurrent lesions. Radiotherapy is useful for patients with inoperable lesions or for elderly patients who are unwilling to undergo surgery. There are limited data to support the use of imiquimod beyond the indications stated by the Food and Drug Administration, which currently preclude its use in high-risk BCC.

PDT is another promising treatment associated with excellent cosmetic results but suboptimal short-term rates of recurrence. These recommendations are similar to those published in a consensus statement by the NCCN in 2005. 5-FU, topical tazarotene, and intralesional interferon alfa-2b are other, uncommon therapeutic options.

Mohs micrographic surgery is the treatment of choice for most high-risk BCCs, particularly in locations where tissue sparing is essential and in clinical situations in which a high risk of recurrence is unacceptable. Patients who have high-risk BCC should be referred to an expert for treatment. More randomized controlled trials are needed to further help guide an evidence based approach to the treatment of BCC.

**Evidence-Based Summary**

| Tx | Conclusion | Level of evidence | References | Title | Year | Location | Single vs. multi-center |
|---|---|---|---|---|---|---|---|
| MMS vs. surgery | Treatment with MMS slightly lowered, recurrence rates for primary and recurrent tumors compared to surgery | II/A | Smeets et al. [54] | Surgical excision vs. Mohs' micrographic surgery for BCC of the face: randomized controlled trial | 2004 | Netherlands | Multi |
| MMS vs. surgery | MMS preferred over surgical excision for treatment of facial recurrent BCCs, but, surgical excision likely suitable in most cases of primary BCCs | II/A | Mosterd et al. [55] | Surgical excision vs. Mohs' micrographic surgery for primary and recurrent BCC of the face: a prospective randomized controlled trial with 5-years' follow-up | 2008 | Netherlands | Multi |
| Surgery vs. XRT | For cosmetic treatment of facial BCC less than 4 cm in diameter, surgery was preferable to radiotherapy | II/A | Avril et al. [56] | BCC of the face: surgery or radiotherapy? Results of a randomized study | 1997 | France | Single |
| Cryosurg vs. surgery | Cosmetic results after SEs were better than after cryosurgery | II/A | Thissen et al. [57] | Cosmetic results of cryosurgery vs. surgical excision for primary uncomplicated BCC of the head and neck | 2000 | Netherlands | Single |
| XRT vs. cryosurg | Cryotherapy not recommended as alternative to radiotherapy in the treatment of BCCs | II/A | Hall et al. [58] | Treatment of BCC: comparison of radiotherapy and cryotherapy | 1986 | UK | Single |
| MAL PDT vs. surgery | Surgery had lower recurrence rates than MAL PDT for primary nodular BCC after 5 years' follow-up but MAL PDT can still effective with a better esthetic outcome | II/A | Rhodes et al. [59] | Five-year follow-up of a randomized, prospective trial of topical methyl aminolevulinate photodynamic therapy vs. surgery for nodular BCC | 2007 | Europe | Multi |
| ALA-PDT vs. surgery | Surgery has superior long-term cure rates compared to ALA PDT for treatment of primary nodular BCCs | II/A | Mosterd et al. [60] | Fractionated 5-aminolaevulinic acid-photodynamic therapy vs. surgical excision in the treatment of nodular BCC: results of a randomized controlled trial | 2008 | Netherlands | Single |
| ALA-PDT vs. cryosurg | ALA-PDT's efficacy is comparable to that of cryosurgery treatment; re-treatment is more often required with ALA-PDT | II/A | Wang et al. [61] | Photodynamic therapy vs. cryosurgery of BCCs: results of a phase III clinical trial | 2001 | Sweden | Single |
| MAL PDT vs. cryosurg | Provides support for use of MAL PDT over cryotherapy as alternative nonsurgical option for primary superficial BCC | II/A | Basset-Seguin et al. [62] | Topical methyl aminolevulinate photodynamic therapy vs. cryotherapy for superficial BCC: a 5 year randomized trial | 2008 | Unknown | Multi |
| Red light laser (monochromatic 630 nm) vs. broadband-lamp light (570–740 nm) using ALA-PDT | No statistically significant difference in cure rates or cosmetic outcomes between light sources, but BL has lower cost and better safety profile | II/A | Soler et al. [63] | Photodynamic therapy of superficial BCC with 5-aminolevulinic acid with dimethylsulfoxide and ethylendiaminetetraacetic acid: a comparison of two light sources | 2000 | Norway | Single |
| Red light laser 60 vs. 120 vs. 180 J/cm² using PDT with verteporfin infusion | A single course of verteporfin PDT using a red light laser source of 180 J/cm² can induce good response rates with favorable esthetic outcomes for patients with multiple NMSCs | II/A | Lui et al. [64] | Photodynamic therapy of multiple nonmelanoma skin cancers with verteporfin and red light-emitting diodes: two-year results evaluating tumor response and cosmetic outcomes | 2004 | North America | Multi |
| Imiquimod 5% cream vs. vehicle cream | Imiquimod 5% cream showed clinical efficacy compared to vehicle in treatment of BCC | II/A | Beutner et al. [65] | Therapeutic response of BCC to the immune response modifier imiquimod 5% cream | 1999 | US | Single |
| Imiquimod 5% cream | Imiquimod 5% cream may be a potentially successful patient-administered treatment option for superficial BCCs | II/A | Marks et al. [66] | Imiquimod 5% cream in the treatment of superficial BCC: results of a multicenter 6-week dose-response trial | 2001 | Australia, New Zealand | Multi |

(continued)

**Evidence-Based Summary** (continued)

| Tx | Conclusion | Level of evidence | References | Title | Year | Location | Single vs. multi-center |
|---|---|---|---|---|---|---|---|
| Imiquimod 5% cream | Topical 5% imiquimod cream is well tolerated and most effective when applied once daily for 7 days/week to nodular BCCs for either a 6 or 12 week period | II/A | Shumack et al. [67] | Efficacy of topical 5% imiquimod cream for the treatment of nodular BCC: comparison of dosing regimens | 2002 | Australia, New Zealand, US | Multi |
| Imiquimod 5% cream 2–3 days/ week with occlusion vs. imiquimod 5% cream 2–3 days/week without occlusion vs. occlusion | Despite acceptable safety profiles for both groups, occlusion did not have a statistically significant effect on efficacy of treatment of superficial or nodular BCC | II/A | Sterry et al. [68] | Imiquimod 5% cream for the treatment of superficial and nodular BCC: randomized studies comparing low-frequency dosing with and without occlusion | 2002 | Europe | Multi |
| Imiquimod 5% cream vs. vehicle cream | Imiquimod 5% cream was effective in treatment of superficial BCC: daily or 5 times a week dosing regimen for a 12-week period demonstrated high efficacy and safety | II/A | Geisse et al. [69] | Imiquimod 5% cream for the treatment of superficial BCC: a double-blind, randomized, vehicle-controlled study | 2002 | US | Multi |
| Imiquimod 5% cream vs. vehicle cream | The difference in clearance rates between two imiquimod dosing groups (5 vs. 7x/week for 6 weeks) was not significant, but 5x/week dosing has a better safety profile | II/A | Geisse et al. [70] | Imiquimod 5% cream for the treatment of superficial BCC: results from two phase III, randomized, vehicle-controlled studies | 2004 | US | Multi |
| Imiquimod 5% cream vs. vehicle cream | Imiquimod 5% cream administered 7x/week for 6 weeks is safe and effective treatment for superficial BCC | II/A | Schulze et al. [71] | Imiquimod 5% cream for the treatment of superficial BCC: results from a randomized vehicle-controlled phase III study in Europe | 2005 | Europe | Multi |
| Imiquimod 5% cream | Imiquimod 5% cream not recommended for nodular BCC. Clinical clearance does not accurately reflect presence or absence of residual disease | II/A | Eigentler et al. [72] | A phase III, randomized, open label study to evaluate the safety and efficacy of imiquimod 5% cream applied thrice weekly for 8 and 12 weeks in the treatment of low-risk nodular BCC | 2007 | Germany | Single |
| 5-FU/epinephrine gel | 5-FU/epi gel is safe and effective for BCC. Best responses with 0.5 mL of 5FU/epi gel 3x weekly for 2 weeks. Response rates support use as nonsurgical alternative in selected patients | II/A | Miller et al. [73] | Nonsurgical treatment of BCCs with intralesional 5-fluorouracil/epinephrine injectable gel | 1997 | US | Multi |
| 5-FU in phosphatidyl choline (PC) cream vs. 5-FU in petrolatum-based cream | Findings may indicate an increase in the short-term clearance of BCC using PC-based vehicle | II/A | Romagosa et al. [74] | A pilot study to evaluate the treatment of BCC with 5-fluorouracil using phosphatidyl choline as a transepidermal carrier | 2000 | US | Single |
| protamine zinc chelate intralesional interferon alfa-2b (single dose of ten million IU vs. one dose of ten million IU per week for 3 weeks) | Three injections of sustained-release protamine zinc preparation of interferon alfa-2b may be practical, cost effective, and cosmetically suitable treatment for some BCCs | II/A | Edwards et al. [75] | The effect of an intralesional sustained-release formulation of interferon alfa-2b on BCCs | 1990 | US | Single |
| intralesional interferon alfa-2b (1.5×10⁶ IU) vs. placebo | Intralesional interferon alfa-2b may be effective nonsurgical alternative treatment for some nodular and superficial BCCs | II/A | Cornell et al. [76] | Intralesional interferon therapy for BCC | 1990 | US | Multi |
| 0.005% mixture of solasodine glycosides (Zycure), vs. vehicle cream | Solasodine glycoside cream is safe therapy for BCC, with a cure rate of 66% at 8 weeks and 78% at 1 year | II/A | Punjabi et al. [77] | Solasodine glycoalkaloids: a novel topical therapy for BCC. A double-blind, randomized, placebo-controlled, parallel group, multicenter study | 2008 | UK | Multi |

# References

1. American Cancer Society. 2008 cancer facts and figures. http://www.cancer.org/downloads/STT/2008CAFF finalsecured.pdf. Accessed 9 March 2009.
2. Barksdale SK, O'Connor N, Barnhill R. Prognostic factors for cutaneous squamous cell and basal cell carcinoma. Determinants of risk of recurrence, metastasis, and development of subsequent skin cancers. Surg Oncol Clin N Am. 1997;6(3):625–38.
3. Roewert-Huber J, Lange-Asschenfeldt B, Stockfleth E, Kerl H. Epidemiology and aetiology of basal cell carcinoma. Br J Dermatol. 2007;157 Suppl 2:47–51.
4. Braun RP, Klumb F, Girard C, Bandon D, Salomon D, Skaria A, et al. Three-dimensional reconstruction of basal cell carcinomas. Dermatol Surg. 2005;31(5):562–6.
5. Owens DM, Watt FM. Contribution of stem cells and differentiated cells to epidermal tumours. Nat Rev Cancer. 2003;3(6):444–51.
6. Diepgen TL, Mahler V. The epidemiology of skin cancer. Br J Dermatol. 2002;146 Suppl 61:1–6.
7. Basal Cell Carcinoma. http://www.skincancer.org/ Basal-Cell-Carcinoma. Accessed 9 March 2009.
8. Lear JT, Smith AG. Basal cell carcinoma. Postgrad Med J. 1997;73:538–42.
9. Staples MP, Elwood M, Burton RC, Williams JL, Marks R, Giles GG. Non-melanoma skin cancer in Australia: the 2002 national survey and trends since 1985. Med J Aust. 2006;184(1):6–10.
10. Richmond-Sinclair NM, Pandeya N, Ware RS, Neale RE, Williams GM, van der Pols JC, et al. Incidence of basal cell carcinoma multiplicity and detailed anatomic distribution: longitudinal study of an Australian population. J Invest Dermatol. 2009;129(2):323–8.
11. Miller DL, Weinstock MA. Nonmelanoma skin cancer in the United States: incidence. J Am Acad Dermatol. 1994;30:774–8.
12. de Vries E, Louwman M, Bastiaens M, de Gruijl F, Coebergh JW. Rapid and continuous increases in incidence rates of basal cell carcinoma in the southeast Netherlands since 1973. J Invest Dermatol. 2004;123: 634–8.
13. Marcil I, Stern R. Risk of developing subsequent NMSC in patients with a history of NMSc: a critical review of the literature and metaanalysis. Arch Dermatol. 2000;136:1524–30.
14. Gallagher RP, Hill GB, Bajdik CD, Fincham S, Coldman AJ, McLean DI, et al. Sunlight exposure, pigmentary factors, and risk of nonmelanocytic skin cancer. I. Basal cell carcinoma. Arch Dermatol. 1995;131(2):157–63.
15. Gallagher RP, Hill GB, Bajdik CD, et al. Sunlight exposure, pigmentary factors, and risk of nonmelanocytic skin cancer. I. Basal cell carcinoma. Arch Dermatol. 1995;131:157–63.
16. Corona R, Dogliotti E, Eric M, et al. Risk factors for basal cell carcinoma in a Mediterranean population: role of recreational sun exposure early in life. Arch Dermatol. 2001;137:1162–8.
17. Kricker A, Armstrong BK, English DR, Heenan PJ. Does intermittent sun exposure cause basal cell carcinoma? A case-control study in Western Australia. Int J Cancer. 1995;60:489–94.
18. Lear JT, Tan BB, Smith AG, et al. Risk factors for basal cell carcinoma in the UK: case-control study in 806 patients. J R Soc Med. 1997;90:371–4.
19. Ron E. Cancer risks from medical radiation. Health Phys. 2003;85(1):47–59.
20. Yu HS, Liao WT, Chai CY. Arsenic carcinogenesis in the skin. J Biomed Sci. 2006;13(5):657–66.
21. Ho WL, Murphy GM. Update on the pathogenesis of post-transplant skin cancer in renal transplant recipients. Br J Dermatol. 2008;158(2):217–24.
22. Nijsten TE, Stern RS. The increased risk of skin cancer is persistent after discontinuation of psoralen+ ultraviolet A: a cohort study. J Invest Dermatol. 2003;121:252–8.
23. Sasson M, Mallory SB. Malignant primary skin tumors in children. Curr Opin Pediatr. 1996;8(4):372–7.
24. Hartevelt M, Bavinck J, Koote A, et al. Incidence of skin cancer after renal transplantation in the Netherlands. Transplantation. 1990;49:506–9.
25. Moloney F, Comber H, Conton P, Murphy G. The role of immunosuppression in the pathogenesis of basal cell carcinoma. Br J Dermatol. 2006;154:790–1.
26. Scrivener Y, Grosshans E, Cribier B. Variations of basal cell carcinomas according to gender, age, location and histopathological subtype. Br J Dermatol. 2002;147:41–7.
27. Sexton M, Jones DB, Maloney ME. Histologic pattern analysis of basal cell carcinoma: study of a series of 1039 consecutive neoplasms. J Am Acad Dermatol. 1990;23:1118–26.
28. Batra RS, Kelley LC. Predictors of extensive subclinical spread in nonmelanoma skin cancer treated with Mohs micrographic surgery. Arch Dermatol. 2002;138: 1043–51.
29. Saldanha G, Fletcher A, Slater DN. Basal cell carcinoma: a dermatopathological and molecular biological update. Br J Dermatol. 2003;148:195–202.
30. Hutchin M. Sustained Hedgehog signaling is required for basal cell carcinoma proliferation and survival: conditional skin tumorigenesis recapitulates the hair growth cycle. Genes Dev. 2005;19:214–23.
31. Gailani MR, Stahle-Backdahl M, Leffell DJ, et al. The role of the human homologue of Drosophila patched in sporadic basal cell carcinomas. Nat Genet. 1996;14: 78–81.
32. Xie J, Murone M, Luoh SM, et al. Activating smoothened mutations in sporadic basal-cell carcinoma. Nature. 1998;391:90–2.
33. Epstein E. Basal cell carcinoma: attack of the hedgehog. Nature. 2008;8:743–54.
34. Kim MY, Park HJ, Baek SC, Byun DG, Houh D. Mutations of the p53 and PTCH gene in basal cell carcinomas: UV mutation signature and strand bias. J Dermatol Sci. 2002;29:1–9.
35. Tilli CM, Van Steensel MA, Krekels GA, Neumann HA, Ramaekers FC. Molecular aetiology and pathogenesis

of basal cell carcinoma. Br J Dermatol. 2005;152: 1108–24.

36. Ziegler A, Leffell DJ, Kunala S, et al. Mutation hotspots due to sunlight in the p53 gene of nonmelanoma skin cancers. Proc Natl Acad Sci USA. 1993;90:4216–20.

37. Rowe D. Comparison of treatment modalities for basal cell carcinoma. Clin Dermatol. 1995;13:617–20.

38. Walling HW, Fosko SW, Geraminejad PA, Whitaker DC, Arpey CJ. Aggressive basal cell carcinoma: presentation, pathogenesis, and management. Cancer Metastasis Rev. 2004;23:389–402.

39. Malone JP, Fedok FG, Belchis DA, Maloney ME. Basal cell carcinoma metastatic to the parotid: report of a new case and review of the literature. Ear Nose Throat J. 2000;79(7):511–5, 518–9.

40. Ting P, Kasper R, Arlette J. Metastatic basal cell carcinoma: report of two cases and literature review. J Cutan Med Surg. 2005;9:10–5.

41. Snow SN, Sahl W, Lo JS, Mohs FE, Warner T, Dekkinga JA, et al. Metastatic basal cell carcinoma. Report of five cases. Cancer. 1994;73(2):328–35.

42. Lo J, Snow S, Reizner G, et al. Metastatic basal cell carcinoma: report of twelve cases with a review of the literature. J Am Acad Dermatol. 1991;24:715–9.

43. Abide J, Nahai F, Bennett R. The meaning of surgical margins. Plast Reconstr Surg. 1984;73(3):492–7.

44. Neville J, Welch E, Leffell D. Management of NMSC in 2007. Nature. 2007;4(8):462–9.

45. Smeets N. Little evidence available on treatments for basal cell carcinoma. Cancer Treat Rev. 2005;31:143–6.

46. National Comprehensive Cancer Network Practice Guidelines in Oncology – Basal Cell Skin Cancer v.1.2009. http://www.nccn.org/professionals/physician_gls/PDF/nmsc.pdf. Accessed 9 March 2009.

47. Silverman M, Kopf A, Grin C, et al. Recurrence rates of treated basal cell carcinomas. Part 1: overview. J Dermatol Surg Oncol. 1991;17:713–8.

48. Brodland D. Features associated with metastasis (basal cell carcinoma). In: Miller S, Maloney M, editors. Cutaneous oncology: pathophysiology, diagnosis, and management. Malden: Blackwell Science; 1998. p. 657–63.

49. Chapter 23: Carcinoma of the skin (excluding eyelid, vulva, and penis). In: Fleming ID, Cooper JS, Henson DE, et al., editors. American Joint Committee on Cancer Staging Manual. 5th ed. Philadelphia: Lippincott-Raven; 1997. p. 157–60.

50. Robinson JK. Follow-up and prevention (basal cell). In: Miller SJ, Maloney ME, editors. Cutaneous oncology pathophysiology, diagnosis, and management. Malden: Blackwell Science; 1998. p. 695–8.

51. Marghoob AA, Slade J, Salopek TG, Kopf AW, Bart RS, Rigel DS. Basal cell and squamous cell carcinomas are important risk factors for cutaneous malignant melanoma. Screening implications. Cancer. 1995;75(2 Suppl):707–14.

52. American Cancer Society. Detailed guide: skin cancer – basal and squamous cell. http://www.cancer.org/docroot/CRI/CRI_2_3x.asp?dt=51. Accessed 9 March 2009.

53. National Cancer Institute: What you need to know about skin cancer. http://www.cancer.gov/pdf/WYNTK/WYNTK_skin.pdf. Accessed 10 March 2009.

54. Smeets NW, Krekels GA, Ostertag JU, Essers BA, Dirksen CD, Nieman FH, et al. Surgical excision vs Mohs' micrographic surgery for basal-cell carcinoma of the face: randomised controlled trial. Lancet. 2004;364(9447):1766–72.

55. Mosterd K, Krekels GA, Nieman FH, Ostertag JU, Essers BA, Dirksen CD, et al. Surgical excision versus Mohs' micrographic surgery for primary and recurrent basal-cell carcinoma of the face: a prospective randomised controlled trial with 5-years' follow-up. Lancet Oncol. 2008;9(12):1149–56.

56. Avril MF, Auperin A, Margulis A, Gerbaulet A, Duvillard P, Benhamou E, et al. Basal cell carcinoma of the face: surgery or radiotherapy? Results of a randomized study. Br J Cancer. 1997;76(1):100–6.

57. Thissen MR, Nieman FH, Ideler AH, Berretty PJ, Neumann HA. Cosmetic results of cryosurgery versus surgical excision for primary uncomplicated basal cell carcinomas of the head and neck. Dermatol Surg. 2000;26(8):759–64.

58. Hall VL, Leppard BJ, McGill J, Kesseler ME, White JE, Goodwin P. Treatment of basal-cell carcinoma: comparison of radiotherapy and cryotherapy. Clin Radiol. 1986;37(1):33–4.

59. Rhodes LE, de Rie MA, Leifsdottir R, Yu RC, Bachmann I, Goulden V, et al. Five-year follow-up of a randomized, prospective trial of topical methyl aminolevulinate photodynamic therapy vs surgery for nodular basal cell carcinoma. Arch Dermatol. 2007; 143(9):1131–6.

60. Mosterd K, Thissen MR, Nelemans P, Kelleners-Smeets NW, Janssen RL, Broekhof KG, et al. Fractionated 5-aminolaevulinic acid-photodynamic therapy vs. surgical excision in the treatment of nodular basal cell carcinoma: results of a randomized controlled trial. Br J Dermatol. 2008;159(4):864–70.

61. Wang I, Bendsoe N, Klinteberg CA, Enejder AM, Andersson-Engels S, Svanberg S, et al. Photodynamic therapy vs. cryosurgery of basal cell carcinomas: results of a phase III clinical trial. Br J Dermatol. 2001;144(4):832–40.

62. Basset-Seguin N, Ibbotson SH, Emtestam L, Tarstedt M, Morton C, Maroti M, et al. Topical methyl aminolaevulinate photodynamic therapy versus cryotherapy for superficial basal cell carcinoma: a 5 year randomized trial. Eur J Dermatol. 2008;18(5):547–53.

63. Soler AM, Angell-Petersen E, Warloe T, Tausjø J, Steen HB, Moan J, et al. Photodynamic therapy of superficial basal cell carcinoma with 5-aminolevulinic acid with dimethylsulfoxide and ethylendiaminetetraacetic acid: a comparison of two light sources. Photochem Photobiol. 2000;71(6):724–9.

64. Lui H, Hobbs L, Tope WD, Lee PK, Elmets C, Provost N, et al. Photodynamic therapy of multiple nonmelanoma skin cancers with verteporfin and red light-emitting diodes: two-year results evaluating tumor response and cosmetic outcomes. Arch Dermatol. 2004;140(1):26–32.

65. Beutner KR, Geisse JK, Helman D, Fox TL, Ginkel A, Owens ML. Therapeutic response of basal cell carcinoma to the immune response modifier imiquimod 5% cream. J Am Acad Dermatol. 1999;41(6): 1002–7.

66. Marks R, Gebauer K, Shumack S, Amies M, Bryden J, Fox TL, et al. Australasian Multicentre Trial Group. Imiquimod 5% cream in the treatment of superficial basal cell carcinoma: results of a multicenter 6-week dose-response trial. J Am Acad Dermatol. 2001;44(5): 807–13.

67. Shumack S, Robinson J, Kossard S, Golitz L, Greenway H, Schroeter A, et al. Efficacy of topical 5% imiquimod cream for the treatment of nodular basal cell carcinoma: comparison of dosing regimens. Arch Dermatol. 2002;138(9):1165–71.

68. Sterry W, Ruzicka T, Herrera E, Takwale A, Bichel J, Andres K, et al. Imiquimod 5% cream for the treatment of superficial and nodular basal cell carcinoma: randomized studies comparing low-frequency dosing with and without occlusion. Br J Dermatol. 2002; 147(6):1227–36.

69. Geisse JK, Rich P, Pandya A, Gross K, Andres K, Ginkel A, et al. Imiquimod 5% cream for the treatment of superficial basal cell carcinoma: a double-blind, randomized, vehicle-controlled study. J Am Acad Dermatol. 2002;47(3):390–8.

70. Geisse J, Caro I, Lindholm J, Golitz L, Stampone P, Owens M. Imiquimod 5% cream for the treatment of superficial basal cell carcinoma: results from two phase III, randomized, vehicle-controlled studies. J Am Acad Dermatol. 2004;50(5):722–33.

71. Schulze HJ, Cribier B, Requena L, Reifenberger J, Ferrándiz C, Garcia Diez A, et al. Imiquimod 5% cream for the treatment of superficial basal cell carcinoma: results from a randomized vehicle-controlled phase III study in Europe. Br J Dermatol. 2005;152(5):939–47.

72. Eigentler TK, Kamin A, Weide BM, Breuninger H, Caroli UM, Möhrle M, et al. A phase III, randomized, open label study to evaluate the safety and efficacy of imiquimod 5% cream applied thrice weekly for 8 and 12 weeks in the treatment of low-risk nodular basal cell carcinoma. J Am Acad Dermatol. 2007;57(4):616–21.

73. Miller BH, Shavin JS, Cognetta A, Taylor RJ, Salasche S, Korey A, et al. Nonsurgical treatment of basal cell carcinomas with intralesional 5-fluorouracil/epinephrine injectable gel. J Am Acad Dermatol. 1997;36(1): 72–7.

74. Romagosa R, Saap L, Givens M, Salvarrey A, He JL, Hsia SL, et al. A pilot study to evaluate the treatment of basal cell carcinoma with 5-fluorouracil using phosphatidyl choline as a transepidermal carrier. Dermatol Surg. 2000;26(4):338–40.

75. Edwards L, Tucker SB, Perednia D, Smiles KA, Taylor EL, Tanner DJ, et al. The effect of an intralesional sustained-release formulation of interferon alfa-2b on basal cell carcinomas. Arch Dermatol. 1990;126(8):1029–32.

76. Cornell RC, Greenway HT, Tucker SB, Edwards L, Ashworth S, Vance JC, et al. Intralesional interferon therapy for basal cell carcinoma. J Am Acad Dermatol. 1990;23(4 Pt 1):694–700.

77. Punjabi S, Cook LJ, Kersey P, Marks R, Cerio R. Solasodine glycoalkaloids: a novel topical therapy for basal cell carcinoma. A double-blind, randomized, placebo-controlled, parallel group, multicenter study. Int J Dermatol. 2008;47(1):78–82.

# Cutaneous Squamous Cell Carcinoma

**3**

### Erica H. Lee, Vicki J. Levine, and Kishwer S. Nehal

Nonmelanoma skin cancer is the most common cancer in the United States, with over one million cases in 2008. Cutaneous squamous cell carcinoma (cSCC) represents approximately 20% of all skin cancer cases and is the second most common skin cancer after basal cell carcinoma (BCC). It is estimated the lifetime risk for developing an SCC in Caucasian males is 9–14% and in women, 4–9% [1]. The incidence of cSCC is increasing with the highest incidence occurring in patients over the age of 85 [2, 3].

Fair skinned individuals with excessive exposure to UV radiation, outdoor occupational, or behavioral exposure and individuals residing near the equator have the highest risk factors for cSCC development. The presence of actinic keratoses and history of a previous nonmelanoma skin cancer are strongly associated with future cSCC development [4]. Ultraviolet B radiation (290–320 nm) is the most common risk factor for the development of cSCC, through activation of the *ras* pathway and p53 tumor suppressor gene mutations [5]. Additional risk factors include immunosuppression, notably organ-transplant recipients, and ionizing radiation (Table 3.1). Organ transplant recipients (OTR) have a 65-fold increase in the risk of developing cSCCs compared to the general population [6]. Most cSCCs develop in areas with the most extensive ultraviolet exposure, such as the lips, ears, and extremities [7]. In men, a disproportionate number of SCCs develop on the scalp, neck, and ear [8].

The precursor lesion of a squamous cell-carcinoma is an actinic keratosis (AK). Actinic keratoses are "precancerous" lesions histologically characterized by partial keratinocyte atypia, whereas SCC in situ has full thickness epidermal keratinocytic atypia. AKs may transform into SCCs with an estimated lifetime risk of 10% [9]. The most common types of squamous cell in situ are Bowen's disease which present on sun-exposed areas and Erythroplasia of Queyrat which occurs on the glans penis of uncircumcised men. Invasive SCC present as pink, smooth or hyperkeratotic papules, plaques or nodules which may be itchy or painful [10]. Verrucous carcinoma is an uncommon variant which presents as an exophytic, verrucous lesion. While these may be locally aggressive, they are less likely to metastasize. Keratoacanthomas present classically as a rapidly developing crater-like nodule

E.H. Lee (✉)
Department of Dermatology Service,
Memorial Sloan-Kettering Cancer Center,
160 East 53rd Street, 2nd floor, New York,
NY 10022, USA

Department of Dermatology, New York University
Medical Center, New York, NY, USA
e-mail: ehlee25@gmail.com

V.J. Levine
Department of Dermatology, New York University
Medical Center, New York, NY, USA

K.S. Nehal (✉)
Department of Dermatology Service,
Memorial Sloan-Kettering Cancer Center,
160 East 53rd Street, 2nd floor, New York,
NY 10022, USA
e-mail: nehalk@mskcc.org

M. Alam (ed.), *Evidence-Based Procedural Dermatology*,
DOI 10.1007/978-0-387-09424-3_3, © Springer Science+Business Media, LLC 2012

**Table 3.1** Risk factors for SCC development

| Ultraviolet radiation (UVA, UVB) |
| --- |
| Ionizing radiation |
| PUVA (psoralen and UVA) |
| Tanning beds |
| Phenotype (skin type) |
| Arsenic exposure |
| Human papillomavirus, notably types 16 and 18 |
| Chronic nonhealing wounds |
| Sites of chronic trauma |
| Chronic inflammatory disorders (discoid lupus, lichen planus) |
| Sites of radiation or chemical exposure |
| Oculocutaneous albinism |
| Xeroderma pigmentosum |
| Genodermatoses |
| Immunosuppression |
| Chronic lymphocytic leukemia (CLL) |
| Organ transplant recipients |
| Cigarette smoking |
| Actinic keratoses |

with a central keratotic core. They are considered by many to be a variant of SCC [11].

Treatment options vary based on the clinical and histologic characteristics of the tumor. Cryotherapy, electrodessication, and curettage may be considered for small, low-risk tumors. Topical therapy with 5-fluorouracil, imiquimod 5% cream and more recently, photodynamic therapy are additional treatment options for low-risk cutaneous SCC. Surgical excision is the treatment option that allows for histopathologic evaluation of the tumor margins. For excision of a well-differentiated, small (≤2 cm in diameter) tumor located on low-risk areas of the body (i.e., trunk, extremities), a surgical margin of 4 mm is usually adequate. If a tumor is poorly differentiated, large (>2 cm) or located in a high-risk area (i.e., face, scalp), a 6 mm margin is recommended [12].

Mohs micrographic surgery or excision with histopathologic assessment of the circumferential and deep tissue margin is the treatment of choice for high-risk tumors. The Mohs technique allows for the entire peripheral and deep margin to be evaluated, decreasing the risk of missing subclinical tumor compared to the standard, bread-loaf tissue processing method in a standard elliptical excision. Radiation is another treatment modality, although it is often reserved for inoperable tumors and nonsurgical candidates. Radiation is also used as an adjunctive treatment following surgery for recurrent or aggressive tumors.

The National Comprehensive Cancer Network (NCCN) publishes treatment and management recommendations for cSCC. In the 2009 Guidelines for SCC (II/A) [13], SCC is divided into low- and high-risk tumors based on multiple clinical and pathologic variables that determine the risk of recurrence (Table 3.2). Primary and adjuvant treatment guidelines are outlined for local low-risk SCC (Fig. 3.1) and local high-risk SCC (Fig. 3.2).

The overwhelming majority of cSCC remains early localized disease while a minority of cases lead to regional and distant metastases. If metastases occur, the regional lymph nodes are involved in 85% of cases and 15% involve distant viscera [14]. A comprehensive evaluation including a detailed history, full body skin, and lymph node examination and histologic evaluation are essential for tumor staging and treatment. As the dermatologic and oncologic communities are managing more SCCs, accurate staging is critical for tumor prognosis and treatment. Unlike other cancers, the evidence for cSCC staging is limited. There is a paucity of randomized controlled studies investigating the prognostic variables of SCCs. The overwhelming evidence is rooted in retrospective and prospective cohort studies and reviews. In this chapter, various staging variables based on consensus documents and existing data will be outlined.

## Consensus Documents

In a dual publication, The British Journal of Plastic Surgery and the British Journal of Dermatology published guidelines for the management of primary cSCC in 2002 and 2003 (III/B) [15, 16]. The factors affecting metastatic potential such as site, tumor size, and diameter, histologic differentiation, host immunosuppression, and previous treatment were briefly discussed. The lack of randomized controlled trials for the treatment of

**Table 3.2** Risk factors for SCC recurrence

| Risk factors for recurrence | | |
|---|---|---|
| H&P | Low risk | High risk |
| Localization/size[a] | Area L < 20 mm<br>Area M < 10 mm<br>Area H < 6 mm[b] | Area L ≥ 20 mm<br>Area M ≥ 10 mm<br>Area H ≥ 6 mm[b] |
| Borders | Well-defined | Poorly-defined |
| Primary vs. recurrent | Primary | Recurrent |
| Immunosuppression | (−) | (+) |
| Site of prior RT or chronic inflammatory process | (−) | (+) |
| Rapidly growing tumor | (−) | (+) |
| Neurologic symptoms | (−) | (+) |
| Pathology | | |
| Degree of differentiation | Well differentiated | Moderately or poorly differentiated |
| Adenoid (acantholytic), adenosquamous (showing mucin production), or desmoplastic subtypes | (−) | (+) |
| Depth: clark level or thickness[c] | I, II, III, or <4 mm | IV, V, or ≥4 mm |
| Perineural or vascular involvement | (−) | (+) |

Reproduced with permission from The NCCN [13]
These guidelines are copyrighted by the NCCN. All rights reserved. These guidelines and illustrations herein may not be reproduced in any form for any purpose without the express written permission of the NCCN
*Note*: All recommendations are category 2A unless otherwise indicated
*Clinical trials*: NCCN believes that the best management of any cancer patient is in a clinical trial. Participation in clinical trials is especially encouraged
*Area H* "mask areas" of face (central face, eyelids, eyebrows, periorbital, nose, lips (cutaneous and vermillion), chin, mandible, preauricular and postauricular skin/sulci, temple, ear), genitalia, hands, and feet
*Area M* cheeks, forehead, scalp, and neck
[a] Must include peripheral rim of erythema
[b] Location independent of size may constitute high risk in certain clinical settings
[c] A modified Preslow measurement should exclude parakeratosis or scale/crust, and should be made from base of ulcer if present

primary lesions, the widely varied biologic behavior of these tumors, and the different experiences of the treating specialists are highlighted as important variables to consider in the interpretation of the available studies. However, surgical excision is emphasized as the treatment of choice in the majority of cases and Mohs micrographic surgery is recommended for high-risk SCCs, especially in difficult anatomic locations.

The American Academy of Dermatology published guidelines of care in 1993 (VI/C) [17]. In an outline form, the clinical appearance of SCC variants, risk factors associated with aggressive behavior, histologic variants, and treatment modalities were discussed.

Guidelines for the management of SCC in organ transplant recipients (OTR) are available from members of the International Transplant Skin Cancer Collaborative (ITSCC) (III/B) [18]. Guidelines for follow-up depend on the number and type of nonmelanoma skin cancer and the rapidity of development in the transplant patient. For example, patients with a history of one SCC are recommended to have skin exams every 3–6 months, whereas patients with multiple NMSCs (number not specified) or high-risk SCCs are examined every 3 months. Multiple treatment algorithms for precursor lesions, low-risk SCC, high-risk SCC, and regional and satellite metastasis are presented to guide management in these challenging patients.

The NCCN is an alliance of the world's 21 leading cancer centers. The NCCN Clinical Practice Guidelines in Oncology provides treatment recommendations based on a review of the most relevant evidence and expert opinion.

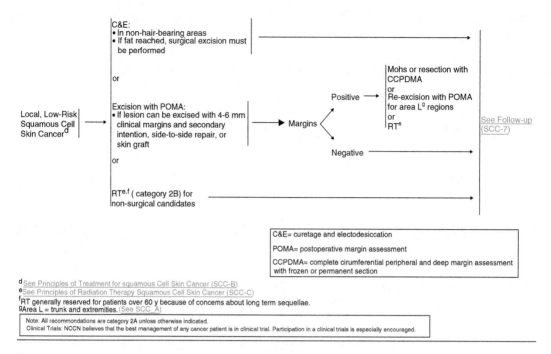

**Fig. 3.1** Treatment algorithm from the NCCN for local, low-risk SCC. Reproduced with permission from The NCCN [13]. These guidelines are copyrighted by the NCCN. All rights reserved. These guidelines and illustrations herein may not be reproduced in any form for any purpose without the express written permission of the NCCN

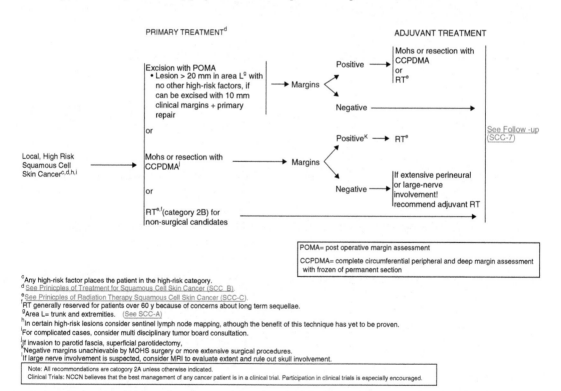

**Fig. 3.2** Treatment algorithm from the NCCN for local, high-risk SCC. Reproduced with permission from The NCCN [13]. These guidelines are copyrighted by the NCCN. All rights reserved. These guidelines and illustrations herein may not be reproduced in any form for any purpose without the express written permission of the NCCN

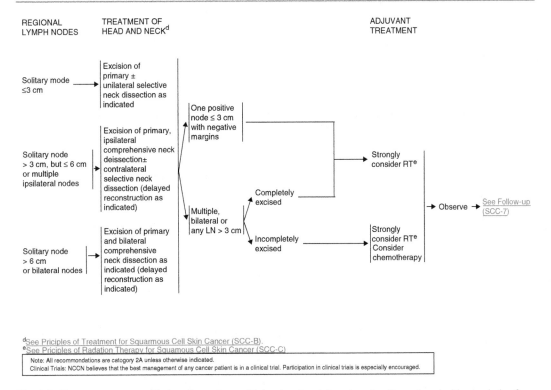

**Fig. 3.3** Treatment recommendations for patients with head and neck lymph nodes. Reproduced with permission from The NCCN [13]. These guidelines are copyrighted by the NCCN. All rights reserved. These guidelines and illustrations herein may not be reproduced in any form for any purpose without the express written permission of the NCCN

Consensus on the most accepted approaches to treatment is presented to serve as a guide for the treating physician to use in the context of each individual case. The categories of evidence are divided into three main categories 1–3, with category 2 subdivided into 2A and 2B based on the level of evidence and whether there is uniform agreement in the consensus panel. In the 2009 Guidelines for Squamous Cell Carcinoma, the recommendations are predominantly Category 2A, or lower level evidence and uniform NCCN consensus (II/A) [13]. Treatment algorithms for local SCC are divided into low- and high-risk tumors based on risk factors for recurrence (see Figs. 3.1 and 3.2). Guidelines for the management of regional lymph nodes are present, using size cutoffs of 3 and 6 cm (Fig. 3.3). For clinical follow-up in local disease, the NCCN recommends a complete skin and regional lymph node exam every 3–6 months for the first 2 years, every 6–12 m for the next 3 years, and then annually thereafter. For regional disease, the guidelines recommend more frequent exams (Fig. 3.4) [13]. These recommendations are continually refined as new significant data becomes available and are updated accordingly by the NCCN.

The American Joint Committee on Cancer (AJCC) systematically stages and classifies cancers to determine prognosis and guide treatment (I/A) [19]. The sixth edition staging system on skin cancers encompassed all nonmelanoma skin cancers, including Merkel cell carcinoma, BCC, and SCC despite significant differences in tumor biology and prognosis. In the seventh edition, published in 2010, a Nonmelanoma Skin Cancer Staging Committee was created to formulate a new staging system for cSCC [20]. The proposed seventh edition separates skin carcinomas into two distinct chapters entitled "Cutaneous Squamous Cell Carcinoma and Other Cutaneous Carcinomas" and "Merkel Cell Carcinoma."

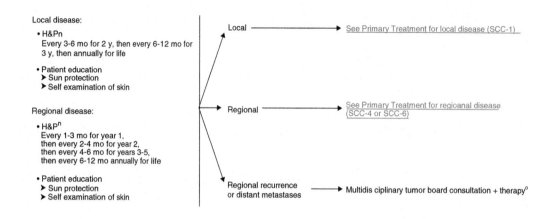

FOLLOW -UP                                          RECURRENCE/DISEASE PROGRESSION

Local disease:

• H&Pn
  Every 3-6 mo for 2 y, then every 6-12 mo for
  3 y, then annually for life

• Patient education
  ➤ Sun protection
  ➤ Self examination of skin

Regional disease:

• H&P[n]
  Every 1-3 mo for year 1,
  then every 2-4 mo for year 2,
  then every 4-6 mo for years 3-5,
  then every 6-12 mo annually for life

• Patient education
  ➤ Sun protection
  ➤ Self examination of skin

Local ──────────→ See Primary Treatment for local disease (SCC-1)

Regional ──────────→ See Primary Treatment for regioanal disease
                      (SCC-4 or SCC-6)

Regional recurrence ──────────→ Multidis ciplinary tumor board consultation + therapy[o]
or distant metastases

[n]Including complete skin and regional lymph node exam.
[o]Consider clinical trials.

Note: All recommendations are catogory 2A unless otherwise indicated.
Clinical Trials: NCCN believes that the best management of any cancer patient is is a clinical trial. Participation in clinical trials is especially encouraged.

**Fig. 3.4** Guidelines for patient follow-up in local and regional disease. Reproduced with permission from The NCCN [13]. These guidelines are copyrighted by the NCCN. All rights reserved. These guidelines and illustrations herein may not be reproduced in any form for any purpose without the express written permission of the NCCN

In the seventh edition staging system of cSCC, the TNM classification is maintained, however with changes in T (tumor) and N (regional lymph node) staging. In the seventh edition, a cutoff of 2 cm is used to differentiate T1 and T2. The most striking change is the addition of evidence-based high-risk tumor features (Table 3.3). These prognosticating tumor variables are a significant addition to the tumor (T) classification and the presence of two or more high-risk features alone can upgrade the T stage regardless of tumor size (Table 3.4).

The evidence supporting many of these variables is largely rooted in retrospective and prospective studies. The collective review of these studies has led to the identification of several significant tumor features including tumor size, thickness, location, and histologic grade. Additional prognostic features, including parotid metastasis are also discussed.

**Table 3.3** High-risk features for the tumor (T) staging in the seventh edition AJCC staging system of cutaneous SCC

| High-risk tumor features |
| --- |
| >2 mm tumor thickness |
| Clark level ≥IV |
| Perineural invasion |
| Anatomic site ear |
| Anatomic site hair-bearing lip |
| Histologic grade (poor or undifferentiated histology) |

Used with the permission of the American Joint Committee on Cancer (AJCC), Chicago, Illinois. The original source for this material is the AJCC Cancer Staging Manual, Seventh Edition (2010) published by Springer Science and Business Media LLC, www.springer.com

## Tumor Size

Tumor size is the maximal clinical diameter of the lesion. A two centimeter diameter is the cutoff differentiating T1 from T2 in the proposed

**Table 3.4** Primary tumor (T) defined by the seventh edition AJCC Staging Manual for cutaneous SCC

| | |
|---|---|
| TX | Primary tumor cannot be assessed |
| T0 | No evidence of primary tumor |
| Tis | Carcinoma in situ |
| T1 | Tumor 2 cm or less in greatest dimension with less than two high-risk features (see Table 3.3) |
| T2 | Tumor greater than 2 cm in greatest dimension or any size tumor with two or more high-risk features (see Table 3.3) |
| T3 | Tumor with invasion of maxilla, mandible, orbit, or temporal bone |
| T4 | Tumor with direct or PNI of skull base or axial skeleton |

Used with the permission of the American Joint Committee on Cancer (AJCC), Chicago, Illinois. The original source for this material is the AJCC Cancer Staging Manual, Seventh Edition (2010) published by Springer Science and Business Media LLC, www.springer.com

seventh edition of the AJCC [20]. Rowe et al., in their 1992 retrospective study evaluated multiple prognostic factors for local recurrence and metastasis (II/A) [21]. In this paper, an extensive review of over 200 studies derived several conclusions. Tumor size greater than 2 cm, tumor depth greater than 4 mm or Clark level IV or V, and poorly differentiated tumors have higher local recurrence and metastatic rates. Tumors 2 cm in diameter or larger had a double rate of local recurrence (15 vs. 7%) and a triple rate for metastasis (30 vs. 9%) compared to tumors less than 2 cm. In a retrospective review of 136 patients by Mullen et al., patients with primary tumors >2 cm in diameter had a 3.8-fold higher risk of recurrence or death (V/B) [22]. Tumors larger than 4 cm were also shown to be strongly associated with nodal metastasis (IV/B) [23].

In a retrospective review of 200 SCC tumors of which 25 were metastatic, tumor size significantly correlated with metastasis ($p < 0.004$), with increasing risk for tumors larger than 2 cm (IV/B) [24]. However, tumors less than 2 cm in size may metastasize as well. In a review of 915 cSCCs from the Netherlands' registry, when compared to matched nonmetastatic controls, the risk of metastasis was significantly higher in tumors with a width of at least 1.5 cm (III/B) [25]. In a prospective study of 266 patients with metastatic SCC,

the median tumor size was 1.5 cm, suggesting size alone is not a good predictor of outcome (V/B) [26].

## Tumor Thickness

The importance of tumor thickness or depth of invasion is highlighted by a study of 673 SCCs by Breuninger et al. that showed metastases were not seen in tumors less than 2 mm in depth (V/B) [27]. A rate of 15% was seen in tumors greater than 6 mm. In 1997, Breuninger et al. showed 44.4% of desmoplastic tumors 5 mm in thickness metastasized (IV/B) [28]. In a prospective study of 193 patients with cSCC of the head and neck, nodal metastases were strongly associated with invasion into the subcutaneous tissue, with 31% of lesions 8 mm or deeper exhibiting nodal metastasis (IV/B) [23]. Brantsch et al. prospectively analyzed risk factors for local recurrence and metastasis in 615 patients. Tumors 2 mm or less in thickness did not metastasize, whereas 4% of tumors 2.1–6 mm thick and 16% of tumors greater than 6 mm in thickness metastasized (IV/B) [29]. The histologic depth of a lesion is also described by the Clark level of invasion. Rowe et al. showed tumors with Clark level IV or V (depth ≥ 4 mm) had higher local recurrence and metastatic rates compared to tumors with a Clark level I to III (II/A) [21].

## Anatomic Location

The anatomic location of the cSCC on the ear and lip is shown to have higher rates of local recurrence and metastasis [21]. In a study evaluating 365 SCCs treated by Mohs micrographic surgery, the highest rates of metastasis were the lips, temple, and dorsal hands (IV/B) [30]. A retrospective case series of 45 cases of cSCC with regional lymph node metastasis, the ear or preauricular area, anterior scalp, and nose were the most common locations (V/B) [31]. In a review of 65 patients in Sweden from 1970 to 1977, the risk of metastasis in tumors on the external ear was 16.4% (V/C) [32]. A retrospective review specifically of lip cancer patients shows tumors larger than 5 cm in diameter and commissure involvement is significantly associated with neck metastasis (V/B) [33]. Although location on the upper or lower lip is occasionally specified, the significance of hair-bearing lip involvement is not clear in these studies. According to the proposed seventh edition cSCC staging system, tumor location on the hair-bearing lip is a high-risk tumor feature [20].

## Histologic Grade

Histologic grade or degree of differentiation also affects prognosis. In 1921, Broders classified squamous cell tumors based on their degree of differentiation into four grades according to the percentage of differentiated to undifferentiated epithelium [34]. In general, well-differentiated tumors are less aggressive. Less differentiated tumors (Grades 2 or higher) have a greater chance of metastasis (V/B) [27]. Eroglu et al. showed in univariate and multivariate analysis, histopathologic grade is a significant risk factor for local recurrence (V/B) [35]. Rowe et al. showed poorly differentiated tumors have two times the local recurrence rate (28.6% compared to 13.6%) and three times the metastatic rate (32.8% compared to 9.2%) [21]. Although poor histologic differentiation is a significant prognostic factor, in their analysis, 63.7% of the tumors that metastasized were well differentiated. Therefore, degree of differentiation alone is not sufficient to prognosticate and stage a tumor.

Desmoplastic SCC is an aggressive histologic subtype characterized by cords of epithelial cells infiltrating a dense, desmoplastic stroma [36]. Desmoplasia is recently regarded as a prognostic factor in the literature. Breuninger et al. prospectively evaluated 594 SCCs of which 44 tumors were identified as desmoplastic based on light microscopy. The tumors were treated with Mohs micrographic surgery and followed for a median of 5.3 years. Desmoplastic SCCs tended to be thicker, more frequently on the ear and associated with a 6 and 10 times higher risk of metastasis and local recurrence, respectively (IV/B) [28].

In a study comparing 51 patients with desmoplastic SCC to 564 patients with nondesmoplastic tumors, 12 desmoplastic tumors (24%) developed a local recurrence compared to only 8 (1%) in the control group. The univariate analysis showed desmoplasia was a significant prognostic factor (IV/B) [37].

The presence or absence of desmoplasia is not routinely reported on histopathology reports and histopathologic evaluation of desmoplasia is subjective. It is important to be aware of its potential implications; however, additional evidence is warranted to further prognosticate the role of desmoplasia in SCC tumors.

## Perineural Invasion

Cutaneous tumors with perineural invasion (PNI) are associated with a higher risk of aggressive behavior, local recurrence, and potential invasion into the bone and central nervous system [38]. Geopfert et al. reviewed 520 patients with 967 cSCC of the face during a 10-year period (IV/B) [39]. Fourteen percent of the tumors showed perineural extension, most commonly involving the maxillary and mandibular branches of the trigeminal nerve. In these cases, 47% recurred vs. 7.3% in the control group and 35% metastasized to the regional nodes compared to 15% in the control group. There was an increase incidence of cervical adenopathy, metastasis, and reduced survival in these patients. In a comparison of 157 nonmetastasizing lower lip SCCs to 30 metastasizing SCCs, PNI was seen in 5 and 41% of tumors, respectively (V/B) [40].

## Lymphovascular Invasion

Evidence suggests lymphovascular invasion may be an important high-risk factor. In a prospective, longitudinal database study by Moore et al., 40% of patients with nodal metastases had lymphovascular invasion compared to only 8% of patients with no nodal involvement. In multivariate analysis (OR 7.54, $p < 0.0001$), lymphovascular invasion was an independent predictor of nodal metastases (IV/B) [23]. In other studies, lymphovascular invasion was not a significant prognostic factor (IV/B) [24, 41]. Additional studies are needed to further delineate the prognostic role of lymphovascular invasion.

## Immunosuppression

Various settings of immunosuppression increase the incidence of SCC such as organ transplantation, long-term use of immunosuppressive agents, and underlying malignancies. The most comprehensive evidence to date is from the organ transplant population. In OTR, SCCs are more aggressive, occur at a higher incidence, and develop at a younger age [42]. In a Norwegian population, the OTR risk was 65-fold higher than the general population, with a 2.9 times greater risk in heart transplant recipients than kidney transplant recipients (V/B) [6]. In a review of 231 cSCCs in 79 OTR, features more commonly seen were acantholytic changes, poor differentiation, increased tumor depth, infiltrative growth pattern, and desmoplasia (V/B) [43]. Southwell et al. retrospectively reviewed 40 patients with metastatic cSCC. Nine immunocompromised patients were identified and shown to have a 7.2 times higher risk of local recurrence, a 5.3 times increased risk of any disease recurrence, and a -year survival of 71 vs. 90% in the immune competent group (IV/B) [44]. In a series of 21 patients with in-transit metastasis by Carucci et al., 15 patients were OTR (V/B) [45]. In this study, the primary tumors were located most commonly on the forehead and scalp and were histologically well-differentiated (81%). After a mean follow-up of 24 months, 33% of the OTR group had no evidence of disease compared to 80% in the non-transplant group; a third succumbed to the tumor while there were no deaths in the control group.

Patients with chronic lymphocytic leukemia (CLL) have an eightfold risk of skin cancer development [46]. In a retrospective case-controlled study of 28 patients by Mehrany et al., the recurrence rate of SCC was seven times higher in patients with CLL ($p = 0.003$). Although this is a small patient group, there was no significant difference in histologic grade or tumor size [47]. Mehrany et al. also retrospectively reviewed 28 patients with CLL and showed CLL patients were more likely to develop and die of a metastasis compared to matched controls [48]. The aggressive behavior of SCC tumors with increased local recurrence and nodal metastasis is further supported by case reports [49].

## Local Recurrence

When evaluating the rate of recurrence or metastasis, it is important to assess if adequate follow-up is performed. Rowe et al. showed that studies with 5 or more years of follow-up had higher local recurrence, metastatic, and mortality rates [21]. In 1996, Eroglu et al. performed univariate and multivariate analyses on 187 patients with locoregional recurrence between 1980 and 1989 in Turkey (V/B) [35]. Local recurrence was seen in 150 patients, regional metastasis in 20, and both recurrence and metastasis in 17 patients. The four factors significant in univariate and multivariate analyses were tumor stage, histopathologic grade, treatment modality, and pre-existing scar tissue. As outlined above, the risk of local recurrence increases in tumors with high-risk features. Several studies characterizing high-risk SCCs are briefly described in Table 3.5.

## Metastatic Potential

The incidence of metastasis from cSCC ranges from 0.5 to 16% [50]. cSCC metastasis typically presents within 1–2 years after diagnosis. However, delayed presentation of up to 8 years is reported [51]. In a retrospective review of 200 patients at the Medical University of South Carolina, invasive SCCs from the tumor registry were compared to nonmetastatic SCC controls (IV/B) [24]. The risk of metastasis increased with tumor size, notably tumors larger than 2 cm. Metastatic SCCs were deeper (Clark level V), more likely to be poorly differentiated, recurrent, and in areas of

**Table 3.5** Studies characterizing high-risk SCCs

| References | Population | Subjects | Time period | Tumor characteristics | Location |
|---|---|---|---|---|---|
| Brantsch et al. [29] | University Tubingen, Germany | 615 pts (63% men)<br>Mean age: 72<br>26 developed metastasis, 9 died | Patient eligibility 1990–2001<br>Follow-up until 31 December, 2005 | ≤2 mm thick: no mets<br>2.1–6 mm: 12 (4%) mets<br>>6 mm: 14 (16%) mets<br>Tumor thickness prognostic factor for mets<br>20 local recurrences, most first year<br>Desmoplasia and thickness<br>>6 mm RF for local recurrence | Metastatic tumors: ear (2), lip (2), and others (5)<br>Ear is a prognostic factor for mets on multivariate analysis |
| Veness et al. [26] | Westmead Hospital, Australia | 266 pts<br>162 w/ parotid ± cervical nodes<br>104 w/ cervical node | Retrospective 1980–2005 | Median size: 15 mm<br>Median thickness: 6 mm<br>46% moderate or poorly differentiated<br>8% PNI<br>5% immunosuppressed | Most common location<br>Ear (20%)<br>Cheek (12%)<br>Frontotemporal scalp (19%) |
| Quaedvlieg et al. [25] | University Hospital of Maastricht | 580 pts<br>73% men<br>582 SCCs of skin<br>63 SCCs of lip<br>68 tumors metastasized (20.6% lip) | 1982–2002<br>Mean f/u: 5.7 years | Multivariate analysis: risk factor for skin mets are tumor diameter, desmoplasia, Clark index. Protective: ±lymphocytic infiltrate RF for lip: plasma cells | Tumor diameter at least 1.5 cm, thickness ≥2 mm, less differentiation, eosinophils, and plasma cells seen more in metastatic tumors |
| Breuninger et al. [28] | University Tubingen, Germany | 445 primary SCCs<br>399 males<br>170 females<br>149 vermillion surface | Prospective<br>Follow-up: 4–10 years | 44 (7.4%) desmoplastic SCCs<br>Tumor thickness greater in desmoplastic SCC<br>Higher metastatic rate in desmoplastic >5 mm thick tumors than "common SCC" of same thickness (44.4 vs. 17.5%) | Desmoplastic SCCs more common on the ear |
| Rowe et al. [21] | Literature review | 71 studies of local recurrence<br>95 observations of metastatic rates<br>38 observations of survival | 1940–1990<br><5 year and >5 year follow-up periods evaluated | Correlates w/ recurrence and mets: ≥2 cm diameter, ≥4 mm depth, Clark IV/V, poor histology, ear, lip, scar carcinoma, previous tx, PNI, and immunocompromised state. Combo tx better for survival in metastasis | Local recurrence and metastatic rates increased with longer f/u and increased each year<br>Mohs is superior to nonMohs tx |

previous radiation. The presence of PNI, small nests and infiltrative strands, acantholysis, and single-cell infiltration was all significantly correlated with metastasis. More than half of the metastases occurred within the first year of diagnosis and treatment (56%).

In a retrospective review by Mullen et al., 136 patients with invasive SCC were identified (V/B) [22]. Factors significantly associated with recurrence-free survival (RFS) included scar carcinoma, tumor diameter >2 cm, nodal disease, and poorly differentiated histology. The RFS curves for large tumor sizes (T2–T4) were worse than for small, T1 tumors (39 vs. 84%) and poorly differentiated tumors had a 2.9 times higher risk of metastasis or death. Nodal disease on presentation was associated with a fivefold risk of recurrence and death and a 5-year RFS of 29% compared to 80% in patients without nodal involvement. Quaedvlieg et al. showed metastatic SCC tumors had a vertical tumor thickness of at least 2 mm, desmoplasia, and an inflammatory response consisting of eosinophils and plasma cells (III/B) [25].

## Parotid Metastasis

Parotid involvement from metastatic SCC is associated with a poor prognosis, particularly if the lesion is in excess of 6 cm or has facial nerve involvement (V/B) [52]. The sixth edition AJCC staging system does not differentiate between cervical lymph node metastasis and parotid metastasis. A staging system that separates parotid involvement from cervical node involvement was recommended several years ago due to the significance of parotid involvement as an independent prognostic factor [53]. Several of these studies are briefly discussed in Table 3.6.

O'Brien et al. from the Royal Prince Alfred Hospital in Sydney prospectively analyzed a series of 87 patients with metastatic SCC (IV/B) [54]. Disease control in the parotid gland decreased with increasing parotid (P) stage and metastatic disease in the neck had a significant influence on survival. The 5-year survival of

patients with neck involvement is less than 50%, whereas patients with only parotid gland disease had a 5-year survival of 80%. Palme et al. retrospectively analyzed 126 patients with metastatic cSCC involving the parotid gland with or without neck disease to assess recurrence and disease-specific survival. The parotid control rate and survival varied significantly with parotid (P) stage (V/B) [55]. A multicenter study of metastatic SCC to the parotid and/or neck showed cumulative disease-specific survival at 5 years was 74%. Survival did not vary significantly based on parotid stage alone; however, early (P1) disease had improved 5-year survival compared to late disease (P2+P3). Neck involvement alone or with parotid involvement worsened survival (V/B) [53].

## Sentinel Lymph Node Biopsy

While sentinel lymph node biopsy (SNLB) is the standard of care for a subset of melanomas, its utility in the evaluation and prognostication of cSCC is not determined. There are multiple studies investigating the role of SNLB in high-risk cSCC patients (V/B) [56–58]. However, due to the lack of controlled studies, definitive conclusions on the role of SNLB in disease-free or overall survival are unclear. Multicenter randomized controlled studies are needed to further define the role of SNLB in cSCC.

## Conclusion

The majority of patients with primary cSCC respond well to standard therapy and have an excellent prognosis. Patients with locally recurrent and metastatic disease have a poorer, long-term prognosis. The evidence demonstrates various tumor variables are critical in understanding tumor biology and patient prognosis. While controlled studies are limited, the evidence supports various cSCC variables have a significant role in the staging, treatment, and management of patients with cSCC.

**Table 3.6** Studies characterizing the role of parotid metastasis

| References | Study type/population | Subjects | Follow-up | Results | Comments |
|---|---|---|---|---|---|
| O'Brien et al. [54] | Prospective Royal Prince Alfred Medical Center, Australia | 87 patients with metastatic SCC to the parotid Parotid stage 1 (P1) = 43 pts, P2 = 35, P3 = 9 | Minimum 2 years | Independent risk factor for survival: positive surgical margins and advanced neck disease | Parotid and neck involvement protends worse prognosis |
| Audet et al. [52] | Retrospective Princess Margaret Hospital, Toronto | 56 pts P1 = 20, P2 = 14, P3 = 22 Treated with surgery, radiation, or surgery + radiation | Minimum 1 year | Survival worse in external beam radiation patients | Combination therapy recommended Poor prognosis in lesions >6 cm and w/ facial nerve involvement |
| Palme et al. [55] | Retrospective Royal Prince Alfred Medical Center, Australia | 126 pts 70 w/ pathology confirmed parotid involvement 51 w/ neck involvement 19 with both | Minimum 2 years | Parotid stage is an independent RF for local control and survival. 5-year survival for P1, 81% vs. P2, 51% and P3, 33% ($p < 0.001$) | Multivariate shows P3 stage and the presence of immunosuppression independently decreased survival |
| Andruchow et al. [53] | Retrospective Multicenter in USA and Australia | 322 pts 217 w/parotid disease 62 w/ neck disease 43 w/parotid and neck disease | Minimum 2 years | | Neck involvement alone or with parotid involvement worsens survival; however, the later was not significant |

*RF* risk factor; *P1* metastatic node up to 3 cm in diameter; *P2* metastatic node >3 cm but <6 cm or multiple nodes; *P3* metastatic node >6 cm or disease involving the facial nerve or skull base

**Evidence-Based Summary**

| Findings | Evidence level |
|---|---|
| Cutaneous SCC predominantly presents as early, local disease, however in some cases, may lead to regional and distant metastasis | |
| The risk of cSCC metastasis increases with tumor size, depth, poor histologic differentiation, and tumor recurrence | (V/B) |
| Cutaneous SCC development on the external ear and lip has higher rates of local recurrence and metastasis | (II/A) |
| The presence of desmoplasia on histopathology is increasingly being regarded as a poor prognostic factor | (IV/B) |
| PNI is associated with a higher risk of aggressive tumor behavior | (IV/B) |
| Organ transplant recipients are at a significantly higher risk of developing an aggressive cSCC | (V/B) |
| There is insufficient evidence establishing a prognostic role of sentinel lymph node biopsy in cSCC | (V/B) |

# References

1. Miller DL, Weinstock MA. Nonmelanoma skin cancer in the United States: incidence. J Am Acad Dermatol. 1994;50:774–8.
2. Gray DR, Suman VJ, Clay RP, Harmsen WS, Roenigk RK. Trends in the population-based incidence of squamous cell carcinoma of the skin first diagnosed between 1984 and 1992. Arch Dermatol. 1997;133:735–40.
3. Holme SA, Malinovszky K, Roberts DL. Changing trends in non-melanoma skin cancer in South Wales, 1988–98. Br J Dermatol. 2000;143:1124–9.
4. English DR, Armstrong BK, Kricker A, et al. Demographic characteristic, pigmentary and cutaneous risk factors for squamous cell carcinoma of the skin: a case-control study. Int J Cancer. 1998;76:628–34.
5. Hussein MR. Ultraviolet radiation and skin cancer: molecular mechanisms. J Cutan Pathol. 2005;32:191–205.
6. Jensen P, Hansen S, Moller B, et al. Skin cancer in kidney and heart transplant recipients and different long-term immunosuppressive therapy regimens. J Am Acad Dermatol. 1999;40:177–86.
7. Buettner PG, Raasch BA. Incidence rates of skin cancer in Townsville, Australia. Int J Cancer. 1998;78:587–93.
8. Salasche SJ. Epidemiology of actinic keratoses and squamous cell carcinoma. J Am Acad Dermatol. 2000;42:4–7.
9. Fuchs A, Marmur E. The kinetics of skin cancer: progression of actinic keratosis to squamous cell carcinoma. Dermatol Surg. 2007;33:1099.
10. Alam M, Ratner D. Cutaneous squamous-cell carcinoma. N Engl J Med. 2001;344:975–82.
11. Beham A, Regauer S, Soyer HP, Beham-Schmid C. Keratoacanthoma: a clinically distinct variant of well differentiated squamous cell carcinoma. Adv Anat Pathol. 1988;5:269.
12. Broadland DG, Zitelli JA. Surgical margins for excision of primary cutaneous squamous cell carcinoma. J Am Acad Dermatol. 1992;27:241–8.
13. NCCN Clinical Practice Guidelines in Oncology. Basal cell and squamous cell skin cancers (Version.1.2009). © 2008 National Comprehensive Cancer Network, Inc. http://www.nccn.org. Accessed 18 Feb 2009.
14. Kwa RE, Campana K, Moy RL. Biology of cutaneous squamous cell carcinoma. Am J Acad Dermatol. 1992;26:1–26.
15. Motley R, Kersey P, Lawrence C. Multiprofessional guidelines for the management of the patient with primary cutaneous squamous cell carcinoma. Br J Plast Surg. 2003;56:85–91.
16. Motley R, Kersey P, Lawrence C. Multiprofessional guidelines for the management of the patient with primary cutaneous squamous cell carcinoma. Br J Dermatol. 2002;146:18–25.
17. Task Force on Cutaneous Squamous Cell Carcinoma. Guidelines of care for cutaneous squamous cell carcinoma. Committee on Guidelines of Care. J Am Acad Dermatol. 1993;28:628–31.
18. Stasko T, Brown MD, Carucci JA, et al. Guidelines for the management of squamous cell carcinoma in organ transplant recipients. Dermatol Surg. 2004;30:642–50.
19. American Joint Committee on Cancer. www.cancer-staging.org. Accessed September 2010.
20. Cutaneous Squamous Cell Carcinoma. In: Edge SB, Byrd DR, Compton CC, editors. AJCC cancer staging manual. 7th ed. New York: Springer; 2010.
21. Rowe DE, Carroll RJ, Day Jr CL. Prognostic factors for local recurrence, metastasis and survival rates in squamous cell carcinoma of the skin, ear, and lip. Implications for treatment modality selection. J Am Acad Dermatol. 1992;26:976–90.

22. Mullen JT, Feng L, Xing Y, et al. Invasive squamous cell carcinoma of the skin: defining a high-risk group. Ann Surg Oncol. 2006;13:902–9.

23. Moore BA, Weber RS, Prieto V, El-Naggar A, et al. Lymph node metastases from cutaneous squamous cell carcinoma of the head and neck. Laryngoscope. 2005;115:1561–7.

24. Cherpelis BS, Marcusen C, Lang PG. Prognostic factors for metastasis in squamous cell carcinoma of the skin. Dermatol Surg. 2002;28:268–73.

25. Quaedvlieg PJF, Cretens DHKV, Epping GG, et al. Histopathological characteristics of metastasizing squamous cell carcinoma of the skin and lips. Histopathology. 2006;49:256–64.

26. Veness MK, Palme CE, Morgan GJ. High-risk cutaneous squamous cell carcinoma of the head and neck. Cancer. 2006;106:2389–96.

27. Breuninger H, Black B, Rassner G. Microstaging of squamous cell carcinomas. Am J Clin Pathol. 1990;94:624–7.

28. Breuninger H, Schaumburg-Lever G, Holzschuh J, Horny HP. Desmoplastic squamous cell carcinoma of skin and vermilion surface: a highly malignant subtype of skin cancer. Cancer. 1997;79:915–9.

29. Brantsch KD, Meisner C, Shonfisch B, et al. Analysis of risk factors determining prognosis of cutaneous squamous-cell carcinoma: a prospective study. Lancet Oncol. 2008;9:713–20.

30. Dinehart SM, Pollack SV. Metastases from squamous cell carcinoma of the skin and lip. An analysis of twenty-seven cases. J Am Acad Dermatol. 1989;21:241–8.

31. Kraus DH, Carew JF, Harrison LB. Regional lymph node metastasis from cutaneous squamous cell carcinoma. Arch Otolaryngol Head Neck Surg. 1998;124:582–7.

32. Afzelius LE, Gunarsson M, Nordgren H. Guidelines for prophylactic radical lymph node dissection in cases of carcinoma of the external ear. Head Neck Surg. 1980;5:361–5.

33. Vartanian JG, Carvalho AL, de Araujo Filho MJ, et al. Predictive factors and distribution of lymph node metastasis in lip cancer patients and their implications on the treatment of the neck. Oral Oncol. 2004;40:223–7.

34. Broders AC. Squamous-cell epithelioma of the Skin. Ann Surg. 1921;73:141–60.

35. Eroglu A, Berberoglu U, Berreroglu S. Risk factors related to locoregional recurrence in squamous cell carcinoma of the skin. J Surg Oncol. 1996;61:124–30.

36. Cassarino DS, DeRienzo DP, Barr RJ. Cutaneous squamous cell carcinoma: a comprehensive clinicopathologic classification. J Cutan Pathol. 2006;33:261–79.

37. Brantsch KD, Meisner C, Schonfisch B, et al. Analysis of risk factors determining prognosis of cutaneous squamous-cell carcinoma: a prospective study. Lancet Oncol. 2008;9:713–20.

38. Feasel AM, Brown TJ, Bogle MA, et al. Perineural invasion of cutaneous malignancies. Dermatol Surg. 2001;27:531–42.

39. Geopfert H, Dichtel WJ, Medina JE, Lindberg RD, Luna MD. Perineural invasion in squamous cell skin carcinoma of the head and neck. Am J Surg. 1984;148:542–7.

40. Frierson Jr HF, Cooper PH. Prognostic factors in squamous cell carcinoma of the lower lip. Hum Pathol. 1986;17:346–54.

41. Czarnecki D, Staples MP, Mar A, et al. Metastases from squamous cell carcinoma of the skin in Southern Australia. Dermatology. 1994;189:52–4.

42. Berg D, Otley CC. Skin cancer in organ transplant recipients: epidemiology, pathogenesis, and management. J Am Acad Dermatol. 2002;47:1–17.

43. Smith KJ, Hamza S, Skelton H. Histologic features in primary cutaneous squamous cell carcinomas in immunocompromised patients focusing on organ transplant patients. Dermatol Surg. 2004;30:634–41.

44. Southwell KE, Chaplin JM, Eisenberg RL, et al. Effect of immunocompromise on metastatic cutaneous squamous cell carcinoma in the parotid and neck. Head Neck. 2006;28:244–8.

45. Carucci JA, Martinez JC, Zeitouni N, et al. In-transit metastasis from primary cutaneous squamous cell carcinoma in organ transplant recipients and nonimmunosuppressed patients: clinical characteristics, management, and outcome in a series of 21 patients. Dermatol Surg. 2004;30:651–5.

46. Manusow D, Weinerman BH. Subsequent neoplasia in chronic lymphocytic leukemia. J Am Med Assoc. 1975;232:267–9.

47. Mehrany K, Weenig RH, Pittelkow MR, et al. High recurrence rates of squamous cell carcinoma after Mohs' surgery in patients with chronic lymphocytic leukemia. Dermatol Surg. 2005;31:38–42.

48. Mehrany K, Weenig RH, Lee KK, et al. Increased metastasis and mortality from cutaneous squamous cell carcinoma in patients with chronic lymphocytic leukemia. J Am Acad Dermatol. 2005;53:1067–71.

49. Hartley BE, Searle AE, Breach NM, et al. Aggressive cutaneous squamous cell carcinoma of the head and neck in patients with chronic lymphocytic leukaemia. J Laryngol Otol. 1996;110:694–5.

50. Dinehart SM, Pollack SV. Metastases from squamous cell carcinoma of the skin and lip. J Am Acad Dermatol. 1989;21:241–8.

51. Weinberg AS, Ogle CA, Shim EK. Metastatic cutaneous squamous cell carcinoma: an update. Dermatol Surg. 2007;33:885–99.

52. Audet N, Palme CE, Gullane PJ, et al. Cutaneous metastatic squamous cell carcinoma to the parotid gland: analysis and outcome. Head Neck. 2004;26:727–32.

53. Andruchow JL, Veness MJ, Morgan GJ, et al. Implications for clinical staging of metastatic cutaneous squamous carcinoma of the head and neck based on a multicenter study of treatment outcomes. Cancer. 2006;106:1078–83.

54. O'Brien CJ, McNeil EB, McMahon JD, et al. Significance of clinical stage, extent of surgery, and pathologic findings in metastatic cutaneous squamous carcinoma of the parotid gland. Head Neck. 2002;24:417–22.

55. Palme CE, O'Brien CJ, Veness MJ, et al. Extent of parotid disease influences outcome in patients with metastatic cutaneous squamous cell carcinoma. Arch Otolaryngol Head Neck Surg. 2003;129:750–3.

56. Wagner JD, Evdokimow DZ, Weisberger E, et al. Sentinel node biopsy for high-risk nonmelanoma cutaneous malignancy. Arch Dermatol. 2004;140: 75–9.

57. Renzi C, Caggiati A, Mannooranparampil TJ, et al. Sentinel lymph node biopsy for high risk cutaneous squamous cell carcinoma: case series and review of the literature. Eur J Surg Oncol. 2007;33:364–9.

58. Ross AS, Schmults CD. Sentinel lymph node biopsy in cutaneous squamous cell carcinoma: a systematic review of the English literature. Dermatol Surg. 2006;32:1309–21.

## Self-Assessment

1. High-risk anatomic locations for SCC include:
   (a) Central face
   (b) Neck
   (c) Ear
   (d) Upper arms
   (e) a+c
   (f) All of the above

2. A 61-year-old male presents with a 1.3 cm keratotic plaque on the right leg diagnosed as a SCC. The lesion was previously treated with curettage and electrodessication several years prior. Which of the following would be the *most* appropriate treatment choice?
   (a) Radiation
   (b) Curettage and electrodessication
   (c) Mohs micrographic surgery
   (d) Combination treatment with photodynamic therapy and curettage

3. In which subset of immunosuppressed patients is the risk for SCC development the *highest*?
   (a) Patients with a hematologic malignancy
   (b) Patients on chemotherapy
   (c) Kidney transplant recipient
   (d) CLL patients
   (e) Heart transplant recipient

4. Which tumor feature is *most* associated with metastasis?
   (a) PNI
   (b) Moderately differentiated tumors
   (c) Lymphovascular invasion
   (d) 1.5 cm tumor size
   (e) Location on the nose

5. Which of the following statements about SCC is true?
   (a) The lifetime risk of developing SCC is higher in women.
   (b) Highest incidence occurs in individuals over the age of 85
   (c) Organ transplant recipients have a 25-fold risk of developing an SCC
   (d) Chronic inflammatory disorders are not a risk factor for SCC development

6. According to the NCCN, the 1-year follow-up recommendation for a patient with an invasive SCC with regional disease is:
   (a) A complete skin exam every 6 months in the first 2 years after diagnosis
   (b) A complete skin and lymph node exam every 4–6 months for the first year
   (c) A complete skin exam every 1–3 months for the first year
   (d) A complete skin and lymph node exam every 1–3 months for the first year

7. Which of the following statements is true?
   (a) The risk of transformation of an AK to SCC is 50%.
   (b) The incidence of SCC metastasis is highest after the second year of diagnosis
   (c) Early parotid stage has improved 5-year survival compared to late parotid stage
   (d) Sentinel lymph node biopsy is the standard of care for high-risk SCC tumors

## Answers

1. e: a+c
2. c: Mohs micrographic surgery
3. e: Heart transplant recipient
4. a: Purineural invasion
5. b: Highest incidence occurs in individuals over the age of 85
6. d: A complete skin and lymph node exam every 1–3 months for the first year
7. c: Early parotid stage has improved 5-year survival compared to late parotid stage

# Melanoma Surgery

**4**

## Joy H. Kunishige and John A. Zitelli

## Introduction

Melanoma is the fifth most common cancer in men and sixth most common cancer in women [1]. Though incidence has doubled over the past decade, mortality is unchanged. It is unclear if true incidence is increasing as a result of environmental and behavioral changes, or if improved awareness and screening explains an artifactual increase [2]. American dermatologists diagnose 80,000 melanomas each year [3]. As experts in melanoma, dermatologists should be familiar with treatment and treatment rationale, particularly when evidenced-based medicine contradicts clinical practice.

J.H. Kunishige (✉)
Zitelli & Brodland Skin Cancer Center, Suite 303, 5200 Centre Avenue, Pittsburgh, PA 15232-1312, USA

Northwest Dermatology, 2500 W. Higgins Road, Suite 1040, Hoffman Estates, IL, USA
e-mail: mohssurg@gmail.com

J.A. Zitelli
Department of Dermatology, University of Pittsburgh Medical Center, 5200 Centre Avenue, Suite 303, Pittsburgh, PA, USA

## Melanoma In Situ and Malignant Melanoma

Melanoma in situ (MIS) refers to malignant melanocytes restricted to the epidermis. Malignant melanocytes have not yet gained the ability to breach and invade below the basement membrane, so MIS cannot metastasize. However, 5% of MIS will become true melanoma. Lentigo maligna (LM) is a form of MIS that occurs on sun-exposed areas of elderly persons, particularly the head and neck. Clinically, it is characterized by a slowly enlarging, irregularly pigmented macule (Fig. 4.1). LM may have a more indolent course than other MIS. In this chapter, the terms LM and MIS are used interchangeably.

Malignant melanoma (MM) is the invasive counterpart to MIS. Malignant melanocytes have either invaded below the basement membrane, or originated and proliferated in the dermis. Melanoma can arise de novo or from a pre-existing nevus. Multiple step-wise genetic mutations drive the development and progression of melanoma. There are several subtypes of melanoma: superficial spreading, nodular, acral lentiginous, and LM melanoma. Regardless of subtype, treatment and prognosis depends on mitotic rate, depth, and sentinel lymph node status.

M. Alam (ed.), *Evidence-Based Procedural Dermatology*,
DOI 10.1007/978-0-387-09424-3_4, © Springer Science+Business Media, LLC 2012

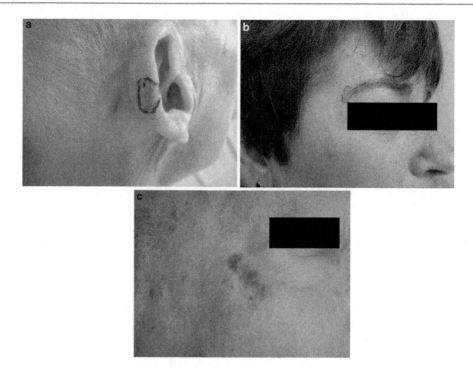

**Fig. 4.1** (a–c) Melanoma in situ, clinical examples

Many publications use the term "early melanoma" for invasive melanoma that is less than 1 or 2 mm thick. Intermediate thickness melanoma usually refers to invasive melanoma that is 2–4 mm thick. Thick melanomas have depth greater than 4 mm and are not discussed here. These cases are treated in concert with general surgery and oncology, and prognosis is poor.

## Clinical Presentation and Demographic Predilection

The characteristics of MIS and LM are discussed above. Superficial spreading melanoma is the most common type of melanoma and occurs between ages 30 and 50 years. It is most frequent on the trunk of men and legs of women. It may demonstrate one of the ABCD characteristics: asymmetry, border irregular or notched, color variation, and diameter greater than 6 mm. Nodular melanoma is the next most common type and occurs during the sixth decade of life. It is typically a black nodule but can be erythematous or skin-colored, i.e.,

"amelanotic melanoma." Acral lentiginous melanoma is the most common type in darker skin, making up 70% of melanomas in blacks and 45% in Asians [4]. Finally, LM and its invasive counterpart, LM melanoma, occur on chronically sundamaged skin of elderly persons as a slowly enlarging brown macule. Risk factors for melanoma include the following: personal or family history of melanoma, presence of many dysplastic nevi, history of sunburns, tendency to burn or inability to tan, light complexion, red hair color, DNA repair defects, and immunosuppression.

## Treatment Options

Complete surgical removal is the best treatment for all melanoma, including MIS. Complete surgical removal can be achieved by standard excision with margins, Mohs micrographic surgery, or staged excision. The general concepts behind these procedures are outlined here, followed by a critical review of the evidence supporting their use. Standard excision with margins means

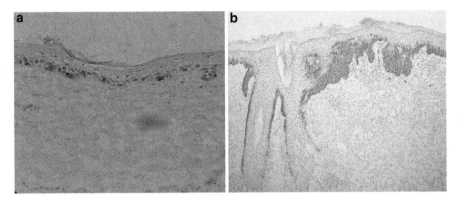

**Fig. 4.2** Melanoma in situ, frozen section with MART-1 immunostain: Negative margin (**a**) and positive margin (**b**)

removing the visible tumor plus an additional margin of "normal skin." This is done to remove any subclinical melanoma extensions not visible to the naked eye. The excised tissue is sent to a pathologist for vertical sectioning, similar to slicing a loaf of bread. A few of the vertical "slices" are examined under the microscope to confirm diagnosis and estimate if the tumor has been completely removed. This is an estimate because less than 1% of the lateral and deep margin is examined. How wide and deep the excision should be is discussed in this chapter.

Unlike standard excision, Mohs micrographic surgery examines 100% of the margin. The technique involves removing the visible tumor, and flattening the resulting specimen so the entire lateral and deep margin lies in one plane. The specimen is then frozen and *horizontal* sections are cut. The entire undersurface of the frozen specimen (the lateral and deep margin) can be examined under the microscope within minutes. Microscopic findings are drawn on a map, which is used to correlate findings to the patient's wound. This process is repeated until the tumor is totally removed. Mohs surgery is commonly used for the removal of cutaneous squamous cell carcinoma and basal cell carcinoma. Because reading melanoma on frozen sections requires meticulous processing, fewer Mohs surgeon routinely perform Mohs surgery for melanoma. Immunostains for melanocytes, such as melanoma antigen recognized by T cells (MART-1), aid interpretation (Fig. 4.2) [5]. Mohs technique not only spares normal tissue but also ensures complete removal of melanoma and its subclinical extensions.

A third surgical alternative is staged excision with paraffin sections. Typically the visible tumor is removed, then a thin square of tissue around the tumor is excised and sent for routine processing. Within days, slides are processed "en face" to visualize the entire periphery. They are usually read by a dermatopathologist, not the dermatologic surgeon. If residual tumor is seen at the margin, then additional tissue can be removed. Throughout this chapter, this will be referred to as "staged excision." This procedure is typically performed by a Mohs surgeon, who is familiar with color coding tissue and repairing defects.

After surgery for melanoma without palpable lymph nodes, there are no further procedures or treatments that improve overall survival. Options to improve disease-free survival are radiation, chemotherapy, interferon, sentinel node biopsy, and if the sentinel node is positive, complete lymph node dissection. If the melanoma patient has palpable lymph node involvement, then complete lymph node dissection is indicated and improves overall survival. Current studies are investigating the role of ultrasound surveillance and sampling of lymph nodes, melanoma vaccines, various chemotherapy regimens, and immunologics.

There is more variability in the way physicians approach MIS. Although surgical removal is the most effective, tumors which are large or close to important structures such as the eye, are treated by some physicians with alternative modalities. Cryosurgery, electrodessication and curettage, laser ablation, radiation, azelaic acid, intralesional 5-fluorouracil, topical imiquimod, and topical tazarotene have been reported for use alone or as adjuvant therapy [6].

## Sentinel Lymph Node Biopsy

Sentinel lymph node biopsy is based on the following theory: metastasizing tumors flow through lymphatics in an organized way, first through the "sentinel" node, then to other lymph nodes in the same basin, then to distant sites in the body. A radioactive substance and blue dye is injected around the tumor, then the first lymph node to pick up radioactive substance or blue dye is identified. This node is deemed the "sentinel lymph node," removed, and sent to pathology for histologic examination. If the sentinel lymph node is found to have tumor, or "micrometastasis," then the patient may opt to remove the remaining lymph nodes (lymph node dissection).

Several studies have shown sentinel lymph node status to be the most powerful prognostic predictor. But, it is unclear how much additional prognostic information it provides beyond what mitotic rate and Breslow depth already projects. Aside from prognosis, proponents of sentinel lymph node biopsy believe all microscopic disease will eventually become palpable disease that can spread, so if the sentinel node is positive, lymph node dissection should be performed. On the contrary, there is growing evidence to suggest microscopic foci [7] do not always progress. The largest study to date is by Morton et al. [8].

The use of sentinel lymph node biopsy is common, though the authors do not feel it should be the standard of care. Currently, patients with melanoma greater than 1 mm thick with nonpalpable lymph nodes are offered sentinel lymph node biopsy, and if positive, are sent for full lymph node dissection. This is sometimes called "elective" because there is no palpable disease, yet other papers refer to this as "therapeutic" because microscopic disease has been found. Prior to sentinel node biopsies, "therapeutic" lymph node dissection referred to removal of the lymph node basin in patients with palpable disease. The controversy over whether sentinel lymph node biopsy should be recommended for all patients with melanoma greater than 1 mm thick is exemplified by conflicting consensus statements: some recommend the procedure while others only recommend the procedure to stratify patients entering a clinical trial. The controversy of sentinel lymph node biopsy is not discussed further here, as the most frequent dilemma for the procedural dermatologist is MIS and thin melanomas. The interested reader can seek the referenced articles for a pro [9, 10] and con [11, 12] opinion.

## Natural History and Prognosis

If left alone, perhaps 5% of LM progress to LM melanoma [13]. Despite the generally slow progression of LM, MIS should be removed completely. Recurrence rates after excision with standard 0.5 cm margins is high, about 6–20% [14–19]. This may be due to the use of vertical sections to evaluate surgical margins, which detects only 58% of positive margins [14]. It is important to obtain true clearance on the first attempt, because when MIS recurs, it may have an invasive component [20]. Mohs micrographic surgery yields lower recurrence rates of 0–5%. Once removed, MIS is virtually cured and associated with a 99% survival rate.

Up to one-fifth of melanomas will become metastatic. The speed at which invasive melanomas acquire mutations to invade more deeply, to invade blood vessels or lymphatics, and to spread to other areas and proliferate is variable. American Joint Committee on Cancer (AJCC) staging is based on tumor depth, mitotic rate, presence of ulceration, lymph node involvement, and metastasis to distant sites. Prognosis is related to stage: Stage I patients have 79–100% 10-year survival while Stage IV patients have 3–15% 10-year survival [21].

## Consensus Documents

The most popular dogma arises from the National Institutes of Health (NIH) Consensus Statement in 1992 – almost 2 decades ago (VI/C). The consensus was based on 2 days of presentations by experts and discussion with the audience. It only addressed management of MIS and early melanoma. For MIS, the panel recommended surgical excision with 0.5 cm margins. This was further defined as a 0.5 cm border of clinically normal skin and a layer of subcutaneous tissue. For thin, invasive melanoma, the panel recommended surgical excision with 1 cm margin and underlying subcutaneous tissue down to, but not including, fascia. The caveat that "the surgical margin should be histologically uninvolved by tumor" pointed to the importance of removing subclinical extension. Regarding Mohs technique as an alternative, they wrote "currently, there is not enough clinical experience utilizing microscopically controlled excision for the treatment of primary melanomas to recommend it as an alternative approach. Mohs surgery may prove a useful technique for certain types and locations of melanoma, but more data are needed." The importance for clinical follow up to detect recurrences and second primary melanomas was highlighted. Elective regional lymph node dissection and imaging were not recommended for early melanoma patients. No recommendations were given for melanoma greater than 1 mm thick [22].

The Dutch Melanoma Working Party issued a consensus report in 1999 (VI/C). The Dutch also recommended 0.5 cm margins for MIS, and 1 cm margins for invasive melanoma with Breslow thickness less than 2 mm. The Dutch addressed deeper tumors as well, and recommended 3 cm margins for melanoma with Breslow thickness 2–4 mm. Excision should be to the fascia. If the subcutis is thin or if fascia was exposed during diagnostic biopsy, then fascia should also be excised. The paper stated that sentinel node biopsy "appears" to be promising, and if positive, lymph node dissection should be performed. Also, isolated regional perfusion for inoperable tumors on extremities and radiation could be used. These experts described adjuvant systemic therapy for melanoma as "experimental." A follow-up period of 5 years was recommended for patients with melanoma less than 1.5 mm thick, and 10 years if melanoma was greater than 1.5 mm thick. Routine blood tests, radiological exam, and ultrasound were not considered worthwhile [23].

The German Cancer Society and German Dermatologic Society's consensus is similar to the Dutch: 0.5 cm margins for MIS, 1 cm margins for melanoma up to 2 mm thick, and 2 cm for deeper tumors (VI/C). The German consensus also states micrographic control of surgical margins may be preferable for facial, acral, or anogenital melanomas [24].

The UK Guidelines are given in terms of the evidence so far published (VI/C to I/A). They recommend 0.2–0.5 cm margins for MIS, 0.75 or 1 cm margins for melanoma less than 1 mm thick, 1 or 2 cm margins for melanomas 1–2 mm thick, and 2 cm margins for melanoma greater than 2 mm thick. Stage II patients with clinically negative nodes may seek sentinel node biopsy for staging but unless evidence emerges for a role in determining outcome, it should not be routine [25].

The Clinical Practice Guidelines for Melanoma in Australia and New Zealand is a large document reviewing evidence and providing "Good Practice Points" (IV/C to I/A). The document recommends 0.5 cm margins for MIS but points out this is "arbitrary," based on Level IV evidence. The document recommends 1 cm margins for melanoma less than 1 mm thick, 1 or 2 cm margins for melanoma that is 1–4 mm thick, and 2 cm margins for melanoma greater than 4 mm thick (based on Level I evidence). Sentinel lymph node biopsy should be considered for patients with melanoma greater than 1 mm thick who want to be "as informed as possible about their prognosis" [26].

The most recent consensus is that by the American Academy of Dermatology (AAD) published in 2011 (VI/C). A work group comprised of 15 melanoma experts (14 from the United States) stated that no prospectively controlled data for melanoma in situ was available, so consensus opinion was rendered. The group recommended 0.5 to 1 cm margins for melanoma in situ, noting wider margins may be necessary for lentigo maligna subtype. Also, careful histologic evaluation of the surgical margins was strongly recommended, which can be achieved using staged excision with peripheral margin examination or Mohs micrographic surgery. The group recommended 1 cm margins for melanomas less than 1 mm thick; 1–2 cm margins for melanoma

**Table 4.1** Consensus recommendations for melanoma surgical margins

| Breslow thickness | NIH Consensus Conference (1992) | Dutch Melanoma Working Party (1999) | UK guidelines (2002) | German guidelines (2008) | Australia and New Zealand (2008) | American Academy of Dermatology (2011) |
|---|---|---|---|---|---|---|
| Melanoma in situ | 0.5 cm | 0.5 cm | 0.2–0.5 cm | 0.5 cm | 0.5 cm | 0.5–1 cm* |
| <1 mm | 1 cm | 1 cm | 1 cm (narrower margins probably safe in lesions <0.75 mm deep) | 1 cm | 1 cm | 1 cm |
| 1–2 mm | No recommendation | 1 cm | 1–2 cm | 1 cm | 1–2 cm | 1–2 cm |
| 2.1–4 mm | No recommendation | 2 cm | 2–3 cm (2 cm preferred) | 2 cm | 1–2 cm | 2 cm |
| >4 mm | No recommendation | 2 cm | 2–3 cm | 2 cm | 2 cm | 2 cm |

*Wider margins may be necessary for lentigo maligna subtype

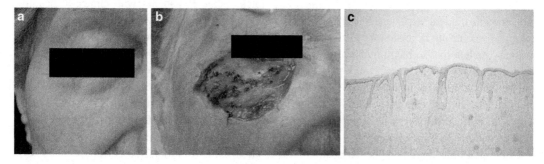

**Fig. 4.3** Lentigo maligna before (**a**) and after (**b**) Mohs micrographic surgery, (**c**) Frozen section with MART-1 immunostain of second stage of Mohs surgery is "positive." In approximately half of melanoma in situ, there is marked subclinical extension that would not be removed with 0.5 cm surgical margins

1.01–2 cm thick; and 2 cm margins for melanoma greater than 2 mm thick [27].

In summary, most dermatologists use a 0.5 cm margin for melanoma in situ based on the opinion of American experts in 1992. More recent consensus statements point out that there are no studies to support the 0.5 cm margin. While there is some variation in the recommended surgical margin for melanoma in situ, recommendations for invasive melanoma are similar (Table 4.1).

## Case Series and Cohort Studies

### Lentigo Maligna

Since the 1992 NIH consensus, multiple case series have shown 0.5 cm margins to be inadequate. Less than half of sizeable LMs are completely extirpated with a 0.5 cm margin [5, 16, 17, 28, 29]. In other words, MIS usually has extensive subclinical extension (Fig. 4.3).

The extent of subclinical extension is demonstrated by Kunishige and Zitelli. They treated 1,120 MISs with Mohs micrographic surgery (IV/B). The minimal surgical margin was 0.6 cm and the total margin was calculated by adding an additional 0.3 cm for each subsequent stage required. Only 86% of MISs would have been successfully excised with 0.6 cm margins, whereas 98.9% would have been successfully excised with 0.9 cm margins [30].

Agarwal-Antal found the 0.5 cm margin to be even more inadequate (IV/B). Polygonal, staged excisions – all 0.5 cm wide – were taken around 92 LMs. Positive areas were further resected with 0.5 cm margins until margins free of tumor were attained. Forty-two percent of patients were tumor-free after one stage, 27% required 1 cm margins, 15% required 1.5 cm margins, 7% required 2 cm margins, and 9% required margins of 2.5 cm or greater to achieve tumor-free margins. If standard excision with 0.5 cm margins had been used, only 42% of the tumors would have cleared [31].

Interestingly, bread-loaf sections of the central portion of these polygonal excisions revealed an invasive component in 16% [31]. Literature review shows one-quarter of biopsy-proven MIS lesions are found to contain invasive melanoma after complete surgical removal and pathologic examination [15]. Mohs technique or staged excisions obviate the need to deliberate over whether a lesion is truly MIS or a focally invasive early melanoma; surgery is not limited to margins predetermined by the initial diagnosis, but is performed until the margin of each particular lesion is clear.

Indeed, Mohs technique or staged excision is the most effective treatment for LM. In contrast to standard excision recurrence rates of 6–20% [15–19], Mohs surgery offers recurrence rates of 0–5%. Bene's study of 167 patients with MIS reported a 1.8% recurrence rate (mean follow-up was 5.3 years) [32] (IV/B). Kunishige's study of 1,120 MISs reported a 0.3% recurrence rate (mean follow-up was 4.7 years) [30] (IV/B). Numerous case series confirm that Mohs surgical technique produces the lowest recurrence rates [15, 28, 29, 32–36] (IV/B).

Nonsurgical treatment includes cryosurgery and topical imiquimod. Recurrence after cryosurgery ranges from 6.6% at 3 years [37] to 34% at 5 years [38] (V/B). There are case reports of successful treatment of LM with imiquimod. However, histopathologic examination often shows incomplete treatment, so clinical improvement may be misleading [39]. A recent literature review of 67 case reports found eight patients developed recurrence, two of which developed LM melanoma (IV/B). Follow-up in these case reports was short, usually less than 12 months [40]. Given the high incidence of invasive disease in lesions initially diagnosed as MIS, cryosurgery and imiquimod are not recommended.

## Early Invasive Melanoma, Intermediate Thickness Melanoma, and High-Risk Melanoma

Since the 1992 NIH consensus, the 1 cm margin for early invasive melanoma less than 1 mm thick has also come into question. Experimental case series using Mohs technique have shown variable extension around melanoma, so 1 cm is sometimes adequate and sometimes inadequate. Several randomized controlled trials investigated narrow vs. wide surgical margin for melanoma, and these are discussed later.

Zitelli used his Mohs experience with melanoma to explore margins for standard excision (VI, B). 184 MIS and 369 melanomas were debulked with a 0.3 cm margin. The first Mohs layer was another 0.3 cm around the debulking defect. Additional 0.3 cm margins were taken as needed to clear the tumors. One Mohs layer, which was equivalent to 0.6 cm margins, was adequate for 83% of the melanomas. 0.9 cm was adequate for 95%; 1.2 cm was necessary for 97%. Margins to remove melanomas on the head, neck, hands, and feet were wider than those on the trunk and extremities. Margins to remove melanomas that were more than 2–3 cm in diameter were wider than for smaller melanomas. About 1.9% of patients had a local recurrence within or near the scar. Based on these results, predetermined surgical margins for excision of melanoma to achieve 97% clearance rate should be: 1 cm for MIS and melanomas on the trunk and proximal extremities smaller than 2 cm in diameter; 1.5 cm for tumors larger than 2 cm in diameter or located on the head, neck, hands, and feet; and finally, 2.5 cm for melanomas larger than 3 cm in diameter. Notably margin recommendations for MIS and melanoma were the same [41].

A second study by the same group validated the use of Mohs for melanoma on the head and neck (VI, B). Three hundred and thirty-one patients with MIS and 294 patients with melanoma of the head and neck were treated with Mohs micrographic surgery. Mean follow-up was 58 months. After stratification by Breslow thickness, 5-year local recurrence rates (Table 4.2), metastasis rates, and disease-specific survival rates were comparable to or better than historical controls [32].

Temple and Arlette have also reported their experience treating melanoma with Mohs (VI, B). They treated 133 MISs and 69 invasive melanomas with Mohs micrographic surgery. The invasive melanomas had mean Breslow depth of 0.92 mm (0.2–3.6 mm). There were no local recurrences, four regional recurrences, and two distant recurrences at a mean follow-up of 29.8 months [42].

Several case series confirm Mohs micrographic surgery is an effective treatment for

**Table 4.2** Local recurrence rates after Mohs micrographic surgery and standard excision [32]

| Thickness | Recurrence rate after Mohs (%) | n | Recurrence rate after standard excision (%) | n | p Value |
|---|---|---|---|---|---|
| MIS | 0.3 ± 0.3 | 331 | 20.0 ± 4.4 | 81 | <0.001 |
| <0.76 mm | 0 | 166 | 7.3 ± 1.9 | 179 | <0.001 |
| 0.76–1.49 mm | 0 | 46 | 4.2 ± 1.0 | 448 | NS |
| 1.50–3.99 | 1.6 ± 1.6 | 64 | 5.3 ± 0.9 | 680 | NS |
| >3.99 | 0 | 18 | 3.9 ± 1.2 | 256 | NS |

invasive melanoma. It is particularly useful for tumors on the head, neck, hands, and feet, where subclinical extension is common and tissue sparing is important.

# Randomized Controlled Trials and Meta-Analyses

## Lentigo Maligna

There are no randomized controlled studies regarding surgical treatment of LM.

## Early Invasive Melanoma

The Swedish Melanoma Study Group performed a prospective, randomized, multicenter study of patients with primary melanoma on the trunk or extremities with tumor thickness between 0.8 and 2 cm (II/A). Patients either received 2 or 5 cm excision margin. Nine hundred and eighty-nine patients were recruited during 1982–1991. The median follow-up was 8 years for recurrent disease, and 11 years for survival. There were no statistically significant differences between the two treatment arms: the hazard ratio for recurrence-free survival was 1.02 (95% confidence interval, 0.8–1.30) for the 2 cm group compared with the 5 cm group. The hazard ratio for overall survival was 0.96 (95% confidence interval, 0.75–1.24) for the 2 cm group compared with the 5 cm group. In total, less than 1% had local recurrence within the scar, 20% had disease recurrence anywhere, and 15% died of melanoma. This study concluded 2 and 5 cm excision margins were equally safe for tumors 0.8–2 mm thick [43].

Two years later, a multicenter European study repeated a similar study with fewer patients but inclusive of thinner tumors (II/A). Three hundred and twenty-six patients with melanoma measuring less than 2.1 mm thick were randomized to excision with either 2 or 5 cm margin. Only 16 of these patients had melanoma on the head and neck. Median follow-up time was 16 years for both estimation of survival and disease recurrence. There were 22 recurrences in the 2 cm arm and 33 recurrences in the 5 cm arm. Median time to disease recurrence was 43 months in the 2 cm arm and 37.6 months in the 5 cm arm. Ten-year disease-free survival rates were 85% for the 2 cm group and 84% for the 5 cm group. For melanoma less than 2.1 mm thick, the authors concluded 2 cm margin was sufficient, and a larger margin did not improve time to recurrence or survival [44].

The WHO Melanoma Trial also looked at patients with melanoma less than 2 mm thick but tried narrower margins (II/A). Six hundred and twelve patients were randomized to receive 1 or 3 cm margins. Facial and acral melanomas were excluded. The subsequent development of metastatic disease involving regional nodes and distant organs was not statistically different in the two groups. Disease-free survival and overall survival rates were also similar in the two groups (mean follow-up was 90 months). Only four patients had a local recurrence as their first relapse. All had undergone narrow excision but each had melanoma with thickness greater than 1 mm. The study concluded 1 cm margins were as effective as 3 cm margins in patients with stage I cutaneous melanoma not thicker than 2 mm [45].

Meta-analysis of the above three trials included 2,087 adults with localized melanoma on the trunk and extremities (I/A). There were no statistically significant differences found between wide (3–5 cm) and narrow (1–2 cm) margins, with respect to local recurrence, disease-free survival, or overall survival. The analysis confirmed that surgical margins around melanoma of the trunk and extremities should be no more than 2 cm [46]. At the time of this publication, no randomized controlled studies have looked at the possibility of using margins less than 1 cm. Also, few melanomas on the head and neck have been included in high-caliber studies (randomized controlled trials).

## Intermediate Thickness and High-Risk Melanoma

The Intergroup Melanoma Surgical Trial compared 2 vs. 4 cm excision margins and published their study in 2001 (II/A). This study is significant because it included thicker tumors (Breslow depth 1–4 mm). Four hundred and sixty-eight patients with melanoma on the trunk or proximal extremity were randomized to receive either a 2 or 4 cm margin. Another 272 patients with melanoma on the head, neck, or distal extremities were excised with a 2 cm margin. Local recurrence was the same for both the 2 and 4 cm groups. Ten-year survival rates were 70% for the 2 cm group and 77% for the 4 cm group. The authors concluded that 2 cm margin was safe for intermediate thickness melanoma. As a side note, the authors found local recurrence did vary by anatomic site: 1.1% for proximal extremity, 3.1% for trunk, 5.3% for distal extremity, and 9.4% for head and neck. Ulceration of the primary melanoma was the most significant prognostic factor heralding local recurrence, and local recurrence was associated with a high mortality rate [47].

A United Kingdom (UK) study by Thomas et al. investigated 1 vs. 3 cm margin for melanoma greater than 2 mm thick (II/A). Nine hundred patients were randomized to receive 1 or 3 cm excision margin. Median follow-up was 60 months. The 1 cm group had more locoregional recurrences (168 vs. 142 recurrences) and the hazard ratio was 1.26 (95% confidence interval,

$1.00–1.59, p = 0.05$). There were also more deaths attributable to melanoma (128 vs. 105 deaths) and the hazard ratio was 1.24 (95% confidence interval, $0.96–1.61, p = 0.1$). Still, overall survival was similar in the two groups (HR for death 1.07, 95% confidence interval, $0.85–1.36, p = 0.6$). The authors stated "a 1 cm margin of excision for melanoma with a poor prognosis (as defined by a tumor thickness of at least 2 mm) is associated with a significantly greater risk of regional recurrence than is a 3 cm margin, but with a similar overall survival rate" [48].

Though the authors of the UK study interpreted their data to show support for 3 cm margins, the confidence interval included 1.00 and the $p$ value was greater than 0.05. When these data were pooled with other studies in a meta-analysis, the borderline benefit of wider margins was not seen. The meta-analysis showed that patients undergoing narrow or wide excision had similar local recurrences, locoregional recurrences, and overall mortality [49] (I/A).

Based on these two studies, patients with melanoma thickness greater than 2 mm can undergo excision with 1 or 2 cm margins. This should result in the same overall survival as larger margins.

## Conclusion

For LM, the lowest recurrence rates are achieved with Mohs micrographic technique. When quality frozen sections with immunostains are not available, staged excision with paraffin sections can be used. Staged excision requires the utmost coordination between the Mohs surgeon, dermatopathologist, and reconstructive surgeon. It also requires more time and effort for all participants, as each stage takes 24 h to 1 week to process. When standard excision is used, older consensus reports recommend 0.5 cm margins. However, this is only adequate half of the time, and 1 cm margins are necessary to achieve 97% clearance. Also 25% of lesions diagnosed as LM may actually be invasive melanoma, which necessitates at least a 1 cm margin. Clearly, the evidence (IV/B) outweighs the old consensus (VI/C) and MIS *should be excised with a 1 cm margin*.

Regarding early invasive melanoma (less than 2 mm thick), most consensus guidelines and the WHO Melanoma Trial support a 1 cm margin. Mohs technique allows narrower margins – though less tissue is taken, the entire margin is examined, and additional tissue can be taken if needed. Mohs technique or staged excision is a particularly good option on the face and distal extremities where preservation of cosmesis and function are important. In fact, most of the data published regarding facial and acral melanoma comes from large case series studies of Mohs technique or staged excision.

Intermediate melanoma (greater than 2 mm thick) is most frequently treated by wide excision with 2 or 3 cm margins. There are two randomized controlled studies that included tumors of this depth: the Intergroup Melanoma Surgical Trial showed 2 cm margins were as effective as 4 cm margins. The UK study concluded that 1 cm margins resulted in more locoregional recurrence but similar overall survival as 3 cm margins. Meta-analysis suggests 1 or 2 cm margins are adequate. In all studies, the smallest margin studied was adequate.

A note on the depth of excision seems warranted. Older consensus papers recommended excision include subcutaneous tissue down to but not including the fascia. More recent consensus from the AAD concedes there is no evidence to guide proper depth so group opinion was then solicited. A simple layer of subcutaneous tissue was recommended for excision of melanoma in situ. Excision down to deep adipose, or to fascia when possible, was recommended for invasive melanoma [27].

These surgical recommendations are summarized in the Evidence-Based Summary. The ability of adjuvant therapy and sentinel lymph node biopsy to prolong overall survival is controversial and beyond the scope of this chapter. Patients with in transit metastasis, palpable lymphadenopathy, or metastatic lung deposits should undergo resection. All melanoma patients and their families should have regular skin examinations to detect additional tumors and recurrences. The use of serum lactate dehydrogenase, chest X-ray, body CT or PET/CT, and brain MRI varies by institution.

**Evidence-Based Summary**

| Findings | Evidence level |
|---|---|
| **Lentigo maligna and melanoma in situ** | |
| Mohs surgery has the lowest recurrence rates | Level IV, B |
| Staged excision is a slower alternative to Mohs surgery with similar efficacy | Level IV, B |
| If standard excision is used, 1 cm margins are necessary to achieve 97% clearance rate | Level IV, B |
| Though consensus panels recommend 0.5 cm margins, this is associated with a low clearance rate of approximately 50% | Level IV, B |
| **Early invasive melanoma (<2 mm thick)** | |
| Consensus panels recommend 1 cm margins | Level VI, C |
| Meta-analysis recommends 1 or 2 cm margins | Level I, A |
| Mohs surgery or staged excision is an effective treatment with survival rates similar to standard excision. In some cases, Mohs surgery allows narrower surgical margins | Level IV, B |
| **Intermediate thickness melanoma (2–4 mm thick)** | |
| Consensus panels recommend 2 or 3 cm margins | Level VI, C |
| Meta-analysis suggests 1 or 2 cm margins are adequate | Level I, A |
| Mohs surgery or staged excision is an effective treatment with survival rates similar to standard excision. In some cases, Mohs surgery allows narrower surgical margins | Level IV, B |

# References

1. National Cancer Institute Common Cancer Types. National Cancer Institute. [Online] [Cited: Jan 14, 2009.] http://www.cancer.gov/cancertopics/commoncancers. Accessed January 2010.
2. Linos E, Swetter SM, Cockburn MG, et al. Increasing burden of melanoma in the United States. J Invest Dermatol. 2009;129(7):1666–74.
3. Salopek TG, Marghoob AA, Slade JM, et al. An estimate of the incidence of malignant melanoma in the United States. Based on a survey of members of the American Academy of Dermatology. Dermatol Surg. 1995;21:301–5.
4. Cress RD, Holly EA. Incidence of cutaneous melanoma among non-Hispanic whites, Hispanics, Asians, and blacks: an analysis of California Cancer Registry data, 1988–93. Cancer Causes Control. 1997;8:246–52.
5. Bricca G, Zitelli JA. Invasive melanoma evaluated by frozen sections. In: Mikhail GR, Snow SN, editors. Mohs micrographic surgery, vol. 19. Madison: The University of Wisconsin Press; 2004. p. 175–82.
6. Silapunt S, Goldberg LH. Lentigo maligna. In: Mikhail GR, Snow SN, editors. Mohs micrographic surgery, vol. 18. Madison: The University of Wisconsin Press; 2004. p. 169–73.
7. de Wilt JH, van Akkooi AC, Verhoef C, Eggermont AM. Detection of melanoma micrometastases in sentinel nodes – the cons. Surg Oncol. 2008;17:175–81.
8. Morton DL, Thompson JF, Cochran AJ, et al. Sentinel-node biopsy or nodal observation in melanoma. N Engl J Med. 2006;355:1307–17.
9. Ross MI, Gershenwald JE. How should we view the results of the multicenter selective lymphadenectomy trial-1 (MSLT-1). Ann Surg Oncol. 2008; 15:670–3.
10. Morton DL, Elashoff R. Sentinel node biopsy: facts to clear the alleged clouds. Arch Dermatol. 2008;144: 685–6.
11. Zitelli JA. An alternative view. Dermatol Surg. 2008;34:544–9.
12. Thomas JM. Time for comprehensive reporting of MSLT-1. Lancet Oncol. 2006;7:9–11.
13. Weinstock MA, Sober AJ. The risk of progression of lentigo maligna to lentigo maligna melanoma. Br J Dermatol. 1987;116:303–10.
14. Kimyai-Asadi A, Katz T, Goldberg LH, et al. Margin involvement after the excision of melanoma in situ: the need for complete en face examination of the surgical margins. Dermatol Surg. 2007;33:1434–41.
15. Dawn ME, Dawn AG, Miller SJ. Mohs surgery for the treatment of melanoma in situ: a review. Dermatol Surg. 2007;33:395–402.
16. McKenna JK, Florell SR, Goldman GD, Bowen GM. Lentigo maligna/lentigo maligna melanoma: current state of diagnosis and treatment. Dermatol Surg. 2006;32:493–504.
17. Zalla MJ, Lim KK, Dicaudo DJ, et al. Mohs micrographic excision of melanoma using immunostains. Dermatol Surg. 2000;26:771–84.
18. Coleman III WP, Davis RS, Reed RJ, et al. Treatment of lentigo maligna and lentigo maligna melanoma. J Dermatol Surg. 1980;6:476–9.
19. Pitman GH, Kopf AW, Bart RS, et al. Treatment of lentigo maligna and lentigo maligna melanoma. J Dermatol Surg Oncol. 1979;5:727–37.
20. DeBloom JR, Zitelli JA, Brodland DG. The invasive growth potential of residual melanoma and melanoma in situ. Dermatol Surg. 2010;36(8):1251–7.
21. Balch CM, Buzaid AC, Soong S, et al. Final version of the American Joint Committee on cancer staging system for cutaneous melanoma. J Clin Oncol. 2001;19:3635–48.
22. NIH Consensus Development Program. National Institutes of Health consensus development conference statement on diagnosis and treatment of early melanoma, January 27–29, 1992. Am J Dermatopathol. 1993;15:34–43.
23. Kroon BBR, Bergman W, Coebergh JWW, et al. Consensus on the management of malignant melanoma of the skin in the Netherlands. Melanoma Res. 1999;9:207–12.
24. Garbe C, Hauschild A, Volkenandt M, et al. Evidence and interdisciplinary consensus-based German guidelines: surgical treatment and radiotherapy of melanoma. Melanoma Res. 2008;18:61–7.
25. Roberts DL, Anstey AV, Barlow RJ, et al. UK guidelines for the management for cutaneous melanoma. Br J Dermatol. 2002;146:7–17.
26. Australian Cancer Network Melanoma Guidelines Revision Working Party. Clinical practice guidelines for the management of melanoma in Australia and New Zealand. Wellington: s.n.; 2008. p. 68–71. Australian Cancer Network Melanoma Guidelines Revision Working Party. Clinical Practice Guidelines.
27. Bichakjian CK, Halpern AC, Johnson TM, et al. Guidelines of care for the management of primary cutaneous melanoma. J Am Acad Dermatol 10.1016/j. jaad/2011.04.031.
28. Huilgol SC, Selva D, Chen C, et al. Surgical margins for lentigo maligna and lentigo maligna melanoma: the technique of mapped serial excision. Arch Dermatol. 2004;140:1087–92.
29. Bub JL, Berg D, Slee A, et al. Management of lentigo maligna and lentigo maligna melanoma with staged excision: a 5-year follow-up. Arch Dermatol. 2004; 140:552–8.
30. Kunishige JH, Zitelli JA. Surgical margins for melanoma in situ. J Am Acad Dermatol. Accepted 2011. In print.
31. Agarwal-Antal N, Bowen GM, Gerwels JW. Histologic evaluation of lentigo maligna with permanent sections: implications regarding current guidelines. J Am Acad Dermatol. 2002;47:743–8.
32. Bene NI, Healy C, Coldiron BM. Mohs micrographic surgery is accurate 95.1% of the time for melanoma in situ: a prospective study of 167 cases. Dermatol Surg. 2008;34:660–4.
33. Bricca GM, Brodland DG, Ren D, et al. Cutaneous head and neck melanoma treated with Mohs micrographic surgery. J Am Acad Dermatol. 2005;52: 92–100.

34. Cohen LM, McCall MW, Zax RH. Mohs micrographic surgery for lentigo maligna and lentigo maligna melanoma: a follow-up study. Dermatol Surg. 1998; 24:673–7.

35. Bienert TN, Trotter MJ, Arlette JP. Treatment of cutaneous melanoma of the face by Mohs micrographic surgery. J Cutan Med Surg. 2003;7:25–30.

36. Clayton BD, Leshin B, Hitchcock MG, et al. Utility of rush paraffin-embedded tangential sections in the management of cutaneous neoplasms. Dermatol Surg. 2000;26:671–8.

37. Kuflik EG, Gage AA. Cryosurgery for lentigo maligna. J Am Acad Dermatol. 2004;31:75–8.

38. Zalaudek I, Horn M, Richtig E, Hödl S, Kerl H, Smolle J. Local recurrence in melanoma in situ: influence of sex, age, site of involvement and therapeutic modalities. Br J Dermatol. 2003;148:703–8.

39. Fleming CJ, Bryden AM, Evans A, et al. A pilot study of treatment of lentigo maligna with 5% imiquimod cream. Br J Dermatol. 2004;151:485–8.

40. Rajpar SF, Marsden JR. Imiquimod in the treatment of lentigo maligna. Br J Dermatol. 2006;155:653–6.

41. Zitelli JA, Brown CD, Hanusa BH. Surgical margins for excision of primary cutaneous melanoma. J Am Acad Dermatol. 1997;37:422–9.

42. Temple CIF, Arlette JP. Mohs micrographic surgery in the treatment of lentigo maligna and melanoma. J Surg Oncol. 2006;94:287–92.

43. Cohn-Cedermark G, Rutqvist LE, Andersson R, et al. Long term results of a randomized study by the Swedish Melanoma Study Group on 2-cm versus 5-cm resection margins for patients with cutaneous melanoma with a tumor thickness of 0.8–2.0 mm. Cancer. 2000;89:1495–501.

44. Khayat D, Rixe O, Martin G, et al. Surgical margins in cutaneous melanoma (2 cm versus 5 cm for lesions measuring less than 2.1-mm thick). Cancer. 2003;97:1941–6.

45. Veronesi U, Cascinelli N. Narrow excision (1-cm margin). A safe procedure for thin cutaneous melanoma. Arch Surg. 1991;126:438–41.

46. Haigh PI, DiFronzo LA, McCready DR. Optimal excision margins for primary cutaneous melanoma: a systematic review and meta-analysis. Can J Surg. 2003;46:419–26.

47. Balch CM, Soong SJ, Smith T, et al. Long-term results of a prospective surgical trial comparing 2 cm vs. 4 cm excision margins for 740 patients with 1–4 mm melanomas. Ann Surg Oncol. 2001;8:101–8.

48. Thomas JM, Newton-Bishop J, A'Hern R. Excision margins in high-risk malignant melanoma. N Engl J Med. 2004;350:757–66.

49. Lens MB, Nathan P, Bataille V. Excision margins for primary cutaneous melanoma: updated pooled analysis of randomized controlled trials. Arch Surg. 2007;142:885–91.

## Self-Assessment

1. The practice of using 0.5 cm margins for excision of melanoma in situ is based on what type of evidence?
   (a) Level I (meta-analysis of randomized controlled trials)
   (b) Level II (at least one randomized controlled trial)
   (c) Level IV (at least one well-designed quasi-experimental study)
   (d) Level V (well-designed nonexperimental descriptive studies)
   (e) Level VI (expert committee opinions or clinical experience)

2. What is the most effective treatment for achieving clear margins with lentigo maligna?
   (a) Surgical excision with 0.5 cm margins
   (b) Mohs technique with frozen section
   (c) Staged excision with paraffin sections
   (d) Imiquimod
   (e) Cryosurgery

3. If you choose to treat lentigo maligna with standard excision, what margin should you use to achieve 97% clearance rate?
   (a) 0.3 cm
   (b) 0.5 cm
   (c) 1 cm
   (d) 1.5 cm
   (e) 2 cm

4. The practice of using 1 cm margins for melanoma less than 2 mm thick is based on what type of evidence?
   (a) Level I (meta-analysis of randomized controlled trials)
   (b) Level II (at least one randomized controlled trial)
   (c) Level IV (at least one well-designed quasi-experimental study)
   (d) Level V (well-designed nonexperimental descriptive studies)
   (e) Level VI (expert committee opinions or clinical experience)

5. There is data to support the use of which surgical margin for excision of melanoma greater than 2 mm thick?
   (a) 1 cm
   (b) 2 cm
   (c) 3 cm
   (d) All of the above
   (e) None of the above

## Answers

1. e: Level VI (expert committee opinions or clinical experience)
   The 1992 NIH Concensus Statement on Early Melanoma recommended 0.5 cm margins for melanoma in situ and 1 cm margins for invasive melanoma less than 1 mm thick. No recommendations were given for invasive melanoma greater than 1 mm thick. It is important to remember that these are just guidelines, and the guidelines are based on the lowest level of evidence (Level VI). Multiple case series (level V evidence) have shown that these margins are not always adequate, particularly for melanoma in situ. In fact, less than 50% of melanoma in situ will be completely removed with a 0.5 cm margin. One centimeter margins are necessary to achieve 97% clearance rate.

2. b or c: Mohs excision with frozen section; Staged excision with paraffin sections.
   Mohs technique with frozen section or staged excision with paraffin sections have been shown to be more effective than surgical excision with 0.5 cm margins in multiple large case series (level V evidence). Whether to use Mohs technique with frozen section or staged excision with paraffin sections probably depends on each institution's ability to obtain high-quality slides. Recurrence rates for lentigo maligna depend on the treatment used: standard excision 6–20%, Mohs surgery 0–5%, cryosurgery 6.6–34%, imiquimod 12%.

3. c: 1 cm
   Margins of 1cm are necessary to achieve 97% clearance rate. Margins of 0.5 clears less than 50% of lentigo maligna, and is associated with a high recurrence rate of 6–20%. This is likely related to the fact that many melanoma in situs have significant subclinical extension not caught by traditional margin examination (bread-loaf sections examine less than 1% of the margin). Of note, 25% of lentigo maligna are actually invasive melanoma so incomplete treatment should be avoided.

4. b: Level II (at least one randomized controlled trial)
   The WHO Melanoma Trial compared 1 vs. 3 cm margins for melanoma less than 2 mm thick. Disease-free survival and overall survival rates were similar in the two groups. Other studies have looked at 2 vs. 5 cm margins for melanoma less than 2 mm thick, and these studies recommend 2 cm margins. Meta-analysis supports the use of 1 or 2 cm margins for melanoma less than 2 mm thick.

5. d: All of the above.
   The Australian consensus recommends 1 cm margins. All other consensus statements and the Intergroup Melanoma Surgical Trial recommend 2 cm margins. A United Kingdom study by Thomas et al. compared 1–3 cm margins and recommended 3 cm margin, which was associated with fewer locoregional recurrences and deaths, but this was not statistically significant and overall survival was similar in both groups. Meta-analysis by Lens et al. suggests wider margins do not improve survival, but this analysis had more patients with melanoma less than 2 mm thick.

# Merkel Cell Carcinoma

**5**

## Conway C. Huang and Christopher K. Bichakjian

## Introduction Regarding Medical Evidence

Currently, definitive information regarding the biologic behavior and optimal management of Merkel cell carcinoma (MCC) is limited given the rarity of this tumor and the lack of prospective, randomized trials, and other high-level medical evidence. The objective of this chapter is to provide those involved in the care of patients with MCC with the best evidence-based recommendations regarding diagnosis, staging, treatment, and follow-up.

A primary reference for this chapter will be the National Comprehensive Cancer Network (NCCN) Clinical Practice Guidelines in Oncology, MCC section. This represents a "best practices" consensus document regarding the management of MCC from a panel of recognized national experts in dermatology, surgical oncology, otorhinolaryngology, dermatopathology, medical oncology, radiation oncology, and hematology/oncology [1]. Although this theoretically is level

C.C. Huang (✉)
Department of Dermatology, University of Alabama at Birmingham, EFH 414, 1530 3RD AVE S, Birmingham, AL 35294-0009, USA
e-mail: chuang@uabmc.edu

C.K. Bichakjian
Department of Dermatology, Cutaneous Surgery and Oncology, University of Michigan, 1910 A. Alfred Taubman Center, Ann Arbor, MI 48109-0314, USA

VI/B evidence, it represents, in fact, a hybrid of recommendations that is primarily based on the highest level medical evidence available and secondarily on expert opinion.

## Introduction Regarding Merkel Cell Carcinoma

MCC is a rare, biologically aggressive cutaneous malignancy. It is believed to arise from Merkel cells which function as mechanoreceptors and resemble cells of the diffuse neuroendocrine system [2]. Based on data from the US Surveillance, Epidemiology, and End Results (SEER) program, the age-adjusted incidence rate was approximately 0.44/100,000 in 2001 (approximately 1,400 cases/year) [3]. This compares with basal cell carcinoma (BCC), squamous cell carcinoma (SCC), and invasive melanoma, with estimated annual US incidences in 2009 of 1.2 million, 400,000, and 70,000, respectively. MCC is 24 times more common in patients >65 years of age than younger individuals, with only 5% of patients being diagnosed before age 50. The vast majority (94%) of patients with MCC are white with a slight male predominance [4].

Exposure to ultraviolet (UV) radiation and immunosuppression are thought to be risk factors for the development of MCC. The facts that most MCCs are located on sun-exposed areas of the skin, that SEER data have shown MCC to be more numerous in geographic locations with higher UV indexes, and that MCC has been associated with concomitant SCC and a history of UV phototherapy, all support an etiologic role of UV radiation [4–6]. The reported increased incidence of MCC at a younger age in solid organ transplant recipients and patients with human immunodeficiency virus, lends support to the association between MCC and immunosuppression [7–9]. Consistent with this association, recent findings have suggested a virus (Merkel cell polyomavirus) as a contributing factor in the pathogenesis of MCC [10].

MCC typically presents as a red to violaceous, firm, and nontender nodule. The differential diagnosis may include BCC, SCC, cyst, pyogenic granuloma, lymphoma, or lipoma. Typical locations for presentation are the head and neck region and extremities which account for 70–90% of all cases [4].

Due to the biologically aggressive and potentially life-threatening nature of MCC, issues of diagnosis, staging, treatment, and follow-up are critical to achieve optimal patient outcomes. In the following sections, these aspects will be covered in more detail.

## Evidence Regarding Histologic Diagnosis

Excisional biopsy is preferred to incisional biopsy in order to maximize the probability of obtaining the most accurate diagnostic and histologic microstaging information and to minimize the possibility of sampling error. Narrow excisional biopsy margins are critical to prevent lymphotome error if subsequent sentinel lymph node biopsy (SLNB) is performed.

Because MCC is histologically composed of small round blue cells, it must be differentiated from metastatic visceral neuroendocrine carcinomas, particularly small cell lung carcinoma (SCLC). In addition to standard hematoxylin and eosin (H&E) staining, CK-20 and TTF-1 immunohistochemical stains should be performed to confirm the diagnosis of MCC (primary cutaneous neuroendocrine carcinoma). This is best interpreted by an experienced dermatopathologist. CK-20, a low-molecular-weight intermediate filament, is a very sensitive (90–100%) marker

for MCC. Because up to 33% of SCLCs and 4% of extrapulmonary small cell carcinomas can also stain positively for CK-20, staining with TTF-1 is highly recommended. TTF-1 is expressed in 83–100% of SCLC and is absent in MCC. Note that since TTF-1 variably stains extrapulmonary small cell carcinomas (3–42%), a negative TTF-1 stain supports but does not confirm the diagnosis of MCC conclusively [11, 12]. Appropriate imaging studies can further help to rule out metastatic visceral neuroendocrine carcinomas. Other immunohistochemical markers of high sensitivity for MCC are synaptophysin, neuron-specific enolase, chromogranin A, neurofilament protein, KIT receptor tyrosine kinase (CD117), BER-EP4, and CAM 5.2 [13]. MCC is invariably negative for S-100 and leukocyte common antigen (CD45) thus distinguishing it from small cell melanoma and lymphoma, respectively.

## Evidence Regarding Staging

Staging is required to help assess prognosis, aid in the counseling of patients, and guide treatment. A new staging system and TNM classification for MCC has recently been adopted by the American Joint Committee on Cancer (AJCC) (Table 5.1). In this system, stages I and II represent localized disease in which stage I signifies a low-risk primary tumor measuring ≤2 cm in diameter, and stage II, a high risk lesion >2 cm. Stages I and II are further subdivided to differentiate between those patients who have been pathologically determined to be node negative by SLNB (I/IIA) and those who have been clinically staged as node negative (I/IIB). Stage III represents regional disease and distinguishes between microscopic metastases detected by SLNB (IIIA) and clinically evident macroscopic nodal disease (IIIB), with in-transit metastases grouped in IIIB. Stage IV signifies distant metastatic disease.

Approximately 70% of patients with MCC present with stage I or II disease, 25% with stage III, and 5% with stage IV [4]. Five-year survival rates range from 30 to 64% with disease stage strongly associated with survival [14, 15]. In one large case series, 5-year survival was 81% for

**Table 5.1** TNM criteria and stage groupings of the new AJCC staging system

| T | N | M | |
|---|---|---|---|
| Tx, primary tumor cannot be assessed | Nx, regional nodes cannot be assessed | Mx, distant metastasis cannot be assessed | |
| T0, no primary tumor | N0, no regional node metastasis[a] | M0, no distant metastasis | |
| Tis, in situ primary tumor | cN0, nodes not clinically detectable[a] | M1, distant metastasis[b] | |
| T1, primary tumor ≤2 cm | cN1, nodes clinically detectable[a] | M1a, distant skin, distant | |
| T2, primary tumor >2 but ≤5 cm | pN0, nodes negative by pathologic exam | subcutaneous tissues or distant lymph nodes | |
| T3, primary tumor >5 cm | pNx, nodes not examined pathologically | M1b, lung | |
| T4, primary tumor invades bone, muscle, fascia, or cartilage | N1a, micrometastasis[c] | M1c, all other visceral sites | |
| | N1b, macrometastasis[d] | | |
| | N2, in-transit metastasis[e] | | |

| Stage | | Stage grouping | | |
|---|---|---|---|---|
| 0 | Tis | N0 | M0 |
| IA | T1 | pN0 | M0 |
| IB | T1 | cN0 | M0 |
| IIA | T2/T3 | pN0 | M0 |
| IIB | T2/T3 | cN0 | M0 |
| IIC | T4 | N0 | M0 |
| IIIA | Any T | N1a | M0 |
| IIIB | Any T | N1b/N2 | M0 |
| IV | Any T | Any N | M1 |

[a] "N0" denotes negative nodes by clinical, pathologic, or both types of examination. Clinical detection of nodal disease may be via inspection, palpation, and/or imaging; cN0 is used only for patients who did not undergo pathologic node staging

[b] Because there are no data to suggest significant effect of M categories on survival in Merkel cell carcinoma, M1a-c are included in same stage grouping

[c] Micrometastases are diagnosed after sentinel or elective lymphadenectomy

[d] Macrometastases are defined as clinically detectable nodal metastases confirmed pathologically by biopsy or therapeutic lymphadenectomy

[e] In-transit metastasis is tumor distinct from primary lesion and located either: (1) between primary lesion and draining regional lymph nodes; or (2) distal to primary lesion

stage I, 67% for stage II, and 52% for stage III. The same series reported an 11% 2-year survival rate for stage IV disease [16]. This association between disease stage and survival is also demonstrated in other studies in which reported 5-year survival rates have ranged from 44 to 68% for stages I and II and from 23 to 42% for stages III and IV [17, 18]. The reported overall recurrence rate ranges from 40 to 45% but has been reported to be as high as 77% on the head and neck [4, 19]. The median time to recurrence is consistently around 8 months with over 90% of recurrences occurring within 2 years of diagnosis [4, 19, 20].

The reported frequency of in-transit, lymph node, and distant metastases ranges widely (20–75%). The most common location of metastasis is the draining lymph node basin (27–60%),

distant skin (9–30%), lung (10–23%), central nervous system (18%), bone (10–15%), and liver (13%) [4, 21]. There is a 3–19% incidence of metastatic MCC with unknown primary at presentation [14].

Most experts recommend an initial chest X-ray to definitively rule out SCLC in combination with appropriate immunohistochemical staining of the primary tumor. The values of CT, MRI, and CT/PET scans are uncertain as they may give false positive or negative results and are only recommended as clinically indicated. No curative treatment is available for stage IV disease, and there is no evidence that the detection and treatment of asymptomatic distant metastatic disease has any impact on survival [22].

The most consistent predictor of survival is lymph node status. No other reliable prognostic indicators have been identified to date. As such, SLNB is considered the most standard of care. The incidence of sentinel lymph node positivity in clinically node negative patients has consistently been reported to be at least in the 20–30% range [22, 23]. Immunohistochemical analysis with CK-20 and pancytokeratins (AE1/AE3) is critical for acceptable sensitivity and specificity in identifying micrometastatic MCC [24, 25]. Numerous studies have confirmed the value of sentinel lymph node status as a prognostic tool. The largest study included 251 patients among whom 5-year survival was 97% for those with a negative SLNB vs. 52% for those with a positive SLNB [16].

## Evidence Regarding Treatment: Localized Disease

There have been no randomized, controlled trials specifically designed to deduce the optimal excisional margin for MCC. Studies on this subject are primarily retrospective in nature and report results inconsistently and in nonstandardized ways that make it challenging to draw any meaningful conclusions. The primary goal is to obtain clear surgical margins. Although wide local excision (WLE) has historically been done with 2–3 cm margins, existing evidence suggests that a 1 cm margin may be adequate for a tumor that is <2 cm in diameter, whereas a 2 cm margin may be indicated for a tumor ≥2 cm. These recommendations are based on a study in which relatively low local recurrence rates (8%) were obtained with surgical margins that averaged 1.1 cm. In this study, margins >1 cm were not superior in preventing recurrence compared to margins <1 cm (9 vs. 10%, $p=0.83$ respectively) [16]. In a different study where Mohs micrographic surgery (MMS) was performed on primary MCCs, a mean margin of 1.7 cm with a median of 1 cm achieved negative margins on a group of tumors with a mean diameter of 1.6 cm. A local recurrence rate of 4–8% was reported in this group [1]. Definitive reconstruction should be delayed until margins are pathologically verified as negative. In cases where primary closure is not possible, split-thickness skin graft or granulation

is recommended to facilitate early detection of a potential local recurrence.

It is currently uncertain whether, or under which circumstances, adjuvant radiotherapy (RT) to the primary site provides a more favorable outcome. Current studies are not standardized in their methods, which makes interpretation of the results problematic and the ability to draw meaningful conclusions difficult. Representative studies that showed no benefit [1, 4, 14, 16] or benefit [15, 17, 26, 27] to adjuvant RT are listed in the references section for interest. The best quality consensus guidelines regarding this issue come from the NCCN practice guidelines in oncology. After WLE of a tumor ≥2 cm in diameter, or when clear surgical margins cannot be obtained or only narrow margins can be employed, strong consideration should be given to adjuvant RT to the primary tumor bed. However, after WLE with clear margins of a tumor <2 cm in diameter, without adverse histologic parameters such as lymphovascular invasion, in an immunocompetent patient, adjuvant RT may likely be omitted. If a patient is deemed inoperable due to highly significant comorbidities or based on primary tumor characteristics, radiation monotherapy as primary treatment for MCC may also be considered [28]. Decisions regarding RT should be made in light of SLNB results and recommendations from a multidisciplinary tumor board consultation [29, 30].

In the setting of clinically localized disease, the primary value of SLNB is early detection of occult nodal disease. When SLNB is positive, additional treatment to the draining nodal basin is indicated. However, the best treatment for micrometastatic disease is still uncertain. Completion lymph node dissection (CLND) has been the most commonly reported treatment in the setting of a positive SLNB and has shown low rates of recurrence in several small case series [23, 31, 32]. For patients with extensive lymph node involvement and/or extracapsular extension, adjuvant RT following CLND should be considered [29]. Radiation therapy has also been reported to be effective as monotherapy for microscopic nodal disease and may be considered as an alternative for those patients for whom

CLND may carry unacceptable morbidity [33]. Failure to treat micrometastatic nodal disease has been shown to result in high recurrence rates in two small series [22, 32]. If SLNB is negative, patients can be spared additional surgery and/or RT, particularly in the axilla and groin. A recent study showed no difference in 3-year recurrence-free survival in those patients with a negative SLNB who either had adjuvant lymph node therapy or not [22]. If the risk of a false negative SLNB is considered significant (for instance for primary tumors on the head and neck) or if SLNB is not performed, irradiating the draining nodal basin should be considered to treat subclinical disease.

When performing SLNB, it is preferable to perform it before or concurrent to any excisional treatment of the primary lesion in order to obtain the most accurate lymphotome mapping. Since excision typically removes significant surrounding tissue, performing SLNB subsequent to excision may result in injection of dye and radioactive tracers into a lymphotome that is not representative of the true lymphotome of the primary tumor. Since MMS is typically not performed in an operating room setting (where SLNB typically occurs), it may be in the patient's best interest to receive standard WLE concurrent to SLNB instead of receiving MMS followed by SLNB. If MMS is particularly indicated for tissue-sparing in such locations as the eyelid or lip, then it is preferable to perform this after SLNB [29, 30].

Available retrospective studies do not suggest a prolonged survival benefit for adjuvant chemotherapy which therefore has no established role in the treatment of localized MCC, unless clinical judgment dictates otherwise.

## Evidence Regarding Treatment: Regional Disease

When clinically evident nodal metastatic disease is detected, without evidence of distant metastases, CLND is considered standard of care with RT as an alternative treatment for those in whom the morbidity of surgery is deemed to be unacceptable. Adjuvant RT following CLND should be considered for those with extensive lymph node involvement and/or extracapsular extension [29].

While earlier studies suggested a potential benefit from adjuvant chemotherapy with or without RT in patients with high risk primary MCC or regional MCC [34], more recent, higher quality studies have not shown a benefit. A recent prospective study in which patients with high risk localized disease received synchronous radiochemotherapy and adjuvant chemotherapy with carboplatin and etoposide did not show a survival benefit [35]. Overall, data are insufficient to assess whether chemotherapeutic regimens improve either relapse-free or overall survival. Given the body of evidence regarding adjuvant chemotherapy in the treatment of high risk localized or regional MCC and the significant morbidity associated with these chemotherapeutic regimens, a blanket recommendation cannot be given to support its use. However, under certain circumstances, adjuvant chemotherapy may be indicated based on clinical judgment. In these instances, similar regimens as recommended for systemic disease are indicated. It should be noted that case series have shown successful treatment of in-transit metastases with hyperthermic isolated limb perfusion with tumor necrosis factor $\alpha$, interferon $\gamma$, and/or melphalan [36, 37].

## Evidence Regarding Treatment: Distant Disease

Best supportive care to include any or all of surgery, RT, and/or chemotherapy is indicated for those patients with distant disease.

The most common chemotherapeutic regimens have been combination therapy with cisplatin or carboplatin plus etoposide. While small series have shown response rates as high as 76–100%, the median duration of response is consistently reported to be approximately 8 months. Response rates to second and third line chemotherapy regimens (such as topotecan, cyclophosphamide, doxorubicin, epirubicin, or vincristine) decrease to 45 and 20% respectively [30]. Factors such as the patient's anticipated lifespan, the patient's performance status, the anticipated toxicity of the selected chemotherapy regimen, the probability of death from toxicity of the selected chemotherapy regimen, and anticipated gain in the patient's lifespan should all be considered when deciding upon chemotherapy.

## Evidence Regarding Follow Up

Proper follow-up should include a complete skin exam and lymph node exam every 1–3 months year 1, every 3–6 months year 2, and annually thereafter. The above time intervals reflect current evidence that the median time to recurrence is 8 months with 90% of recurrences occurring with 24 months [16, 30].

## Evidence-Based Summary

|  | Level of evidence |
|---|---|
| **Histologic diagnosis** | |
| Excisional biopsy with narrow margins is preferred to incisional biopsy | VI/C |
| Appropriate immunopanel should include cytokeratin-20 (CK-20) and thyroid transcription factor-1 (TTF-1) to differentiate between primary cutaneous MCC and metastatic visceral neuroendocrine carcinoma | IV/B |
| Appropriately experienced dermatopathologists should perform the histopathologic interpretation | VI/C |
| **Staging** | |
| Thorough history and physical exam including a complete skin and lymph node exam | (VI/C) |
| Imaging (CT, MRI, PET/CT) may be indicated to distinguish between primary cutaneous MCC and metastatic visceral neuroendocrine carcinoma or to rule out distant metastatic disease based on clinical suspicion | (VI/C) |
| SLNB for clinically node-negative patients | (III/B) |
| **Treatment** | |
| Localized disease (clinically node negative) | |
| Wide local excision (WLE) with or without adjuvant radiation therapy (RT) to primary site | |
| One-to-two cm margins to investing fascia of muscle or pericranium with clear pathologic margins should be obtained whenever possible. Alternative excisional techniques include Mohs micrographic surgery (MMS) utilizing frozen sections, modified MMS where final tangential margins are sent for permanent sections, or complete circumferential and peripheral deep-margin assessment using permanent sections. When using MMS-based techniques, emphasis is on tumor extirpation, not on tissue sparing | (VI/B) |
| SLNB | |
| *Positive* | |
| Completion lymph node dissection (CLND) and/or adjuvant RT | (III/B) |
| May consider adjuvant chemotherapy | (III/B) |
| *Negative* | |
| Observation of nodal basin or adjuvant RT if high risk of false negative | (III/B) |
| Regional disease (clinical lymphadenopathy) | |
| Fine needle aspirate (FNA) to include at least CK-20 and pancytokeratins (AE1/AE3) | (VI/B) |
| FNA positive | |
| Imaging studies (CT, MRI, and/or PET/CT) as indicated | (VI/C) |
| *No distant disease* | |
| CLND with or without adjuvant RT. | (III/B) |
| Finding | |
| May consider adjuvant chemotherapy | (III/B) |
|  | (continued) |

**Evidence-Based Summary** (continued)

|  |  |
|---|---|
| *Distant disease* | |
| See below section on distant disease | |
| FNA negative | |
| Consider open lymph node biopsy if clinical suspicion remains | (VI/C) |
| *Open biopsy positive* | |
| See FNA positive | (VI/C) |
| *Open biopsy negative* | |
| Observation | |
| Distant disease | |
| Best supportive care to include any or all of the following: surgery, RT, and/or chemotherapy | |
| **Follow-up** | |
| Year 1: Every 1–3 months, year 2: every 3–6 months, annually thereafter | |
| Follow-up to include complete skin and lymph node exam and imaging studies as indicated | |

# References

1. Boyer JD, Zitelli JA, Brodland DG, D'Angelo G. Local control of primary Merkel cell carcinoma: review of 45 cases treated with Mohs micrographic surgery with and without adjuvant radiation. J Am Acad Dermatol. 2002;47:885–92.
2. Ferringer T, Rogers HC, Metcalf JS. Merkel cell carcinoma in situ. J Cutan Pathol. 2005;32:162–5.
3. Hodgson NC. Merkel cell carcinoma: changing incidence trends. J Surg Oncol. 2005;89:1–4.
4. Medina-Franco H, Urist MM, Fiveash J, Heslin MJ, Bland KI, Beenken SW. Multimodality treatment of Merkel cell carcinoma: case series and literature review of 1024 cases. Ann Surg Oncol. 2001;8:204–8.
5. Lunder EJ, Stern RS. Merkel cell carcinomas in patients treated with methoxysalen and ultraviolet A radiation. N Engl J Med. 1998;339:1247–8.
6. Miller RW, Rabkin CS. Merkel cell carcinoma and melanoma: etiological similarities and differences. Cancer Epidemiol Biomarkers Prev. 1999;8:153–8.
7. Buell JF, Trofe J, Hanaway MJ, Beebe TM, Gross TG, Alloway RR, et al. Immunosuppression and Merkel cell cancer. Transplant Proc. 2002;34:1780–1.
8. Penn I, First MR. Merkel's cell carcinoma in organ transplant recipients: report of 41 cases. Transplantation. 1999;68:1717–21.
9. Engels EA, Frisch M, Goedert JJ, Biggar RJ, Miller RW. Merkel cell carcinoma and HIV infection. Lancet. 2002;359:497–8.
10. Feng H, Shuda M, Chang Y, Moore PS. Clonal integration of a polyomavirus in human Merkel cell carcinoma. Science. 2008;319:1049–50.
11. Hanly AJ, Elgart GW, Jorda M, Smith J, Nadji M. Analysis of thyroid transcription factor-1 and cytokeratin 20 separates Merkel cell carcinoma from small cell carcinoma of the lung. J Cutan Pathol. 2000;27:118–20.
12. Cheuk W, Kwan MY, Suster S, Chan JK. Immunostaining for thyroid transcription factor 1 and cytokeratin 20 aids the distinction of small cell carcinoma from Merkel cell carcinoma, but not pulmonary from extrapulmonary small cell carcinomas. Arch Pathol Lab Med. 2001;125:228–31.
13. Gruber SB, Wilson LD. Merkel cell carcinoma: In: Cutaneous oncology: pathophysiology, diagnosis, and management. Malden: Blackwell Science; 1998. p. 710–21.
14. Veness MJ, Perera L, McCourt J, Shannon J, Hughes TM, Morgan GJ, et al. Merkel cell carcinoma: improved outcome with adjuvant radiotherapy. Aust N Z J Surg. 2005;75:275–81.
15. Lewis KG, Weinstock MA, Weaver AL, Otley CC. Adjuvant local irradiation for Merkel cell carcinoma. Arch Dermatol. 2006;142:693–700.
16. Allen PJ, Bowne WB, Jaques DP, Brennan MF, Busam K, Coit DG. Merkel cell carcinoma: prognosis and treatment of patients from a single institution. J Clin Oncol. 2005;23:2300–9.
17. Eng TY, Boersma MG, Fuller CD, Cavanaugh SX, Valenzuela F, Herman TS. Treatment of Merkel cell carcinoma. Am J Clin Oncol. 2004;27:510–5.
18. McAfee WJ, Morris CG, Mendenhall CM, Werning JW, Mendenhall NP, Mendenhall WM. Merkel cell carcinoma: treatment and outcomes. Cancer. 2005;104:1761–4.
19. Gillenwater AM, Hessel AC, Morrison WH, Burgess MA, Silva EG, Roberts D, et al. Merkel cell carcinoma of the head and neck: effect of surgical excision and radiation on recurrence and survival. Arch Otolaryngol Head Neck Surg. 2001;127:149–54.
20. Eng TY, Naguib M, Fuller CD, Jones WE, Herman TS. Treatment of recurrent Merkel cell carcinoma: an analysis of 46 cases. Am J Clin Oncol. 2004;27:576–83.
21. Muller A, Keus B, Neumann N, Lammering G, Schnabel T. Management of Merkel cell carcinoma:

case series of 36 patients. Oncol Rep. 2003;10: 577–85.

22. Gupta SG, Wang LC, Penas PF, Gellenthin M, Lee SJ, Nghiem P. Sentinel lymph node biopsy for evaluation and treatment of patients with Merkel cell carcinoma: the Dana-Farber experience and meta-analysis of the literature. Arch Dermatol. 2006;142:685–90.

23. Hill AD, Brady MS, Coit DG. Intraoperative lymphatic mapping and sentinel lymph node biopsy for Merkel cell carcinoma. Br J Surg. 1999;86:518–21.

24. Schmalbach CE, Lowe L, Teknos TN, Johnson TM, Bradford CR. Reliability of sentinel lymph node biopsy for regional staging of head and neck Merkel cell carcinoma. Arch Otolarnygol Head Neck Surg. 2005;131:610–4.

25. Su LD, Lowe L, Bradford CR, Yahanda AI, Johnson TM, Sondak VK. Immunostaining for cytokeratin 20 improves detection of micrometastatic Merkel cell carcinoma in sentinel lymph nodes. J Am Acad Dermatol. 2002;46:661–6.

26. Meeuwissen JA, Bourne RG, Kearsley JH. The importance of postoperative radiation therapy in the treatment of Merkel cell carcinoma. Int J Radiat Oncol Biol Phys. 1995;31:325–31.

27. Jabbour J, Cumming R, Scolyer RA, Hruby G, Thompson JF, Lee S. Merkel cell carcinoma: assessing the effect of wide local excision, lymph node dissection, and radiotherapy on recurrence and survival in early stage disease – results from a review of 82 consecutive cases diagnosed between 1992 and 2004. Ann Surg Oncol. 2007;14:1943–52.

28. Mortier L, Mirabel X, Fournier C, Piette F, Lartigau E. Radiotherapy alone for primary Merkel cell carcinoma. Arch Dermatol. 2003;139:1587–90.

29. National comprehensive cancer network practice guidelines in oncology, v.1.2009, Merkel cell carcinoma. http://www.nccn.org/professionals/physician_gls/f_guidelines.asp.

30. Bichakjian CK, Lowe L, Lao CD, Sandler HM, Bradford CR, Johnson TM, et al. Merkel cell carcinoma: critical review with guidelines for multidisciplinary management. Cancer. 2007;110:1–12.

31. Messina JL, Reintgen DS, Cruse CW, Rappaport DP, Berman C, Fenske NA, et al. Selective lymphadenectomy in patients with Merkel cell carcinoma (cutaneous neuroendocrine) carcinoma. Ann Surg Oncol. 1997;4:389–95.

32. Mehrany K, Otley CC, Weenig RH, Phillips PK, Roenigk RK, Nyugen TH. A meta-analysis of the prognostic significance of sentinel lymph node status in Merkel cell carcinoma. Dermatol Surg. 2002;28:113–7.

33. Schmalbach CE, Lowe L, Teknos TN, Johnson TM, Bradford CR. Reliability of sentinel lymph node biopsy for regional staging of head and neck Merkel cell carcinoma. Arch Otolaryngol Head Neck Surg. 2005;131:610–4.

34. Poulsen M, Rischin D, Walpole E, Harvey J, Mackintosh J, Ainslie J, et al. High risk Merkel cell carcinoma of the skin treated with synchronous carboplatin/etoposide and radiation: a Trans-Tasman radiation oncology group study – TROG 96:07. J Clin Oncol. 2003;21:4371–6.

35. Poulsen MG, Rischin D, Porter I, Walpole E, Harvey J, Hamilton C, et al. Does chemotherapy improve survival in high risk stage I and II Merkel cell carcinoma of the skin? Int J Radiat Oncol Biol Phys. 2006;64:114–9.

36. Gupta AS, Heinzman S, Levine EA. Successful treatment of in-transit metastases from Merkel's cell carcinoma with isolated hyperthermic limb perfusion. South Med J. 1998;91:289–92.

37. Olieman AFT, Lienard D, Eggermont AM, Kroon BBR, Lejeune FJ, Hoekstra HJ, et al. Hyperthermic isolated limb perfusion with tumor necrosis factor alpha, interferon gamma, and melphalan for locally advanced nonmelanoma skin tumors of the extremities: a multicenter study. Arch Surg. 1999;134: 303–7.

## Self-Assessment

1. Given the gravity of a diagnosis of MCC, accurate initial diagnosis is critical to facilitate appropriate and timely treatment. Which of the following is false:
   (a) Incisional biopsy is preferred to excisional biopsy with narrow margins.
   (b) CK-20 is a sensitive marker for MCC, but it also stains positively in small cell lung carcinomas and extrapulmonary small cell carcinomas.
   (c) TTF-1 is a sensitive marker for small cell lung carcinomas and is absent in MCC.
   (d) For the highest probability of accurate diagnosis, appropriately experienced dermatopathologists should perform the histopathologic interpretation.

2. Correct staging of MCC is important to help determine prognosis and proper treatment. Which of the following is false:
   (a) The most consistent predictor of survival is lymph node status.
   (b) In the most recent staging system that was adopted from the AJCC, key clinical characteristics are tumor diameter, clinical node status, pathologic node status, and in-transit or distant metastatic disease.
   (c) In addition to an initial CXR to rule out SCLC along with appropriate immunohistochemical staining of the primary tumor, additional imaging studies such as CT, MRI, and CT/PET scans are indicated as part of a staging work-up.
   (d) No curative treatment is currently available for stage IV disease, and there is no evidence that detection and treatment of asymptomatic distant metastatic disease has any impact on survival.

3. The majority of the time, MCC presents as localized disease. Which of the following statements is true concerning the treatment of localized disease?
   (a) Appropriate treatment of localized disease consists of wide local excision with 1–2 cm margins and postoperative radiotherapy.
   (b) Appropriate treatment of localized disease consists of wide local excision with 1–2 cm margins and antecedent or concurrent SLNB with CLND and/or adjuvant radiotherapy if positive or observation with or without postoperative radiotherapy if negative.
   (c) Postoperative radiotherapy has been definitively shown to be of benefit in the treatment of localized disease.
   (d) SLNB can be performed either before or after wide local excision with equal accuracy.

4. For less fortunate patients, MCC will present as regional or distant disease. Which of the following statements is true concerning the treatment of regional or distant disease?
   (a) For regional disease, FNA is indicated with appropriate imaging studies if positive. If no distant disease is detected, CLND is considered standard of care with adjuvant radiotherapy for extensive lymph node involvement/extracapsular extension.
   (b) For regional disease, when an FNA is negative, open lymph node biopsy is not appropriate.
   (c) There is evidence definitively substantiating a benefit from chemotherapy in the treatment of regional or distant disease.
   (d) For distant disease, effective life-prolonging measures consist of wide local excision of the primary tumor, SLNB with CLND if positive, postoperative radiotherapy, and chemotherapy.

5. All patients with MCC will require close follow-up due to the propensity for MCC to locally recur and/or metastasize. Which of the following statements regarding follow-up for MCC is false?

   (a) Follow-up schedules for MCC are determined by the fact that the median time to recurrence is 8 months with 90% of recurrences occurring in 24 months.

   (b) At each follow-up visit the following should be performed: a complete skin exam.

   (c) An appropriate follow-up schedule is every 1–3 months for the first year, every 3–6 months for the second year, and annually thereafter.

   (d) The NCCN practice guidelines (listed in the references) are an excellent resource to stay current on the latest in consensus and evidence-based treatment recommendations regarding MCC and other skin cancers such as BCC, SCC, and dermatofibrosarcoma protuberans.

## Answers

1. a: Incisional biopsy is preferred to excisional biopsy with narrow margins.

2. c: In addition to an initial CXR to rule out SCLC along with appropriate immunohistochemical staining of the primary tumor, additional imaging studies such as CT, MRI, and CT/PET scans are indicated as part of a staging work-up.

3. b: Appropriate treatment of localized disease consists of wide local excision with 1–2 cm margins and antecedent or concurrent SLNB with CLND and/or adjuvant radiotherapy if positive or observation with or without postoperative radiotherapy if negative.

4. a: For regional disease, FNA is indicated with appropriate imaging studies if positive. If no distant disease is detected, CLND is considered standard of care with adjuvant radiotherapy for extensive lymph node involvement/extracapsular extension.

5. b: At each follow-up visit the following should be performed: a complete skin exam.

# Photodynamic Therapy

## Yue (Emily) Yu

## Introduction

At the dawn of the twentieth century, Hermann von Tappeiner, then director of the Institute of Pharmacology at the University of Munich, first coined the term "photodynamic reaction [1]," later revised to photodynamic therapy (PDT), to describe the interaction of light, oxygen, and a photosensitizer inside a diseased tissue to achieve a therapeutic effect. The photosensitizing chemical in the target tissue absorbs light of an appropriate wavelength and the "excited" molecule then interacts with oxygen in the tissue, resulting in the formation of singlet oxygen ($^1O_2$) and other free radicals that are cytotoxic. When the photosensitizer accumulates preferentially in diseased vs. normal cells, the therapeutic index is improved.

Current FDA-approved PDT drug/device combinations consist of two intravenously delivered photosensitizers (photofrin and verteporfin) used with red light but only rarely for dermatologic

disease and two topically applied pro-drugs, δ-aminolevulinic acid (ALA) and methyl aminolevulinate (MAL) (Table 6.1). Discussion throughout this chapter concerns topical ALA-PDT or MAL-PDT that avoid the drawback for the available systemic photosensitizing drugs of prolonged generalized phototoxicity.

It is essential to choose an appropriate light source for PDT to ensure adequate photosensitizer excitation and tissue penetration. Absorption peaks for protoporphyrin IX (PpIX), the principal active metabolite of ALA and MAL, are at 400–410 (Soret band, maximum), 505, 540, 580, and 635 nm (Fig. 6.1). The intensity of photoactivation depends on the efficiency of incident photons and the number of absorbable photons that reach the photosensitizer in the target tissue, as well as on the local concentration of the photosensitizer [2]. Long wavelengths penetrate deeper into the tissue (Fig. 6.2), but their advantage for the treatment of thicker lesions is counterbalanced by how strongly the photosensitizer absorbs at these long wavelengths. For example, for PpIX, a dose of 10 $J/cm^2$ at 410 nm (blue light) is roughly equivalent to 200–300 $J/cm^2$ at 635 nm (red light) [3]. No single light source is ideal for every indication. Choice may be based on the proposed clinical indication, convenience, compactibility, treatment time, and cost.

Y. (Emily) Yu (✉)
Department of Dermatology, Boston University
School of Medicine, 609 Albany Street-J507,
Boston, MA 02118, USA
e-mail: yue.yu@bmc.org

**Table 6.1** Comparison of topical ALA vs. MAL for PDT

| Compound | Aminolevulinic acid (ALA) | Methyl aminolevulinate (MAL) |
|---|---|---|
| Final active metabolite | Protoporphyrin IX | Protoporphyrin IX |
| Preparation | Solution | Peanut oil based cream |
| Brand name | Levulan (DUSA Pharmaceuticals) | Metvix (Galderma) |
| Approval in | USA | Europe, Australia, New Zealand, and USA[a] |
| Approved for | AKs only | AKs, BD, sBCCs, and nBCCs |
| Co-approved light source | Blue light (417 ± 5 nm) | Red light (570–670 nm) |
| Approved protocol | 14–18 h incubation, no occlusion | 3 h incubation under occlusion |

[a]Approved in 2008 in USA, not yet marketed in USA

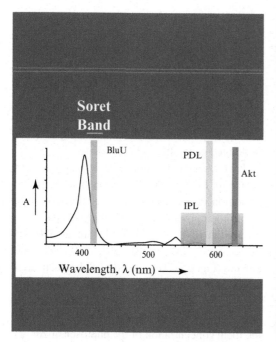

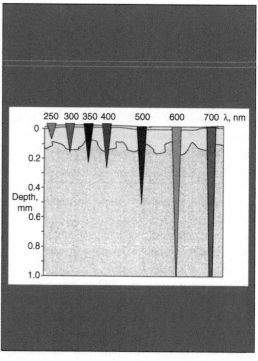

**Fig. 6.1** Absorption (activation) spectrum for porphyrins with frequently used PDT light sources superimposed. *Blu U* Blu U therapeutic illuminator, the DUSA device FDA-approved for use with topical ALA (*left most bar*); *IPL* intense pulsed light; *PDL* pulsed dye laser (*middle bar*); *Akt* aktilite, the Galderma device FDA-approved for use with topical MAL (*right most bar*)

**Fig. 6.2** Influence of wavelength on light penetration in human skin (left most wavelength (250 nm) is *purple* and right most wavelength (700 nm) is *red*). Reproduced from Kochevar et al. [42] with permission

Some investigators have included PDT pretreatment of lesional skin with desferrioxamine (DFO), an iron chelating agent that results in higher PpIX concentration by blocking its metabolism to heme in a step catalyzed by ferrous oxide ions, but no study has yet demonstrated an improved clinical outcome from this modification,

despite more intense tissue fluorescence, indicative of a higher PpIX concentration [4].

In this chapter, we review accepted and emerging indications for topical PDT, including focal treatment for actinic keratoses (AKs), "field therapy" for AKs, nonmelanoma skin cancer (NMSC) treatment and prevention, and cosmetic photorejuvenation.

## Prior Evidence-Based Consensus Reports

Workshops held by the British Photodermatology Group in November 2000 and the International Society for Photodynamic Therapy in Dermatology in January 2005 provided evidence-based recommendations for using PDT for AKs and NMSCs [5, 6] (Table 6.2). Both sets of recommendations were based on MEDLINE searches of MAL-PDT and ALA-PDT for premalignant and malignant indications, considering safety, efficacy, cosmesis, and patient preference. On the basis of evidence data published through 2005,

PDT was recommended as a first-line treatment for AKs, Bowen's disease (BD), and superficial basal cell carcinoma (sBCC) [6]. MAL-PDT was also recommended for nodular basal cell carcinoma (nBCC), particularly for lesions <2 mm deep [6]. The groups concluded that there was insufficient evidence to advocate routine use of PDT for the treatment of squamous cell carcinoma (SCC) or for the prevention of NMSCs in immunosuppressed patients or patients with Gorlin syndrome. The following sections review by indication the published experience with ALA-PDT and MAL-PDT in order to update and reinforce those evidence-based recommendations.

**Table 6.2** Recommendations and supporting data for PDT in the treatment of premalignant and malignant skin lesions

| Lesions | Number of studies | Evidence grading system[a] | First-line treatment (yes/no) | Comments |
|---|---|---|---|---|
| AK | Six open studies in BPG and 11 open label/randomized studies in ISPTD | IA | Yes | Response rates comparable with topical 5-FU and cryotherapy, superior cosmetic response compared to cryotherapy |
| SCCis (Bowen's disease) | Thirteen open and 3 randomized studies in BPG and 4 randomized studies in ISPTD | IA | Yes | Response rates comparable with cryotherapy or 5-FU, but with fewer adverse events; particularly recommended for large or multiple lesions, those in poor healing sites, and for penile, digital and facial lesions |
| SCC | Three open label studies at both BPG and ISPTD | VB | No | Not recommended for routine use |
| sBCC | Twelve open label, retrospective and randomized studies in ISPTD | IA | Yes | Particularly for large, extensive and multiple lesions; for MAL-PDT, demonstrated long term efficacy based on 5 year follow up data |
| nBCC | Twelve retrospective, open label, and randomized studies in ISPTD | IA | Yes (MAL-PDT) | MAL-PDT effective and reliable treatment option for nBCC (<2 mm deep) with good cosmetic outcome and long term efficacy based on 5 year follow up data; topical ALA-PDT less effective |
| NMSC prevention in immunosuppressed patients | Few case reports and randomized studies in ISPTD | IIA | No | Maybe considered as a method of preventing new AKs, SCCs, and BCCs in immunosuppressed patients |
| BCC prevention in Gorlin syndrome | Only few case reports in ISPDT | VB | No | Insufficient evidence |

[a]Scoring system of the consensus meetings has been converted to the evidence grading system employed in this book

## PDT for AKs

AKs are cutaneous neoplasms present in up to 40–60% of whites older than 40 years and 80% of whites older than 60 years, whose presence is associated with the development of SCCs at rates up to 6–10% during a 10-year period in patients having multiple lesions [7]. Many therapies for AKs exist, including ablative procedures (e.g., electrodessication and curettage (ED&C), cryotherapy, and medium-depth chemical peeling) and topical chemotherapy (e.g., fluorouracil, imiquimod, and diclofenac) [8, 9]. Recently, PDT was introduced as a third category of AK therapy.

Summarizing the literature regarding treatment of AKs is complicated by variation in topical photosensitizers (ALA vs. MAL), incubation time, light source, treatment protocols, and follow-up times. Initial topical PDT studies predominantly used red light, but randomized studies done by Jeffes et al. [10] and Piacquadio et al. [11] demonstrated that shorter wavelengths (blue light) were also safe and effective in treating multiple nonhyperkeratotic AKs of the face and scalp.

The FDA-approved protocol specifies a 14–18 h delay between ALA application and blue light exposure, which was demonstrated to be sufficient for therapeutic photosensitization and restricts only to clinically apparent AKs, with clearance rate of 88% of thin AKs and 78% of moderately thick AKs after one treatment [10]. Subsequently, topical PDT has been shown to be effective in the treatment of multiple AKs with short incubation time (1–3 h) and broad area application [12]. The advantages of broad-area topical PDT for the treatment of AKs include efficacy (as effective as conventional therapy) for visible lesions, tolerability, lack of scarring or depigmentation, an office-based complete treatment that eliminates the need for patient compliance, probable decreased incidence of AKs in the future because of treating subclinical lesions, and improved appearance of photoaged skin that contributes to high patient satisfaction.

MAL enjoys wide popularity particularly in Europe for the treatment of AKs and NMSCs. MAL is said to offer improved skin penetration compared to ALA as a result of enhanced lipophilicity and deeper penetration of red light compared

to blue light. Compared to conventional treatments (e.g., cryotherapy) for AKs, MAL-PDT showed comparable efficacy, but superior cosmetic outcomes [13]. In a first randomized side to side comparison study using ALA vs. MAL in the treatment of scalp AKs [14], both ALA-PDT and MAL-PDT resulted in a significant reduction in scalp AKs without significant difference in efficacy. However, PDT employing an overnight ALA incubation is more painful than PDT employing a 3 h MAL incubation under occlusion in the treatment of extensive scalp AKs.

A large number of clinical studies have demonstrated safety and efficacy using ALA- or MAL-PDT in the treatment of AKs (Table 6.3), with reported lesion cure rates for AKs in the range of 70–100%. Overall, the face, scalp, and thin AKs (grade 1) responded better than the hands, forearms, trunk, and hyperkeratotic AKs (grade 3). PDT provided excellent cosmetic results and well-tolerated photosensitivity.

## PDT for BD and SCC

BD (or SCC in situ) typically presents as red, scaly or crusted plaques on the lower legs of elderly patients (although they can appear anywhere on the skin), with approximately 3% developing into invasive carcinoma, one-third of which may metastasize [15].

BD can be treated effectively by destruction (e.g., cryotherapy and ED&C), radiotherapy, topical chemotherapy (e.g., 5-FU), or surgical excision [15]. An important feature of any therapy for BD should be high efficacy coupled with good tolerability at poor healing sites (particularly the lower leg in elderly patients with poor vascular status). For large and numerous lesions, or lesions in anatomically difficult areas, conventional methods may be unsatisfactory. ALA-PDT or MAL-PDT offers a nonscarring treatment option for BD (Table 6.4). In addition, several randomized studies establish that PDT for BD is comparable in efficacy and tolerability to other modalities such as 5-FU and cryotherapy. A randomized clinical study by Morton et al. [16] showed treatment of BD using ALA-PDT to be at least as effective as cryosurgery, and to be associated with

**Table 6.3** Selected studies of ALA- or MAL-PDT for treatment of AKs

| Case series or cohort study (references) | Number of patients | Protocol | Results | Comments |
|---|---|---|---|---|
| Szeimies [43] (V/B) | 10 | One treatment of 10% ALA for 6 h under occlusion, irradiation with red light (580–740 nm, 150 J/cm$^2$) | Complete remission (CR) in 71% of AK localized on the head without notable side effects at 3 months | Initial pilot study demonstrated potential of good efficacy and tolerability in the treatment of AK using topical ALA-PDT |
| Jeffes et al. [44] (IV/B) | 40 | ALA (10–30%) under occlusion for 3 h, irradiated with an argon pumped dye laser (630 nm, 10–150 J/cm$^2$) | Three weeks after a single treatment, clearing of 91% of nonhypertrophic AKs on the face/scalp and 45% on the trunk/extremities; no significant differences using 10, 20, or 30% ALA, but all were more effective than vehicle alone | Lesions on the face and scalp responded better than lesions on the trunk and extremities, and hypertrophic AKs responded poorly |
| Goldman and Atkin [45] (IV/B) | 32 | 20% ALA with 15–20 h incubation followed by exposure to blue light (1,000 s, 10 J/cm$^2$) to individual target lesions treated or to entire affected area | Rapid resolution of multiple AK lesions. Side effects were influenced by a number of factors: use of analgesic and topical anesthetic agents, body region treated, focal vs. broad area treatment, and light exposure time | One of the first studies investigating 20% ALA-PDT using blue light in the treatment of AKs |
| Alexiades-Armenakas and Geronemus [46] (III/B) | 41 | Single application of 20% ALA for 3 or 14–18 h, followed by long pulsed dye laser (LP PDL) at 595 nm | After one treatment 99.5, 83.1, and 85% of 2,620 lesions on the head, 949 on the extremities, and 53 on the trunk cleared at 10 days. At 8 months, 90.3, 100, and 65% were clear. No difference in safety or efficacy was found between the 3 vs. 14–18-h incubation times. Biopsy of nonresponding lesions demonstrated many to be SCC and other non-AK neoplasms | Treatment of AKs using LP PDL (595 nm) at nonpurpuric parameters following topical application of ALA is safe and effective |
| Tschen et al. [47] (IV/B) | 110 | Same protocol as Piacquadio et al. [11] (II/A), followed for 12 months; 11 centers with a total of 968 lesions enrolled (6–12 discrete AKs on the face or the scalp) | CR in the first and second months, one ALA-PDT treatment (baseline): 76 and 72%, respectively. 60% of the patients received a second ALA-PDT treatment if target AKs still present at month 2. CR peaked at 86% at month 4 then decreased to 78% at month 12. The overall 12-month recurrence rate was 24% (162/688). Of the 162 recurrent lesions, 16 were lost to follow-up, 7 spontaneously cleared, and 139 were biopsied. Of the 139 lesions biopsied, 91% were AKs, 7% were SCCs, 0.7% were BCCs, and 1% were other non-AK diagnoses | Consistent with previous phase III multicenter trials [11], ALA-PDT is effective and safe for the treatment of AKs of the face and scalp. ALA-PDT treatment for AKs produced long-term clearance of AKs with about one-fifth recurring within 12 months |

(continued)

**Table 6.3** (continued)

| Case series or cohort study (references) | Number of patients | Protocol | Results | Comments |
|---|---|---|---|---|
| Randomized control study (references) | | | | |
| Touma et al. [12] (II/A) | 18 | ALA application to the entire face randomized to 1, 2, or 3 h incubation before exposure to 10 J/cm$^2$ of blue light | Significant reduction in AKs and several photodamage parameters both 1 and 5 months after a single treatment. 11/18 patients had complete resolution of their AKs 1 month after treatment. 7/10 patients followed at 5 months showed complete resolution. ALA application times (1–3 h) did not affect the results. One week of 40% urea vs. vehicle cream before treatment had no effect on results. 3% lidocaine vs. vehicle cream alone 45 min before light exposure did not affect discomfort during light exposure | First study investigating the efficacy of short incubation time, broad area application of ALA-PDT using blue light for facial AKs and photodamage |
| Kurwa et al. [48] (II/A) | 17 | Right and left hands were randomized to receive a 3-week course of 5-FU bid or ALA-PDT (4 h incubation, red light 580–740 nm, 150 J/cm$^2$) | No statistically significant difference in reduction in lesional area at 4 weeks between ALA-PDT (73%) and 5-FU (70%) or in the overall pain or erythema associated with treatment | ALA-PDT is comparable to 5-FU in efficacy and tolerability for treatment of AKs on the dorsal hands |
| Radakovic-Fijan et al. [49] (II/A) | 27 | Patients with at least three mild or moderate AKs on the scalp or face 4 h occlusion with 20% ALA, followed by high-pressure metal halide lamp (600–750 nm) with 70, 100, or 140 J/cm$^2$ (one AK per dose) | Rate of CR was 81–92% at 1 month and 69–81% at 3 months with no significant difference among the three light doses at either time points. PDT-induced pain was also comparable among groups | ALA-PDT with red light at irradiation dose of 70 J/cm$^2$ (and possibly even less) is as effective as up to twice that dose in the treatment of mild to moderate AKs on the scalp and face |
| Smith et al. [50] (II/A) | 36 | AKs on the face or scalp randomized to either ALA-PDT (1 h incubation followed by blue light or pulsed dye laser) or 5-FU (bid ×4 weeks) | At 1 month, ≥75% of AKs cleared in 75, 42, and 75% of pts receiving ALA (blue light), ALA (laser light), and 5-FU, respectively | ALA-PDT blue light is as effective as 5-FU for AKs |
| Jeffes et al. [10] (II/A) | 36 | At least four nonhypertrophic AKs on the face or scalp, AKs per pt treated with vehicle or 20% ALA (14–18 h incubation) followed by blue light, 2, 5, or 10 J/cm$^2$. Repeat treatment if no response at week 8 | At week 8, CR 66% (88% with optimal light dose of 10 J/cm$^2$) vs. 17% with ALA- vs. vehicle-PDT ($P<0.001$) regardless of light dose. At 16 weeks, CR 85 vs. 25% (increased significantly from 66 to 85% statistically due to retreatment at week 8). Thin AKs (grade 1) responded better than slightly thicker (grade 2) AKs | First study examining the safety and efficacy of PDT using topical 20% ALA and nonlaser, fluorescent blue light to treat multiple AKs on the face and scalp |

| Study | n | Methods | Results | Conclusions |
|---|---|---|---|---|
| Piacquadio et al. [11] (II/A) | 243 | Randomized in a 3:1 ratio to 20% ALA or vehicle (14–18 h incubation) followed by blue light at 10 J/cm$^2$. Lesions remaining at week 8 were re-treated. 96% of patients completed the study | Lesional CR at weeks 8 and 12 were 83 and 91%, for ALA and 31 and 25%, for vehicle ($P<0.001$); at weeks 8 and 12, 77 and 89% of ALA-PDT patients were ≥75% clear; 66 and 73% were 100% clear | Demonstrated that ALA-PDT with blue light is a highly effective therapy for facial and scalp AKs during a 12-week follow-up period |
| Pariser et al. [51] (II/A) | 80 | Randomized into MAL- or placebo-PDT (3 h occlusion) followed by red light (570–670 nm, 75 J/cm$^2$). Repeat treatment 1 week later | CR at 3 months significantly higher with MAL-PDT (82%) vs. placebo-PDT (21%). 91% of patients documented excellent or good cosmetic outcome, with 73% preferring MAL-PDT to previous therapies | MAL-PDT is an effective, safe, and well-tolerated treatment for AKs, with excellent cosmetic outcome |
| Szeimies [13] (II/A) | 202 | Randomized to MAL-PDT with red light (3 h occlusion, 570–670 nm at 75 J/cm$^2$) vs. cryotherapy (2×). Repeat treatment at 1 week for lesions not on the face or scalp | Lesion CR 69% for PDT and 75% for cryotherapy. 98% of patients treated with MAL-PDT and 91% of patients treated with cryotherapy graded cosmetic outcome excellent or good ($P=0.035$) | MAL-PDT has comparable response rate to that of cryotherapy in the treatment of AKs, but with significantly better cosmetic outcome |
| Moloney [14] (II/A) | 16 | Right and left frontoparietal scalp AKs randomized to MAL-PDT (3 h occlusion) or ALA-PDT (5 h occlusion) as first or second treatment 2 weeks apart | Reduction of AKs with ALA-PDT of 6.2±1.9 vs. 5.6±3.2 with MAL-PDT ($P=0.588$). Better CR with ALA-PDT in 6 patients (40%), MAL-PDT in 1 patient (6.7%) and no difference in 8 patients (53.3%). Greater pain intensity in ALA-treated side at all time points: (3–16 min). Duration of discomfort persisted longer with ALA vs. MAL-PDT ($P=0.044$) | Both ALA-PDT and MAL-PDT resulted in a significant reduction in scalp AKs without significant difference in efficacy. However, ALA-PDT was more painful than MAL-PDT |
| Pariser et al. [52] (II/A) | 96 | Randomized to MAL vs. vehicle (3 h occlusion), followed by red light(630 nm, 37 J/cm$^2$) with repeated treatment 1 week later | MAL-PDT was superior to vehicle-PDT in both lesion complete response (86.2 vs. 52.2%) and patient complete response (59.2 vs. 14.9%); $P<0.0001$ for both | MAL-PDT under red light-emitting diode light is an appropriate treatment alternative for multiple AK lesions |

**Table 6.4** Selected studies of ALA- or MAL-PDT for treatment of NMSCs

| Case series or cohort study (references) | Number of patients, type of lesions | Protocol | Results | Comments |
|---|---|---|---|---|
| Stables et al. [53] (V/B) | 3 pts with BD | 20% ALA applied under occlusion for 4 h followed by 250 W quartz-tungsten-halogen lamp (400–700 nm, 125 J/cm²) | At 3 months, >90% CR. Repeat biopsies at 6–12 months showed no residual epidermal dysplasia but slight superficial scaring | All maintained a CR response 12–26 months after a second treatment |
| Morton et al. [54] (V/B) | 38 pts with 40 BD patches >20 mm; 10 pts with ≥3 BD patches; 18 pts with 73 large/multiple BCCs | 20% ALA applied (4–6 h incubation), irradiated with red (630 ± 15 nm, ~125 J/cm²) | 88% of both large BD patches and BCCs cleared following 1–3 ALA-PDT treatment, respectively (4 recurred within 12 and 34 months); 98 and 90% multiple BD patches and BCCs, respectively cleared following 1 or 2 treatments of ALA-PDT (4 and 2 recurrence over 12–41 months) | ALA-PDT is an effective tissue-sparing modality with good cosmesis, and can be considered as a first-line therapy for large and/or multiple areas of BD and superficial BCCs less than 2 mm thick |
| Britton et al. [55] (V/B) | 13 pts with BD | 20% ALA under occlusion for 4 h, irradiated using PDL (585 nm, 10 J/cm²) | 82% CR at 1 year; one lesion required a second treatment, with 0% recurrence rate | PDL is an effective light source for ALA-PDT of BD |
| Wennberg et al. [56] (V/B) | 37 patients with 190 sBCCs; 6 with 10 nBCCs, and 5 with 18 BDs | 20% ALA under occlusion for 3 h, irradiated with red light (620–670 nm, 75 or 100 J/cm²) | 92% sBCC, 20% nBCC, and 78% BDs cleared in 6 months | PDT is effective in the treatment of sBCCs with good cosmesis, regardless of lesion size |
| Haller et al. [57] (V/B) | 6 patients with 26 sBCCs | 20% ALA under occlusion for 4 h, illuminated with red light (630 ± 15 nm, 120–134 J/cm²). Repeat treatment 7 days later | At 1 month, 100% CR. Only one lesion relapsed (4%) 16 months post-PDT, with excellent cosmetic results | Double treatments with ALA-PDT are effective for sBCC, particularly those located in anatomically difficult or cosmetically sensitive sites |
| Thissen et al. [26] (V/B) | 23 patients with 24 nBCCs | 20% ALA under occlusion for 6 h, irradiated with red light (630–635 nm, 120 J/cm²). Three months after PDT, all lesions biopsied for residual tumor | 92% nBCCs showed a complete response on clinical and histopathological examination | ALA-PDT red light is safe, effective, and nonsurgical treatment of nBCCs, with excellent cosmetic results |
| Soler et al. [25] (V/B) | 48 patients with 119 nBCCs (≥2 mm thick) | Debulking and topical application of DMSO, followed by 20% ALA(3 h) and halogen light (550–700 nm, 100 J/cm²) | CR 92 and 95% at 3–6 months and at 12–26 months, respectively. 5% recurred. 91% with good to excellent cosmetic results | Curettage and DMSO as pretreatment improves ALA-PDT treatment of nBCCs |
| Wolf et al. [20] (V/B) | 13 patients with 9 AKs, 6 SCCs, 37 sBCCs, 10 nBCCs, 8 metastases of MM | 20% ALA applied under occlusion for 4–8 h before exposure to red light | Complete response after a single treatment: 9/9 AKs, 5/6 early invasive SCCs, 36/37 sBCCs, 1/10 nBCCs, 0/8 metastases of MM | ALA-PDT is effective for superficial epithelial skin tumors |

| Study | Patients | Treatment | Results | Conclusions |
|---|---|---|---|---|
| Calzavara-Pinton et al. [58] (V/B) | 85 patients with 50 AKs, 23 sBCCs, 30 nBCCs, 4 pigmented BCCs, 12 superficial SCCs, 6 nodular SCCs, 6 BD and 4 KA | 20% ALA under occlusion for 6–8 h, irradiated with 630 nm red dye laser light. Every other day treatment until complete disappearance or treatment interrupted in the case of a partial response if, after two additional treatments, no further improvement was observed | All AKs, sBCCs, BD, and KAs showed a complete response. 91.6% superficial SCCs, 80.0% nBCCs and 66.7% nodular SCCs responded completely. All four pigmented BCCs were resistant to the therapy. Final response rates: 84.0% AKs, 86.9% sBCCs, 50% nBCCs, 83.3% superficial SCCs, 33.3% nodular SCCs, 100% BDs, and 100% KAs | ALA-PDT is effective and safe for superficial skin tumors. Its use in the treatment of nodular and heavy pigmented tumors is less effective |
| Svanberg et al. [21] (V/B) | 21 patients with 55 sBCCs and 25 nBCCs, 3 patients with 10 BDs, and 2 patients with 4 CTCL | 20% ALA under occlusion for 4–6 h, followed by pulsed frequency doubled Nd:YAC laser (630 nm, 60 J/cm²) | 100% sBCCs, 64% nBCCs, and 90% BDs responded after a single laser treatment; and 100% nBCC responded after one additional treatment. 2/4 CTCL plaques resolved after two treatments, with follow-up between 6 and 14 months | ALA-PDT is very effective for sBCCs and BD, also effective for nBCCs, and may be an alternative treatment for CTCL lesions |
| Fink-Puches et al. [59] (V/B) | 47 patients with 95 sBCCs and 35 sSCCs | 20% ALA under occlusion for 4 h before exposure to either UVA or different wavebands of polychromatic visible light (full spectrum visible light, >515, >570, >610 nm) | CR 86% for sBCCs and 54% for superficial SCCs without statistical significant differences in different wave bands. At 8–9 months, recurrence rate 44% sBCCs and 69% superficial SCCs, respectively. At 36 months, the projected disease-free rate was 50% for BCC vs. 8% for SCC ($P < 0.001$) | Long-term results for ALA-PDT with polychromatic light in the treatment of superficial NMSCs are poor, particularly for SCCs |
| Fijan et al. [22] (V/B) | 49 patients with 34 sBCCs, 22 nBCCs, 43 AKs, and 10 BDs | 20% ALA with 3% DFO , applied under occlusion for 20 h. Irradiated with a halogen lamp with a red filter (300 J/cm²) | After 1× ALA-PDT, 81.4% AKs, 88.2% sBCCs, 31.8% nBCCs, 30% BDs showed complete remission | PDT with ALA-DFO is effective in the management of AKs and NMSCs |
| Dijkstra et al. [60] (V/B) | 38 patients (3 NBCNS, 1 with multiple BDs (>50% of the scalp), 34 with 35 sBCCs, 10 nBCCs, 4 large AKs and 5 BDs) | ALA applied for 8 h, followed by irradiation with blue light (400–450 nm, 10–20 J/cm²) with 30 min exposure time | Complete remission both clinically and histologically after a single treatment in 82% sBCCs (100% after a second treatment), 50% nBCCs, 1/4 AKs (partial remission 3/4), and 90–100% BDs | ALA-PDT blue light is an effective treatment for premalignant and malignant skin lesions; especially useful when there are multiple lesions or large patches |
| de Haas et al. [61] (V/B) | 164 patients (32 pts with 70 AKs, 90 pts with 430 sBCCs, 16 pts with 20 nBCCs, and 26 pts with 32 BDs) | ALA-PDT using a twofold illumination scheme (ALA applied for 4 h, and irradiated with two light fractions of 20 and 80 J/cm² separated by a 2-h interval) | Overall CR of 95% for all lesions, with complete response rate of 98% AKs, 97% sBCCs, 84% BDs, and 80% nBCC after 2 years. Cosmetic outcome was good to excellent in 95% of the treated lesions | ALA-PDT using a twofold illumination scheme led to high complete response rates at 2 years and is effective treatment for AKs and superficial NMSCs |

(continued)

**Table 6.4** (continued)

| Case series or cohort study (references) | Number of patients, type of lesions | Protocol | Results | Comments |
|---|---|---|---|---|
| Wolf et al. [30] (V/5) | Two patients with MF lesions | 20% ALA-PDT using a broad-spectrum red light source (40 J/cm²) | Both patients cleared after 4–5 ALA-PDT treatments | ALA-PDT can be effective treatment for MF lesions |
| Recio et al. [62] (V/5) | Two patients with unilesional MF | 20% ALA under occlusion for 4 h, followed by C-Beam laser 585 nm (8 J/cm², 0.45 ms without cooling); treatment repeated 3× at monthly intervals | Both patients showed clinical remission, and biopsy-confirmed histological regression. No recurrence at 24-month follow-up | ALA-PDT can be effective treatment of unilesional MF |
| Markham et al. [63] (V/5) | 1 patient with tumor stage MF | 20% ALA under occlusion for 4 h, then irradiated with Waldmann PDT lamp (580–740 nm, 20 J/cm²) | Tumor stage MF lesions cleared after five consecutive treatments over 12 weeks. Biopsy-confirmed clearance of original infiltrate of malignant T cells | ALA-PDT is beneficial for tumor stage MF |

| Randomized control study (references) | # of patients | Protocol | Results | Comments |
|---|---|---|---|---|
| Morton et al. [16] (II/A) | 19 patients with 40 BDs | Randomized to cryotherapy (20 s, 1 cycle) or ALA-PDT (20% ALA under 4 h occlusion and red light (630 nm, 125 J/cm²). All patients were reviewed at 2-month intervals for 12 months and treatments repeated if required | CR of 50 and 75% in cryotherapy and ALA-PDT, respectively, after one treatment (P=0.08). Cryotherapy was associated with ulceration (5/20), infection (2/20), and recurrent disease (2/20). No such complications occurred following PDT | ALA-PDT with a nonlaser light source is at least as effective as cryotherapy in the treatment of BD with fewer adverse effects, excellent cosmesis, and a lower recurrence rate |
| Salim et al. [17] (II/A) | 40 patients with BDs | Randomized to ALA-PDT (20% ALA with 4 h incubation, followed by red light (630 nm, 100 J/cm²)) or 5-FU (daily during week 1 and bid during weeks 2–4) | Initial CR 88 vs. 67% after ALA-PDT and 5-FU, respectively. At 12 months, complete clinical clearance rates of 82 and 48%, respectively (P=0.006, odds ratio 4.78). Side effects are more favorable in the ALA-PDT group | ALA-PDT can be considered as one of the first-line therapies in BDs, with superior efficacy to 5-FU and fewer adverse events |
| Morton et al. [64] (II/A) | 16 patients with 61 BDs | Randomized to ALA-PDT (20% ALA under 4 h occlusion) followed by irradiation with either red (630±15 nm) or green (540±15 nm) light. Repeat treatment after 2 months if necessary | Initial CR 94% (red light) vs. 72% (green light) (P=0.002). At 12 months, 2 and 7 recurrences in the red light and green light group reducing the clearance rates to 88 and 48%, respectively. Treatments were well tolerated in both groups | Green light was less effective than red light, at a theoretically equivalent dose with ALA-PDT, in the treatment of BDs |
| Wang et al. [65] (II/A) | 88 patients, one BCC from each patient | Randomized to 20% ALA-PDT (6 h incubation under occlusion followed by frequency doubled Nd:YAG laser (635 nm, 5 kHz, 100 ns) or cryotherapy (2 cycles). The follow-up period was 1 year | Histological recurrence rates 25% for ALA-PDT vs. 15% for cryosurgery. Clinical recurrence rates 5% for ALA-PDT and 13% for cryosurgery. Additional treatments needed in 30% PDT group vs. 3% cryosurgery group. The healing time was considerably shorter and the cosmetic outcome significantly better with PDT | ALA-PDT has comparable efficacy with cryosurgery as treatment for BCCs, but with better cosmetic outcome. Retreatments were more often required with PDT than with cryosurgery |

| Study | Patients | Protocol | Results | Conclusion |
|---|---|---|---|---|
| Mosterd et al. [66] (II/A) | 149 patients with 173 nBCCs | Randomized to ALA-PDT (debulking, 4 h incubation, 2× red light same day) or surgical excision (3-mm margin), followed by histological examination | At 3 months, CR 94% with ALA-PDT vs. 98% with surgical excision ($P=0.27$). A 3-year interim analysis showed cumulative incidence of failure was 2.3% for surgical excision and 30.3% for PDT ($P<0.001$) | Surgical excision proved to be significantly more effective than treatment with ALA–PDT |
| Morton et al. [67] (II/A) | 229 patients with histologically confirmed SCCis (6–40 mm) and no evidence of progression | Randomized to MAL-PDT placebo-PDT (3 h incubation followed by red light (570–670 nm, 75 J/cm²), repeated 1 week later), or standard therapies (cryotherapy (1×) or 5-FU (daily first wk, then bid wk 2–4)). Retreatment if partial response at 3 months | At 3 months, the clinically lesion CR: 93, 21, 86, and 83% in the MAL-, placebo-PDT, cryotherapy, and 5-FU group, respectively. At 12 months, 80, 67, and 69% in the MAL-PDT, cryotherapy, and 5-FU group, respectively, with a statistically significant difference between MAL-PDT and the combined standard therapy group ($P=0.04$). Recurrence rates in the MAL-PDT group (15%), compared to placebo-PDT group (50%) or cryotherapy group (21%), and similar to 5-FU group (17%). Cosmetic outcome at 3 months was good to excellent in 94% of patients treated with MAL-PDT vs. 66% with cryotherapy vs. 76% with 5-FU, and was maintained at 12 months | MAL-PDT is an effective treatment option for SCCis, with sustained lesion response rates at 12 months higher than those for cryotherapy (statistically significant) and for 5-FU (not statistically significant), with excellent overall cosmesis |
| Rhodes et al. [27] (II/A) | 101 patients with biopsy proven and previously untreated nBCCs | Randomized consecutively to MAL-PDT (two treatments 1 week apart, 3 h occlusion followed red light (570–670 nm, 75 J/cm²)) or surgical excision (≥5 mm margins) Patients were followed for 24 months | At 3 month, complete lesion response 91 vs. 98% for MAL-PDT and excision, respectively ($P=0.25$). At 12 months, 83 vs. 96% ($P=0.15$). At 24 months, 5 vs. 1 lesion had recurred in MAL-PDT and excision, respectively. Both clinician and pts favored MAL-PDT over surgery at all time points (3, 12, and 24 months) for cosmetic outcomes | Treatment of nBCCs with MAL-PDT is as effective as excision surgery at 3 months |
| Rhodes et al. [28] (II/A) | 66 patients (31 treated with MAL-PDT and 35 treated with surgery) from original study [27] completed the 5-year follow up evaluation | Same protocol as above study [27], with a 5-year follow-up evaluating recurrence rates in primary nBCCs with MAL-PDT vs. surgery | At 5 years, recurrence rates of 14 vs. 4% in MAL-PDT vs. excision groups ($P=0.09$). Estimated sustained lesion complete responses rates were 76% for MAL-PDT compared with 96% for surgery ($P=0.01$). More patients treated with MAL-PDT (87%) than surgery (54%) had an excellent or good cosmetic outcome ($P=0.007$) | Trend for higher recurrence with MAL-PDT compared to excision at 5-year follow-up, but supported MAL-PDT in the treatment of nBCCs given its moderately low 5-year lesion recurrence rate, particularly when better cosmesis was a priority |

fewer adverse effects. An overlapping group of investigators reported similar advantages for ALA-PDT compared to 5-FU in a subsequent randomized study [17].

SCCs in Caucasians result most often from chronic sun exposure. They arise from AKs and may be difficult or impossible to distinguish clinically from hypertrophic AKs. Risk of metastasis is lower than for SCCs arising in the setting of radiation dermatitis or nonhealing ulcers, but all SCCs must be regarded as potentially dangerous lesions. PDT for treatment of cutaneous SCC is not well studied, but appears far less satisfactory than for BD. A study conducted by Calzavara-Pinton et al. assessed the efficacy, prognostic features, tolerability, and cosmetic outcome of MAL-PDT for the treatment of BD and SCC [18] (V/B). They enrolled 55 patients with a total of 112 biopsy-proven BD or SCC lesions. MAL cream (160 mg/g) was applied under occlusion for 3 h prior to illumination with a light-emitting diode source (wavelength range $635 \pm 18$ nm; light dose 37 J/cm$^2$) and second treatment was given 7 days later. The overall complete response rates were 73.2% at 3 months and 53.6% at 2 years. However, complete response rates for BD (SCCis) were 87.8% at 3 months and 70.7% at 2 years; while those for microinvasive SCCs (Clark level II) and invasive SCCs (Clark level III–IV) were significantly lower, 80.0 and 45.2%, respectively at 3 months and 57.5 and 25.8%, respectively at 2 years. Clinical thickness, atypia, and lesion depth were significant predictors of the response at 3 months when using a univariate analysis ($P < 0.001$), but multivariate logistic regression analysis revealed that cell atypia was the only statistically significant independent predictor of the treatment outcome at 3 months. The authors concluded that MAL-PDT may represent a valuable, effective, and well-tolerated treatment option with good cosmetic outcome for BD and microinvasive SCC. By contrast, its use for nodular lesions, particularly if poorly differentiated keratinocytes are present, should be avoided. The authors recommended that primary PDT treatment of SCC should be reserved for early disease and must employ multiple treatments (at least two PDT treatment sessions). However, PDT may be an attractive alternative for large lesions, sites associated with significant morbidity after surgical excision, and for patients unwilling or unable to undergo conventional treatment.

## PDT for Basal Cell Carcinoma (BCC)

BCCs are the most common cutaneous malignancies with more than a million cases per year in the USA. They typically occur in sun-exposed skin, particularly on the face [19]. Traditionally BCCs are treated by surgery, ED&C, cryosurgery, or radiotherapy, all scarring forms of therapy with a recurrence rate of 5–10% [19]. Microscopically controlled excision or Mohs surgery offers a higher cure rate, but entails greater cost and use of medical resources. Thus, it is desirable to find more efficient treatments that yield cosmetically appealing results.

Superficial BCCs, also termed multicentric BCCs, typically present as well-circumscribed erythematous patches or thin plaques that rarely penetrate more than 100 μm into the dermis. These lesions respond very well to both ALA-PDT and MAL-PDT, yielding excellent cosmetic results (Table 6.4). Compared to sBCCs, nBCCs show a much lower response rate to ALA-PDT or MAL-PDT in multiple reported series [20–22], even after initial curettage to decrease lesional thickness [20], although repeated treatment sessions may improve the results [23]. One explanation for the poor response of nBCCs is that either the ALA or the light (or both) cannot penetrate deep enough into the tumor [24]. Two studies have suggested that partial debulking to reduce the thickness of the tumor improves ALA-PDT outcome in the treatment of nBCCs [25, 26], although this procedure is associated with the risk of scarring.

Few randomized studies, summarized in Table 6.4, have compared the efficacy of ALA- or MAL-PDT to other modalities such as cryotherapy and surgical excisions in the treatment of BCCs. In a multicenter, randomized, prospective study with a 5-year follow-up, comparing the efficacy and cosmesis of MAL-PDT with standard excisional surgery in the treatment of primary nodular BCCs

[27, 28], MAL-PDT was as effective as excisional surgery, as determined by clinical complete response rate at 3 months. There was a trend for higher recurrence with MAL-PDT compared to excision after 5 years (14 vs. 4%, $P=0.09$), but MAL-PDT showed better cosmetic outcomes as assessed by both clinicians and patients, supporting a role for MAL-PDT in the treatment of nBCCs given its moderately low 5-year lesion recurrence rate, particularly when better cosmesis was a priority.

## PDT in Cutaneous T Cell Lymphoma (CTCL)

ALA-PDT is particularly attractive for the treatment of mycosis fungoides (MF) lesions in which activated and malignant T lymphocytes express the transferrin receptor (CD71) at high levels. Because transferrin is involved in iron transport, CD71 expression correlates with low intracellular iron levels, and favors accumulation of PpIX, as described above. Therefore, CD71$^+$ status may predict selectivity of PDT for discrete lesions of CTCL [29]. Wolf et al. reported two patients with MF in whom prolonged remission (8 and 14 months) of MF plaques was observed after 4–5 treatments using topical 20% ALA and filtered red light [30]. In a second report, complete remissions lasting 6 and 14 months were noted in 2 of 4 CTCL lesions subjected to multiple ALA-PDT treatments [21] (Table 6.4). Based on these limited data, PDT cannot be recommended as first-line therapy for CTCL, but may be considered as alternative therapy for certain lesions.

## PDT in Melanoma

In one study, lutenizing texaphyrin, a photosensitizer activated by very deeply penetrating 752 nm red light, destroyed subcutaneous melanoma metastases in phase I trials [31]. In contrast, Wolf et al. [20] reported eight cutaneous metastases of malignant melanoma that did not respond to ALA-PDT. At present, PDT should not be considered a treatment option for cutaneous melanoma,
but might offer palliation for small cutaneous and subcutaneous metastases of advanced melanoma in some settings.

## PDT for Skin Cancer Prevention in High Risk Groups

Nevoid basal cell carcinoma syndrome (NBCCS), or Gorlin syndrome, is a rare autosomal dominant genodermatosis characterized by the appearance of multiple BCCs and caused by mutations of the tumor suppressor gene (PTCH) that negatively regulates the hedgehog signaling pathway [32, 33]. NBCCS patients typically develop multiple BCCs at an early age [34] and undergo numerous surgical procedures that, over time, disfigure them. Therefore, these patients are the excellent candidates for BCC treatment with nonsurgical modalities such as PDT, with the goal of decreasing the need for multiple surgeries. As well, they are ideal candidates for prophylactic treatments employing broad area ALA-PDT. Only a few case reports in the literature evaluate the efficacy of ALA-PDT in the management of NBCCS [23, 35, 36], but they suggest multiple benefits, including a reduced number and size of patients' presenting BCCs, improved appearance ("remodeling") of previous surgical scars, and a decreased rate of new tumor development.

A second setting with a high risk of skin cancer is chronic radiation dermatitis, now seen most often in patients treated with ionizing radiation in childhood for acne, tinea capitis, or other benign dermatoses [37]. Such patients not only typically develop numerous NMSCs, but may also experience poor healing in the damaged skin. In a small number of such patients, the authors have observed positive responses to ALA-PDT.

Increased risk of NMSC is also a recognized complication of long-term immunosuppression in organ transplant recipients. Within 5 years of solid organ transplantation, up to 40% of patients develop premalignant skin lesions such as AKs and 90% have warts, many of which are atypical and in sun-exposed areas. The development of such keratotic lesions is associated with a 100-fold increased risk of developing SCC and up to a tenfold increased risk of BCC, compared to age-matched controls [38]. The risk of developing NMSCs increases with graft survival time and duration of immunosuppressive therapy. Together these factors contribute to a tenfold increase in mortality due to SCC in transplant patients compared with the general population, highlighting the need for prevention and early treatment of premalignant lesions, minimizing progression to invasive NMSCs. Although various therapies are available, most incur considerable discomfort, scarring, and less than optimal cosmetic outcome [38]. Several studies suggest that PDT may be an effective and well-tolerated modality, not only for treatment, but also for prevention of AKs and NMSCs in the high risk transplant populations (Table 6.5).

## PDT in Photorejuvenation

Photoaging is characterized by wrinkling, coarse skin texture, pigmentary alterations, telangiectases, and often AKs. It is a nearly universal cosmetic problem for fair skinned middle-aged and elderly individuals. It is also the context in which skin cancer arises and cancer-predisposing mutations in genes such as the p53 tumor suppressor are commonly observed, even in the absence of clinical AKs [39].

Photodynamic photorejuvenation was first discussed in the literature in 2002 [40]. Since then, several case studies and split-face comparison studies using short incubation broad area ALA-PDT with IPL (red light) vs. IPL alone, a commonly employed skin rejuvenation treatment, have shown that the ALA-PDT-IPL combination is safe and more effective for facial rejuvenation than IPL treatment alone (Table 6.6), providing significantly greater improvement in global photodamage, mottled pigmentation, and fine lines. Similar improvement in photoaging was reported after a single ALA-PDT treatment using blue light (417 nm, 10 J/cm$^2$) at one- and 5-month follow-up visits [12] (Table 6.2).

More recently, Orringer et al. examined cellular and molecular changes that occur after PDT of photodamaged human skin [41]. Twenty-five volunteers aged 54–83 years with clinically apparent photodamage of the forearms were enrolled in the study. ALA was applied (under occlusion) for 3 h, followed by pulsed-dye laser therapy using nonpurpura-inducing settings to focal areas on the forearms. Serial biopsy specimens were obtained in 24 subjects taken at baseline and various times after treatment. The authors found that epidermal proliferation was stimulated as demonstrated immunohistochemically by >5-fold increases in Ki67 on day 2 ($P < 0.05$) and a slight increase in epidermal thickness sustained for at least 1 month ($P < 0.05$) after treatment. Collagen production assayed at the mRNA and protein levels was more than doubled for at least 1 month ($P < 0.05$). The authors concluded that ALA-PDT/PDL produces statistically significant molecular changes previously associated with improved appearance of the photoaging skin following resurfacing procedures [41]. The peaks in type I and III procollagen gene expression were roughly twice those produced with PDL treatment alone, reported earlier by the same group, suggesting that the photodynamic reaction enhances tissue response, consistent with the clinical experience of other investigators (Table 6.6).

## Conclusions

In the past decade, topical PDT has been employed for multiple indications. Unlike systemically administered hematoporphyrin derivatives, PpIX generated from the prodrugs ALA and its methyl ester (MAL) do not cause long-lasting generalized cutaneous photosensitization. Because of its safety and efficacy, topical PDT has received regulatory approval for AKs, BD, and basal cell carcinoma in many countries and is widely considered a first-line treatment for many cutaneous tumors. Although approved only for focal treatment of lesional skin, off-label short incubation protocols that greatly decrease the burning and stinging associated with intense porphyrin photosensitization have permitted broad area treatment that appears to offer tremendous advantages in the prevention of cutaneous malignancies and management of photoaging.

**Table 6.5**  Selected studies of ALA- or MAL-PDT for skin cancer prevention and treatment in high risk groups

| Case study (references) | # of patients | Protocol | Results | Comments |
|---|---|---|---|---|
| Itkin and Gilchrest [35] (V/B) | 2 NBCCS patients (age 21 and 47) | 20% ALA-PDT applied 1–5 h prior to blue light (417 nm, 10 J/cm²) on the face, and 67% of sBCC on the lower extremities. One course: 2× ALA-PDT 1 week apart. Each patient underwent two courses of ALA-PDT 2–4 months apart | Complete CR: 89% sBCCs, 31% nBCCs on the face, and 67% of sBCC on the lower extremities. No new BCCs developed during the 8-month follow-up period in areas treated with excellent cosmetic outcome | First report of broad application of ALA-PDT with blue light in treatment and prevention of skin cancers in NBCCS patients |
| Oseroff et al. [36] (V/B) | 3 children (age 6, 10, and 17) with NBCCS involving 12–25% of their BSA | 20% ALA (24 h under occlusion) prior to illumination with red light from two different sources under general anesthesia | After 4–7 sessions, with individual areas receiving 1–3 treatments, 85–98% overall clearance, and excellent cosmetic outcomes without scarring. Responses were durable up to 6 years | First report of broad application of ALA-PDT with red light in treatment and prevention of skin cancers in NBCCS patients |
| Gilchrest et al. [23] (V/B) | 7 NBCCS patients | ALA-PDT using a broad area, blue light (417 nm, 10 J/cm²) 1 h incubation protocol. Repeated treatment at 3–6 month intervals, with average 3-year follow-up | In all seven patients, multiple BCCs disappeared with ALA-PDT and no BCC that resolved has recurred. The number of BCCs dropped from hundreds per year prior to the therapy to only occasional BCCs | The incidence of new BCCs is greatly reduced when broad area ALA-PDT is performed on a regular basis, several times annually in NBCCS patients |
| Dragieva [68] (III/B) | 20 transplant recipients and 20 immunocompetent controls, with histologically proven AKs and BDs | Single or two consecutive treatments of topical ALA-PDT (20% ALA 5 h incubation followed by illumination with 75 J/cm² of visible light). Clinical response was evaluated at 4 and 12 weeks after treatment | The overall complete response rates in TR at 4, 12, and 48 weeks were 0.86, 0.68, and 0.48, respectively, while those in control group were 0.94. 0.89, and 0.72, respectively. The cure rates were comparable at 4 weeks but were significantly lower in TR than in controls at 12 and 48 weeks (P<0.05). Treatment was well tolerated | ALA-PDT is an effective and safe treatment for AK and BD in immunosuppressed TR, with initial response rates comparable with those in immunocompetent patients |
| Randomized control (references) | | | | |
| Dragieva et al. [69] (II/A) | 17 transplant recipients with 129 mild to moderate AKs | Two lesional areas/pt were randomized for 2× MAL- vs. placebo- (3 h incubation) PDT (600–730 nm, 75 J/cm²) 1 week apart. Evaluated at weeks 4, 8 and 16 after treatment | At 16 week, clinically complete response in 13/17, partial response 3/17, no response 1/17 in MAL-PDT treated areas vs. no response in all placebo-PDT treated areas. The overall lesion complete response rate was 56/62 for MAL-PDT and 0/67 for placebo-PDT (P=0.0003) | MAL-PDT is a safe and effective treatment for AKs in transplant recipients, particularly in patient with widespread and numerous lesions |
| Wulf et al. [70] (II/A) | 27 renal transplant patients with total of 263 lesions (AKs or other skin lesions). All patients have received immunosuppressive therapy for more than 3 years | For each patient, the two contralateral areas (5 cm diameter) were randomized to treatment (MAL-PDT, 3 h incubation followed by red light (570–670 nm, light dose 75 J/cm²)) or no treatment (control) | The mean time to occurrence of a new skin lesion (AK, BCC, keratoacanthoma, SCC or warts) was significantly longer in the treated area than the control area (9.6 vs. 6.8 months, P=0.034). At the end of 12-month follow up period. 62 vs. 35% of the patients were free from new lesions in treated vs. control areas | MAL-PDT is a promising preventative treatment for new premalignant or malignant skin lesions in immunosuppressed patients |
| Wennberg et al. [71] (II/A) | 81 transplant recipients with 889 lesions (90% AKs) | Each patient (two 50 cm² area) randomized to treatment (MAL-PDT, 3 h incubation, red light (630 nm 37 J/cm²)) vs. control areas (lesion-specific treatment, 83% cryotherapy). Two treatments 1 week apart, with additional single treatments at 3, 9, and 15 months. All visible lesions were given lesion-specific treatment 21 and 27 months | At 3 months, MAL-PDT significantly reduced the occurrence of new lesions (65 vs. 103 lesions in the control area; P=0.01), mainly AK (46% reduction, P=0.006). This effect was not significant at 27 months (253 vs. 312; P=0.06). Hypopigmentation assessed by the investigator was less evident in the treatment than control areas (16 vs. 51%, P=0.001) at 27 months | Repeated field using topical MAL-PDT may prevent new AK in transplant recipients |

**Table 6.6** Selected studies of ALA-PDT in photorejuvenation

| References | # of patients | Protocol | Results | Comments |
|---|---|---|---|---|
| Ruiz-Rodriguez et al. [40] (V/B) | 17 patients (Fitzpatrick skin types II–III) with a combination of AKs (total of 38 AKs) and diffuse photodamage | 20% ALA under occlusion for 4 h prior to pulsed-light device (615 nm cutoff filter, 40 J/cm², 4 ms double-pulse mode). Two treatments at 1-month interval | At 1 months, resolution of 76.3% AKs and adjacent photodamaged skin. At 3 months, with 2× ALA-PDT-IPL treatments, 91% AKs disappeared with excellent cosmetic results | Photodynamic photorejuvenation was first introduced in this study |
| Avram and Goldman [72] (V/B) | 17 patients | 1 h ALA incubation and IPL activation | 68% AK resolution, 55, 48, and 25% improvement in telangiectasias, pigmentary changes, and skin texture after a single treatment, respectively. Minimal change in fine wrinkles | ALA-PDT-IPL effective treatment in photorejuvenation |
| Alster et al. [73] (II/A) | 10 patients with mild to moderate photodamage | Randomized to ALA-PDT-IPL on one facial half and IPL alone on the contralateral side. Two treatments were delivered at 1-month intervals | Higher clinical improvement scores on the combination ALA-PDT-IPL treated areas in all facets of photorejuvenation, with excellent cosmetic results | ALA-PDT-IPL more effective in photorejuvenation compared to IPL alone. |
| Gold et al. [74] (IV/B) | 16 patients enrolled, 13 patients completed | One side of each patient's face received ALA-PDT-IPL (30–60 min), and the other side received IPL alone. Therapeutic course: 3× treatments at 1-month intervals | At 3 months, greater improvement in the ALA-PDT-IPL side vs. IPL side for all aspects of photodamage: crow's feet (55 vs. 29.5%), tactile skin roughness (55 vs. 29.5%), hyperpigmentation (60.3 vs. 37.2%), telangiectasia (84.6 vs. 53.8%), and AK clearance (78 vs. 53.6%) | Treatment with short contact ALA-PDT-IPL brought about greater improvement in photodamaged skin and greater clearance of AK lesions than IPL alone. |
| Dover et al. [75] (II/A) | 20 patients | A series of three split-face treatments 3 weeks apart: half of the face pretreated with ALA (30–60 min incubation) followed by IPL treatment while the other half was treated with IPL alone (515–1,200 nm, 23–28 J/cm²). Two additional full-face treatments with IPL alone 3 weeks apart to all subjects | ALA-PDT-IPL resulted in more improvement in photoaging (80 vs. 45%, $P=0.008$), mottled pigmentation (95 vs. 60%, $P=0.008$), and fine lines (60 vs. 25% patients; $P=0.008$) than IPL alone. The final investigator cosmetic evaluations ($P=0.0002$) and subject satisfaction scores ($P=0.005$) were significantly better for the ALA pretreated side | ALA-PDT-IPL resulted in greater improvement in photorejuvenation than IPL alone. |

Evaluation of the PDT literature is challenging due to the multiple treatment protocols (focal/broad area, ± curettage, one vs. multiple sessions), photosensitizers, incubation times, light source employed, and follow-up times, as well as inconsistent outcome measures. Nevertheless, well-designed, randomized studies summarized above clearly support the safety and efficacy of PDT in the treatment of AKs and several types of NMSCs.

PDT heralds a revolution in nonsurgical approaches to NMSCs. Surgery, whether conventional or micrographically controlled, requires a high level of skill, is often time-consuming and expensive, and always scars. Multiple well-designed, randomized studies demonstrate good to excellent efficacy of PDT in the treatment of BDs and BCCs after one or two sessions, with an acceptable recurrence rate. Critically, patients overwhelmingly favor PDT over surgery or other destructive modalities. Therefore, PDT offers a safe, effective, convenient, and nonscarring treatment modality for many superficial NMSCs.

Most importantly, PDT offers the prospect of reducing the development of both premalignant and malignant skin lesions in patients at high risk by virtue of severe photodamage, genetic predisposition, or iatrogenic immunosuppression. Aside from sun avoidance and sunscreen use, there is currently no other approach to this unmet medical need. Hopefully, this as yet insufficiently documented potential benefit of broad area PDT will become better established in the coming years.

## Evidence-Based Summary

| Findings | Evidence level |
|---|---|
| PDT (either ALA or MAL) should be considered as first-line treatment for AKs, with comparable response rates, but superior comesis to topical 5-FU or cryotherapy | I/A |
| PDT (either ALA or MAL) should be considered as a first-line therapy for BDs, with similar efficacy as cryotherapy or 5-FU, but fewer adverse events | I/A |
| PDT is currently not recommended for routine use in the treatment of SCC | V/B |
| PDT (either ALA or MAL) should be considered as a first-line therapy for sBCC, particularly for large, extensive, and multiple lesions; MAL-PDT demonstrated long-term efficacy based on 5-year follow-up data | I/A |
| MAL-PDT is effective and reliable treatment option for nBCC (<2 mm deep) with good cosmetic outcome and long-term efficacy based on 5-year follow-up data | I/A |
| PDT cannot be recommended as first-line therapy, may be considered as an alternative treatment option for certain lesions of CTCL or MM | V/B |
| PDT may be considered as a method of preventing new AKs and NMSCs in immunosuppressed patients | II/A |
| PDT may be considered as a method of preventing BCCs in patients with Gorlin syndrome | V/B |
| ALA-PDT in combination with IPL provides significantly greater improvement in the treatment of facial photoaging than treatment with IPL alone | II/A |

# References

1. Szeimies RM, Dräger J, Abels C, Landthaler M. History of photodynamic therapy in dermatology. In: Calzavara-Pinton PG, Szeimies RM, Ortel B, editors. Photodynamic therapy and fluorescence diagnosis in dermatology. Amsterdam: Elsevier; 2001. p. 3–16.
2. Kennedy JC, Pottier RH, Pross DC. Photodynamic therapy with endogenous protoporphyrin IX: basic principles and present clinical experience. J Photochem Photobiol B. 1990;6:143–8.
3. Farah JB, Ralston J, Zeitouni NC, Oseroff AR. ALA-PDT treatment of pre-skin cancer. In: Goldman MP, editor. Photodynamic therapy. Philadelphia: Elsevier; 2005. p. 53–63.
4. Choudry K, Brooke RC, Farrar W, Rhodes LE. The effect of an iron chelating agent on protoporphyrin IX levels and phototoxicity in topical 5-aminolaevulinic acid photodynamic therapy. Br J Dermatol. 2003; 149(1):124–30.
5. Morton CA, Brown SB, Collins S, Ibbotson S, Jenkinson H, Kurwa H, et al. Guidelines for topical photodynamic therapy: report of a workshop of the British Photodermatology Group. Br J Dermatol. 2002;146:552–67.
6. Braathen LR, Szeimies RM, Basset-Seguin N, Bissonnette R, Foley P, Pariser D, et al. International Society for Photodynamic Therapy in Dermatology. Guidelines on the use of photodynamic therapy for nonmelanoma skin cancer: an international consensus. J Am Acad Dermatol. 2007;56:125–43.
7. Salasche SJ. Epidemiology of actinic keratoses and squamous cell carcinoma. J Am Acad Dermatol. 2000;42(1 Pt 2):4–7.
8. Drake LA, Ceilley RI, Cornelison RL, et al. Guidelines of care for actinic keratoses. J Am Acad Dermatol. 1995;32:95–8.
9. Stockfleth E, Kerl H. Guidelines for the management of actinic keratoses. Eur J Dermatol. 2006;16:599–606.
10. Jeffes EW, McCullough JL, Weinstein GD, Kaplan R, Glazer SD, Taylor JR. Photodynamic therapy of actinic keratoses with topical aminolevulinic acid hydrochloride and fluorescent blue light. J Am Acad Dermatol. 2001;45:96–104.
11. Piacquadio DJ, Chen DM, Farber HF, Fowler Jr JF, Glazer SD, Goodman JJ, et al. Photodynamic therapy with aminolevulinic acid topical solution and visible blue light in the treatment of multiple actinic keratoses of the face and scalp: investigator-blinded, phase 3, multicenter trials. Arch Dermatol. 2004;140:41–6.
12. Touma D, Yaar M, Whitehead S, Konnikov N, Gilchrest BA. A trial of short incubation, broad-area photodynamic therapy for facial actinic keratoses and diffuse photodamage. Arch Dermatol. 2004;140:33–40.
13. Szeimies RM, Karrer S, Radakovic-Fijan S, Tanew A, Calzavara-Pinton PG, Zane C, et al. Photodynamic therapy using topical methyl 5-aminolevulinate compared with cryotherapy for actinic keratosis: a prospective, randomized study. J Am Acad Dermatol. 2002;47:258–62.
14. Moloney FJ, Collins P. Randomized, double-blind, prospective study to compare topical 5-aminolaevulinic acid methylester with topical 5-aminolaevulinic acid photodynamic therapy for extensive scalp actinic keratosis. Br J Dermatol. 2007;157:87–91.
15. Cox NH, Eedy DJ, Morton CA. Therapy Guidelines and Audit Subcommittee, British Association of Dermatologists. Guidelines for management of Bowen's disease: 2006 update. Br J Dermatol. 2007; 156(1):11–21.
16. Morton CA, Whitehurst C, Moseley H, et al. Comparison of photodynamic therapy with cryotherapy in the treatment of Bowen's disease. Br J Dermatol. 1996;135:766–71.
17. Salim A, Leman JA, McColl JH, Chapman R, Morton CA. Randomized comparison of photodynamic therapy with topical 5-fluorouracil in Bowen's disease. Br J Dermatol. 2003;148:539–43.
18. Calzavara-Pinton PG, Venturini M, Sala R, Capezzera R, Parrinello G, Specchia C, et al. Methylaminolaevulinate-based photodynamic therapy of Bowen's disease and squamous cell carcinoma. Br J Dermatol. 2008;159(1):137–44.
19. Telfer NR, Colver GB, Morton CA. British association of dermatologists. Guidelines for the management of basal cell carcinoma. Br J Dermatol. 2008;159(1):35–48.
20. Wolf P, Rieger E, Kerl H. Topical photodynamic therapy with endogenous porphyrins after application of 5-aminolevulinic acid: an alternative treatment modality for solar keratoses, superficial squamous cell carcinomas, and basal cell carcinomas? J Am Acad Dermatol. 1993;28:17–21.
21. Svanberg K, Andersson T, Killander D, et al. Photodynamic therapy of non-melanoma malignant tumours of the skin using topical d aminolevulinic acid sensitization and laser irradiation. Br J Dermatol. 1994;130:743–51.
22. Fijan S, Honigsmann H, Ortel B. Photodynamic therapy of epithelial skin tumours using delta-aminolaevulinic acid and desferrioxamine. Br J Dermatol. 1995;133:282–8.
23. Gilchrest BA, Brightman LA, Thiele JJ, Wasserman DI. Photodynamic therapy for patients with basal cell nevus syndrome. Dermatol Surg. 2009;35(10):1576–81.
24. Morton CA, MacKie RM. Photodynamic therapy for basal cell carcinoma: effect of tumour thickness and duration of photosensitizer application on response. Arch Dermatol. 1998;134:248–9.
25. Soler AM, Warloe T, Tausjo J, Berner A. Photodynamic therapy by topical aminolevulinic acid, dimethylsulphoxide and curettage in nodular basal cell carcinoma: a one-year follow-up study. Acta Derm Venereol. 1999;79:204–6.
26. Thissen MR, Schroeter CA, Neumann HA. Photodynamic therapy with delta-aminolaevulinic acid for nodular basal cell carcinomas using a prior debulking technique. Br J Dermatol. 2000;142: 338–9.
27. Rhodes LE, de Rie M, Enström Y, Groves R, Morken T, Goulden V, et al. Photodynamic therapy using topical

methyl aminolevulinate versus surgery for nodular basal cell carcinoma: results of a multicenter randomized prospective trial. Arch Dermatol. 2004;140:17–23.

28. Rhodes LE, de Rie MA, Leifsdottir R, Yu RC, Bachmann I, Goulden V, et al. Five-year follow-up of a randomized, prospective trial of topical methyl aminolevulinate photodynamic therapy vs surgery for nodular basal cell carcinoma. Arch Dermatol. 2007; 143:1131–6.

29. Rittenhouse-Diakun K, Van Leengoed H, Morgan J, et al. The role of transferring receptor (CD71) in photodynamic therapy of activated and malignant lymphocytes using the heme precursor or delta-aminolevulinic acid (ALA). Photochem Photobiol. 1995;61:523–8.

30. Wolf P, Fink-Puches R, Kerl H. Photodynamic therapy for mycosis fungoides after topical photosensitization with 5-aminolevulinic acid. J Am Acad Dermatol. 1995;33:541.

31. Kalka K, Merk H, Mukhtar H. Photodynamic therapy in dermatology. J Am Acad Dermatol. 2000;42: 389–413.

32. Hahn H, Wicking C, Zaphiropoulous PG, et al. Mutations of the human homolog of Drosophila patched in the nevoid basal cell carcinoma syndrome. Cell. 1996;85(6):841–51.

33. Johnson RL, Rothman AL, Xie J, et al. Human homolog of patched, a candidate gene for the basal cell nevus syndrome. Science. 1996;272(5268):1668–71.

34. Gorlin RJ. Nevoid basal cell carcinoma (Gorlin) syndrome. Genet Med. 2004;6(6):530–9.

35. Itkin A, Gilchrest BA. Delta-Aminolevulinic acid and blue light photodynamic therapy for treatment of multiple basal cell carcinomas in two patients with nevoid basal cell carcinoma syndrome. Dermatol Surg. 2004;30:1054–61.

36. Oseroff AR, Shieh S, Frawley NP, Cheney R, Blumenson LE, Pivnick EK, et al. Treatment of diffuse basal cell carcinomas and basaloid follicular hamartomas in nevoid basal cell carcinoma syndrome by wide-area 5-aminolevulinic acid photodynamic therapy. Arch Dermatol. 2005;141:60–7.

37. Karagas MR, McDonald JA, Greenberg ER, Stukel TA, Weiss JE, Baron JA, et al. Risk of basal cell and squamous cell skin cancers after ionizing radiation therapy. J Natl Cancer Inst. 1996;88:1848–53.

38. Berg D, Otley CC. Skin cancer in organ transplant recipients: epidemiology, pathogenesis, and management. J Am Acad Dermatol. 2002;47:1–17.

39. Liang SB, Ohtsuki Y, Furihata M, Takeuchi T, Iwata J, Chen BK, et al. Sun-exposure- and aging-dependent p53 protein accumulation result in growth advantage for tumour cells in carcinogenesis of nonmelanocytic skin cancer. Virchows Arch. 1999;434:193–9.

40. Ruiz-Rodriguez R, Sanz-Sánchez T, Córdoba S. Photodynamic photorejuvenation. Dermatol Surg. 2002;28:742–4.

41. Orringer JS, Hammerberg C, Hamilton T, Johnson TM, Kang S, Sachs DL, et al. Molecular effects of photodynamic therapy for photoaging. Arch Dermatol. 2008;144(10):1296–302.

42. Kochevar IE, Taylor CR, Krutmann J. Fundamentals of cutaneous photobiology and photoimmunology. In: Wolff K, Austen KF, Goldsmith LA, et al., editors. Fitzpatrick's dermatology in general medicine. New York: McGraw-Hill; 2007. p. 803.

43. Szeimies RM, Karrer S, Sauerwald A, Landthaler M. Photodynamic therapy with topical application of 5-aminolevulinic acid in the treatment of actinic keratoses: an initial clinical study. Dermatology. 1996;192: 246–51.

44. Jeffes EW, McCullough JL, Weinstein GD, Fergin PE, Nelson JS, Shull TF, et al. Photodynamic therapy of actinic keratosis with topical 5-aminolevulinic acid: a pilot dose-ranging study. Arch Dermatol. 1997;133: 727–32.

45. Goldman M, Atkin D. ALA/PDT in the treatment of actinic keratosis: spot versus confluent therapy. J Cosmet Laser Ther. 2003;5:107–10.

46. Alexiades-Armenakas MR, Geronemus RG. Laser-mediated photodynamic therapy of actinic keratoses. Arch Dermatol. 2003;139:1313–20.

47. Tschen EH, Wong DS, Pariser DM, Dunlap FE, Houlihan A, Ferdon MB. Photodynamic therapy using aminolaevulinic acid for patients with nonhyperkeratotic actinic keratoses of the face and scalp: phase IV multicentre clinical trial with 12-month follow up. Br J Dermatol. 2006;155:1262–9.

48. Kurwa HA, Yong-Gee SA, Seed PT, et al. A randomized paired comparison of photodynamic therapy and topical 5-fluorouracil in the treatment of actinic keratoses. J Am Acad Dermatol. 1999;41:414–8.

49. Radakovic-Fijan S, Blecha-Thalhammer U, Kittler H, Hönigsmann H, Tanew A. Efficacy of 3 different light doses in the treatment of actinic keratosis with 5-aminolevulinic acid photodynamic therapy: a randomized, observer-blinded, intrapatient, comparison study. J Am Acad Dermatol. 2005;53:823–7.

50. Smith S, Piacquadio D, Morhenn V, Atkin D, Fitzpatrick R. Short incubation PDT versus 5-FU in treating actinic keratoses. J Drugs Dermatol. 2003;2: 629–35.

51. Pariser DM, Lowe NJ, Stewart DM, Jarratt MT, Lucky AW, Pariser RJ, et al. Photodynamic therapy with topical methyl aminolevulinate for actinic keratosis: results of a prospective randomized multicenter trial. J Am Acad Dermatol. 2003;48:227–32.

52. Pariser D, Loss R, Jarratt M, Abramovits W, Spencer J, Geronemus R, et al. Topical methyl-aminolevulinate photodynamic therapy using red light-emitting diode light for treatment of multiple actinic keratoses: a randomized, double-blind, placebo-controlled study. J Am Acad Dermatol. 2008;59(4):569–76.

53. Stables GI, Stringer MR, Robinson DJ, Ash DV. Large patches of Bowen's disease treated by topical aminolaevulinic acid photodynamic therapy. Br J Dermatol. 1997;136:957–60.

54. Morton CA, Whitehurst C, McColl JH, Moore JV, MacKie RM. Photodynamic therapy for large or multiple patches of Bowen's disease and basal cell carcinoma. Arch Dermatol. 2001;137:319–24.

55. Britton JE, Goulden V, Stables G, Stringer M, Sheehan-Dare R. Investigation of the use of the pulsed dye laser in the treatment of Bowen's disease using 5-aminolaevulinic acid phototherapy. Br J Dermatol. 2005;153:780–4.

56. Wennberg AM, Lindholm LE, Alpsten M, Larko O. Treatment o superficial basal cell carcinomas using topically applied deltaaminolaevulinic acid and a filtered xenon lamp. Arch Dermatol Res. 1996;288:561–4.

57. Haller JC, Cairnduff F, Slack G, Schofield J, Whitehurst C, Tunstall R, et al. Routine double treatments of superficial basal cell carcinomas using aminolaevulinic acid-based photodynamic therapy. Br J Dermatol. 2000;143:1270–5.

58. Calzavara-Pinton PG. Repetitive photodynamic therapy with topical delta-aminolaevulinic acid as an appropriate approach to the routine treatment of superficial non-melanoma skin tumours. J Photochem Photobiol B. 1995;29:53–7.

59. Fink-Puches R, Soyer HP, Hofer A, Kerl H, Wolf P. Long-term follow-up and histological changes of superficial nonmelanoma skin cancers treated with topical delta-aminolevulinic acid photodynamic therapy. Arch Dermatol. 1998;134:821–6.

60. Dijkstra AT, Majoie IM, van Dongen JW, van Weelden H, van Vloten WA. Photodynamic therapy with violet light and topical 6-aminolaevulinic acid in the treatment of actinic keratosis, Bowen's disease and basal cell carcinoma. J Eur Acad Dermatol Venereol. 2001;15:550–4.

61. de Haas ER, de Vijlder HC, Sterenborg HJ, Neumann HA, Robinson DJ. Fractionated aminolevulinic acid-photodynamic therapy provides additional evidence for the use of PDT for non-melanoma skin cancer. J Eur Acad Dermatol Venereol. 2008;22:426–30.

62. Recio ED, Zambrano B, Alonso ML, de Eusebio E, Martín M, Cuevas J, et al. Topical 5-aminolevulinic acid photodynamic therapy for the treatment of unilesional mycosis fungoides: a report of two cases and review of the literature. Int J Dermatol. 2008;47(4):410–3.

63. Markham T, Sheahan K, Collins P. Topical 5-aminolaevulinic acid photodynamic therapy for tumour-stage mycosis fungoides. Br J Dermatol. 2001;144(6):1262–3.

64. Morton CA, Whitehurst C, Moore JV, MacKie RM. Comparison of red and green light in the treatment of Bowen's disease by photodynamic therapy. Br J Dermatol. 2000;143:767–72.

65. Wang I, Bendsoe N, Klinteberg CA, Enejder AM, Andersson-Engels S, Svanberg S, et al. Photodynamic therapy vs. cryosurgery of basal cell carcinomas: results of a phase III clinical trial. Br J Dermatol. 2001;144:832–40.

66. Mosterd K, Thissen MR, Nelemans P, Kelleners-Smeets NW, Janssen RL, Broekhof KG, et al. Fractionated 5-aminolaevulinic acid-photodynamic therapy vs. surgical excision in the treatment of nodular basal cell carcinoma: results of a randomized controlled trial. Br J Dermatol. 2008;159(4):864–70.

67. Morton C, Horn M, Leman J, Tack B, Bedane C, Tjioe M, et al. Comparison of topical methyl aminolevulinate photodynamic therapy with cryotherapy or fluorouracil for treatment of squamous cell carcinoma in situ: results of a multicenter randomized trial. Arch Dermatol. 2006;142:729–35.

68. Dragieva G, Hafner J, Dummer R, Schmid-Grendelmeier P, Roos M, Prinz BM, et al. Topical photodynamic therapy in the treatment of actinic keratoses and Bowen's disease in transplant recipients. Transplantation. 2004;77:115–21.

69. Dragieva G, Prinz BM, Hafner J, Dummer R, Burg G, Binswanger U, et al. A randomized controlled clinical trial of topical photodynamic therapy with methyl aminolaevulinate in the treatment of actinic keratoses in transplant recipients. Br J Dermatol. 2004;151:196–200.

70. Wulf HC, Pavel S, Stender I, Bakker-Wensveen CA. Topical photodynamic therapy for prevention of new skin lesions in renal transplant recipients. Acta Derm Venereol. 2006;86:25–8.

71. Wennberg AM, Stenquist B, Stockfleth E, Keohane S, Lear JT, Jemec G, et al. Photodynamic therapy with methyl aminolevulinate for prevention of new skin lesions in transplant recipients: a randomized study. Transplantation. 2008;86:423–9.

72. Avram DK, Goldman MP. Effectiveness and safety of ALA-IPL in treating actinic keratoses and photodamage. J Drugs Dermatol. 2004;3(1 Suppl):S36–9.

73. Alster TS, Tanzi EL, Welsh EC. Photorejuvination of facial skin with topical 20% 5-aminolevulinic acid and intense pulsed light treatment: a split-face comparison study. J Drugs Dermatol. 2005;4:35–8.

74. Gold MH, Bradshaw VL, Boring MM, Bridges TM, Biron JA. Split-face comparison of photodynamic therapy with 5-aminolevulinic acid and intense pulsed light versus intense pulsed light alone for photodamage. Dermatol Surg. 2006;32:795–801.

75. Dover JS, Bhatia AC, Stewart B, Arndt KA. Topical 5-aminolevulinic acid combined with intense pulsed light in the treatment of photoaging. Arch Dermatol. 2005;141:1247–52.

## Self-Assessment

1. PDT requires which of the following components?
   (a) Photosensitizing drugs
   (b) Activating wavelength of light
   (c) Oxygen
   (d) All of the above

2. Topical PDT is strongly recommended for which of the following indications? (choose all that apply)
   (a) AKs, grade 1
   (b) AKs, grade 3
   (c) sBCCs
   (d) Melanoma in situ
   (e) SCC in situ
   (f) MF

3. Advantages of broad area PDT compared to conventional surgical excision for small basal cell carcinomas include: (choose all that apply)
   (a) Higher 5-year cure rate
   (b) Better cosmesis
   (c) Lower cost
   (d) Possible reduction in incidence of new tumors

4. The characteristic of PDT that best determines treatment-associated patient discomfort: (choose one only)
   (a) MAL vs. ALA as the topically applied drug
   (b) Length of MAL or ALA incubation
   (c) Wavelength of light source
   (d) Pretreatment of the skin with DFO

5. Identify the following statements as true (T) or false (F):
   (a) ALA-PDT and MAL-PDT use different photosensitizers. T/F
   (b) MAL-PDT is effective only when red light is employed. T/F
   (c) Blue light photons are better absorbed by protoporphyrin than red light photons. T/F
   (d) Red light photons penetrate more deeply into skin on average than blue light photons. T/F

## Answers

1. d: All of the above
2. a, c, & e: AKs, grade 1, sBCCs, and SCC in situ
3. b, c, & d: Better cosmesis, lower cost, and possible reduction in incidence of new tumors
4. b: Length of MAL or ALA incubation
5. (a) False
   (b) False
   (c) True
   (d) True

# Treatment of Precancers with Topical Agents

Bahar Firoz and Arash Kimyai-Asadi

## Introduction and Definition of Procedures to Be Discussed

Actinic keratosis (AK), also termed solar keratosis and senile keratosis, is a very common lesion of the skin and is a potential precursor to squamous cell carcinoma (SCC). Estimates of AK progression to invasive SCC range from less than 1 to16% [1]. SCC of the skin has the potential to metastasize and may account for up to 20% of deaths from skin cancer [2]. With the incidence of nonmelanoma skin cancer on the rise, treatment for AKs has been recommended to reduce the development of invasive SCC, to lower healthcare expenditure, and for patient well-being [3, 4]. The likelihood of an invasive SCC evolving from one AK lesion has been estimated to occur at a rate of 0.075–0.096% per lesion per year. For a person with the average number of AKs, or 7.7 AKs, SCC would develop at a rate of 10.2% over 10 years. Other estimates quote even higher rates for untreated lesions, from 13 to 20% over a 10-year period [4].

AKs are usually diagnosed clinically, and appear as red–brown macules, papules, or plaques with scale which may be significantly hyperkeratotic. They may appear in conjunction with other signs of solar damage, specifically telangiectasias, solar lentigines, rhytides, and poikiloderma. Histologically, AKs exhibit varying degrees of intraepidermal keratinocytic atypia. Clinical and histological subtypes of AKs include the classic variant already described, hyperplastic (or hyperkeratotic), pigmented, lichenoid, atrophic, bowenoid, "cutaneous horn," and actinic cheilitis.

Much like nonmelanoma skin cancer, AKs are thought to develop due to ultraviolet light exposure and resulting DNA mutations. They also occur more frequently in fairer skinned individuals but can be seen in all races. Most AKs occur in sun-exposed areas such as the head, lower lip, neck, dorsal hands, forearms, and upper chest. Increasing age, male gender, a history of AKs, and nonmelanoma skin cancer are other risk factors for developing AKs. High-risk AKs are mainly associated with immunosuppression. Organ-transplant recipients have a 250-fold higher risk of developing AKs and a 100-fold higher risk of developing invasive SCCs [5]. While approximately 40% of immunosuppressed patients develop invasive SCC, only 6–16% of immunocompetent individuals with AKs show this progression [5].

B. Firoz (✉)
Department of Dermatology, University of Texas Health Science Center San Antonio, MC 7876, CTRC 3rd Floor Grossman, 7979 Wurzbach, San Antonio, TX 78229, USA
e-mail: bahar.firoz@gmail.com

A. Kimyai-Asadi
Dermsurgery Associates, 7515 South Main Street, Suite 290, Houston, TX 77030, USA

M. Alam (ed.), *Evidence-Based Procedural Dermatology*,
DOI 10.1007/978-0-387-09424-3_7, © Springer Science+Business Media, LLC 2012

Several treatment modalities have been employed to treat AKs in an attempt to prevent progression to invasive SCC. The modalities which will be discussed and evaluated in this chapter include topical sunscreen, cryosurgery with liquid nitrogen, topical 5 and 0.5% 5-fluorouracil (5-FU) (Efudex and Carac), topical 5% imiquimod cream (Aldara), topical diclofenac with sodium hyaluronate gel (Solaraze), and chemical peels including trichloroacetic acid and Jessner's solution applied to affected skin.

Topical sunscreens are applied to the skin and ideally block both UVA and UVB ultraviolet radiation, theoretically preventing the formation of AKs. Topical 5FU is a chemotherapeutic antimetabolite that interferes with DNA synthesis and is approved by the United States Food and Drug Administration (US FDA) for treatment of AKs. This effect is thought to target rapidly dividing tumor cells. Topical 5% imiquimod cream is a newer topical agent, also approved by the US FDA for AK treatment. It is a topical immunomodulator, and is a toll-like receptor-7 agonist, activating antigen-presenting cells to produce interferon, other cytokines, and chemokines. These cytokines stimulate the nonspecific innate immune response and help direct the acquired immune response. Side effects include burning, erythema, and crusting. The mechanism of action of topical diclofenac with sodium hyaluronate gel is not completely understood; however, it is thought to be related to NSAID inhibition of the cyclo-oxygenase pathway and a possible reduction in the end products of arichodonic acid metabolism. Common side effects include dermatitis, pruritus, and xerosis.

Cryosurgery is a destructive method that utilizes liquid nitrogen (−196°C) to freeze and thereby destroy both normal and dysplastic cells, and eliminate diseased epidermis by creating a separation of the epidermis from the dermis. Side effects include pain, blistering, hypopigmentation, and scar. Chemical peels are also an ablative modality, and chemically destroy the epidermis and variable depths of the dermis depending on the type of peel. Peels are typically applied to the general affected area, as opposed to spot-treatment of individual lesions. Side effects include pain, infection, hypopigmentation, and scar.

# Consensus Documents Regarding Procedure

Several consensus documents exist regarding AKs and the treatments employed to eliminate them. The American Academy of Dermatology (AAD) committee on the guidelines of care and task force on AKs published guidelines of care for AKs in 1995 [6]. They defined AKs as common premalignant skin tumors which show varying degrees of epidermal atypia and that may progress to SCC. They estimated that 60% of predisposed persons older than 40 years have at least one AK. Without treatment for AKs, they assert that a significant number of patients will develop one or more invasive SCCs. They also comment on several risk factors for the development of AKs, including but not limited to "fair skin, excessive UV exposure whether occupational or recreational, ionizing radiation, geographic latitude, reflectants, immunosuppression, and certain genodermatoses." They list several treatment modalities, and recommend consideration be given to size, location, duration, change in growth pattern, previous treatment, and certain anatomic locations such as the scalp and ear [6].

The European Dermatology Forum has also published guidelines for the management of AKs in 2006 [5]. They assert that AKs "should be classified as in situ SCC" [5]. They mention UV exposure with or without iatrogenic exposure to psoralens and human papilloma virus as risk factors for the development of AKs. They quote a 15% prevalence rate of AKs in men and 6% in women based on a UK study. They quote a prevalence of 11–26% in the USA and 37–55% in Australia. They also mention that organ-transplanted patients have a 250-fold higher risk of developing AKs and a 100-fold higher risk of developing invasive SCCs. They also state that 40% of immunosuppressed patients develop invasive SCCs whereas only 10% of immunocompetent patients with AKs show this type of progression. Before discussing treatment modalities, they also recommend evaluating the duration and course of lesions, whether the AKs are solitary or multiple, patient age, co-morbid conditions, the patient's mental condition, anticipated patient compliance, pre-existing skin cancers, and particularly immunosuppression. They discuss that although cryotherapy is widely used, controlled studies are missing. Complete responses differ from 75 to 98% and recurrence rates are estimated from 1.2 to 12% at 1-year follow-up. Chemical peeling is recommended for extensive facial AKs, and the efficacy depends on the agent used and is quoted to be around 75% with a recurrence rate at 1 year between 25 and 35%. Imiquimod is discussed with impressive remission rates and low recurrence rates, with potential side effects including the "lighting-up" of subclinical AKs, local irritant skin reactions, and fever-like symptoms. Topical 5-FU also boasts impressive remission rates, particularly for localized disease, and potential severe irritant dermatitis may be minimized with "pulse" therapy. Diclofenac in hyaluronic acid gel also shows AK remission in a few randomized controlled trials when applied for 60 or 90 days with minimal side effects. Finally, they recommend regular follow-up.

The British Association of Dermatologists has also published guidelines for the management of AKs in 2006 [7]. In contrast to the European guidelines, they define AKs as "focal areas of abnormal keratinocyte proliferation with low risk of progression to invasive squamous cell carcinoma…and higher potential for spontaneous regression." The authors discuss several factors to help determine the choice for therapy, based on efficacy, ease of use, morbidity, and cost–benefit analysis. They conclude that "there is good evidence that 5% 5-FU cream used twice daily for 3 weeks is effective at reducing AKs on the face and back of hands by about 70% for up to 12 months. There is insufficient RCT evidence to support or refute the efficacy of alternative regimens and formulations, although one RCT suggests that a single night-time application for 3 months for AKs on the back of hands is effective. Imiquimod has been more rigorously assessed with modern RCT design and may produce a similar pattern of side-effects and response to 5-FU. Diclofenac gel is a relatively mild agent that reduces the AK count but there are no follow-up data beyond 1 month. Topical tretinoin has some efficacy on the face, with partial clearance of AKs, but may need to be used for up to a year at a time to optimize benefit. Sun block, emollient, and 2% salicylic acid ointment may reduce the AK count by a similar amount" [7].

## Case Series and Cohort Studies

### Medium-Depth Chemical Peels

Two patients were treated successfully with trichloroacetic acid peels for extensive AKs on the face and scalp. No long-term follow-up was provided (V/B) [8]. Seventy percent glycolic acid plus 35% trichloroacetic acid was compared to Jessner's plus 35% trichloroacetic acid when applied to the right versus the left face in 13 patients. AKs, fine wrinkling, and solar lentigines were evaluated prospectively with a 60-day follow-up. Improvement was clinically noted for both peels (IV/B) [9].

Eight patients with severe facial actinic damage were treated on the left face with Jessner's and 35% trichloroacetic acid and on the right face with twice daily application of 5% 5-FU cream for 3 weeks. Clinical evaluation was performed at 1, 6, 12, and 32 months and included AK counts, random skin biopsies, and sun exposure surveys. A 78% reduction in the mean number of clinical AKs was observed at 12 months for both treatments, but the mean number of AKs increased between 12 and 32 months. They suggest 18-month follow-up in all AK patients (IV/B) [10].

Sixteen men with actinic damage were treated with 40% trichloroacetic acid peels and evaluated at 6 weeks and 6 months after treatment. Half were pretreated and post-treated with topical tretinoin. Examiners assessed clinical outcome using photographs, and patients used a self-assessment tool. The peel, both with and without tretinoin, produced improvements in actinic damage, although quantitative measures are lacking in this study (V/B) [11].

### Cryosurgery

A retrospective study investigating cryosurgery for the treatment of AKs evaluated cure rates in 70 patients with 1,018 lesions. Follow-up ranged from 1 to 8.5 years and demonstrated a cure rate of 99%. No histologic confirmation of AK resolution was obtained (III/A) [12].

In a prospective, multicentered, nonblinded study, which was a subsidiary of a randomized controlled trial, 90 adult patients with 421 AKs were treated with cryotherapy. Lesions of 5 mm or greater in size on the face and scalp were evaluated based on clinical diagnosis only, and freeze-thaw cycles of differing lengths were employed depending on the treatment center. At 3-month follow-up, lesions were assessed for complete response and cosmetic outcome. There was a 57% complete clearance rate in the intention to treat population. Complete response was 39% for freeze times less than 5 s, 69% for freeze times greater than 5 s, and 83% for freeze times greater than 20 s (III/B) [13].

## Randomized Controlled Trials (RCTs) and Meta-Analyses

### Sunscreen

A blinded, RCT undertaken during one summer in Australia between September 1991 and March 1992 evaluated the effect of sunscreen with sun-protection factor of 17 vs. vehicle cream on AKs in 431 subjects aged 40 years or older. AKs were diagnosed clinically, although a subsample had biopsies for verification and there was 81% concordance between clinical and histologic diagnosis. Subjects kept daily diaries, recording the application of cream and were asked to avoid sun and use of other sunscreen products during the study. Patients were evaluated over 7 months, and 25% of the AK lesions present at baseline had remitted in the sunscreen group compared to 18% in the vehicle cream group. The mean number of AKs increased by 1 per subject in the vehicle cream group, whereas it decreased by 0.6 per subject in the sunscreen group (II/A) [14].

### Cryotherapy

In a multicenter, randomized, controlled, open study, the efficacy of cryotherapy vs. methyl aminolevulinate photodynamic therapy (MAL-PDT) of facial and scalp AKs was assessed via right–left comparison. One hundred and twenty-one patients with 1,343 lesions, the majority (98%) on the extremities, were evaluated at 12 and 24 weeks. Information on the duration of the freeze cycle was unavailable, but depended on the study site; the mean total freezing time for cryotherapy was 20 s. At the end of the study, MAL-PDT showed a 78% mean percent reduction in AK compared to 88% for cryotherapy (II/A) [15].

A randomized trial compared cryosurgery (20–40 s per lesion), topical 5-FU applied twice daily for 4 weeks, and 1 or 2 courses of imiquimod 3 times weekly applied overnight for 4 weeks with a 12-month follow-up period. Seventy-five patients with AKs diagnosed clinically and confirmed histologically were enrolled. Initial clearance of lesions 6–8 weeks after therapy completion, as evaluated clinically, was 96% (23/24) for 5-FU, 85% (22/26) for imiquimod, and 68% (17/25) for cryosurgery. When confirmed histologically, clearance was 73% in the imiquimod group vs. 67% for 5-FU and only 32% for cryosurgery. Twelve-month follow-up showed high rates of recurrence and new lesions in the 5-FU and cryosurgery arms. The sustained clearance rate for individual lesions at 12 months was 73% for imiquimod, 54% for 5-FU, and 28% for cryosurgery. Evaluating the entire treatment field, sustained clearance at 12 months was 73% for imiquimod, 33% for 5-FU, and 4% for cryosurgery. They conclude imiquimod resulted in superior cosmetic and sustained clearance rates, although the overall number in each group was small (II/A) [16].

In one study, 193 patients with 699 AKs, the majority on the face and scalp (92%), were randomized to receive either cryotherapy with liquid nitrogen or photodynamic therapy (PDT) using topical methyl 5-aminolevulinate cream and red light. Lesions were graded as thin, moderate, and thick. In patients receiving cryotherapy, markedly hyperkeratotic lesions were curetted first in 36% of lesions. Lesion response was assessed at 3 months after initial treatment and classified as complete or noncomplete response. The overall lesion complete response rate was 69% for PDT and 75% for cryotherapy, and the highest response rates were noted in thin lesions. Since at least one-third of lesions treated with cryotherapy were curetted first, it is difficult to compare this study to other studies involving cryotherapy alone (II/A) [17].

## Topical Diclofenac with Sodium Hyaluronate Gel

A meta-analysis was performed using three double-blind placebo-controlled trials comparing 3% diclofenac in 2.5% sodium hyaluronate gel (DHA) vs. hyaluronate gel vehicle alone (HAV) in a total of 364 patients pooled across studies and a treatment duration of 60 days. AKs were located on the head and extremities. Outcomes evaluated at 30 days post-treatment included target lesion number score indicating complete resolution and cumulative target lesion number score indicating resolution of target lesions and new lesions in the treatment area. Intention to treat analysis showed that DHA significantly improved the total lesion score compared to HAV, with an OR = 3.72 (2.05–6.74). DHA also significantly improved the cumulative target lesion score compared to HAV, with an OR = 4.09 (2.55–6.56). Overall, 40% had complete resolution of target lesions with an average treatment length of 75 days. Thirty-nine percent had no lesions at all (resolution of both target lesions and new lesions), with average treatment duration of 78 days. Common side effects included pruritus, contact dermatitis, dry skin, rash, and scaling. None of the studies had histologic verification of the AK diagnosis, and none compared DHA to other modalities used in the treatment of AKs. Follow-up longer than 30 days, more studies, and subgroup analysis regarding efficacy of DHA for thick lesions are needed in future studies (I/A) [18].

## 5-FU

A meta-analysis investigating the efficacy of 5-FU for AKs of the face and scalp included six studies, 146 patients, with variable follow-up times ranging from 1 to 11 months. 5, 1, and 0.5% formulations of 5-FU were included. The meta-analytical average complete clinical response rate for 5-FU across these studies was 52.2% (SD = 18%).

In one study, at 11-month follow-up, complete clearance was seen in 86.4% of the 5% 5-FU group compared to 0% in the 1% 5-FU group. Two other studies showed differing results with 5% 5-FU applied twice daily over 2 weeks, with only complete clearance of facial AKs in 6.7% of subjects at 1-month follow-up compared with 100% of subjects in another study. Two separate studies investigating 0.5% 5-FU showed complete clearance rates at 4-week follow-up of 57.8 and 47.5% in patients with facial AKs who were treated for 4 weeks (I/A) [19].

Thirty-six patients with four or more clinically diagnosed AKs were randomly assigned to receive 5% 5-FU cream twice daily for 2–4 weeks or 5% imiquimod cream twice weekly for 16 weeks in a physician blinded study. Evaluations were performed at baseline and every 4 weeks until 24 weeks. At week 24, the total AK count was reduced by 94% from baseline with 5-FU compared to 66% with imiquimod. Complete clearance of AKs was 84% in the 5-FU group compared to 24% in the imiquimod group. Erythema levels were initially higher in the 5-FU group but were comparative to imiquimod by week 16. Limitations of this study include twice weekly application of imiquimod which may be a substandard regimen, small sample size, clinical diagnosis of AK made by one evaluating physician without histologic confirmation, and failure to perform an intent to treat analysis (II/A) [20].

Twenty patients with a clinical diagnosis of AK on the scalp and/or face were randomized into two groups. Thirteen patients applied 5% 5-FU twice daily for 3 weeks and were compared to seven patients who applied the same cream twice daily for 1 day per week for 12 weeks. Follow-up was performed at weeks 3, 12, 24, and 52 and clinical photographs and a lesion count were performed. The difference in lesion count at each follow-up was statistically significantly different between both groups. The groups had the same median lesion count at baseline (17.5), but in the first group the lesion count fell and remained at zero after week 12, whereas the second group fell to 6 at week 12, 5.5 at week 24, and 3 at week 52. In conclusion, applying 5% 5-FU twice daily for 3 weeks has superior efficacy than pulse therapy (II/A) [21].

## Imiquimod 5% Cream

A meta-analysis of five short-term, double-blind, randomized-controlled trials evaluating imiquimod 5% cream for the treatment of AK was performed. One thousand two hundred and ninety-three patients were pooled across studies, of which 90% comprised men. All studies diagnosed AKs clinically, except for two which confirmed diagnoses histologically. All studies compared imiquimod 5% cream with vehicle cream, applied 2 or 3 times weekly for 12–16 weeks. Complete clearance occurred in 50% of patients with imiquimod, compared to 5% with vehicle. The number needed to treat (NNT) for one patient to have AKs completely cleared after 12–16 weeks was 2.2 (2.0–2.5). The NNTs for topical diclofenac were 3.7 and 2.0 for 5-FU. Most adverse events were local, specifically erythema, scabbing, and flaking. Optimal frequency and duration of treatment still needs to be determined, and long-term effectiveness beyond 12–16 weeks still needs to be addressed. Only one study followed patients with complete clearance after imiquimod treatment and was able to examine 82% of patients at 16 months after treatment. Twenty-five percent of patients treated 3 times weekly showed recurrence, compared to 43% who were treated twice weekly, and 47% who were treated with vehicle cream (I/A) [1].

A randomized controlled trial specifically addressed the use of imiquimod 5% cream 3 times weekly compared to vehicle alone for 16 weeks in kidney, heart, and liver transplant patients. Forty-three patients with histologically confirmed AKs were assessed and 34 patients completed the study. Follow-up was performed 8 weeks after the completion of therapy and a punch biopsy was obtained to verify lesion resolution. Complete clearance rates for individual AKs were 62% in patients who applied imiquimod, and 0% in vehicle patients. In fact, overall lesion clearance rate for vehicle patients was −99%, showing a large increase in overall lesion count from baseline. Common adverse reactions included application site reactions followed by fatigue, headache, diarrhea, nausea, rash, and leukopenia. No patients experienced rejection of the transplanted organ (II/A) [22].

## Conclusions

In summary, several effective treatment modalities exist for the treatment of AKs. The least rigorous studies have investigated the use of chemical peels for AKs. Most of the literature regarding chemical peels comprises case series or cohort studies, with small sample sizes of 16 patients or less. Only one study evaluated patients 1 year later, and found a 78% reduction in mean AK count by 12 months. AK counts increased between 12 and 32 months, requiring regular follow-up in patients with AKs.

Cryotherapy also has less rigorous studies investigating the efficacy for treatment of AKs. Nonstandardized freezing techniques make it difficult to interpret results. A randomized trial comparing cryotherapy to 5-FU and imiquimod revealed that cryotherapy had the poorest initial clinical clearance at 6–8 weeks after treatment, as well as the worst histologic clearance rates and sustained clearance rates. A separate prospective study showed a 57% complete clearance rate at 3-month follow-up, with the best clearance rates in patients treated with freeze cycles of 20 s or more. Another randomized controlled trial comparing cryotherapy to MALA-PDT showed a mean 88% clearance rate of AKs at 6 months after cryotherapy, although 98% of lesions were on the extremities and the freeze cycles varied.

The evidence that sunscreens provide a modest reduction in the development of AKs is nicely delineated in a blinded, randomized, placebo-controlled trial in which AK diagnosis was verified histologically. Over 7 months of follow-up, patients using sunscreen had a 25% reduction in AKs compared to 18% in the placebo group.

5-FU has several studies evaluating its efficacy for AKs although dosing, follow-up, and cream strength vary between studies. In one randomized trial comparing cryotherapy, 5% 5-FU, and imiquimod, 5-FU had the highest initial clearance of lesions 6–8 weeks after therapy completion, at 96% in a group of 24 patients. This clearance rate was only 67% for 5-FU after histologic confirmation. Twelve-month follow-up showed a sustained clearance rate for individual lesions of only 54%. A meta-analysis pooled six randomized studies together, and concluded that overall complete clearance rate with varying strengths of 5-FU was 52.2%. Application regimens were also investigated, and superior clearance rates were found when 5-FU was applied twice daily for 2–4 weeks as compared to pulse therapy. In conclusion, 5-FU is effective for the treatment of AKs, and twice daily dosing for 2–4 weeks shows superior results to other dosing regimens. Five percent 5-FU is also more effective

than 0.5%. Most studies only have short-term follow-up, and retreatment is recommended since lesions tend to recur by 1 year in studies with longer length of follow-up.

Imiquimod has the most rigorous studies as well as the highest number of blinded, randomized-controlled trials investigating its efficacy for AKs. The follow-up period is not greater than 6 months, however. Application of imiquimod shows optimal results with 3 times weekly application for 12–16 weeks. A meta-analysis reported 50% complete clearance rates for imiquimod. Finally, imiquimod is the only modality tested in organ transplant recipients and there is a complete clearance of 62% at 8-week follow-up.

**Evidence-Based Summary**

| Findings | Evidence level |
| --- | --- |
| Sunscreen is an effective preventive measure against AKs | II/A |
| Chemical peels are an effective field treatment for AKs | IV/B |
| Cryotherapy is an effective spot treatment for clinically visible AKs and longer freeze cycles improve efficacy | II/A |
| 3% diclofenac in 2.5% sodium hyaluronate gel is a topical agent with few side effects when applied twice daily for a minimum of 60 days; follow-up longer than 30 days is lacking | I/A |
| 5% 5-FU is an effective field treatment for clinically visible and invisible AKs when applied twice daily for 2–4 weeks; significant side effects may occur | II/A |
| Imiquimod is an effective field treatment for clinically visible and invisible AKs applied 2 or 3 times weekly for 12–16 weeks; increased efficacy with 3 times weekly application and significant side effects may occur | I/A |
| Imiquimod is the only treatment modality for AKs evaluated in high-risk organ transplant recipients | II/A |

# References

1. Hadley G, Derry S, Moore RA. Imiquimod for actinic keratosis: systematic review and meta-analysis. J Invest Dermatol. 2006;126(6):1251–5.
2. Szeimies RM, Gerritsen MJ, Gupta G, Ortonne JP, Serresi S, Bichel J, et al. Imiquimod 5% cream for the treatment of actinic keratosis: results from a phase III, randomized, double-blind, vehicle controlled, clinical trial with histology. J Am Acad Dermatol. 2004;51: 547–55.
3. Lebwohl M, Dinehart S, Whiting D, Lee PK, Tawfik N, Jorizzo J, et al. Imiquimod 5% cream for the treatment of actinic keratosis: results from two phase III, randomized, double-blind, parallel group, vehicle-controlled trials. J Am Acad Dermatol. 2004;50: 714–21.
4. Rigel DS, Cockerell CJ, Carucci J, et al. Actinic keratosis, basal cell carcinoma, and squamous cell carcinoma. In: Bolognia J, Jorizzo J, Rapini RP, editors. Dermatology. 2nd ed. Amsterdam: Elsevier; 2008. p. 1645–51.
5. Stockfleth E, Kerl H. Guideline subcommittee of the European Dermatology Forum. Guidelines for the management of actinic keratoses. Eur J Dermatol. 2006;16(6):599–606.
6. Drake LA, Ceilley RI, Cornelison RL, Dobes WL, et al. Guidelines of care for actinic keratoses. J Am Acad Dermatol. 1995;32:95–8.
7. de Berker D, McGregor JM, Hughes BR. British Association of Dermatologists Therapy Guidelines and Audit. Guidelines for the management of actinic keratoses. Br J Dermatol. 2007;156(2):222–30.
8. Brodland DG, Roenigk RK. Trichloroacetic acid chemoexfoliation (chemical peel) for extensive premalignant actinic damage of the face and scalp. Mayo Clin Proc. 1988;63(9):887–96.
9. Tse Y, Ostad A, Lee HS, et al. A clinical and histologic evaluation of two medium-depth peels. Glycolic acid versus Jessner's trichloroacetic acid. Dermatol Surg. 1996;22(9):781–6.
10. Witheilder DD, Lawrence N, Cox SE, et al. Long-term efficacy and safety of Jessner's solution and 35% trichloroacetic acid vs. 5% fluorouracil in the treatment of widespread facial actinic keratoses. Dermatol Surg. 1997;23:191–6.
11. Humphreys TR, Werth V, Dzubow L, et al. Treatment of photodamaged skin with trichloroacetic acid and topical tretinoin. J Am Acad Dermatol. 1996;34:638–44.
12. Lubritz RR. Cryosurgery cure rate of actinic keratoses. J Am Acad Dermatol. 1982;7(5):631–2.
13. Thai KE, Fergin P, Freeman M, et al. A prospective study of the use of cryosurgery for the treatment of actinic keratoses. Int J Dermatol. 2004;43(9): 687–92.
14. Thompson SC, Jolley D, Marks R. Reduction of solar keratoses by regular sunscreen use. N Engl J Med. 1993;329(16):1147–51.
15. Kaufmann R, Spelman L, Weightman W, et al. Multicentre intraindividual randomized trial of topical methyl aminolaevulinate-photodynamic therapy vs. cryotherapy for multiple actinic keratoses on the extremities. Br J Dermatol. 2008;158(5):994–9.
16. Krawtchenko N, Roewert-Huber J, Ulrich M, et al. A randomized study of topical 5% imiquimod vs. topical 5-fluorouracil vs. cryosurgery in immunocompetent patients with actinic keratoses: a comparison of clinical and histological outcomes including 1-year follow-up. Br J Dermatol. 2007;157 Suppl 2:34–40.
17. Szeimies RM, Karrer S, Radakovic-Fijan S. Photodynamic therapy using topical methyl 5-aminolevulinate compared with cryotherapy for actinic keratosis: a prospective, randomized study. J Am Acad Dermatol. 2002;47(2):258–62.
18. Pirard D, Vereecken P, Melot C, et al. Three percent diclofenac in 2.5% hyaluronan gel in the treatment of actinic keratoses: a meta-analysis of the recent studies. Arch Dermatol Res. 2005;297:185–9.
19. Gupta AK, Davey V, Mcphail H. Evaluation of the effectiveness of imiquimod and 5-fluorouracil for the treatment of actinic keratosis: critical review and meta-analysis of efficacy studies. J Cutan Med Surg. 2005;9(5):209–14.
20. Tanghetti E, Werschler P. Comparison of 5% 5-fluorouracil cream and 5% imiquimod cream in the management of actinic keratoses on the face and scalp. J Drugs Dermatol. 2007;6(2):144–7.
21. Jury CS, Ramraka-Jones VS, Gudi V, Herd RM. A randomized trial of topical 5% 5-fluorouracil (Efudix cream) in the treatment of actinic keratoses comparing daily with weekly treatment. Br J Dermatol. 2005;153(4):808–10.
22. Ulrich C, Bichel J, Euvrard S, Guidi B, Proby CM, van de Kerkhof PC, et al. Topical immunomodulation under systemic immunosuppression: results of a multicentre, randomized, placebo-controlled safety and efficacy study of imiquimod 5% cream for the treatment of actinic keratoses in kidney, heart, and liver transplant patients. Br J Dermatol. 2007;157 Suppl 2:25–31.

## Self-Assessment

1. How much higher risk do patients with organ transplants have for developing actinic keratoses ?
    (a) 50%
    (b) 100%
    (c) 150%
    (d) 200%
    (e) 250%

2. Imiquimod is an agonist for which toll-like receptor ?
    (a) TLR 3
    (b) TLR 4
    (c) TLR 7
    (d) TLR 8

3. In one study evaluating AKs in patients who did and did not use sunscreen, what was the percent reduction in AKs after 7 months ?
    (a) 25%
    (b) 18%
    (c) 10%
    (d) 5%
    (e) 1%

4. Which treatment modality for AKs has been evaluated in organ transplant recipients ?
    (a) Cryotherapy
    (b) 5-FU
    (c) Imiquimod
    (d) Chemical peels
    (e) Sunscreen

5. AK recurrence rates are equivalent when using imiquimod 5% cream twice weekly compared to 3 times weekly
    (a) True
    (b) False

6. Twice daily application of 5-FU for 2–4 weeks shows increased AK clearance rates when compared to pulse therapy
    (a) True
    (b) False

7. In one study evaluating cryotherapy for complete clearance of AKs, how many seconds were necessary to achieve a complete clearance rate of 83%?
    (a) 3 s
    (b) 5 s
    (c) 10 s
    (d) 20 s

## Answers

1. e: 250%
2. c: TLR 7
3. a: 25%
4. c: Imiquimod
5. b: false
6. a: true
7. d: 20 s

# Reconstruction: Flaps, Grafts, and Other Closures

**8**

Gabriel J. Martinez-Diaz and Hayes Gladstone

## Introduction

Flaps and grafts have been used for facial reconstruction for centuries. For a dermatologic surgeon, there are many methods available for closing surgical defects. The methods range from simple side-to-side closure to more advanced closures that involve adjacent tissue transfer. In deciding the method for closure, the dermatologic surgeon must consider the patient, the type of tumor, the location of the wound, and the local tissue characteristics and availability.

When faced with a defect, the dermatologic surgeon goes through an algorithm or a "reconstructive differential diagnosis" [1]. (VI/C) There are several cardinal rules of closure. The reconstruction must not distort fixed anatomic structures. The scar should be as minimal or camouflaged as possible. As a corollary, the reconstruction should restore the cosmetic unit to as close to the precancer appearance as possible. Finally, maintaining simplicity will generally result in the most elegant result. First, can the defect heal by second intent?

If the defect is in a concavity such as the temple, then this may be the best option. If the result will be unsightly, is a primary closure appropriate? If the reservoir of skin is not sufficient which will result in excessive tension, or if the linear scar will be long, a flap may be more appropriate. A flap may be also required in cases where there is exposed tendon, cartilage, or bone, as well as in wounds with poorly vascularized areas. The most common flaps used in dermatologic surgery are as follows: advancement, rotation, transposition, and interpolation staged flaps. There are some instances when the skin mobility is poor, or a flap may produce an obvious scar, or the defect is superficial, when performing a full thickness skin graft is advantageous. An elderly woman with a superficial nasal tip defect may benefit from this type of skin graft. The resulting scar can easily be optimized with derma-sanding, or covered with makeup.

More than 1,000,000 new cases on nonmelanoma skin cancers are diagnosed and treated annually in the United States. More than 80% of these cancers occur on the head and neck. Most are effectively treated and cured by physicians using modalities including excision, electrodessication and curettage, cryosurgery, and radiation therapy. Subsets of these skin cancers, however, result in significant functional and cosmetic morbidity and, on occasion, mortality. These difficult tumors are best treated with Mohs micrographic surgery, which provides the highest possible cure

G.J. Martinez-Diaz
Department of Dermatology, University of Pittsburgh, Pittsburgh, PA, USA

H. Gladstone (✉)
Division of Dermatologic Surgery,
Department of Dermatology, Stanford University,
Redwood City, CA, USA
e-mail: hbglad@gmail.com

M. Alam (ed.), *Evidence-Based Procedural Dermatology*,
DOI 10.1007/978-0-387-09424-3_8, © Springer Science+Business Media, LLC 2012

rates while it maximizes the preservation of normal tissue. Following excision, many of these cancers leave significant soft tissue and sometimes structural defects. Many techniques from skin grafting to complex facial flaps have been developed by dermatologic surgeons and plastic surgeons to repair these defects. Each cosmetic unit of the head and neck presents its own challenging and unique anatomy when considering the appropriate reconstruction options.

While most of the above recommendations are based on anecdotal experiences of dermatologic, plastic, and head and neck surgeons, there is limited data on what are the best options in terms of evidence based data from clinical studies on reconstruction with flaps, grafts, and other closure techniques. This chapter's aim is to provide the practicing procedural dermatologist with an overview of the relevant evidence-based medical literature that supports clinical indications or contraindications of different reconstructive methods.

## Soft Tissue Facial Reconstruction Evidence-Based Medicine

The evidence for soft tissue facial reconstruction has been largely anecdotal. Though it is challenging to quantify the number of evidence-based reconstructive studies, in a PubMed search for "Flaps and Mohs Surgery," 277 articles appear. When the term "studies" is added, the number decreases to 62. Another search including terms such as "Facial Flaps and dermatology" yields 158 articles. However, when the term "studies" again is added, there are only 15 publications. Being more specific by combining "Mohs surgery and nasal reconstruction" results in 132 articles. Yet when the term "studies" is added, the number of articles decreases to 32. These searches are inclusive from 1979 to the present. There is also the question of what constitutes a study. Though facial reconstruction by its nature cannot be as rigorous in its studies (very difficult to perform a randomized double blind trial) as other aspects of medicine, most of these reports possess no objective data.

## Flap Types (Table 8.1)

### Advancement Flaps

The advancement flap involves the linear advancement of tissue in one direction. This flap can be used to close a variety of defects, ranging from small defects on the scalp or extremities to large, complicated defects involving cosmetic units on the face. The movement of the advancement flap must be balanced by the blood supply of the flap. The excision of Burow's triangles along various aspects of the advancement flap can increase movement and improve cosmesis of the flap. Advancement flaps are versatile and useful basic flaps for repairing defects [2] (V/C).

The evidence of advancement flaps for reconstruction of the ear is limited to case series studies. In a small, nonrandomized study of 12 patients with skin tumors on the ear rim, Goldberg et al. found that the postauricular cutaneous advancement flap provided excellent cosmetic results in all but one patient, who experienced minimal superficial necrosis of the flap [3] (V/C).

In addition to helical rim advancement, flaps have been successfully used in upper eyelid reconstruction surgery. Upper eyelids are difficult to reconstruct primarily due to their complicated anatomy and specialized functions. In a series of eight patients aged 17–72 years, Demir et al. used an orbicularis oculi myocutaneous advancement flap to reconstruct upper eye lids of eight [4] (V/C). Most of these patients were followed up to 3 years after surgery, and included assessment of position, closure, length of palpebral rim, eyelid opening, esthetic balance, presence of corneal erosion, entropion, levator function, and donor-site morbidity. The flap was viable in every patient, without total or partial necrosis. No patient required surgical revision or experienced recurrence. Unfortunately, there was no objective criteria used for esthetic outcomes.

Upper lip reconstruction after the removal of a malignancy can be accomplished in a myriad of ways. A poll of a select group of surgeons ($n = 122$) demonstrated variability in their choice of upper lip reconstruction options. The cheek

**Table 8.1** Summary of one-stage flaps studies

| References | Flap | Anatomic location | Sample size (N) | Main findings |
|---|---|---|---|---|
| Martin et al. [5] | Advancement | Upper lip | 122 | Surgeons' choice of upper lip reconstruction options varied, although the nasolabial flap was found to be the least-chosen option. Trends in choices based upon experience and comfort level were demonstrated |
| Moore et al. [12] | Rotation | Head and neck | 33 | Compound cervicofacial and cervicothoracic rotation flaps provide a straightforward, reliable, and efficient means to reconstruct complex defects of the face, lateral skull base, and neck, with the potential for excellent cosmetic results |
| McGeorge [16] | Rhombic | Head and neck | 104 | No dog-ear formation was found in any of the cases. Rhombic flap has been found to be simple to design, and also practical with a wide variety of wound shapes and anatomic sites successfully closed. The modified rhombic flap is a very versatile, safe method, of wound repair and is particularly well suited to Mohs' excision surgery |
| Zitelli [17] | Bilobed | Nose | 400 | Four hundred consecutive surgical wounds on the nose were studied for wound management. The most commonly used flap was the bilobed double transposition flap that is especially useful for reconstruction of defects on the lower third of the nose. While the standard design often results in tissue protrusions or pincushioning, improvements in the design are outlined herein to achieve the best results for defects on the nose |

advancement flap was the first choice with 34.4%, followed by Abbe flap (31.2%), myocutaneous rotation flap (20.5%), and nasolabial flap (13.9%), with the nasolabial flap being statistically the least popular ($p < 0.01$). Trends in choices based upon years of operative experience and comfort level were demonstrated [5] (VI/C).

Recently, the bilateral cheek-to-nose advancement flap has been used as an alternative to the paramedian forehead flap in patients with prominent nasolabial folds and prominent cheek tissue laxity, who require closure of Mohs surgery defects on the nasal dorsum and sidewall. Sand et al. reported 12 patients that were treated with the advancement flap and evaluated after 2 weeks and 6 months [6] (V/C). The patients' subjective and the surgeons' objective evaluation after 6 months was either completely satisfied or not satisfied. The bilateral cheek-to-nose advancement flap

appears to be a reliable tool in the interventional portfolio of the reconstructive surgeon.

## The Rotation Flap

The rotation flap is a workhorse flap for many surgeons in reconstructing facial defects after Mohs micrographic surgery. The rotation flap is defined by its arc-like incision, which distributes skin tension. While the motion is an arc, there is an element of the advancement of tissue in this flap. A burow's triangle is often created at the distal portion of this incision, which aids in releasing the flap. Wide undermining is important in helping to mobilize the rotation flap. Conventionally, the length of the incision should be 3–4 times the diameter of the defect. However, given the face and scalp's vascularity, this rule

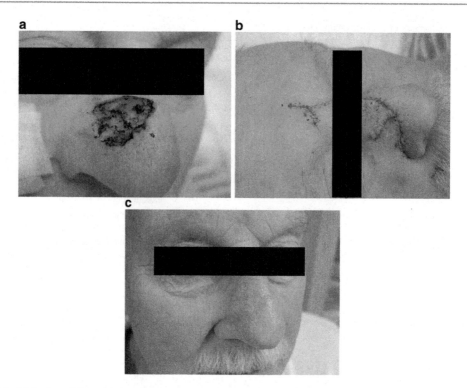

**Fig. 8.1** (**a**) 3 × 4 cm defect of the medial cheek and upper lip, (**b**) reconstructing this complex defect with a combination rotation and advancement flap, (**c**) postoperative result at 1 month

can be bent. Because this flap can recruit large amounts of skin from distant sites, it can be used for large defects. The Mustarde flap for large cheek defects is an example. Yet, this rotational arc can also release skin from adjacent sites with minimal distortion; this flap can be used for small defects in very sensitive areas. The Tenzel flap for lower lateral eyelid defects takes advantage of this quality. Multiple rotation flaps can be used to close large defects particularly on the scalp where the skin may not be as elastic. This flap is mostly used where there are curved RSTL's. These cosmetic units include the cheek, chin, temple scalp, the distal third of the nose (Fig. 8.1a–c) (Peng flap), the and upper lip (Karapanzic flap).

There have been many descriptions of the rotation flap in the literature. Most of these examples are reported as case studies. There have been few substantial case series, and objective studies are rare. For the cheek rotation flap, a case series of 30 patients followed complications, which included a 10% rate of nerve palsy [7] (V/C). Yet 93% of the patients were satisfied with their results. There were any independent evaluations of images.

In terms of specific technique, a comparison was performed between a subcutaneous approach and a deeper dissection [8] (V/B). This retrospective study involved 32 patients, which were followed for a mean of 32 months. All the patients underwent the subcutaneous approach. Patient demographics were included, and 97% were satisfied with the outcome. Complications such an ectropian and paresthesias were reported though not truly quantified. The authors compared their subcutaneous approach to the deep approach as reported in the literature so a true comparison by the same surgical team was impossible. A composite version of the rotation flap was evaluated in seven patients [9] (V/C). It included a table of all of seven patients' results as well as photo evaluation by two surgeons, though it is not clear if these were independent evaluators. There were no ratings by the patients. Because the study is small, conclusions are difficult to formulate.

Other case series include another variation of the facelift rotation flap [10] (V/C). The authors reported three cases and that there were good results and no complications. A dog ear version of the rotation flap was reported by Schmidt and Mellette [11] (VI/C). There were four pre and post images of this technique but no other objective evidence.

Moore et al. evaluated large cervicorotation flaps in the head and neck in 33 patients. Complications were evaluated. Interestingly, there was a 100% flap survival in the 17 patients who engaged in tobacco abuse. Yet, there were not objective criteria for measuring esthetic outcomes. Photos of three results were shown, though only one long term [12] (V/C).

For the scalp, there have been many case reports on using the rotation. In some patients, these flaps for reconstruction have been modified from the hair restoration literature. There have also been several reviews of the indications and technique of using the rotation flap to close medium and large defects on the scalp. Yet, there are very few series evaluating the actual results through quantifiable evidence. A modification of the "Banana Peel" for scalp reconstruction typifies the literature [13] (VI/C). It is a very creative technique for large scalp defects, but the series consists of only four patients. There is neither any independent evaluation of images nor are subjective ratings by patients.

## Transposition Flaps

Transposition flaps such as banner, bilobed, and rhombic flaps are useful for closure of most medium to large defects on the head and neck. These flaps are designed to transpose the flap over normal skin to repair the defect. The main drawbacks of these flaps can be lack of movement due to "torquing" the skin as well as pincushioning that result in elevation of the flap (Fig. 8.2a–d).

In a prospective study examining the reliability and cosmetic outcome of a Z-transposition flap with mucosal advancement for repairing partial thickness defects of the lower lip measuring less than 50% the lower lip length, the authors found that all 11 patients healed uneventfully with good cosmetic results and flap reliability. The Z-transposition flap is an acceptable alternative for reconstructing partial thickness defects of the lower lip [14] (VI/C).

## Rhombic

Rhombic flaps are very versatile and can be used commonly on the scalp, eyelid, nose cheek, chin, and temporal defects. The excision is performed using a rhombus with 60 and 120° angles. The donor flap bisects the 120° angle. The flap is drawn to place the donor site incision within normal facial rhytides. This can be determined easily by identifying the area of skin with maximal extensibility. A modification of this technique that simplifies the design was described by McNay et al. [15] (VI/C), though this was reported as a surgical pearl without objective evidence.

A series of 104 cases was assessed by photographic and clinical record perioperatively and at 6 months of postoperative follow-up. They found no dog-ear formation in any of the cases. Other complications were minimal [16] (V/C).

## Bilobed

Bilobed flaps use two lobes to borrow skin to close the defect. The primary lobe is transposed into the defect while the secondary lobe fills the new defect. The secondary defect is closed first which aids in transposing the primary lobe. Bilobed flaps are used in cosmetic units that have less mobile adjacent skin such as the nose. The flaps are designed on a 45–90° axis to the primary defect, and are elevated in the subcutaneous plane. These flaps may result in pincushioning – which may lead to secondary revisions.

In 1989, Zitelli described a new design of the bilobed flap for defects on the distal third of the nose. It reduced the angle of each lobe rotation along an arc to 45° [17] (V/C). Of the 400 nasal reconstructions in this series, 60 were repaired with flaps. Twenty of these flaps used the modified bilobed design. The author reported that there were no incidences of necrosis or pincushioning, though there were two instances of superficial slough.

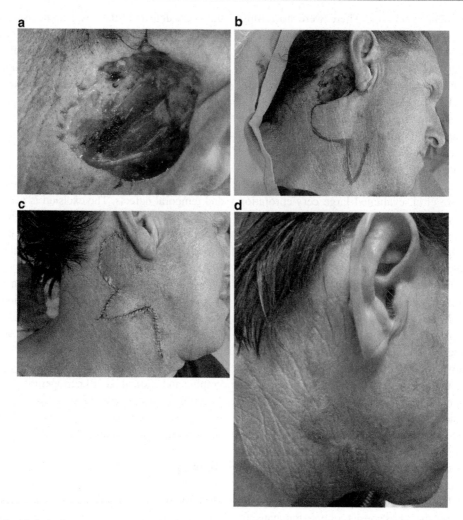

**Fig. 8.2** (a) A 4×5 cm postauricular defect, (b) marking the bilobed flap, (c) bilobed flap inset, (d) postoperative result at 2 months

None of the patients required surgical revision. The scar results were rated as good to excellent.

In a retrospective review of 171 patients who underwent bilobed flap repairs of the distal nose, Moy et al. [18] (V/C) found a 3% incidence of infection, 7% incidence of partial flap necrosis, and 5% incidence of "trapdooring" and contour distortion.

More recently, Dinehart reported that designing a "rhombic" bilobed flap where the lobes were angulated resulted in excellent results in 9 of 10 patients [19] (V/C). None of the patients experienced trapdooring. Though there was not any objective data in this report, another study

described a similar angular design or a "diamond" bilobed based on computer generated finite element modeling, which resulted in potentially a lesser risk for pincushioning [20] (V/C).

## Island Pedicle

The island pedicle flap is a random pattern advancement flap well suited to reconstruct a variety of small to intermediate-sized soft tissue wounds. Utilizing a well-preserved central vascular pedicle, complications are infrequent. However, its mobility is constrained by the length of its pedicle. The random pattern island pedicle flap is a versatile and robust flap used to repair a variety of soft tissue wounds in a single-stage procedure with reproducible operative outcomes [21] (VI/C).

Optimal esthetic reconstruction of cutaneous defects following excisional surgery is largely dependent on the availability of regional donor tissue that shares a likeness of the original tissue in color, texture, sebaceous quality, and thickness. The island pedicle flap is a useful tool in facial reconstruction because it minimizes regional anatomic distortion, and in many instances optimizes tissue match. Leonhardt and Lawrence [22] (V/C) reviewed four locations where the island pedicle flap is particularly well suited. Through careful planning and implementation, the island pedicle flap may be used on the nasal tip, the nasal ala, the upper cheek, and the upper lip for closures with much success. Myocutaneous island pedicle flaps for nasal reconstruction have been described [23] (V/C). Bi-level undermining creating a sling island pedicle was reported in 61 patients. The authors noted eight patients who required dermabrasion and one who had alar notching. Otherwise the results were excellent, though there were not rating scales by independent physicians or quantifiable subjective evaluations by patients [24] (V/C). In 2005, Asgari and Odland described their technique in eight patients [25] (V/C). They noted that 7/8 patients had excellent functional and esthetic outcomes. Images of four patients were shown.

## Staged Flaps (Table 8.2)

### Postauricular Flaps

Postauricular staged flaps use skin from the posterior part of the ear and the retroauricular aspect of the scalp to repair defects in the helical rim and the anterior surface of the ear [26] (VI/C). It provides good coverage and cosmesis in medium-to-large defects on the helix and adjacent anti-helix, with or without the loss of small amounts of cartilage [27] (VI/C).

Few satisfactory closure options exist for large anterior auricular defects. Humphrey et al. [28] (VI/C) described the use of the postauricular (revolving door) island pedicle flap for closure of large defects on the scapha, antihelix, and helix.

Mohs micrographic surgery for excision of basal cell carcinoma was performed on the anterior auricular surface of two patients. Both defects were closed using a posterior auricular island flap that was advanced through cartilage with excellent cosmetic results. The postauricular (revolving door) island pedicle flap is a good closure option for large anterior auricular defects lacking perichondrium and not easily repaired by other methods. A variation of this flap based on the superficial temporal artery and its parietal branch was described in 52 patients. It was also used mainly for superior helical rim defects. According to the authors, there were more complications and the results were good, though there were no objective criteria [29] (V/C).

Johnson and Fader [30] (V/C) reported using the staged retroauricular flap for helical rim and anti-helix defects in 26 consecutive patients. There were no major complications, though two patients required a z plasty and one a skin graft to release postoperative ear pinning. The authors noted that both they and the patients felt that the results were good to excellent. However, there were no numeric evaluation scales.

## Melolabial Flaps

The melolabial flap is a versatile technique for reconstruction of defects of the central face. Variations of this flap may be used to reconstruct the lower eyelids, the nose, the upper and lower lip, chin, and malar regions. In a case series [31] (V/C), Younger discussed the indications, technical considerations, and avoidance of complications when using this flap in ten bilateral cadaver dissections of the melolabial area, in conjunction with 70 reconstructive cases that used this flap. The results of this study revealed that this two staged flap's viability is compromised by previous radiation and smoking. According to the author, alternate methods of reconstruction of the central face should be used in patients who have a history of these problems [31].

While it is versatile, it is most commonly used to repair alar defects. The melolabial flap can be performed in a single stage. Zitelli [32] (V/C) described his technique in 32 patients. He outlined a number of steps including the use of periosteal

**Table 8.2** Summary of two-stage flaps studies

| References | Flap | Anatomic location | Sample size (N) | Main findings |
|---|---|---|---|---|
| Cordova et al. [29] | Island flap | Ear and head | 52 | Superior pedicle retroauricular island flap can be considered as a first choice option to repair nonmarginal losses of substance of the upper half of the ear. Because of its wide arc of rotation, it can also be used for superficial marginal defects of the helix and in selected cases of temporal region defects |
| Younger [31] | Melolabial | Melolabial | 80 | Melolabial flap viability is compromised by previous radiation and smoking. Consequently, alternate methods of reconstruction of the central face should be used in patients who have a history of these problems |
| Zitelli [32] | Nasolabial | Nasolabial | 32 | An improved technique used in 32 patients is presented, which allows use of this procedure as a single-stage rather than the more commonly seen two-stage procedure. None of the 32 patients presented required a second-stage procedure to correct trapdoor defects or to recreate natural folds or creases |
| Rifaat [41] | Abbe | Lower lip | 17 | Lower lip reconstruction aims to restore function and appearance with the best results obtained by utilizing residual normal lip tissues incorporating potentially innervated muscle fibers. With larger defects, reconstruction is less than optimal, but every effort should be taken to obtain an adequate sphincter function and lip continence to saliva, both of which are the most important goals to achieve in lip reconstruction |

and suspension sutures to recreate the nasal crease. None of the patients required a revision [32]. In 2001, Lindsey [33] (V/C) conducted a retrospective study on 105 patients who underwent a one stage melolabial flap for nasal reconstruction. While there were no major complications, there were 29 instances of minor complications from hematomas, infections, and trapdooring.

## Paramedian Forehead Flaps

The forehead flap is perhaps the oldest reconstructive method for resurfacing extensive nasal defects. It was first used in the Indian subcontinent over 3,000 years ago. It has evolved from a midline wide flap to a paramedian flap with a trunk of no more than a centimeter in width. The robustness of this flap is due to its excellent collateral supply of blood vessels in addition to the supratrochlear artery. This has been confirmed in cadavers' studies [34, 35] (VI/C). It is often used in conjunction with cartilage grafts. Along with the

requisite internal lining, it provides an excellent vascular supply for the cartilage [36] (VI/C). The result is an approximate reproduction of the nasal architecture before the tumor extirpation [37] (VI/C) (Fig. 8.3a–c).

Forehead flaps are divided at 3 weeks, even though they have been reported to be taken down successfully at 1 week. Somoano and Gladstone conducted a study of 35 consecutive patients who had paramedian forehead flaps. Twenty-six flaps were taken down at 1 week and contoured at 3 weeks. There were no flap failures, and the patients overwhelmingly preferred the 1-week flap division from a quality of life perspective [38] (V/C). On the other extreme, Menick described his technique of completely dividing the flap at 6 weeks [39] (VI/C).

In a retrospective review, Arden et al. [40] (V/C) qualitatively and quantitatively described esthetic and functional outcomes following Mohs ablative surgery involving the alar subunit, using

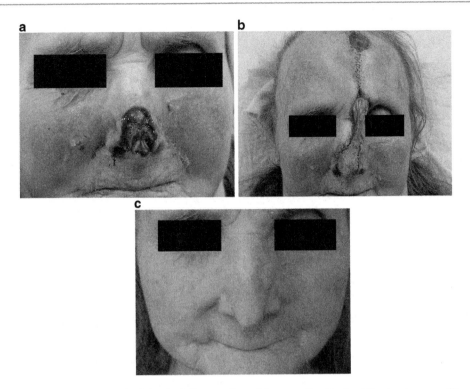

**Fig. 8.3** (**a**) Nasal tip and supratip defect including cartilage, (**b**) paramedian forehead flap inset over cartilage graft, (**c**) postoperative result at 3 months

a paramedian or subcutaneous melolabial island flap in 38 patients. Objective measures (alar rim thickness, donor scar width and length), subjective assessment (seven esthetic parameters) by three academic otolaryngologists, and patient satisfaction questionnaires were evaluated. Questionnaire results demonstrated a significant difference ($p = 0.026$) in donor site rating favoring melolabial group responses. Objective scar measurements and subjective ratings of textural quality and alar notching also favored melolabial reconstructions. More favorable esthetic and functional outcomes are seen with single subunit cutaneous alar defects reconstructed with the melolabial island flap than with deep composite or extensive unilateral nasal defects reconstructed with the paramedian forehead flap [40] (VI/C).

## Abbe Flap

Full-thickness defects involving more than 40% of either the upper or the lower lip generally require a 2-staged cross lip flap known as the Abbe Estlander flap. This flap transfers functional orbicularis oris muscle. The Abbe flap is used to reconstruct defects in the opposite lip and consists of a full-thickness segment of the lip with a pedicle on the vermilion border based on the labial artery. For most defects, the flap is one half to two-thirds the size of the defect. The secondary defect is closed primarily. The Abbe flap is usually divided at 3 weeks.

Clinical factors such as size and location, but also surgeon experience and comfort level, may influence decisions in reconstructive methods. After polling a group of plastic surgeons [5], investigators found that nasolabial flap was found to be the least-chosen option in regards to upper lip reconstruction. Cheek advancement flap was the first choice in 34.4%, followed by Abbe flap (31.2%), myocutaneous rotation flap (20.5%), and nasolabial flap (13.9%), with the nasolabial flap being statistically the least popular. For surgeons with more than 20 years' experience and those with less than 10 years' experience, the

Abbe flap was the most common first choice (38.9 and 32.4%, respectively). For surgeons with 11–20 years experience, the cheek advancement flap was the most common first choice (46.2%) [5]. From 2002 to 2005, Rifaat reported 17 lip reconstructions due to squamous cell carcinoma [41] (V/C). The most common type of closure was a karapandzic flap. Two of the patients underwent an Abbe cross lip procedure. There were no complications or microstomia. The author reported the results to be satisfactory and good in these two patients. Interestingly, only the simplest

closures – wedge advancement – in this series were rated as "excellent."

## Grafts (Table 8.3)

Grafts commonly employed for cutaneous surgery are split-thickness skin grafts (STSGs), full-thickness skin grafts (FTSGs), free cartilage grafts, and composite grafts. The most common grafts used by dermatology surgeons are full thickness skin grafts. They can be used for

**Table 8.3** Summary of graft studies

| References | Graft | Anatomic location | Sample size (N) | Main findings |
|---|---|---|---|---|
| Johnson and Zide [44] | Full-thickness | Face | 30 | Not many complications were seen except for rare surface necrosis and depression of the grafted site, and the esthetic results were generally satisfactory when full-thickness skin grafts are used in facial reconstructions |
| Kuijpers et al. [45] | Full-thickness | Nose | 30 | Grafts treated with azithromycin had a significant longer survival. Smoking had a significant negative effect on the survival of the graft. Systemic antibiotics with an accurate bacterial spectrum should be advised in full thickness skin graft reconstruction after surgery for nonmelanoma skin cancer of the nose. Smoking should be strongly discouraged |
| Wines et al. [46] | Split-thickness | Ear | 272 | Split thickness skin grafting was the preferred method of reconstruction. The histopathology of the lesions and the size of the post-Mohs defect did not influence the choice of technique, except for lesions less than 1 cm in which healing by secondary intention was favored. Tumor size, type, and aggressiveness did not influence repair technique choice. Surgeon preference was therefore the principle factor dictating method of reconstructive technique following Mohs micrographic surgery |
| Keck et al. [48] | Composite | Ear | 19 | Composite ear grafts may provide good functional and esthetic results when combined with overlying skin flaps in reconstruction of partial nasal defects. Even though composite ear grafts used for restoration of the inner nasal lining may be deformed or absorbed and impairment of nasal airway patency or esthetic result may be postoperatively observed, the combination of composite ear grafts with locoregional transposition flaps provides additional reconstructive options for selected nasal defects |

shallow defects such as on the nasal tip; however, color match and skin texture are always issues with full thickness skin grafts. Split thickness skin grafts are used for larger shallow defects, and generally have a higher survival rate than full thickness skin grafts because of lesser metabolic demands. STSG's on the face may have poor esthetic outcomes. Composite and free cartilage grafts are used mainly for nasal defects. The former is commonly used to recreate the nasal subsurface framework while the latter is often used to reconstruct an alar rim defect. Because the free graft is sewn into the defect, and must reestablish its vascular supply, it will have a significantly decreased survival rate if there is tobacco abuse [42] (VI/C).

## Full Thickness Skin Grafts

FTSGs consist of the complete epidermis and partial dermis. FTSGs are relatively easy to harvest and to secure to their recipient sites. FTSGs rarely match as well as a local skin flap because of regional differences in skin thickness, texture, color, and actinic damage. FTSGs tend to be more prone to necrosis than STSGs, yet FTSGs tend to contract less. Defects that are well suited to be repaired with FTSGs include, but are not limited to those located in the nasal tip, dorsum, ala, and sidewall, as well as on the lower eyelid and ear [43] (VI/C).

Johnson and Zide [44] (V/C) reviewed the use of FTSGs for closure of facial defects. Their study included 30 patients who had FTSGs after removal of premalignant or malignant facial skin lesions. Their most commonly used graft harvest sites included the preauricular or periauricular region (15), neck (three), supraclavicular region (three), forehead (two), adjacent area (Burow's) (six), and eyelid (one). No hematomas or infections occurred in the donor sites. Four patients developed a dark crust that ultimately sloughed off the graft site. In two of these cases, the final graft site was shiny and contracted, whereas in the other two the graft sites healed perfectly. Color was good to excellent in most cases when grafting was intended as the final reconstructive effort. Graft depression was noted occasionally.

FTSGs offer a reliable alternative to the use of flaps in selected cases [44].

Full thickness grafts on the nose do not always heal without problems. Partial or entire necrosis of the graft is likely to lead to less favorable cosmetic results and prolonged wound care. Kuijpers et al. [45] (II/B) evaluated the effect of systemic antibiotics on the survival of full thickness grafts on the nose. Through a randomized, controlled trial, the authors compared azithromycin with standard treatment in 30 patients, who underwent a full thickness graft reconstruction of a surgical defect on the nose after surgery for NMSC. Grafts treated with azithromycin showed a significantly higher survival rate 86.6 vs. 36.2% of the patients ($p=0.002$). Of all the variables analyzed, only smoking had a significant ($p<0.001$) negative effect on the survival of the graft. Systemic antibiotics with an accurate bacterial spectrum should be advised in full thickness skin graft reconstruction after surgery for nonmelanoma skin cancer of the nose. Smoking should be strongly discouraged.

## Split Thickness Grafts

In a retrospective analysis of 272 patients with conchal bowl tumors, split thickness skin grafting was the preferred method of reconstruction. The histopathology of the lesions and the size of the post-Mohs defect did not influence the choice of technique, except for lesions less than 1 cm in which healing by secondary intention was favored. Tumor size, type, and aggressiveness did not influence repair technique choice. Surgeon preference was therefore the principle factor dictating method of reconstructive technique following Mohs micrographic surgery [46] (V/C).

In a randomized clinical trial undertaken to compare the healing time of STSG donor sites in elderly patients using cultured epidermal allografts vs. nonadherent dressings, Phillips et al. [47] (V/C) found that cultured allografts can accelerate healing in STSG donor compared with nonadherent dressings. Fresh-cultured epidermal grafts were used in ten STSG donor sites in nine patients ranging in age from 63 to 87 years. In each patient, half the donor site was allografted and the other half treated with nonadherent dressings. Biopsy specimens were taken from allografted areas in three patients 2 months after the grafting procedure, for multilocus DNA analysis. The mean time to complete healing was 8.4 days in allografted sites compared with 15.3 days in control sites. There was no evidence of survival of cultured allogeneic cells in allografted areas. Cultured allografts do not survive permanently on the wound bed [47].

## Composite Grafts

Composite ear grafts may provide good functional and esthetic results when combined with overlying skin flaps in reconstruction of partial nasal defects. In a case series of 19 patients, Keck et al. [48] (V/C) only found postoperative deformation in three transplanted composite grafts. Relative shrinkage was observed in 5 of 19 composite grafts, whereas complete loss of the composite graft was seen in only one patient. Postoperative follow-up ranged from 8 to 15 months with an average follow-up of 10 months. Nasal airway obstruction was observed in the patients with deformity or loss of composite graft (4 of 15 patients), and an unsuccessful esthetic result was seen only in the patient with total composite graft failure (1 of 19 transplanted grafts). Composite ear grafts, when used in conjunction with transposition flaps, provide additional reconstructive options for specific nasal defects – albeit it comes with some risks [48].

## Free Grafts

Van der Eerden described a cohort of 13 patients seen in one institution and received free cartilage grafts in combination with secondary intention healing for reconstruction of the alar subunit and lateral nasal wall defects after Mohs surgery for cutaneous cancer [49] (V/C). Follow-up ranged 6–49 months, with a mean of 17 months. The authors reported that wound healing by secondary intention were uneventful, and patients and physicians had satisfactory responses to the results. The minor complications experienced by three patients included, minor esthetic faults (hypertrophic scars and alar notching). One patient had a functional complaint of nasal blockage on the side that was surgically treated.

## Conclusion

It is clear from the literature that dermatologic surgeons, facial plastic surgeons, oculoplastic surgeons, oral-maxillo facial surgeons, and plastic surgeons are very creative in repairing facial defects after skin cancer removal preferably by Mohs micrographic surgery. However, the very large majority are single case reports. While these innovations propel the specialties forward, it does not necessarily give the reader confidence that these techniques can be reproduced with similar esthetic results as well as minimal adverse effects. In short, there is no evidence.

There is a small percentage of case series of the various closure techniques, which have been highlighted in this chapter. They demonstrate reproducibility and often will tabulate complications. Yet, only a handful includes any objective evaluation. There are reports that the results are "good to excellent" yet there is not an independent panel evaluating digital images on a numeric scale. There is not a subjective score by the patients. In many instances, there are only one set of before and after images, which can be assumed to be the surgeon's best result. While double blind studies and "p values" are difficult in facial reconstruction since there unlikely to be two types of reconstructions to be compared, we have offered a number of recommendations:

- Larger numbers – more multicenter studies may be merited.
- Digital image evaluation by an independent panel. Photos are not perfect because of their two dimensional quality, but if enough of them are evaluated, it will provide better evidence.
- Patient evaluation based on a numeric rating scale.
- Include the complication rate.

- More before and after photos.
- Step by step illustration of the method.
- Long term follow up – at least 1 year.
- When possible, a 3D evaluation of the result.

A better mix of case reports and case series with quantifiable data as well as potentially comparing different techniques for grafting or challenging areas such as the distal aspect of the nose, eyelids, lips, and ears will allow us to consistently provide the best results and improve patient care.

# References

1. Gladstone HB, Stewart D. An algorithm for the reconstruction of complex facial defects. Skin Therapy Lett. 2007;12(2):6–9.
2. Krishnan R, Garman M, Nunez-Gussman J, Orengo I. Advancement flaps: a basic theme with many variations. Dermatol Surg. 2005;31(8 Pt 2):986–94.
3. Goldberg LH, Mauldin DV, Humphreys TR. The postauricular cutaneous advancement flap for repairing ear rim defects. Dermatol Surg. 1996;22(1):28–31.
4. Demir Z, Yuce S, Karamursel S, Celebioglu S. Orbicularis oculi myocutaneous advancement flap for upper eyelid reconstruction. Plast Reconstr Surg. 2008;121(2):443–50.
5. Martin TJ, Zhang Y, Rhee JS. Options for upper lip reconstruction: a survey-based analysis. Dermatol Surg. 2008;13:13.
6. Sand M, Boorboor P, Sand D, Altmeyer P, Mann B, Bechara FG. Bilateral cheek-to-nose advancement flap: an alternative to the paramedian forehead flap for reconstruction of the nose. Acta Chir Plast. 2007; 49(3):67–70.
7. Rashid M, Sarwar SR, Hameed S, Masood T. Experience with lateral cheek rotation flap for the reconstruction of medial cheek soft tissue defects. J Pak Med Assoc. 2006;56(5):227–30.
8. Austen Jr WG, Parrett BM, Taghinia A, Wolfort SF, Upton J. The subcutaneous cervicofacial flap revisited. Ann Plast Surg. 2009;62(2):149–53.
9. Delay E, Lucas R, Jorquera F, Payement G, Foyatier JL. Composite cervicofacial flap for reconstruction of complex cheek defects. Ann Plast Surg. 1999;43(4): 347–53.
10. Flynn TC, McDonald WS, Chastain MA. The "facelift" flap for reconstruction of cheek, lateral orbit, and temple defects. Dermatol Surg. 1999;25(11):836–43.
11. Schmidt DK, Mellette Jr JR. The dog-ear rotation flap for the repair of large surgical defects on the head and neck. Dermatol Surg. 2001;27(10):908–10.
12. Moore BA, Wine T, Netterville JL. Cervicofacial and cervicothoracic rotation flaps in head and neck reconstruction. Head Neck. 2005;27(12):1092–101.
13. Frodel Jr JL, Ahlstrom K. Reconstruction of complex scalp defects: the "Banana Peel" revisited. Arch Facial Plast Surg. 2004;6(1):54–60.
14. Trokel Y, Finn R. TZ-transposition flap: an alternate method of lower lip reconstruction for partial thickness defects. J Oral Maxillofac Surg. 2006;64(9):1381–4.
15. McNay AT, Ostad A, Moy RL. Surgical pearl: modified rhombic flap. J Am Acad Dermatol. 1997;37(2 Pt 1): 256–8.
16. McGeorge BC. Modified rhombic flap for closure of circular or irregular defects. J Cutan Med Surg. 1998;3(2):74–8.
17. Zitelli JA. The bilobed flap for nasal reconstruction. Arch Dermatol. 1989;125(7):957–9.
18. Moy RL, Grossfeld JS, Baum M, Rivlin D, Eremia S. Reconstruction of the nose utilizing a bilobed flap. Int J Dermatol. 1994;33(9):657–60.
19. Dinehart SM. The rhombic bilobed flap for nasal reconstruction. Dermatol Surg. 2001;27(5):501–4.
20. Gladstone H. A computer generated diamond bilobed may result in decreased pincushioning. In: Annual meeting of the American College of Mohs Micrographic Surgery. Denver; 2000.
21. Braun Jr M, Cook J. The island pedicle flap. Dermatol Surg. 2005;31(8 Pt 2):995–1005.
22. Leonhardt JM, Lawrence N. Back to basics: the subcutaneous island pedicle flap. Dermatol Surg. 2004; 30(12 Pt 2):1587–90.
23. Papadopoulos DJ, Pharis DB, Munavalli GS, Trinei F, Hantzakos AG. Nasalis myocutaneous island pedicle flap with bilevel undermining for repair of lateral nasal defects. Dermatol Surg. 2002;28(2):190–4.
24. Willey A, Papadopoulos DJ, Swanson NA, Lee KK. Modified single-sling myocutaneous island pedicle flap: series of 61 reconstructions. Dermatol Surg. 2008;34(11):1527–35.
25. Asgari M, Odland P. Nasalis island pedicle flap in nasal ala reconstruction. Dermatol Surg. 2005;31(4): 448–52.
26. Lewin M. Formation of the helix with a postauricular flap. Plast Reconstr Surg. 1950;5(5):432–40.
27. Cochran Jr JH, Shinn JB. The postauricular flap in helical injuries. Laryngoscope. 1979;89(8):1347–50.
28. Humphreys TR, Goldberg LH, Wiemer DR. The postauricular (revolving door) island pedicle flap revisited. Dermatol Surg. 1996;22(2):148–50.
29. Cordova A, Pirrello R, D'Arpa S, Moschella F. Superior pedicle retroauricular island flap for ear and temporal region reconstruction: anatomic investigation and 52 cases series. Ann Plast Surg. 2008;60(6):652–7.
30. Johnson TM, Fader DJ. The staged retroauricular to auricular direct pedicle (interpolation) flap for helical ear reconstruction. J Am Acad Dermatol. 1997;37(6): 975–8.
31. Younger RA. The versatile melolabial flap. Otolaryngol Head Neck Surg. 1992;107(6 Pt 1):721–6.
32. Zitelli JA. The nasolabial flap as a single-stage procedure. Arch Dermatol. 1990;126(11):1445–8.

33. Lindsey WH. Reliability of the melolabial flap for alar reconstruction. Arch Facial Plast Surg. 2001;3(1):33–7.
34. Shumrick KA, Smith TL. The anatomic basis for the design of forehead flaps in nasal reconstruction. Arch Otolaryngol Head Neck Surg. 1992;118(4):373–9.
35. Reece EM, Schaverien M, Rohrich RJ. The paramedian forehead flap: a dynamic anatomical vascular study verifying safety and clinical implications. Plast Reconstr Surg. 2008;121(6):1956–63.
36. Burget GC, Menick FJ. Nasal support and lining: the marriage of beauty and blood supply. Plast Reconstr Surg. 1989;84(2):189–202.
37. Brodland DG. Paramedian forehead flap reconstruction for nasal defects. Dermatol Surg. 2005;31(8 Pt 2): 1046–52.
38. Somoano B, Gladstone HB. Accelerated takedown of the paramedian forehead flap at one week. J Am Acad Dermatol. 2011;65(1):97–105.
39. Menick FJ. A 10-year experience in nasal reconstruction with the three-stage forehead flap. Plast Reconstr Surg. 2002;109(6):1839–55; discussion 56–61.
40. Arden RL, Nawroz-Danish M, Yoo GH, Meleca RJ, Burgio DL. Nasal alar reconstruction: a critical analysis using melolabial island and paramedian forehead flaps. Laryngoscope. 1999;109(3):376–82.
41. Rifaat MA. Lower lip reconstruction after tumor resection; a single author's experience with various methods. J Egypt Natl Canc Inst. 2006;18(4):323–33.
42. Adams DC, Ramsey ML. Grafts in dermatologic surgery: review and update on full- and split-thickness skin grafts, free cartilage grafts, and composite grafts. Dermatol Surg. 2005;31(8 Pt 2):1055–67.
43. Ratner D. Skin grafting. From here to there. Dermatol Clin. 1998;16(1):75–90.
44. Johnson T, Zide MF. Freehand full-thickness grafting for facial defects: a review of methods. J Oral Maxillofac Surg. 1997;55(10):1050–6.
45. Kuijpers DI, Smeets NW, Lapiere K, Thissen MR, Krekels GA, Neumann HA. Do systemic antibiotics increase the survival of a full thickness graft on the nose? J Eur Acad Dermatol Venereol. 2006;20(10): 1296–301.
46. Wines N, Ryman W, Matulich J, Wines M. Retrospective review of reconstructive methods of conchal bowl defects following mohs micrographic surgery. Dermatol Surg. 2001;27(5):471–4.
47. Phillips TJ, Provan A, Colbert D, Easley KW. A randomized single-blind controlled study of cultured epidermal allografts in the treatment of split-thickness skin graft donor sites. Arch Dermatol. 1993;129(7): 879–82.
48. Keck T, Lindemann J, Kuhnemann S, Sigg O. Healing of composite chondrocutaneous auricular grafts covered by skin flaps in nasal reconstructive surgery. Laryngoscope. 2003;113(2):248–53.
49. van der Eerden PA, Verdam FJ, Dennis SC, Vuyk H. Free cartilage grafts and healing by secondary intention: a viable reconstructive combination after excision of nonmelanoma skin cancer in the nasal alar region. Arch Facial Plast Surg. 2009;11(1):18–23.

## Self-Assessment

1. When considering the repair of a defect, which is the first option to consider?
   (a) Primary closure
   (b) Advancement flap
   (c) Second intent
   (d) Full thickness skin graft

2. For upper lip reconstruction, one study showed that most surgeons preferred which flap?
   (a) Nasolabial flap
   (b) Myocutaneous rotation flap
   (c) Abbe flap
   (d) Cheek advancement flap

3. For a lower full thickness eyelid defect, the most preferred flap to use is?
   (a) Mustarde flap
   (b) Peng flap
   (c) Tenzel flap
   (d) Karapanzic flap

4. In Zitelli's study of bilobed flaps, how many incidences of pincushioning were reported?
   (a) 0
   (b) 5
   (c) 10
   (d) 13

5. Myocutaneous island pedicle flaps are best utilized in which anatomic region?
   (a) Cheek
   (b) Forehead
   (c) Lower lip
   (d) Nose

6. What factor was shown to compromise the viability of the two staged melolabial flap?
   (a) Coumadin
   (b) Diabetes
   (c) Previous radiation treatment
   (d) Alcohol use

7. Full thickness skin grafts showed a higher rate of survival when which drug was taken postoperatively?
   (a) Aspirin
   (b) Azithromycin
   (c) Keflex
   (d) Famvir

## Answers

1. c: Second intent
2. d: Cheek advancement flap
3. c: Tenzel flap
4. a: 0
5. d: Nose
6. c: Previous Radiation treatment
7. b: Azithromycin

# Prevention and Treatment of Scars

# 9

Brenda LaTowsky, Jennifer L. MacGregor,
Jeffrey S. Dover, and Kenneth A. Arndt

## Introduction

Scarring is a challenge that every procedural dermatologist encounters. It affects patients of all ages and all demographics. Left untreated, scars never go away, and rarely improve spontaneously. Even with treatment, complete resolution is near impossible. It is difficult to find another complaint that is so tied to the patient's emotional well-being. However, if success – meaning improvement, not resolution – is met, the self-satisfaction and patient appreciation is great.

The most common type of scarring a procedural dermatologist is asked to treat is acne scarring. Because of the difficult nature of acne scars,

B. LaTowsky (✉)
Skin Care Physicians, 1244 Boylston Street, Suite 103,
Chestnut Hill, MA 02467, USA

Paradise Valley Dermatology, Phoenix, AZ, USA
e-mail: blatowsky@yahoo.com

J.L. MacGregor
SkinCare Physicians, 1244 Boylston Street, Suite 103,
Chestnut Hill, MA 02467, USA

Division of Dermatology, Georgetown University
Hospital, Washington, DC, USA

J.S. Dover • K.A. Arndt
SkinCare Physicians, 1244 Boylston Street, Suite 103,
Chestnut Hill, MA 02467, USA

Section of Dermatologic Surgery and Cutaneous
Oncology, Yale University School of Medicine,
New Haven, CT, USA

Dartmouth Medical School, Hanover, NH, USA

just about every type of laser and light device has been used in an attempt to treat acne scars. Numerous chemical and surgical techniques have also been described, with varying reports of success. Newer techniques are also being utilized in an attempt to combat this universal problem.

Jacob et al. defined a simple classification system for atrophic acne scars that is useful when considering treatment options, as the different types of acne scarring respond selectively to treatment. Figure 9.1 shows the different types of acne scars. Width, depth, and three-dimensional shape are used to categorize scars as ice pick, boxcar, and rolling. Ice pick scars are usually less than 2 mm in width and depth. The scar is a sharply marginated epithelial tract that extend to the deep dermis or subcutaneous tissue. The width of the scar tends to taper as it goes deeper, but the depth is typically below the target of non-surgical treatment modalities. Rolling scars, on the contrary, are wide, depressed scars with a base that appears to be identical to normal skin. There are fibrous attachments from below that are responsible for the difficulty in treating this type of scar. Therefore, treatment of rolling scars cannot focus on the surface of the skin and must affect the subdermis. Boxcar scars are depressions with sharply demarcated borders; the skin appears to have a step-off. They may be shallow or deep, which affects the treatment modality chosen to treat them [1].

Hypertrophic scars are defined as an abnormal wound-healing process that results in scars that may be raised and discolored, usually red or pink.

M. Alam (ed.), *Evidence-Based Procedural Dermatology*,
DOI 10.1007/978-0-387-09424-3_9, © Springer Science+Business Media, LLC 2012

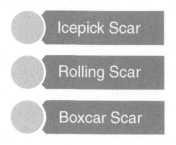

**Fig. 9.1** Classification of atrophic acne scars [1]

These scars are sometimes pruritic. The margins of the scar do not exceed the margins of the original wound. Keloids are scars that infiltrate into surrounding tissue, beyond the original margins of the wound. They are often painful and/or pruritic [2].

Realistic expectations are crucial before the patient undergoes treatment for acne scarring. Clear communication in consultation educates the patient that the skin will never attain its original texture. Additionally, in the experience of the authors, most scars require a 50% improvement before the eyes of friends and families can visualize a difference. The personality of the patient should tailor the treatment plan: is the patient more likely to endure a series of treatments with minimal downtime or fewer treatments with more downtime? What are the appropriate modalities for each preference? For these reasons, reviewing evidence-based literature is crucial when evaluating treatment options for patients.

# Recent Review Articles Regarding the Treatment and Prevention of Scars

## Keloids and Hypertrophic Scars

A recent review by Wolfram et al. summarizing therapeutic management for hypertrophic scars and keloids emphasizes that prevention of the scar is of upmost importance. Patients who are prone to keloids or have any history of abnormal wound healing should approach surgical procedures with caution. Care should be taken that wounds have little or no tension. Ideally, incisions

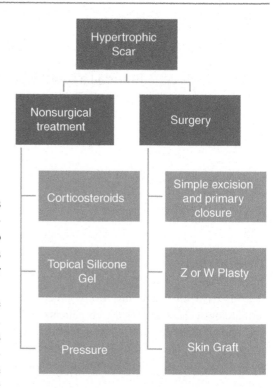

**Fig. 9.2** Summary of treatment recommendations for hypertrophic scars [2]

should not cross joint spaces. High risk areas, such as the chest, should be avoided. Incisions should follow skin creases whenever possible. Especially on the face, subcutaneous sutures should only be used when necessary to alleviate tension.

Treatment options for hypertrophic scars can be summarized in Fig. 9.2. Hypertrophic scars may be treated with topical or intralesional corticosteroids, topical silicone gel or pressure therapy. However, surgery is the most effective and definitive treatment. Scars that have been subjected to factors that contribute to poor wound healing, such as infection or delayed closure can undergo simple re-excision. Performing a Z- or W-plasty changes the direction of the scar and thereby reduces tension. Advantages to these methods of surgical repair are that the limbs of the repair, especially the W-plasty, can be concealed by natural skin creases or rhytides. If the wound cannot be closed by primary repair, skin grafts may be required.

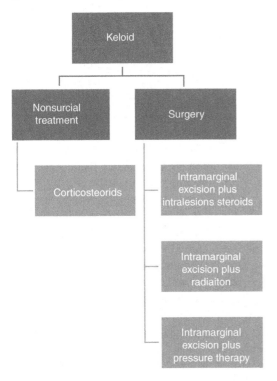

**Fig. 9.3** Summary of treatment recommendations for keloids [2]

Treating keloids and hypertrophic scars with surgery in a susceptible individual warrants a cautious approach: the patient may have the same wound healing response and develop a recurrence. Keloids should be surgically debulked rather than excised; treatment should be coupled with adjuvant measures so that keloid recurrence can be prevented (Fig. 9.3). Kauh et al. combined surgical excision with intralesional corticosteroid injection. The combination resulted in the downregulation of type I collagen gene expression without compromising wound healing (IV, B) [3]. If this approach is taken, sutures may be left in place for 2–3 days longer than normal to prevent dehiscence. Additional adjuvant therapy includes pressure, especially for ear lobe keloids. Topical silicone gel sheeting can be applied after reepithelialization. Daily application at least 12 h/day is recommended [2].

Radiation as a monotherapy for keloids is ineffective, but coupled with surgery the efficacy rate is between 65 and 99% (IV/B) [4, 5]. The minimum effective dose has been reported as 900 cGy. Other parameters such as the timing of radiation, fractionation, duration of treatment, and scar location are less important. A Japanese study examining effectiveness of surgical excision and postoperative irradiation reported a recurrence rate of 21.2% overall with no recurrence observed in the craniofacial area. The study concluded that surgical excision plus electron beam radiation started within a few days is beneficial in both controlling scar quality and preventing recurrence (V/B) [6]. Cryotherapy can also be used to induce direct physical damage to hypertrophic scars and keloids.

The carbon dioxide laser ($CO_2$) and the pulsed dye laser (PDL) have been reported to be efficacious in the treatment of keloids, although laser therapy is probably inferior to surgical modalities. Alster reported improvement in keloids in 14 patients after treatment with the 585-nm PDL. Pulse duration was 0.45 ms and fluence ranged from 6.5 to 7.25 $J/cm^2$. A 57% clinical improvement was noted after one treatment and 83% in clinical improvement was noted after the second treatment. Improvement was maintained at 6-month follow up (IV/B) [7]. However, in a controlled study, Chan et al. reported no esthetic benefit in 27 hypertrophic scars in Chinese patients after 3–6 treatments with the 585-nm PDL. Symptoms such as pruritus were improved in the treated side (III/B) [8].

Intralesional corticosteroids are probably the most commonly used, easiest, and most effective nonsurgical option in the treatment of hypertrophic scars and keloids. Topical and intralesional steroids tend to result in flattening of the scars, but not resolution. A triamcinolone (TA) concentration of 5–10 mg/mL injected with a 25–27 gauge needle into the upper dermis may be used for a developing hypertrophic scar. Treatments should be repeated every 3–6 weeks until the scar is stable or if side effects such as tissue atrophy, hypopigmentation, or telangiectasia develop. Preexisting keloids should be treated with intralesional injections of TA at a dose of 40 mg/mL mixed with equal parts 2% lidocaine for at least three treatment sessions with 1-month intervals. Hyaluronidase may be mixed in the syringe to help disperse the injection [2].

**Table 9.1** Examples of topical or injectables reported to improve acne scars [10]

| |
|---|
| Vitamins A, E, and C |
| Zinc |
| Hyaluronidase |
| Cyclosporine |
| Honey |
| Onion extract |
| 5-Fluorouracil |
| Bleomycin |
| Retinoids |
| Verapamil |
| Pepsin |
| Hydrochloric acid |
| Fomalin |

5-fluorouracil (5-FU) affects the rapidly proliferating fibroblasts in hypertrophic scars and keloids. Intralesional injection seems to be effective in hypertrophic scars, but there are mixed results in studies with keloids. Side effects include purpura and even ulceration. Faster and improved efficacy with fewer side effects using 5-FU with concomitant intralesional steroids has been reported. PDL may be combined with 5-FU for enhanced therapeutic response (III/B) [2, 9].

Studies regarding topical therapies are inconsistent, with limited evidence and a small number of patients evaluated. Examples include imiquimod 5% cream, onion extract, interferons, and immunotherapy including tacrolimus and sirolimus. In general, surgical, intralesional, and light-based therapies are preferred over topical modalities. Occasionally, topical therapies may be used as adjunctive treatments for hypertrophic scars and keloids; the reader is encouraged to consult outside sources for the most recent evidence-based literature, as new modalities and reports tend to appear rapidly within the literature. Table 9.1 lists examples of topical treatments that have been reported to improve scars [10].

## Acne Scarring

A review by Rivera published in 2008 divides the management of acne scarring into medical management, surgical management, procedural management, tissue augmentation, and light, laser, and energy therapy [10]. Medical management includes topical or injectable substances (Table 9.1). Retinoids have the most supporting evidence in topical management and seem to improve scar architecture by altering the dermal elastic and collagen content [11, 12]. Intralesional steroids are commonly used for hypertrophic scars and keloids and may require several treatments at monthly intervals. The effectiveness of silicone dressings and pressure therapy are controversial for acne scarring [10].

Surgical management of acne scarring (Fig. 9.4) includes punch excision, elliptical excision, punch elevation, skin grafting, subcision, and debulking. The majority of surgery is done on icepick, deep boxcar, and deep rolling scars. Ice pick scars smaller than 3.5 mm may be treated with punch excision; larger lesions are treated with elliptical excisions. Laser resurfacing may be performed as an adjunct after punch excision and may enhance results. Punch excision can even be performed the same day as resurfacing, without increased risk of complications (IV/B) [13]. Depressed boxcar scars can be treated with punch elevation. This technique is optimized by ensuring that the base of the scar has a smooth surface that will match the surrounding skin. Rolling and depressed boxcar scars can be treated by subcision over several sessions using a tri-bevel needle to release the tethering connections and to induce trauma, leading to connective tissue deposition. Rarely electrodessication can be useful in reshaping edges of the scar. Procedures and evidence grading used for acne scarring are outlined in Table 9.2.

Superficial chemical peels include alpha hydroxy acid, beta hydroxyacid, Jessner's solution, modified Jessner's solution, resorcinol, and <10% trichloroacetic acid (TCA). Medium-depth chemical peels include 10–40% TCA with or without Jessner's solution. Deep chemical peels include phenol or croton oil. Although reports of efficacy exist [14, 15] (V–VI/C), in the experience of the authors, superficial and medium chemical peels do not significantly improve acne scars when compared with other available modalities. Deep chemical peels can be useful – especially focal application. The chemical reconstruction of skin scars (CROSS) technique originally described

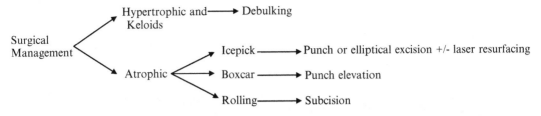

**Fig. 9.4** Surgical approach in the treatment of scars [10]. Adapted from Rivera [10]

**Table 9.2** Procedural management in acne scarring and evidence-based grading

| | |
|---|---|
| Cryosurgery | VI/C |
| Electrodessication | VI/C |
| Radiation | IV/B |
| Chemical peels | V/C [14, 15] |
| Microdermabrasion | VI/C [19] |
| Dermabrasion | VI/C |

Adapted from Rivera [10]

**Table 9.3** Tissue augmentation and evidence-based grading for acne scars

| | |
|---|---|
| Collagen (Zyderm, Zyplast) | VI, C |
| ArteFill and Artecoll | VI, C |
| Autologous fat | V, B |
| Silicone | V, B |
| Hyaluronic acid | VI, C |
| Polyacrylamides (outline, evolution, bio-alcamid, argiform, aquamid) | VI, C |
| Poly-L-lactic acid (NewFill, Sculptra) [23] | VI, C |
| Calcium hydroxyapatite (Radiesse) | III, B |
| Dextran beads (Reviderm Intra) | VI, C |
| Polyoxyethylene and polyoxypropylene polymer (ProFill) | VI, C |
| Plasma, gelatin, epsilon-aminocaproic acid, lidocaine (Fibrel) | VI, C |

Adapted from Rivera [10]

by Lee et al. involves focal application of 50–100% TCA directly to icepick and rolling acne scars rather than the entire face (IV/B) [16]. Blinded physician assessment revealed a 50–70% improvement in 90% of patients after 3–6 treatments. Increasing the strength of the TCA resulted in increased efficacy and increased patient satisfaction: 82% of patients treated with 65% TCA were satisfied with results compared to a 94% satisfaction in the patients treated with 100% TCA. The CROSS technique was subsequently shown to increase epidermal and dermal thickness as well as dermal collagen content at TCA concentrations of 50, 65, and 100% (but not 30%). These findings were significantly better than the simple application of TCA to normal skin (III/B) [17]. Clinical improvement is proportional to the number of treatments [16]. Fabbrocini et al. confirmed (in three patients) that 50% TCA is also effective using the CROSS technique (IV/B) [18].

Microdermabrasion may be used for superficial scars with variable results over several treatment sessions. The more abrasive crystals, such as aluminum oxide, or diamond-tipped abrasive devices are more efficacious than the less expensive and less aggressive methods. The authors do not routinely recommend microdermabrasion to patients, although anecdotal reports in the literature do exist (VI/C) [19]. Dermabrasion can be

extremely effective but results rely heavily on the operator. It may be used alone for superficial scars and for improvement of deeper scars or in combination therapy with surgical modalities. Because of the need for adnexal structures for the healing process, dermabrasion is not recommended for keloids, hypertrophic scars, or scars on the back, chest, or neck. The authors rarely use dermabrasion because of other modalities that are safer, with comparable efficacy.

Table 9.3 lists the substances that may be used to physically fill the atrophic scars. Autologous fat has been reported to have a durability of 65% at 3 months, 50% at 6 months, 40% at 9 months, and 30% at 12 months. Resorption in areas of fibrotic acne scars may be due to decreased vascularity and, thus, viability (V, B) [20]. Adding adipose-derived stem cells to the injected fat has been reported to increase survival of the grafts, as indicated by increased weight (2.5 times the fat-only injected group), greater volume and less fibrous grafts (V, B) [21]. Silicone has been shown to be safe in humans. Its efficacy, safety, and longevity for acne scarring have been reported by Barnett and Barnett in a report with five patients who have 30-year follow-up post-treatment (V/B) [22]. Poly-L-lactic acid (Sculptra, Sanofi-Aventis, Bridgewater, NJ) has been used in a single-center, open-label prospective study in 20 patients with moderate to severe acne or varicella scars. Investigator-assessed reductions in acne scar size and severity were significant ($p < 0.0001$) during the course of seven treatments. Subject-rated reduction in scar severity was also significant ($p = 0.0078$) (IV/B) [23].

Laser therapy is divided into ablative and nonablative. Ablative devices include the carbon-dioxide laser ($CO_2$), erbium-yttrium-aluminum-garnet (Er/YAG), and fractionated $CO_2$ lasers. Traditional resurfacing is useful for hypertrophic, boxcar, and (far less so) keloids. Walia and Alster report 60 patients who experienced an average improvement in severe atrophic acne scars of 69% at 1 month, 67% at 6 months (the decrease was attributed to resolution of edema with the temporary revisualization of some lesions), 73% at 12 months, and 75% at 18 months. Neocollagenesis and remodeling continued the entire 18-month follow-up period (IV/B) [24]. The Er/YAG does not penetrate as deeply and therefore thermal damage leading to scar improvement is less. A study including 158 patients performed by Woo et al. treated 83 patients with short-pulsed Er/YAG (Derma 20, ESC Medical Systems, Haifa, Israel), 35 patients with variable-pulsed Er/YAG ($CO_3$, Cynosure, Wayland, MA) and 40 with dual-mode Er/YAG (Contour, Sciton, Inc, Palo Alto, CA). Good to excellent results were achieved with all examined Er/YAG lasers for ice pick and shallow boxcar scars. Good to excellent results for rolling scars were achieved only with dual-mode Er/YAG treatment. Dual-mode Er/YAG also improved deep boxcar scars more effectively than the other modalities (rating of good). A long-pulse duration resulting in increased thermal energy may be necessary for successful treatment of rolling and deep boxcar scars (IV/B) [25].

Erbium fractional photothermolysis (Fraxel Re:Store™, Reliant technologies, Mountain View, CA) is a relatively new technology reported to be useful in the treatment of scars. Alster et al. treated 53 patients with more than one session of fractional photothermolysis. Ninety-one percent of patients were reported to have a 25–50% improvement after a single treatment; 87% of patients undergoing three treatments had 51–75% improvement. Results were maintained at 6-month follow-up (IV/B) [26].

Because of the less aggressive nature of nonablative lasers, the devices are more effective in the treatment of atrophic, rolling, or hypertrophic scars rather than ice pick, boxcar, or keloids scars. The 532-nm KTP laser (Aura KTP, Laserscope, San Jose, CA, USA) is used for the treatment of acne and therefore is able to prevent scar formation (III/B) [27]. The 585-nm PDL probably decreases vascularity and induces collagen alterations. Treatment of argon-laser scars with the 585-nm PDL showed an improvement in both hypertrophic and atrophic scars (IV/B) [28, 29].

The 1,064-nm neodymium/YAG (Nd/YAG) laser targets vascular lesions more than pigment and is also effective on scars; the mechanism may be similar to the PDL. In a small study that treated nine patients with a short-pulsed 1,064 Nd/YAG (Vantage, Cutera, Brisbane, CA) with eight treatments at 2-week intervals, all scars improved. Laser parameters were 0.3 ms pulse duration, 14 J/$cm^2$, 7 Hz and 5-mm spot size. Physician assessment at 1–2 month follow-up showed a 29% average improvement; self-assessment ranged from 10 to 50% improvement in all but one patient. Patient satisfaction was high (IV/B) [30]. Another study treated 12 patients with mild to moderate acne scarring every 4–6 weeks for a total of five treatments using a long-pulsed 1,064-nm Nd/YAG (Quantum DL, Lumenis Corp., Yokneam, Israel) The laser is a triple-pulse laser (7.0/7.0/7.0-ms pulse duration, 70-ms delay), and patients were treated with an energy fluence of 120 J/$cm^2$. Patient satisfaction was 8.6 out of 10. Photographs were evaluated by independent dermatologists and the improvement was rated as only mild to moderate (one patient was graded by one physician as having no improvement). There was a significant histological increase in dermal collagen (IV/B) [31].

The 1,320-nm Nd/YAG laser (Cooltouch, ICN Pharmaceuticals, Inc., Costa Mesa, CA) penetrates to the deep papillary and mid-reticular dermis. It seems to be most useful for atrophic acne scars: in a report of 12 patients with atrophic vs. mixed acne scars, those with the atrophic scars experienced the most improvement (1.7 vs. 1.3 for physician rating of improvement of atrophic vs. mixed on a 10-point scale, respectively), but the trend was not statistically significant. The mean acne scar improvement was 1.5 points on physician assessment and 2.2 points on patient assessments ($p = 0.01$). The authors conclude that the type rather than the extent of scarring is the best predictor of clinical response to the 1,320-nm Nd/YAG laser (IV/B) [32].

The 1,450-nm diode laser (Smoothbeam, Candela Corp., Wayland, MA) is primarily used for acne treatment, and may also be important in preventing scars. A split-face study evaluating the laser in the treatment of acne noted that acne scarring improved in 83% of patients. The investigators treated half the face with a single pass of double-stacked pulses and the other half was treated with a double pass of single pulses. The improvement in scars was rated as 1 (using a 0–3 scale) on both sides (V/B) [33].

The 1,540 erbium (Er)/glass laser (Aramis-Quantel, Quantel Medical, Clermont Ferrand, France) penetrates to the papillary dermis to stimulate collagen regeneration and tightening. The results from treatment with this laser may be gradual (occurring over 6 months). A review on several studies noted progressive improvement after a series of four treatments over a 6-month period of time. Responders tend to show a 20–30% improvement in acne scarring (IV/B) [34].

Nonlaser light and energy sources include intense pulsed light (IPL), radiofrequency, and plasma. It has been indicated by histological examination that IPL increases fibrosis in the superficial papillary dermis and fibroblasts throughout the dermis (IV, B) [35]. The light source has also been reported to improve nonfacial hypertrophic scars, resulting in a 45% improvement after the first treatment and a 65% improvement after the second treatment. In this study, the 595-nm PDL also showed similar improvement in the scars and led the authors to conclude that the IPL is an alternative, one that is

perhaps less painful, to the PDL for the treatment of nonfacial hypertrophic scars (III, B) [36]. Radiofrequency (Thermotherapy) has been studied as a modality in the treatment of acne. One study reported the incidental finding of improved acne scarring (TheraCool TC, Thermage, Inc., Hayward, CA) (V, C) [37]. Plasma uses radiofrequency to temporarily excite nitrogen gas, creating energy that diffuses as heat into the dermis. Residual thermal damage may ultimately lead to collagen remodeling. One study reported a 34% reduction in depth of acne scarring at 10 days, 26% reduction at 3 months, 23% reduction in depth at 6 months, but no significant change in clinical findings between 6 months and 2 years (IV/B) [38]. Therefore, this modality may result in temporary improvement of scars, but long-lasting effects are absent.

## Case Series and Cohort Studies

### 1,320-nm Nd/YAG

A prospective study evaluating eight patients with facial acne scars were treated with 6 monthly treatments with the 1,320-nm Nd/YAG laser (Cooltouch). Patients were treated with three nonoverlapping passes at the following settings: fluences of 14–18 J/cm$^2$ during the first two passes and fluences of 13–17 J/cm$^2$ during the third pass. The peak surface temperature was 44°C. Changes in acne scars were assessed by two nontreating, nonblinded physicians by comparing baseline photographs to those taken at 5 months and 1 year after treatment and using a six-point grading scale (0 = no improvement, 5 = maximum improvement). The mean improvement was 3.9 points at 5 months ($p = 0.002$) and 4.3 points at 1 year ($p = 0.011$). Patients also graded their improvement, which was statistically significant at 5 months (improvement of 3.6 points, $p = 0.002$). No adverse effects were reported. The authors concluded that the 1,320-nm Nd/YAG is safe and efficacious in improving the appearance of acne scarring. Of note, this study was sponsored by the company that manufactures the Cooltouch and the laser was also provided at a reduced cost (IV/B) [39].

Bhatia et al. performed a retrospective study with 34 patients with Fitzpatrick skin types (FST) II–IV after they had received six treatments of the 1,320-nm Nd/YAG (Cooltouch) for photoaging or acne scarring. Posttreatment questionnaires were given 3–12 months after the final treatment. The patients rated their improvement on a scale from 0 to 10 (0 = no improvement, 10 = maximum improvement). The mean improvement was 5.4 in the acne scarring group (statistically significant over the photoaging group, $p < 0.04$). The patients in the acne scarring group also reported a textural improvement of 36% (compared to 27% of patients treated for photoaging). Discomfort was associated with the treatment. Overall satisfaction with the treatment was 58.8%. The authors noted that long-term follow up (6-months or greater) may have resulted in greater perceived improvement (V/B) [40].

## 1,450-nm Diode

Twenty patients were treated with three treatments at 4 week intervals with the 1,450-nm diode laser (Smoothbeam, Candela Corp., Wayland, MA). The study was a randomized, split-face trial with the primary endpoint of measuring acne lesion and sebum reduction. One side of the face was randomized to receive a higher fluence than the contralateral side. Treatment settings were as follows: 14 vs. 16 J/cm², 6 mm spot size and dynamic cooling device (DCD) was set at 40 ms at 14 J/cm² and 45 ms at 16 J/cm². The improvement was noted by physicians to increase over time, especially for the higher fluences, and was 25–50% at the 6-month follow-up. Subjective improvement in acne scarring and sebum production was noted in all patients. Almost 80% of subjects reported continued improvement in acne scars at 3-month follow-up: 93.3% reported continued improvement in acne scars at the 6-month follow-up; 85.9% of patients noted continued improvement at the 12-month follow-up (V/B) [41]. Another study used the Smoothbeam to treat 57 Asian patients with FST IV–V for 4–6 treatments. Fluences were 11–12 J/cm², pulse duration was 250 ms, DCD spray duration was 50 ms and

**Table 9.4** Quartile grading system used for acne scarring

| | |
|---|---|
| 1 | 1–25% improvement |
| 2 | 26–50% improvement |
| 3 | 51–75% improvement |
| 4 | >76% improvement |

repetition rate was 1 Hz. Scars were treated with a single nonoverlapping pass. The mean physician assessment ranging from 5 to 6.6% improvement in acne scars 6 months after the final treatment. There was not a correlation between scar improvement and number of treatments received. Notably, 40% of patients reported no to very minimal clinical improvement. Postinflammatory hyperpigmentation (PIH) was noted in 39% of patients. Pain was also significant, with 55% of patients rating the pain as moderate, and 5% rating the pain as severe. The authors noted that icepick and deep boxcar scars tended to be resistant to treatment (IV/B) [42].

## 1,550-nm Fractional Photothermolysis

Fractional photothermolysis has changed the prognosis of acne scarring. The 1,550-nm Er-doped fractional photothermolysis nonablative laser (Fraxel, Reliant technologies, Inc., San Diego, CA) was the first device that was reported to significantly improve acne scarring. Geronemus found an average level of improvement of 41% in 17 patients by topographical analysis after five treatments with the Fraxel laser spaced 1–3 weeks apart. A posttreatment questionnaire revealed 100% of patients were satisfied with the treatment and the perceived improvement was 48% (IV/B) [43]. Alster et al., as described in discussion above, reported a 51–75% improvement in 87% of patients after treatment with the Fraxel laser. The fluences used ranges from 8 to 16 J/cm² at densities of 125–250 microthermal zones (MTZ) per cm². Eight to ten passes were performed with total energies of 4–6 kJ per session. Patients were treated at 4 week intervals and three treatments were performed. Patients were evaluated based on a quartile scale (Table 9.4) with photographs

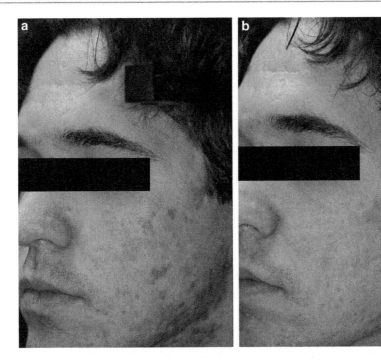

**Fig. 9.5** Patient with acne scarring at baseline (**a**) and after six treatments with 1,550-nm fractionated photothermolysis (Fraxel Re:Store™, Reliant technologies, Mountain View, CA) (**b**). There is market improvement of boxcar and icepick scarring. Photographs courtesy of Paul Friedman, MD

taken at baseline, before each treatment session and 6 months after the final treatment. Clinical improvement was found to increase proportionally to each treatment session. One patient with FST V developed transient PIH using a higher density (250 MTZ/cm$^2$) and this did not recur with use of a lower density (125 MTZ/cm$^2$). Acneiform eruptions occurred as a result of 5% of treatment sessions and the eruptions were treated with doxycycline (IV/B) [26].

An upgraded model of the Fraxel allows for higher energies and densities (Fraxel Re:Store, Reliant technologies). Chrastil et al. studied the higher fluences allowed using the newer model. Twenty nine patients were treated with 2–6 treatments with the second-generation Fraxel at fluences ranging from 35 to 40 J/cm$^2$. Patients had FST ranging from I to V. Treatment levels ranged from 7 to 10, which corresponded with a treatment density of 20–35%. The patients were evaluated by three independent physicians using baseline and posttreatment photography using a four-point scale. The majority (18 of 29) patient achieved a 50–75% improvement in facial and back acne scarring. Five patients achieved an improvement of greater than 75% in acne scarring (Fig. 9.5). No significant adverse effects were noted (IV/B) [44].

Fractional photothermolysis has also been reported to improve hypopigmented surgical scars. A small pilot study with seven patients who had hypopigmented surgical scars were treated with 2–4 treatments with the Fraxel laser. The fluence ranged from 7 to 20 J/cm$^2$ and a total density of 1,000–2,500 MTZ/cm$^2$ was used. Digital photographs at baseline and at 4 weeks after the last treatment were used to evaluate the patients on a four-point scale by independent physicians. Six of the seven patients had a 51–75% improvement in hypopigmentation. Overall the texture of the scars was improved. The patient's degree of satisfaction paralleled the physician's assessment of

**Table 9.5** Vancouver scar scale

| Pigmentation | |
|---|---|
| 0 | Normal color (resembles nearby skin) |
| 1 | Hypopigmentation |
| 2 | Hyperpigmentation |
| Vascularity | |
| 0 | Normal |
| 1 | Pink (slight increase blood supply) |
| 2 | Red (significant increase in local blood supply) |
| 3 | Purple (excessive local blood supply) |
| Pliability | |
| 0 | Normal |
| 1 | Supple (flexible with minimal resistance) |
| 2 | Yielding (giving way to pressure) |
| 3 | Firm (solid/inflexible, not easily moved, resistant to manual pressure) |
| 4 | Banding (rope-like, blanches with extension of scar, does not limit range of motion) |
| 5 | Contracture (permanent shortening of scar producing deformity or distortion; limits range of motion) |
| Height | |
| 0 | Normal (flat) |
| 1 | <2 |
| 2 | >2 and <5 |
| 3 | >5 |

improvement. All patients reported improvement in hypopigmentation lasting greater than 3 months after the last treatment (IV/C) [45].

Prevention of thyroidectomy scars was studied using a 1,550-nm fractional erbium glass laser (MOSAIC, Lutronic Corp., Princeton Junction, NJ). Twenty-seven South Korean patients were treated with four treatments at 1-month intervals starting 2–3 weeks after thyroidectomy. Independent patients who underwent thyroidectomy but were not treated with laser were used for controls. The fluence used was 10 mJ and the density was 1,500 spot/cm². Evaluation was performed 6 months after the final treatment using the Vancouver Scar Score (VSS) (Table 9.5) and a clinical assessment using a four-point scale by three independent physicians. Scars were improved in the treatment group, which had a mean VSS of 1.52 (vs. a score of 3.0 for the untreated group). The mean global assessment was 3.15 in the treated group vs. 2.07 in the untreated group. Although a limitation of the study was the unrelated control group, the authors concluded that low-level stimulation of

healing tissue could results in the prevention of hypertrophic scars (III/B) [46].

Fractionated $CO_2$ resurfacing is one of the newest technologies used to treat acne scars (Fig. 9.6a, b). A prospective study treated 13 patients with FST I–IV with moderate to severe acne scars with 2 or 3 treatments with a 30 W $CO_2$ laser (Fraxel Re:Pair® laser, Reliant Technologies, Inc, Mountain View, CA) at 1–2-month intervals. Maximum energies of 70–100 mJ were used for acne scar regions (cheeks, forehead, chin); treatments of the eyelids were limited to 20–30 mJ. Densities ranged from 100 to 400 mJ per pass, with total treatment densities of 200–1,200 MTZ/cm² (densities were reduced in sensitive areas such as the nose and upper and lower eyelids). Clinical improvement was graded by the patient and investigator on a quartile scale at 1 and 3 months following final treatment. Topographic measurements were also taken (using PRIMOS, GFM, Teltow, Germany) at baseline and 3 months after the final treatment. Patients demonstrated an overall texture improvement and improvement of atrophy rated by both investigator and subjects as

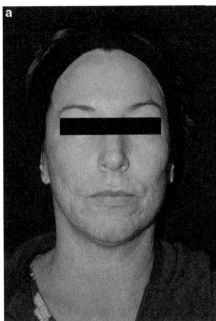
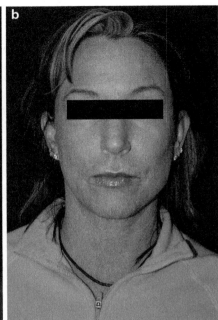

**Fig. 9.6** Patient with acne scars at baseline (**a**) and 2 weeks after fractioned $CO_2$ (Fraxel Re:Pair™) (**b**). The fluence used on the cheeks and perioral regions was 50 mJ. A fluence of 30 mJ on the eyelids and jawline was used. A fluence of 40 mJ was used on the forehead. Density used was 40%. The patient experienced an approximate improvement of 65% at 2-week follow-up. Photographs courtesy of Michael Kaminer, MD

26–50%. Topographical analysis showed significant improvement in deeper acneiform scars, ranging from 47.6 to 79.9%, with an overall mean of 66.8%. The authors note that higher energy levels corresponded with higher improvement scores. No delayed pigmentary changes were noted, but transient PIH was noted in three patients (IV/B) [47].

## Randomized Controlled Trials and Meta-Analyses

### Prevention of Scarring

A Cochrane review on silicon gel sheeting for preventing and treating hypertrophic and keloid scars reviewed 15 trials involving 615 people. The trials compared the efficacy of silicon gel sheeting with control, nonsilicon gel sheeting, Vitamin E, laser, intralesional TA, and nonadhesive silicon gel sheeting. Prevention studies showed that the silicon gel sheeting reduced the incidence of hypertrophic scarring in patients prone to scarring (RR 0.46, 95% CI 0.21–0.98). The sheeting may also produce a significant reduction in scar thickness (RR −1.99, 95% CI −2.13 to −1.85) and color improvement (RR 3.05, 95% CI 1.57–5.96). Overall, the authors concluded that the studies were "of poor quality and very susceptible to bias." It was also determined that weak evidence exists for using silicon gel sheeting in preventing abnormal scarring in susceptible individuals, but "poor quality of research means a great deal of uncertainty prevails" (I/C) [48].

A blinded, prospective, randomized clinical trial in 31 patients assessed the role of botulinum toxin in facial wound healing. Botulinum toxin was injected into musculature adjacent to a forehead surgical wound within 24 h and was compared to placebo injection. Photographs were graded by facial plastic surgeons using a 10-point visual analog scale. The follow-up period was 2 years. The botulinum toxin-treated patients scored a median of 8.9, vs. 7.2 for the placebo group ($p=0.003$). The authors concluded that botulinum-toxin induced immobilization of forehead wounds enhances healing (II/A) [49].

A randomized controlled comparative study examined postoperative corticosteroid injections vs. radiation therapy in the prevention of earlobe keloid recurrence after excision. Thirty-one keloids were treated with postoperative radiation or corticosteroid injection and followed for 12 months. Six keloids recurred: two after postoperative radiation treatment and four after postoperative corticosteroid injection. The difference was not statistically significant, but the authors conclude that postoperative radiotherapy is simpler and may have been more effective in preventing earlobe keloids recurrences (II/A) [50].

## Striae Distensae

The effect of fractional photothermolysis on striae rubra and striae alba was studied in a randomized controlled study. Twenty female patients received six treatments using a 1,550-nm erbium-doped fiber laser (Fraxel Re:Store) at 2–3 week intervals. The control was site-matched nontreated striae. Clinical response was assessed by the patient and investigator at 1-, 2-, and 3-month follow-up intervals. Baseline and 3-month follow-up photographs were graded on a quartile system by four independent dermatologists. The results from the independent evaluators were as follows: overall improvement of 26–50% in 5/8 (63%) of patients, improvement in dyschromia of less than 25% in 4/8 (50%) of patients, improvement in texture of 26–50% in 4/8 (50%) of patients. No adverse effects were noted. The authors conclude that fractional photothermolysis is safe and effective in the treatment of striae distensae (III/B) [51].

A randomized controlled trial treated striae rubra (two patients) and striae distensae (nine patients) with the 1,450-nm diode laser (Smoothbeam laser) in Asian patients with FST IV–VI. The striae on the contralateral side served as the untreated control. The patients were randomized to the following treatment settings: 4, 8, or 12 $J/cm^2$. Three treatments were performed at 6-week intervals. Photographs taken at baseline and after each treatment were graded by blinded nontreating physicians. Two months after the last treatment, no improvement was noted between the treated and untreated striae. Additionally, PIH occurred in seven (64%) of patients. The authors concluded that the Smoothbeam laser is not useful in the treatment of striae in patients with skin types IV–VI (III/B) [52].

## Hypertrophic Scars and Keloids

A meta-analysis was conducted by Leventhal et al. in 2006 using PubMed databases through October 2005. The search excluded studies composed solely of African American or Asian patients, studies that used nonclinical outcome measures or studies that included burn injuries. Each study was graded in an attempt to standardize the analysis. Based on the 70 included studies of all combined treatment modalities, the authors concluded that there is a 70% chance of improvement in keloids and hypertrophic scars with treatment. However, this finding fell within the confidence interval (CI 49–91%). Therefore, improvement of hypertrophic scars and keloids after treatment was not statistically significant from improvement due to chance. The mean amount of improvement achieved was reported to be approximately 60% and there was no difference in improvement rates between treatments. This analysis suggests that current modalities in the treatment of keloids and hypertrophic scars are not likely to result in scar improvement, but the meta-analysis is limited by the quality of the studies and varied clinical endpoints. Different treatment parameters in each study results in factors that could not be controlled, such as anatomical sites, duration of scar formation, prior therapies, dosages and dosing schedules. It is also possible that clinical benefit diminished over the follow-up periods, which were varied (I/B) [53].

A randomized controlled trial in 2007 studied the pulse width of a 595-nm flashlight-pumped PDL on keloidal and hypertrophic sternotomy scars. Sternotomy scars were divided into two segments in 19 patients with FST III–V and each segment was randomized to a different pulse width: 0.45 or 40 ms. Fluence was set at 7 J/cm$^2$. Three treatments were performed at 4-week intervals. Scar volume, height, erythema, and pliability were measured and evaluated at weeks 0, 4, 8, and 24. The 0.45 ms pulse width was more effective than the 40 ms pulse width (after the third treatment a scar volume resolution of 24.4 vs. 16.9%, respectively). No side effects, including pigmentary changes, were reported (II/A) [54]. The authors note that improvement in this study with Asian patients was not as effective as that reported in Caucasian patients. They discuss the results of the study by Alster (discussed above) that reported improvement of 83% after two treatments in patients with FST I–II (IV/B) [7].

Another study on sternotomy scars was a randomized controlled study comparing intralesional traimcinolone (TA), 5-flurouracil (5-FU), and 585-nm PDL. Ten patients had the keloids and hypertrophic scars divided into five segments, which were randomly treated with: 585-nm PDL with fluence of 5 J/cm$^2$, intralesional TA (20 mg/mL), intralesional 5-FU (50 mg/mL), and intralesional TA 1 mg/mL with mixed 5-FU (45 mg/mL). One segment of the keloid was the untreated control. Scar height, erythema, and pliability were evaluated before and every 8 weeks after treatment. Additionally, biopsies were sent for histologic analysis at week 32. All treated areas were found to be significantly improved; the intralesional treatments responded more rapidly to therapy and had more improvement in induration than the PDL alone. The texture of the scar improved more in the PDL-treated segments. Scar erythema did not significantly improve over control. The segments that received the intralesional corticosteroid alone had a 50% incidence of hypopigmentation, telangiectasia, or skin atrophy. The authors concluded that all therapies were comparable in efficacy, with intralesional steroid monotherapy having an increased risk of adverse reactions (III/B) [55].

A randomized trial including 45 patients, FST II–IV, with hypertrophic scars and keloids compared the efficacy of bleomycin tattoo to cryotherapy combined with intralesional TA. The tattoo technique was performed after anesthetizing with lidocaine. Bleomycin (1.5 IU/mL, maximum of 10 IU per session) was "dripped" onto the lesion and then punctures were made with a 25-gauge needle. Approximately, 40 punctures were made per 5 mm$^2$. Cryotherapy was performed with cotton wool swabs using one freezing cycle lasting 30 s, and TA (40 mg/mL, 0.1–1 mL and no more than 80 mg per session) was injected. Four treatments were performed at 1 month intervals and lesion size, symptoms, color, and thickness were assessed at each visit. The mean improvement was 88.3% in the group treated with bleomycin and 67.3% in the group treated with cryotherapy and intralesional TA ($p=0.001$). Improvement was statistically significant in patients who were younger than 30 years of age, but not in those who were older than 30. In the group receiving cryotherapy and intralesional steroids, the response of the smaller lesions (less than 100 mm$^2$) response were superior compared to larger lesions. Hyperpigmentation was noted in 75% of the patients in the bleomycin group. The authors conclude that bleomycin could be a good option for patients with large keloids and hypertrophic scars in covered areas (II/A) [56].

Interestingly, a double-blinded study showed superiority of cryosurgery over intralesional TA in the treatment of early, vascular acne keloids. The authors demonstrate that 85% of early, and in particular vascular, keloids respond to treatment. Cryosurgery was reported to have a superior response over intralesional TA, particularly in early, vascular lesions (I/A) [57].

## Surgical Scars and Acne Scars

### 532-nm Neodymium/Yttrium-Aluminum-Garnet (Nd/YAG)

In 2001, Bernstein et al. conducted a randomized, controlled trial of patients treated for mild-severe lip rhytids and mild-moderate acne scarring on the cheeks with the 532-nm, 2 ms pulse duration, frequency-doubled Nd/YAG laser. Twenty-two patients with FST I–III (11 with photoaging and 11 with acne scaring) were included and an average of three treatments was performed at 3–6 week intervals. Patients were asked to assess the percentage of improvement 3 months after treatment, and a blinded investigator attempted to identify the treated side of the face by examination. Patients treated for facial acne scarring reported an average improvement of 53.6% (vs. 51.4% for upper lip rhytids). No adverse effects were reported (II/A) [58].

## 585-nm and 595-nm PDL

A randomized, controlled study treated 11 patients with 12 postoperative scars to determine if PDL could affect the appearance and texture of postoperative scars. One half of the scar received three treatments with the 585-nm PDL starting on the day of suture removal and the other half was the untreated control. Treatments were given at 1 month intervals and the treatment parameters were as follows: 0.45 ms pulse width, 10-mm spot size, 3.5 J/cm$^2$, and 10% overlap. FST I–IV was included in the study. A blinded examiner evaluated the scars using the VSS for pigmentation, vascularity, pliability, and height. Scars were also blindly evaluated for cosmetic appearance using a visual analog scale. No purpura was noted at this low fluence. There was a significant improvement in the treated scars in all parameters for the VSS and also the cosmetic appearance of the scars (7.3 vs. 5.2 on a 11-point scale). The authors concluded that three treatments with these subpurpuric settings resulted in improvement of surgical scars on the day of suture removal (II/A) [59].

A 595-nm cryogen-cooled PDL (VBeam, Candela Corporation, Wayland, MA) was used to evaluate efficacy on surgical scars starting on the day of suture removal. Sixteen patients with FST I to IV were treated at 4–8 week intervals for three treatment sessions. The surgical scars were greater than 2 cm, and the half of the scar served as the untreated control. Treatment settings were as follows: fluence of 8 J/cm$^2$, 7 mm spot size, pulse width of 1.5 and 30 ms spray duration with 10 ms delay. The VSS was used to evaluate the scars by a blinded examiner. Additionally, the same evaluator graded the cosmetic appearance on a 0 (worst) to 10 (best) scale. There was significant improvement in the treated portion of the scar using the VSS (60% improvement of treated vs. negative 3% improvement of untreated

control). The most significant improvement was found in the vascularity and pliability of the scars. The overall cosmetic appearance of the treated portion of the scars were rated an average of two points higher than the untreated portion. Some minor purpura was noted. The authors noted that decreasing the fluence to a subpurpuric level may decrease treatment side effects while maintaining efficacy (II/A) [60].

Alam et al. conducted a randomized controlled trial with 17 patients. Surgical scars were treated with a 595-nm PDL (Vbeam, Candela Corporation, Wayland, MA) at the time of suture removal (2 weeks after excision). The control was either half of the scar that remained untreated or a separate scar of the same size. Settings were: 7 J/cm$^2$, 7 mm spot size, 1.5 ms pulse duration and 30-ms spray, 20-ms delay of dynamic cooling. Pulses were delivered with 10% overlap. Blinded evaluators graded pictures of the scars at 6 week follow up; no difference in clinical appearance was found in the treated vs. untreated scars (scars were graded on visibility of the incision, erythema, hyperpigmentation, hypopigmentation, induration, and atrophy). The authors concluded that a single PDL treatment does not impact appearance of surgical scars; they theorized that minimum benefit may be between 1 and 3 treatments of PDL (II/A) [61].

## 1,064-nm Nd/YAG

A randomized, controlled comparative trial evaluating the 1,064-nm Nd/YAG and the 1,320-nm Nd/YAG nonablative lasers for acne scars was published in 2005. Twelve patients (11 with facial acne scarring and one with back acne scarring) with FST I to III were randomly selected to have half of the face or back treated with the Lyra 1,064-nm Nd/YAG (Laserscope Corporation, San Jose, CA) or the CoolTouch II 1,320 nm Nd/YAG (ICN Pharmaceuticals, Inc., Costa Mesa, CA). Three treatments were performed at 4 week intervals. Settings for 1,064-nm laser were 10 mm spot size, 40-ms pulse duration, and fluence of 24 J/cm$^2$. Three passes were performed over the treatment area. Parameters for the 1,320-nm laser were as follows: 10 mm spot, 250 µs pulse duration, fluences of 12–20 J/cm$^2$ precooling and 10 and 17 J/cm$^2$ postcooling with means of 14 and 12 J/cm$^2$, respectively. Two passes were performed with precooling (targeted therapeutic temperature was 45°C) and one pass was performed with postcooling (targeted therapeutic temperature of less than 42°C). Acne scarring was graded on a three-point scale by three independent observers (mild, moderate, and severe: "mild referred to a few slightly depressed scars, and severe indicated many deep depressions"). Two subjects had mild, seven had moderate, and three had severe acne scarring. Follow up was at 6 months and photographs were taken. Baseline and 6-month follow up photographs were evaluated by three investigators using an 11 point scale. No long-term adverse effects occurred, but the 1,320-nm laser was found to produce greater pain and swelling. The average investigator-related improvement in acne scars was 28% with the 1,064-nm Nd/YAG (30–40% improvement in 58% of subjects, 11–29% improvement in 42% of subjects) and 22% with the 1,320-nm laser (30–40% improvement in 42% of patients and 11–29% improvement in 42% of patients and 10% or less improvement in 16% of patients). The patients also performed grading of the acne scars and reported a 37% improvement with the 1,064-nm laser and a 39% improvement with the 1,320-nm laser. Investigators postulated the higher patient improvement ratings with the 1,320-nm laser were due to the increased amount of pain and the false pretense that pain corresponds to efficacy. The limitations of the study include the small sample size, and lack of statistical significant results (II/A) [62].

Another randomized, split-faced comparative study compared the 585-nm PDL and a 1,064-nm Nd/YAG laser for the treatment of acne scars. Eighteen Asian patients with FST IV–V were treated in four session with PDL or Nd/YAG at 2-week intervals. One side of the face was randomized to PDL treatment (Cynergy, Cynosure Inc., Westford, MA) with treatment settings of 10–11 J/cm$^2$, a 40 ms pulse duration with 7 mm spot size (subpurpuric settings). The contralateral side was treated with the 1,064-nm long-pulsed Nd/YAG laser (Cynergy) at a fluence of 50–70 J/cm$^2$, 50–100 ms pulse duration and a 7 mm spot size. Two passes with the laser were performed and forced air cooling was used for epidermal protection. Two nontreating blinded dermatologists assessed the patients as having 18.3% improvement in the PDL-treated scars and an 18.7% improvement in the 1,064-nm Nd/YAG-treated scars. Improvements were statistically significant from baseline, but no significant difference was found between the two groups. Histologic evaluation showed increased collagen in both treatment groups. There was no difference in patient satisfaction between the two laser treatments. The authors note that the lasers were most effective at treating superficial boxcar and rolling scars and were less effective at treating deep boxcar, deep rolling, and ice-pick scars. However, the ice pick scars tended to respond better to PDL and deep boxcar scars responded better to Nd/YAG (differences were not statistically significant) (II/A) [63].

## 1,320-nm Nd/YAG

Please see the earlier discussion of the randomized controlled trial comparing the 1,064 nm laser to the 1,320 nm laser for the treatment of acne scars on the face and back (II/A) [62].

Please see the discussion below regarding the randomized controlled trial by Tanzi and Alster comparing the 1,450-nm diode laser and the 1,320-nm Nd/YAG laser in the treatment of atrophic facial scars (II/A) [64].

## 1,450-nm Diode

Tanzi and Alster published a report in 2004 comparing the 1,450-nm diode with the 1,320-nm Nd/YAG for the treatment of atrophic facial scars. The study was a randomized, controlled, prospective clinical and histological study. Twenty patients with FST I–V with mild to moderate facial acne scars underwent three treatments at 4-week intervals: one half of the face was randomly assigned to receive the CoolTouch 1,320-nm laser and the other half was treated with the 1,450-nm diode laser (Smoothbeam, Candela Corp., Wayland, MA). The settings for the 1,450-nm diode laser were as follows: fluence ranging from 8 to 14 J/cm$^2$ (average of 11.8 J/cm$^2$), 6 mm spot, DCD level two (10 ms precool, 30 ms intraoperative cool, 10 ms postcool) with a single, nonoverlapping pass. The 1,320-nm Nd/YAG laser was used with the following settings: fluence of 12–17 J/cm$^2$

(average of 14.8 J/cm$^2$), 10 mm spot size, postir-radiation skin surface temperature between 39 and 45°C. Two nonoverlapping passes were performed with the 1,320-nm Nd/YAG to produce a clinical endpoint of transient erythema and edema without vesiculation. Independent dermatologists evaluated patients using a quartile scale based on photographs taken before each treatment and at 1, 3, 6, and 12 months after the final treatment. Six patients also had skin biopsies of scars at the above time intervals, and the histopathology was examined by a dermatopathologist. Textural changes were also assessed sign a three-dimensional microtopography skin imaging system (PRIMOS, GFM, Teltow, Germany). At the 12-month visit, patients also ranked their satisfaction with the treatment using an 11-point scale. A modest improvement in clinical scaring was greatest at the 6-month visit; mean clinical score difference was 1.67 for the 1,320-nm Nd/YAG and 1.81 for the 1,450-nm diode laser (the 1,450-nm diode laser had higher average clinical scores at each visit). Histologic evaluation showed increased dermal collagen after both treatment modalities at 6 months; further increase in collagen did not occur at 12 months. Skin surface texture was improved (average decrease in mean roughness was 26.14 after 1,450-nm diode and 19.89 μm after 1,320-nm Nd/YAG) 6 months after the last treatment. Side effects were limited to PIH in four patients after treatment with the 1,450-nm diode and two patients after treatment with the 1,320-nm Nd/YAG (not statistically significant). The PIH resolved in all patients within 6 weeks with the use of topical bleaching agents. Patient satisfaction was 4.6 on the 1,320-nm Nd/YAG side (patients noted lack of significant improvement) and 5.7 on the 1,450-nm diode side (patients noted pain during treatment). The authors noted that an additional pass with the 1,320-nm Nd/YAG with a final skin temperature of 45–48°C may have been more efficacious. The authors concluded that both nonablative lasers were safe and efficacious for patients who are not candidates for or are unwilling to undergo ablative resurfacing (II/A) [64].

## CO$_2$ and Erbium/YAG Resurfacing

A Cochrane review on laser resurfacing for facial and acne scars searched databases (to 1,999) as well as used information from experts and commercial laser manufacturers. No randomized controlled trials comparing resurfacing to another laser or to placebo were found. There were four randomized controlled trials: one split-face trial comparing CO$_2$ alone vs. CO$_2$ followed by erbium, two comparing different types of CO$_2$ laser in each of the four facial quadrants and one that compared two (out of the six available) types of Er/YAG. The other 23 studies that were included were "poor quality case series with small numbers of acne-scarred patients." Of these 23 case series, 17 involved CO$_2$ and five used Er/YAG. The authors concluded that there is a lack of evidence supporting laser resurfacing (CO$_2$ and Er/YAG) for the treatment of acne scars. They emphasize the need for randomized controlled studies comparing CO$_2$ and Er/YAG (I/A) [65].

A review of laser resurfacing of the skin for the improvement of facial acne scarring published in the British Journal of Dermatology also found that there were no controlled trials, and the 14 case series reviewed on the effects of the carbon dioxide or erbium/YAG laser were of poor quality. No standard scale was used to measure scar improvement. No validated measure of patient satisfaction was used. Improvement was often based on clinical judgment and often without blinded assessment. However, overall evidence supported laser resurfacing using the carbon dioxide laser and the erbium/YAG laser: efficacy ranged from 25 to 90%. Pigmentary changes are common side effects (affecting up to 44% of patients), although resolution of the abnormalities often occurred within several weeks. The authors conclude that good quality randomized controlled trials are needed with standardized scarring scales and validated patient outcome measures to accurately assess the effectiveness of laser resurfacing in patients with facial acne scarring (I/C) [66].

## Miscellaneous Techniques

In 2007, Weiss published an IRB-approved prospective, placebo-controlled Phase III clinical trial using autologous cultured living fibroblast injection for facial contour deformities. Ten US sites treated 151 patients with: acne scars ("boxcar and craterform type"), nasolabial and melolabial folds, periorbital, vermillion and glabellar lines and forehead wrinkles. Three treatments of live fibroblasts or placebo were administered to at 1–2-week intervals. Patients were evaluated using a 7-point photoguide at 1, 2, 4, 6, 9, and 12 months after the first injection. The primary efficacy endpoint was a 2-point shift in at least one treated area 4 months after the first treatment. Six months after treatment, patients were unblinded and placebo-treated patients were given the option of fibroblast injection (all requested treatment). Participants receiving fibroblasts were followed for 12 months. The proportion of responders was higher in the live fibroblast group than in the placebo group throughout the study, and reaching statistical significant at 6 months (81 vs. 36.4%). At 9 months the fibroblast group showed a response rate of 75% and at 12 months the response rate was 81.6%. The improvements seen in the placebo group were theorized to be secondary to subcision and injection of the placebo media. The authors state "the clinical effect of fibroblast injection was particularly pronounced among patients treated for acne scars. In this subgroup, the response rate at 6-month follow-up was 48.4%, compared with 7.7% for placebo, a statistically significant difference ($p < 0.05$)" (II/A) [67].

## Conclusions

Tables 9.6 and 9.7 review recent evidence-based therapies for treating scars, and the Evidence-Based Summary located at the end of the chapter reviews the evidence grading of important treatment modalities in scarring. Preventing scars, whether they are hypertrophic, keloid, surgical,

**Table 9.6** Summary of recent studies in the treatment of hypertrophic scars and keloids

| References | Design | N = | F/u | Results |
|---|---|---|---|---|
| Hypertrophic scars | | | | |
| Alster [7] | Prospective | 14 | 6 months | A 57–83% clinical improvement was seen in the scars after 1 or 2 585-nm PDL treatments, respectively. Fluence used was 6.5–7.25 J/cm²; pulse width was 0.45 s. Optical profilometry measurements for texture was obtained from five of the patients before and after treatment: return of skin markings approximating those of normal skin observed after treatments. Results maintained at follow-up |
| Chan et al. [8] | Controlled, prospective | 56 (71 scars) | 12 months | Two groups treated with 585-nm PDL: prevention group (scars in high-risk areas within 6-months of injury) and treatment group (hypertrophic scars). Half of scar treated at 8-week intervals for maximum period of 12 months, the other half served as a control. Settings were: 8 J/cm², 5-mm spot and 1.5 µs pulse duration. There was a significant degree of lightening of the treated scars, but scar thickness and viscoelasticity was not significantly better than controls. Subjects reported a 54 and 66% improvement in scars in prevention group and treatment group, respectively |
| Striae distensae | | | | |
| Stotland et al. [51] | Controlled (site-matched) | 20 | 3 months | Overall improvement using nonablative fractional photothermolysis of 26–50% in 5/8 patients, <25% improvement dyschromia 4/8 patients, texture improvement of 26–50% in 4/8 patients |
| Keloids | | | | |
| Kauh et al. [3] | Controlled, prospective | 6 | 2 weeks | Intralesional TA 10 mg/mL injected immediately postop and 2 weeks after excision of keloid (control). Biopsies taken 2 weeks after excision. Pro-α1 (I) collagen mRNA was downregulated and histological analysis of collagen fibers showed thinner and less dense bundles in the immediate treatment group vs. control. Clinical correlation was not performed |
| Klumpar et al. [4] | Prospective | 126 | 12 years | Keloids treated with excision, then radiation therapy. Efficacy of orthovoltage and electron beam radiation also compared. Control rates (no recurrence) of 72–92%. Higher recurrence rates noted at infected sites and in patients with a family history. Electron beam radiation offers no advantage over orthovoltage as effective as electron beam radiation |

(continued)

**Table 9.6** (continued)

| References | Design | N = | F/u | Results |
|---|---|---|---|---|
| Kovalic and Perez [5] | Prospective | 113 | 9.75 years | Radiation to keloids showed a control rate of 73%. Lesions that were >2 cm, had been treated previously and present in males had an increased recurrence rate. No advantage to starting radiation within 1 day of surgery. Mean time to recurrence rate was 12.8 months |
| Sclafani et al. [50] | Randomized controlled comparative | 31 | 12 months | Postop radiation vs. ILK to prevent earlobe keloids recurrence: Recurrence in 2/16 keloids treated with radiation and in 4/12 keloids treated with ILK |
| Keloids and hypertrophic scars | | | | |
| Akita et al. [6] | Prospective | 38 | 4.4 ± 2.2 years | Keloids were excised, repaired with 3-layer closure, then treated with electron beam irradiation. The post-treatment scars had significantly improved pigmentation, pliability, height and vascularity as compared to the original keloid: 2.6 vs. 1.0, 3.7 vs. 1.7, 2.9 vs. 1.3, and 2.7 vs. 1.3, respectively. Durometer readings (measuring firmness) were significantly lower post-treatment: 15.2 vs. 7.7. The recurrence rate was 21.2% overall with none in craniofacial locations |
| Asilian et al. [9] | Randomized, prospective, single-blinded | 60 | 12 week | Comparison of: Group 1: TA, 10 mg/mL. Group 2: TA + 5-FU (0.1 mL of 40 mg/mL TAC was added to 0.9 mL of 5-FU with concentration 50 mg/mL). Group 3: TA + 5-FU + 585-nm PDL, 5–7.5 $J/cm^2$ at the first, fourth, and eighth weeks. All injections administered weekly × 8 weeks. Lesions were assessed for erythema, pruritus, pliability, height, length, and width. At the 8- and 12-week follow-up visits, all groups showed an acceptable improvement in nearly all measures, but in comparison between groups, these were statistically more significant in the TAC + 5-FU and TAC + 5-FU + PDL groups ($p < 0.05$ for all). At the end of the study, the erythema score was significantly lower, and itch reduction was statistically higher in the TAC + 5-FU + PDL group ($p < 0.05$ for both). Patients in Group 3 reported the most improvement. Good to excellent responses were reported by the blinded observer as follows: 15% in Group 1, 40% in Group 2, and 70% in Group 3 ($p < 0.05$) |
| Leventhal et al. [53] | Meta-analysis | N/A | N/A | Seventy treatment series evaluated; 70% improvement with any type of treatment; however not statistically significant over chance alone. No statistically significant difference between treatment modalities. Mean amount of expected improvement was 60%. Therefore, according to this review, most treatments offer "minimal likelihood of improvement" |
| Manuskiatti et al. [54] | Randomized, controlled, comparative | 19 | | Keloidal or hypertrophic sternotomy scars treated with a 595-nm PDL at a fluence of 7 $J/cm^2$ in pts with FST IV–V. One half of scar randomly treated with pulse width of 0.45 and the other half treated with pulse width of 40 ms every 4 weeks for a total of three treatments. Scar volume, height, erythema, and pliability were measured at weeks 0, 4, 8, and 24. Segments treated with a 0.45-ms pulse width showed significantly greater improvement and higher elasticity than those treated with 40-ms pulses. No difference was seen in scar erythema |
| Manuskiatti and Fitzpatrick [55] | Randomized, controlled, comparative | 10 | 2 months | Comparison of ILK, 5-FU, ILK + 5-FU, 585 nm PDL and untreated control. Clinical improvements occurred and were similar in all treated segments except control. Increased SE in ILK alone |
| Naeini et al. [56] | Randomized, comparative | 45 | 3 months | Group A treated with bleomycin tattoo, group B treated with cryotherapy and ILK. Four treatments at 1 month sessions showed greater than 88% improvement in both groups in small (<100 $mm^2$) lesions; larger lesions responded significantly better to bleomycin. Hyperpigmentation occurred in >75% of patients tx with bleomycin |
| Layton et al. [57] | Randomized, controlled, double-blinded, comparative | | | Intralesional triamcinolone was compared to cryosurgery for the treatment of acne keloids. 85% of keloids showed a moderate to good flattening response. Cryosurgery was superior to ILK, especially in newer, vascular keloids |

**Table 9.7** Summary of recent studies in the treatment of acne and surgical scars

| References | Design | Patient # | F/u | Results |
|---|---|---|---|---|
| **TCA** | | | | |
| Lee et al. [16] | Prospective | 65 | 6 months | Of patients treated by CROSS technique with 65 and 100% TCA, 82 and 94%, respectively, had a good clinical response; improvement correlated with number of treatments |
| Cho et al. [17] | Prospective, controlled | 5 | 6 weeks | Histometric analysis of simple TCA application vs. CROSS technique for atrophic scars. Untreated scars served as controls. Epidermal and dermal thickness and neocollagenesis statistically higher with CROSS technique, and results improved with increasing concentrations |
| Fabbrocini et al. [18] | Prospective | 5 | 8 week | Patients and investigators reported improvement s/p 50% TCA using CROSS technique (vs. 100% TCA previously reported); histologically increased collagen and elastin in dermis |
| **Surgery and laser** | | | | |
| Grevelink and White [13] | Prospective, single-blinded | 21 | | FST I–III with mild-severe facial acne scarring treated with a combination of laser skin resurfacing and punch excision of acne scars in the same treatment session. Photographs evaluated by one blinded and one nonblinded assessor: clinical improvement was 25–50% in FST I, 50–75% in FST II, and 50–75% in FST III. Subjective improvement was 25–50% in FST I, 50–75% in FST II and 75–100% in FST III. No wound dehiscence, evidence of infection, or hypertrophic scarring of treated areas noted on follow-up |
| **Laser** | | | | |
| Walia and Alster [24] | Prospective (clinical), blinded histological | 60 | 18 months | Independent clinical assessments and blinded histological assessments made at months 1, 6, 12, 18 after $CO_2$. Average improvement was 69, 27, 73, and 75%, respectively. Histologic analysis showed increased collagenesis and dermal remodeling throughout the follow-up period |
| Woo et al. [25] | Prospective, comparative | 158 | 6 months | Improvement in atrophic vs. mixed types of acne scars were evaluated using a short-pulsed Er:YAG, a variable-pulsed Er:YAG, and a dual-mode Er:YAG. Shallow boxcar and ice-pick scars achieved a rating of good to excellent (>51% improvement). Rolling and deep boxcar scars achieved best results (rating of fair to good, 26–75% improved) using a long-pulse duration with the Er:YAG |
| Bernstein et al. [58] | Randomized, controlled | 22 | 3 months | 532 nm, 2 ms pulse-duration, frequency-doubled Nd:YAG laser used for mild-to-deep lip wrinkles and mild-moderate acne scarring; one half of lip (wrinkles) or cheek (acne scarring) treated, other side was untreated control, 3 treatments at 3–6 week intervals performed. Subjects reported an average improvement of 53.6% for facial acne scarring |
| Lipper and Perez [30] | Prospective | 9 | 6–12 months | FST I–V, 8 treatments at 2-week intervals with 1,064-nm Nd:YAG (Vantage): 14 $J/cm^2$, 0.3 ms, 5-mm spot, 7 Hz, 2,000 pulses per side of face. Three physicians rated photographs as 29.36% improved. 89% of patients rated their acne scars as greater than 10% improved. 5 pts reported moderate scar improvement at 6–12 months (laser upgrade was provided to the authors at a reduced price) |
| Keller et al. [31] | Prospective | 12 | 6 months | FST II–V, 5 treatments at 4-week intervals with 1,064-nm Nd:YAG (quantum): 120 $J/cm^2$, 7.0/7.0/7.0-ms pulse duration, 70-ms delay, 6 mm spot, three passes over scar. Three independent dermatologists graded 50% of patients with moderate improvement. Subjects reported a mean satisfaction score of 8.6 on scale of 0–10. Histometric analysis showed increase in dermal collagen ($p < 0.5$) |
| Rogachefsky et al. [32] | Prospective | 12 | 6 months | FST I–III, pts were divided into a group with atrophic acne scars and a group with mixed acne scars. A 1,320-nm Nd:YAG (CoolTouch) was used to treat. Parameters were: 10 mm spot, 13–22 $J/cm^2$ (first two passes 16–22 $J/cm^2$, third pass 13–17 $J/cm^2$), 50-ms macropulse. Three treatments performed at 4 week intervals. Mean scar improvement on 10-point scale was 1.5 points for physician assessment and 2.2 points for patient assessment. Atrophic scars improved the most, but this trend was not statistically significant (study funded in part by CoolTouch Lasers) |

(continued)

**Table 9.7** (continued)

| References | Design | Patient # | F/u | Results |
| --- | --- | --- | --- | --- |
| Uebelhoer et al. [33] | Prospective | 11 | 3 months | Three treatments at 3-week intervals with 1,450-nm diode laser (Smoothbeam) with settings of: 11 $J/cm^2$ (or lower as tolerated) with one-half of face receiving a single-pass with stacked double pulses and the other half receiving a double pass of single pulses. Primary endpoint was acne improvement (57.6 and 49.8% reduction, respectively). 83% of pts had improvement of acne scars, which was graded a mean of 1 on a scale of 0–3. No difference in scar improvement between the two sides (laser provided by and study funded by Candela Corp) |
| Jih et al. [41] | Prospective | 20 | 12 months | Pts with FST II–VI received three treatments with 1,450-nm diode laser (Smoothbeam) at 3–4 week intervals. Physicians and patients graded acne scaring improvement as: <25% improved at 3 months after last treatment, 25–50% improved at 6-month follow-up, with further improvement noted at 12-month followup for scars treated at a fluence of 16 $J/cm^2$ but not 14 $J/cm^2$. All patients noted improvement of acne scars at 12-months follow-up visit |
| Chua et al. [42] | Prospective | 57 | 6 months | Asian pts with FST IV–V treated with 4–6 treatments with 1,450-nm diode laser (Smoothbeam). Improvements based on patient's assessment vs. physician's assessments were: 15.7 vs. 6.6% for four treatments, 20 vs. 7.9% for five treatments, 17.3 vs. 5.0% for six treatments, respectively. There was significant pain with laser treatments, and hyperpigmentation occurred in 29% of patients |
| Fournier and Mordon [34] | Review | N/A | N/A | Review of pts tx with 1,540-nm Er:glass laser (Aramis-Quantel). Mild (20–30%) improvement noted over a period of 6 months after the last treatment |
| Nouri et al. [59] | Randomized, controlled | 11 | 4 weeks | Compared three treatments with 585-nm PDL of surgical scars vs. untreated control. Treatments initiated the day of suture removal. An improvement of VSS and cosmesis in scars noted in treated scars vs. untreated |
| Conologue and Norwood [60] | Randomized, controlled | 16 | 1 months | Pts with FST I–IV had three treatments of surgical scars with 595-nm PDL at 4–8-week intervals with half of the scar serving as untreated control starting the day of suture removal. Assessment by blinded examiner using VSS and overall cosmetic assessment on 11-point scale (0–10). Final evaluation of 60% of treated side vs. −3% using the VSS; treated portions scored 2 points higher in overall cosmetic appearance |
| Alam et al. [61] | Randomized, controlled | 17 | 6 week | Compared single treatment of 595-nm PDL of surgical scars vs. untreated controls on day of suture removal. No clinical difference found between the two groups |
| Lee et al. [63] | Randomized, controlled, split-face, comparative | 18 | 2 months | Patients treated with 585-nm PDL and 1,064-nm Nd:YAG (Cynergy) (split-face) for four treatments, 2 weeks apart. Both lasers resulted in improvement in acne scars (18.3 and 18.7%, respectively), but the improvement was not statistically significant between the two groups. Collagen production as assessed histologically was increased in both groups |
| Yaghmai et al. [62] | Randomized, controlled, split-face, comparative | 12 | 6 months | Comparison of the 1,064-nm laser to the 1,320-nm laser for the nonablative treatment of acne scars of face and back. There was 28% improvement in scars using the 1,064-nm laser; 22% improvement using the 1,320-nm laser. Prolifometric studies demonstrated comparable improvement. No statistical significance achieved between the two groups |
| Tanzi and Alster [64] | Randomized, controlled, split-face, comparative | 20 | 12 months | Comparison of the 1,450-nm diode laser (Smoothbeam) to the 1,320-nm Nd:YAG laser (Cooltouch) for the treatment of facial acne scars. After three treatments, mild to moderate improvement in the majority of patients. Although both lasers offered improvement, "the 1,450-nm diode laser showed greater clinical scar response at the parameters studied" |

(continued)

**Table 9.7** (continued)

| References | Design | Patient # | F/u | Results |
|---|---|---|---|---|
| Sadick and Schecter [39] | Prospective | 8 | 12 months | Patients treated with three passes of the 1,320-nm Nd:YAG (Cooltouch). Six treatments at monthly intervals performed. Improvement in acne scarring 3.9 points at 5 months ($p=0.002$) and 4.3 points ($p=0.011$) at 1 year. Patient-rated improvement was statistically significant at 5 months (3.6 points, $p=0.002$) |
| Bhatia et al. [40] | Retrospective | 34 | 12 months | Patients treated for photoaging or acne scars interviewed 3–12 months after a series of 6 treatments with the 1,320-nm Nd:YAG. Patient satisfaction with treatment for acne scarring was 62% (patient satisfaction higher for acne scarring than photoaging). Textural improvement reported to be 31% |
| Geronemus [43] | Prospective | 17 | | Pilot study: 5 treatments with1,550-nm erbium-doped laser (Fraxel) administered at 1–3 week intervals. Mean improvement levels in acne scars using digital photography was 25–50% |
| Alster et al. [26] | Prospective | 53 | 6 months | Three treatments with Fraxel 1 month apart in FST I–V with fluences 8–16 J/cm$^2$, densities 150–250 MTZ/cm$^2$. 87% of patients achieved a 51–75% clinical improvement in acne scars |
| Chrastil et al. [44] | Prospective | 29 | 1–6 months | Two-6 Fraxel treatments 1 month apart in FST I–V using second-generation device with fluences 35–40 J/cm$^2$, density of 20–35%. 18 patients achieved 51–75% clinical improvement, 5 patients achieved >75% improvement |
| Glaich et al. [45] | Prospective | 7 | 3 months | Two-4 treatments with Fraxel administered 1 month apart in hypopigmented surgical scars. Independent physicians graded patients on a 4-point scale 1 month after final tx. 6 pts experienced a 51–75% improvement in pigmentation, 1 pt had 26–50% improvement. Texture was improved in all pts |
| Choe et al. [46] | Prospective, controlled | 27 | 6 months | Korean pts with thyroidectomy scars tx with 1,550-nm fractional erbium glass laser (MOSAIC) compared with patients with untreated thyroidectomy scars. Four treatments at 1-month intervals were given, starting 2 or 3 weeks after surgery. VSS scores and clinical appearance as graded by three independent physicians were improved in treated group (VSS score of 1.52 vs. 3.00 and clinical assessment of 3.15 vs. 2.07 based on 4-point scale for treatment group and untreated group, respectively) |
| Chapas et al. [47] | Prospective | 13 | 14 months | Pts with FST I–IV with moderate-severe acne scarring treated with 2–3 treatments fractional $CO_2$ resurfacing (Fraxel Re:Pair). Clinical and topographical improvement evaluated. Both investigator and patients rated improvement 26–50% in both overall texture and improvement of atrophy. Mean topographical improvement of 66.8% |
| Pinski and Roenigk [20] | Prospective | 43 | Mean 26 months | Patients treated with autologous fat transplantation and clinically assessed. Durability of 65% at 3 months, 50% at 6 months, 40% at 9 months and 30% at 12 months. Higher resorption noted in fibrotic acne scars |
| Mosely et al. [21] | Prospective, controlled, but in mice | | | Longevity and volume of the autologous fat graft was enhanced using fresh donor stem cells from the adipose tissue of mice. 6 months after transplantation, the fat with freshly isolated stem cells had a weight 2.5 times greater than the fat graft–only group ($p=0.021$). Cultured adipose-derived stem cells were greater in maintaining graft volume than fat only. At 6 months grafted fat with fresh stem cells maintained its adipocyte-rich appearance, whereas the grafted tissue without cell supplementation group had a more fibrous tissue appearance |
| Barnett and Barnett [22] | Prospective | 5 | 30 | Five patients with acne scarring treated with liquid silicone using monthly microdroplet, multiple injection approach. Authors report that liquid silicone is safe, effective, precise and permanent |
| Weiss et al. [67] | Randomized, multicenter, controlled, phase III clinical trial | 151 | 12 months | Patients injected with live autologous fibroblasts in rhytides, folds and acne scars. Primary endpoint was 2-point improvement on 7-point scale. Higher number of responders to treatment throughout trial, but statistically significant at 6-month follow-up. Responders for acne scars vs. placebo particularly impressive at 6-month mark (48.4 vs. 7.7%) |

or acne scars is important because of the difficult nature of their treatment. Once a scar has formed, the treatment is dependent on the subtype. Hypertrophic scars tend to respond to simple surgical excision, or excision with W- or Z-plasty revision to relieve tension. Keloids respond well to surgical debridement, then radiation. Multiple adjuvant modalities such as pressure, intralesional TA or 5-FU, and PDL treatments can augment hypertrophic and keloid response.

Surgical techniques are usually required to correct icepick and/or localized deep atrophic scars. Nonablative light sources can help some-what with atrophic scars, but tend not to be as effective as ablative resurfacing. However, there are no randomized controlled studies comparing ablative vs. nonablative resurfacing. Nonablative and ablative fractional photothermolysis holds great promise in the treatment of acne scars; further technologies and randomized controlled trials. For example, comparative analyses of ablative vs. nonablative fractionated photothermolysis treatments would be extremely useful. As new technologies emerge, critical studies will be required to evaluate what advantage, if any, will be gained over existing modalities.

| Evidence-Based Summary | |
| --- | --- |
| Prevention of scars | Evidence level |
| PDL starting day of suture removal, >1 treatment | III/A |
| Hypertrophic scars and keloids | |
| Surgery and intralesional TA | IV/B |
| Surgery and radiation | IV/B |
| Cryotherapy (esp. vascular lesions) | I/A |
| PDL | II/A–III/B |
| 5-FU + PDL | III/B |
| PDL + intralesional TA or 5-FU | III/B |
| Topicals (Table 9.1) | V/C |
| Bleomycin tattooing | II/A |
| Acne scarring | |
| Surgery + laser resurfacing | IV/B |
| Chemical peels | V–VI/C |
| CROSS | III–IV/B |
| Microdermabrasion | VI/C |
| Autologous fat | V/B |
| Silicone | V/B |
| Poly-L-lactic acid | IV/B |
| Laser resurfacing | I/B |
| Er fractional photothermolysis | IV/B |
| $CO_2$ fractional photothermolysis | IV/B |
| 532-nm Nd/YAG | II/A |
| 585-nm and 595-nm PDL | II/A–IV/B |
| 1,064-nm Nd/YAG | II–IV/B |
| 1,320-nm Nd/YAG | II/A |
| 1,450-nm diode | II/A |
| 1,540-nm Er/glass | IV/B |
| IPL | III/B |
| Thermotherapy | V/C |
| Plasma (short-term effects) | IV/B |
| Fibroblasts | II/A |

# References

1. Jacob CI, Dover JS, Kaminer MS. Acne scarring: a classification system and review of treatment options. J Am Acad Dermatol. 2001;45:109–17.
2. Wolfram D, Tzankov A, Pulzi P, Piza-Katzer H. Hypertrophic scars and keloids – a review of their pathophysiology, risk factors and therapeutic management. Dermatol Surg. 2009;35:17–81.
3. Kauh YC, Rouda S, Mondragon G. Major suppression of pro-alpha1(I) type I collagen gene expression in the dermis after keloid excision and immediate intrawound injection of triamcinolone acetonide. J Am Acad Dermatol. 1997;37:586–9.
4. Klumpar DI, Murray JC, Anscher M. Keloids treated with excision followed by radiation treatment. J Am Acad Dermatol. 1994;31:225–31.
5. Kavalic JJ, Perez CA. Radiation therapy following keloidectomy: a 20-year experience. Int J Radiol Oncol Biol Phys. 1989;17:77–80.
6. Akita S, Akino K, Yakabe A, Imaizumi T, Tanaka K, Anraku K, et al. Combined surgical excision and radiation therapy for keloid treatment. J Craniofac Surg. 2007;18:1164–9.
7. Alster TS. Improvement of erythematous and hypertrophic scars by the 585-nm flashlamp-pumped pulsed dye laser. Ann Plast Surg. 1994;32:186–90.
8. Chan HH, Wong DS, Ho WS, Lam LK, Wei W. The use of pulsed dye laser for the prevention and treatment of hypertrophic scars in Chinese persons. Dermatol Surg. 2004;30:987–94.
9. Asilian A, Darougheh A, Shariati F. New combination of triamcinolone, 5-fluorouracil, and pulsed-dye laser for treatment of keloid and hypertrophic scars. Dermatol Surg. 2006;32:907–15.
10. Rivera AE. Acne scarring: a review and current treatment modalities. J Am Acad Dermatol. 2008;59:659–76.
11. Harris DW, Buckley CC, Ostler LS, Rustin MHA. Topical retinoic acid in the treatment of fine acne scarring. Br J Dermatol. 1991;125:81–3.
12. Berardesca E, Gabba P, Farinelli N, Borroni G, Rabbiosi G. In vivo tretinoin-induced changes in skin mechanical properties. Br J Dermatol. 1990;122:525–9.
13. Grevelink JM, White VR. Concurrent use of laser skin resurfacing and punch excision in the treatment of facial acne scarring. Dermatol Surg. 1998;24:527–30.
14. Al-Waiz MM, Al-Shargi AI. Medium-depth chemical peels in the treatment of acne scars in dark-skinned individuals. Dermatol Surg. 2002;28:383–7.
15. Atzori L, Brundu MA, Orru A, Biggio P. Glycolic acid peeling in the treatment of acne. J Eur Acad Dermatol Venereol. 1999;12:119–22.
16. Lee JB, Chung WG, Kwahck H, Lee KH. Focal treatment of acne scars with trichloroacetic acid: chemical reconstruction of skin scars method. Dermatol Surg. 2002;28:1017–21.
17. Cho SB, Park CO, Chung WG, Lee KH, Lee JB, Chung KY. Histometric and histochemical analysis of the effect of trichloroacetic acid concentration in the chemical reconstruction of skin scars method. Dermatol Surg. 2006;32:1231–6.
18. Fabbrocini G, Cacciapuoti S, Fardella N, Pastore F, Monfrecola G. Cross technique: chemical reconstruction of skin scars method. Dermatol Ther. 2008;21 Suppl 3:S29–32.
19. Bhalla M, Gurvinder TP. Microdermabrasion: reappraisal and brief review of the literature. Dermatol Surg. 2006;32:809–14.
20. Pinski KS, Roenigk HH. Autologous fat transplantation. Long term follow-up. J Dermatol Surg Oncol. 1992;18:179–84.
21. Moseley TA, Zhu M, Hedrick MH. Adipose-derived stem and progenitor cells as fillers in plastic and reconstructive surgery. Plast Reconstr Surg. 2006;118S:21S–8.
22. Barnett JG, Barnett CR. Treatment of acne scars with liquid silicone injections: 30-year perspective. Dermatol Surg. 2005;31:1542–9.
23. Beer K. A single-center, open-label study on the use of injectable poly-L-lactic acid for the treatment of moderate to severe scarring from acne or varicella. Dermatol Surg. 2007;33 Suppl 2:S159–67.
24. Walia S, Alster RS. Prolonged clinical and histological effects from $CO_2$ laser resurfacing of atrophic acne scars. Dermatol Surg. 1999;25:926–30.
25. Woo SH, Park JH, Kye YC. Resurfacing of different types of facial acne scar with short-pulsed, variable-pulsed, and dual-mode Er:YAG laser. Dermatol Surg. 2004;30:488–93.
26. Alster TS, Tanzi EL, Lazarus M. The use of fractional laser photothermolysis for the treatment of atrophic scars. Dermatol Surg. 2007;33:295–9.
27. Baugh WP, Kucaba WD. Nonablative phototherapy for acne vulgaris using the KTP 532 nm laser. Dermatol Surg. 2005;31:1290–6.
28. Dierickx C, Goldman MP, Fitzpatrick RE. Laser treatment of erythematous/hypertrophic and pigmented scars in 26 patients. Plast Reconstr Surg. 1995;95:84–90.
29. Alster TS, Kurban AK, Grove GL, Grove MJ, Tan OT. Alteration of argon laser-induced scars by the pulsed dye laser. Lasers Surg Med. 1993;13:368–73.
30. Lipper GM, Perez M. Nonablative acne scar reduction after a series of treatments with a short-pulsed 1,064-nm neodymium:YAG laser. Dermatol Surg. 2006;32:998–1006.
31. Keller R, Junior WB, Valente NYS, Rodrigues CJ. Nonablative 1,064-nm Nd:YAG laser for treating atrophic facial acne scars: histologic and clinical analysis. Dermatol Surg. 2007;33:1470–6.
32. Rogachefsky AS, Hussain M, Goldberg DJ. Atrophic and a mixed pattern of acne scars improved with a 1,320-nm Nd:YAG laser. Dermatol Surg. 2003;29:904–8.

33. Uebelhoer NS, Bogle MA, Dover JS, Arndt KA, Rohrer TE. Comparison of stacked pulses versus double-pass treatments of facial acne with a 1,450-nm laser. Dermatol Surg. 2007;33:552–9.

34. Fournier N, Mordon S. Nonablative remodeling with a 1,540 nm erbium:glass laser. Dermatol Surg. 2005; 31:1227–36.

35. Goldberg DJ. New collagen formation after dermal remodeling with an intense pulsed light source. J Cutan Laser Ther. 2000;2:59–61.

36. Bellew SG, Weiss MA, Weiss RA. Comparison of intense pulsed light to 595-nm long-pulsed pulsed dye laser for the treatment of hypertrophic surgical scars: a pilot study. J Drugs Dermatol. 2005;4:448–52.

37. Ruiz-Esparza J, Gomez JB. Nonablative radiofrequency for active acne vulgaris: the use of deep dermal heat in the treatment of moderate to severe acne vulgaris (thermotherapy): a report of 22 patients. Dermatol Surg. 2003;29:333–9.

38. Potter MJ, Harrison R, Ramsden A, Bryan B, Andrews P, Gault D. Facial acne and fine lines: transforming patient outcomes with plasma skin regeneration. Ann Plast Surg. 2007;58:608–13.

39. Sadick NS, Schecter AK. A preliminary study of utilization of the 1320-nm Nd:YAG laser for the treatment of acne scarring. Dermatol Surg. 2004;30:995–1000.

40. Bhatia AC, Dover JS, Arndt KA, Stewart B, Alam M. Patient satisfaction and reported long-term therapeutic efficacy associated with 1,320 nm Nd:YAG laser treatment of acne scarring and photoaging. Dermatol Surg. 2006;32:346–52.

41. Jih MH, Friedman PM, Goldberg LH, Robles M, Glaich AS, Kimyai-Asadi A. The 1450-nm diode laser for facial inflammatory acne vulgaris: dose-response and 12-month follow-up study. J Am Acad Dermatol. 2006;55:80–7.

42. Chua SH, Ang P, Khoo LS, Goh CL. Nonablative 1450-nm diode laser in the treatment of facial atrophic acne scars in type IV to V Asian skin: a prospective clinical study. Dermatol Surg. 2004;30:1287–91.

43. Geronemus RG. Fractional photothermolysis: current and future applications. Lasers Surg Med. 2006;38:169–76.

44. Chrastil B, Glaich AS, Goldberg LH, Friedman PM. Second-generation 1,550-nm fractional photothermolysis for the treatment of acne scars. Dermatol Surg. 2008;34:1327–32.

45. Glaich AS, Rahman Z, Goldberg LH, Friedman PM. Fractional resurfacing for the treatment of hypopigmented scars: a pilot study. Dermatol Surg. 2007;33:289–94.

46. Choe JH, Park YL, Kim BJ, Kim MN, Rho NK, Park BS, et al. Prevention of thyroidectomy scar using a new 1,550-nm fractional erbium-glass laser. Dermatol Surg. 2009;35:1–7.

47. Chapas AM, Brightman L, Sukal S, Hale E, Daniel D, Bernstein LJ, et al. Successful treatment of acneiform scarring with $CO_2$ ablative fractional resurfacing. Lasers Surg Med. 2008;40:381–6.

48. O'Brien L, Pandit A. Silicon gel sheeting for preventing and treating hypertrophic and keloid scars (review). Cochrane Database Syst Rev. 2009(1):CD003826.

49. Gassner HG, Brissett AE, Otley CC, Boahene DK, Boggust AJ, Weaver AL, et al. Botulinum toxin to improve facial wound healing: a prospective, blinded, placebo-controlled study. Mayo Clin Proc. 2006;81: 1023–8.

50. Sclafani AP, Gordon L, Chadha M, Romo III T. Prevention of earlobe keloid recurrence with postoperative corticosteroid injections versus radiation therapy: a randomized, prospective study and review of the literature. Dermatol Surg. 1996;22:569–74.

51. Stotland M, Chapas AM, Brightman L, Sukal S, Hale E, Karen J, et al. The safety and efficacy of fractional photothermolysis for the correction of striae distensae. J Drugs Dermatol. 2008;7:857–61.

52. Tay YK, Kwok C, Tan E. Non-ablative 1,450-nm diode laser treatment of striae distensae. Lasers Surg Med. 2006;38:196–9.

53. Leventhal D, Furr M, Reiter D. Treatment of keloids and hypertrophic scars: a meta-analysis and review of the literature. Arch Facial Plast Surg. 2007;9: 139–40.

54. Manuskiatti W, Wanitphakdeedecha R, Fitzpatrick RE. Effect of pulse width of a 595-nm flashlamp-pumped pulsed dye laser on the treatment response of keloidal and hypertrophic sternotomy scars. Dermatol Surg. 2007;33:152–61.

55. Manuskiatti W, Fitzpatrick RE. Treatment response of keloidal and hypertrophic sternotomy scars: comparison among intralesional corticosteroid, 5-fluorouracil, and 585-nm flashlamp-pumped pulsed-dye laser treatments. Arch Dermatol. 2002;138:1149–55.

56. Naeini FF, Najafian J, Ahmadpour K. Bleomycin tattooing as a promising therapeutic modality in large keloids and hypertrophic scars. Dermatol Surg. 2006; 32:1023–30.

57. Layton AM, Yip J, Cunliffe WJ. A comparison of intralesional triamcinolone and cryosurgery in the treatment of acne keloids. Br J Dermatol. 1994;130: 498–501.

58. Bernstein EF, Ferreira M, Anderson D. A pilot investigation to subjectively measure treatment effect and side-effect profile of non-ablative skin remodeling using a 532 nm, 2 ms pulse-duration laser. J Cosmet Laser Ther. 2001;3:137–41.

59. Nouri K, Jimenez GP, Harrison-Balestra C, Elgart GW. 585-nm pulsed dye laser in the treatment of surgical scars starting on the suture removal day. Dermatol Surg. 2003;29:65–73.

60. Conologue TD, Norwood C. Treatment of surgical scars with the cryogen-cooled 595-nm pulsed dye laser starting on the day of suture removal. Dermatol Surg. 2006;32:13–20.

61. Alam M, Pon K, Van Laborde S, Kaminer MS, Arndt KA, Dover JS. Clinical effect of a single pulsed dye laser treatment of fresh surgical scars: randomized controlled trial. Dermatol Surg. 2006;32:21–5.

62. Yaghmai D, Garden JM, Bakus AD, Massa MC. Comparison of a 1,064 nm laser and 1,320 nm laser for the nonablative treatment of acne scars. Dermatol Surg. 2005;31:903–9.
63. Lee DH, Choi YS, Min SU, Yoon MY, Suh DH. Comparison of a 585-nm pulsed dye laser and a 1064-nm Nd:YAG laser for the treatment of acne scars: a randomized split-face clinical study. J Am Acad Dermatol. 2009;60(5):801–17.
64. Tanzi EL, Alster AS. Comparison of a 1450-nm diode laser and a 1320-nm Nd:YAG laser in the treatment of atrophic facial scars: a prospective clinical and histological study. Dermatol Surg. 2004;30:152–7.
65. Jordan R, Cummins CCL, Burls A, Seukeran DDC. Laser resurfacing for facial acne scars (review). Cochrane Database Syst Rev. 2009(1): CD001866.
66. Jordan R, Cummins C, Burls A. Laser resurfacing of the skin for the improvement of facial acne scarring: a systematic review of the evidence. Br J Dermatol. 2000;142:413–23.
67. Weiss RA, Weiss MA, Beasley KL, Munavalli G. Autologous cultured fibroblast injection for facial contour deformities: a prospective, placebo-controlled, phase III clinical trial. Dermatol Surg. 2007; 33:263–8.

## Self-Assessment

1. When evaluating a scar, it is useful to classify it to determine the most effective treatment. Which of the following types of scars are included in the atrophic acne-scarring classification scheme?
   (a) Icepick
   (b) Picker's scar
   (c) Boxcar
   (d) Rolling
   (e) Hypertrophic scar
   Jacob et al. described a classification system for atrophic acne scars. When evaluating a patient with atrophic acne scars, it is useful to classify the scars because treatment methods should be influenced by the types of scarring. Picking at acne lesions can result in different types of scarring; the etiology does not provide any information about the treatment method that should be used. Hypertrophic scars and keloids can result from acne, but they are not atrophic acne scars.

2. When treating keloids and hypertrophic scars, the most effective approach is:
   (a) Surgical debulkment
   (b) External beam radiation
   (c) Laser treatment
   (d) Intralesional corticosteroid
   (e) A combined approach
   Taking steps to prevent keloids and hypertrophic scars is the most critical aspect of their formation. However, once present, the literature supports a combination approach that is to be individually tailored to each patient. For example, surgical debulkment is usually combined with external beam radiation; intralesional corticosteroids can be combined with intralesional 5-fluorouracil or bleomycin. Injections are often combined with laser treatment, such as the pulsed-dye laser, for enhanced results.

3. What topical modality is best backed by evidence-based medicine as a treatment for acne scars?
   (a) 5-Fluorouracil
   (b) Retinoids
   (c) Onion extract
   (d) Silicone sheeting
   (e) Pressure therapy
   Retinoids have the most supporting evidence in the topical management of scars. Scar architecture is improved by retinoid alteration of the dermal elastic and collagen content. Although the other choices have reports in the literature claiming efficacy, retinoids continue to be first-line based on available evidence-based information.

4. What seems to be the best method(s) to treat icepick scars?
   (a) Punch excision
   (b) Retinoids
   (c) Laser resurfacing
   (d) Dermal fillers
   (e) Nonablative laser treatment
   (f) Focal application of 50–100% TCA
   Punch excision can be combined with ablative laser resurfacing, even on the same day, when treating icepick scars. Additionally, the CROSS technique, described by Lee et al., has been reported to be efficacious. This technique involves only focal treatment of the scars, which can minimize downtime.

5. What nonablative laser is the most effective treatment for scars, including atrophic acne scars, surgical scars and hypopigmented scars?
   (a) 1,450-nm diode
   (b) 1,320-nm Nd/YAG
   (c) 1,550-nm fractional erbium
   (d) 532-nm KTP laser
   (e) 585/595-nm pulsed dye laser

   Although all of the listed lasers have evidence supporting their use in the treatment of atrophic acne scars, the 1,550-nm fractional erbium device (Fraxel) has shown dramatic results and has become the first-line nonablative device when treating atrophic acne scars. Although randomized clinical trials are lacking, this device has also been reported to be efficacious in the treatment of surgical and hypopigmented scars.

6. What laser is the most effective treatment for striae distensae?
   (a) 1,450-nm Diode
   (b) 1,320-nm Nd/YAG
   (c) 1,550-nm fractional erbium
   (d) 532-nm KTP laser
   (e) 10,600-nm fractional $CO_2$ resurfacing

   Fractional photothermolysis has been reported in a randomized controlled study to be effective for striae distensae. A randomized controlled trial using the 1,450-nm diode laser for the treatment of striae distensae and striae rubra showed this device to be ineffective.

7. According to the available evidence, the PDL (585/595-nm) can be used to improve the appearance of surgical scars:
   (a) With one treatment, starting the day of suture removal
   (b) With three treatments, starting the day of suture removal
   (c) With three treatments, 1 year after suture removal
   (d) With six treatments, starting 1 month after suture removal

   The PDL has been shown to improve the appearance of surgical scars after three treatments, starting on the day of suture removal. A study by Alam et al. showed no improvement in surgical scars after one treatment on the day of suture removal.

# Answers

1. a, c, and d: Ice pick, boxcar, and rolling.
2. e: A combined approach
3. b: Retinoids
4. a, c, and f: Punch excision, laser resurfacing, and focal application of 50–100% TCA
5. c: 1,550-nm fractional erbium
6. c: 1,550-nm fractional erbium
7. b: With three treatments, starting the day of suture removal

# Prevention and Treatment of Procedure-Associated Infection

# 10

## Douglas Fife

## Introduction

Wound infection is a dreaded complication in Dermatologic Surgery, which is associated with increased cost and patient morbidity. Wound infection occurs when an inoculum of virulent pathogens is deposited at the wound site and overwhelms the host defenses, causing a variety of problems, including pain, dehiscence, abscesses, poor healing, or even sepsis. Wound infection is defined by the CDC as an infection at the site of a procedure within 30 days of the procedure [1]. Infection can occur in any procedure in which the skin barrier is compromised, including excisional surgery, Mohs micrographic surgery, biopsies, all type of reconstructions, chemical peels, dermabrasion, laser resurfacing, liposuction, blepharoplasty, injections, or other procedures [2]. Most infections are bacterial; however, viral, fungal, and mycobacterial infections may occur. Some dermatologic procedures have a higher risk of infection than others due to their location on the body, surface area of involvement, risk of contamination, duration of procedure, or other characteristics (Table 10.1). Other risk factors such as the patient's host defenses and pre and postoperative care may increase the risk of post-surgical infection and should be considered by

the surgeon (Table 10.2). The risk of surgical infection can be conceptualized according to the equation in Fig. 10.1.

It is important to note that the majority of large, well-designed studies evaluating interventions to prevent surgical wound infection are from the "traditional" surgery literature (General Surgery, Orthopedic Surgery, Otolaryngology, Neurosurgery, and Plastic Surgery, and Gynecologic Surgery), usually involving procedures performed in the operating room of a hospital and involving a postoperative stay. In contrast, the vast majority of dermatologic surgical procedures are in the outpatient setting under local anesthesia. Most dermatologic surgical procedures fall into the category of class I (Clean) or class II ("clean-contaminated") wounds [3, 9] (Table 10.3). The rate of infection for dermatologic procedures overall is low (0.5–5% quoted) but is not well studied [10–12]. While in the general surgical literature Class II wounds have an average infection rate of 10% (Haas), the quoted rate of infection in dermatologic surgery is 2–5% [3, 13]. This apparent discrepancy between the rates of infection in dermatologic surgery compared to other Class II wounds may be accounted for by multiple reasons, including the small, superficial nature of many wounds in dermatologic surgery (such as shave biopsies or curettage) compared to Class II wounds in ENT or general surgery; different methods of defining or diagnosing wound infection [5] (VI/C); the relatively rich blood supply of the face, which is the most common site of dermatological surgical

D. Fife (✉)
Surgical Dermatology & Laser Center, 9280 W. Sunset Road, Suite 310, Las Vegas, NV 89117, USA
e-mail: dfife@surgical-dermatology.com

M. Alam (ed.), *Evidence-Based Procedural Dermatology*,
DOI 10.1007/978-0-387-09424-3_10, © Springer Science+Business Media, LLC 2012

**Table 10.1** List of dermatologic surgical procedures stratified by risk of infection [3–5]

| Moderate | Flaps on the nose, skin grafts, surgical site on the lower extremity, procedures which breach a mucosal surface, procedures on inflamed or infected skin |
|---|---|
| Low-moderate | Mohs surgery and reconstruction, excisional surgery with repair, blepharoplasty, chemical peels, laser resurfacing |
| Low | Biopsy, curettage and dessication, liposuction, procedures which involve injection of a sterile material into the skin (botulinum toxin, intralesional triamcinolone, soft tissue fillers, sclerotherapy) |

**Table 10.2** Risk factors for wound infection [3, 5–7]

- Site within or close to oral, nasal, or anal mucosa, lower extremities, flaps on the nose
- Type of procedures (total resurfacing, skin grafts, large flaps), see Table 10.1
- Larger depth or surface area of wound
- Poor postoperative care
- Prolonged duration of surgical procedure
- Breaks in aseptic technique
- Presence of a hematoma, seroma, foreign body material, or damaged or nonviable tissue
- Grossly contaminated wound
- Patient risk factors
  - Immunocompromise
    - Disease (HIV, leukemia/lymphoma, others)
    - Advanced age or malnourishment
    - Corticosteroids or other immunosuppressive medications
    - Radiation therapy
  - Diabetes
  - Smoking
  - Low albumin
  - Elevated BMI
  - Vascular insufficiency
    - Atherosclerosis/poor perfusion
    - Smoking, diabetes, hypertension
    - Venous insufficiency, with accompanying edema/stasis
  - Infection/colonization with pathogenic organisms at distant sites (MRSA nasal colonization, abscesses, orolabial herpes simplex infection)

procedures; the overall clinical status of patients undergoing surgery, or other reasons. To maintain focus on wound prevention in the specific setting of dermatologic surgery, the dermatologic surgery literature will be reviewed, as well as studies from the traditional surgical literature, which may apply to dermatologic surgical procedures.

This chapter will focus on studies evaluating specific interventions, which can be implemented to prevent or treat wound infections. Interventions may be grouped into four categories: prophylactic antibiotics, preoperative preparation of the patient, protocol/attire worn by the surgical team, and postoperative wound care (Table 10.4). Each of these will be addressed in a separate section, and the studies of varying quality will be presented for each of these categories. Finally, evidence relating to the treatment of surgical site infections will be addressed.

## Prophylactic Systemic Antibiotics

Systemic antibacterial, antiviral, and antifungal agents decrease the population of pathogenic organisms in tissue. They are used perioperatively with the two main objectives: To prevent surgical site infections and to prevent bacteremia resulting in endocarditis or prosthetic joint infection. The timing of administration of prophylactic systemic antibiotics has varied; they have been given in the days preceding surgery, immediately preoperatively, or postoperatively. Some authors call postoperative antibiotic administration "treatment" instead of "prophylaxis" [5]. Controversy exists over the timing of antibiotic administration, the antibiotic of choice in different situations, and the appropriate dosage. Systemic antiviral and antifungal medications are important in laser resurfacing and other procedures in which the epidermal barrier is compromised, which may be complicated by the growth of organisms these agents target. Herpes simplex

**Fig. 10.1** Risk of surgical site infection [8] (VI/C)

$$\frac{\text{Dose of bacterial contamination } \mathbf{X} \text{ virulence}}{\text{Resistance of the host patient}} = \text{Risk of surgical site infection}$$

**Table 10.3** Wound classifications [3, 9]

| Wound class | Infection rate (%) | Description |
| --- | --- | --- |
| Class I (clean) | 1–4 | Noncontaminated skin, sterile surgical technique |
| Class II (clean-contaminated) | 5–10 | Minor breaks in aseptic technique, or wounds involving oral or nasal mucosa, axilla, or perineum wounds |
| Class III (contaminated) | 6–25 | Major breaks in sterile technique, traumatic wounds, or acute nonpurulent inflammation |
| Class IV (infected) | >25 | Gross contamination or devitalized tissue |

**Table 10.4** Interventions utilized to prevent wound infection

Prophylactic systemic antibiotics
  For prevention of wound infection
  For prevention of infective endocarditis or hematogenous joint infection
Preoperative preparation of patient
  Preoperative antiseptic skin preparation
  Antibacterial washes prior to surgery to decrease skin colonization
  Shaving vs. not shaving the skin, including timing of shaving
Attire worn/protocol of surgical team
  Hand washing
  Facemasks
  Strict aseptic surgical technique
  Sterile vs. nonsterile gloves in Mohs and other dermatologic procedures
Postoperative wound care
  Postoperative dressings
  Topical antibiotics
  Other wound care

virus (HSV) reactivation is an especially difficult problem after resurfacing procedures such as laser resurfacing, dermabrasion, or chemical peels, with the quoted rates of reactivation in untreated patients from 0 to 33% [14–19].

## Prophylactic Systemic Antibiotics: Consensus Documents

Maragh et al., in their 2008 article "Antibiotic Prophylaxis in Dermatologic Surgery: Updated Guidelines" published in the *Journal of the American Academy of Dermatology*, emphasize that the overall infection rate in dermatologic surgery is low, and that prophylactic antibiotics should be administered for the following two purposes: First, the prevention of bacterial endocarditis and hematogenous prosthetic joint infection, and second for the prevention of surgical site infections. They point out that that for dermatologic surgery oral administration of antibiotics is more reasonable than parenteral, and that the optimal time to administer antibiotics is 60 min prior to surgery. They stress that the site of surgery is the most important determining factor of which antibiotic to administer. Two grams of oral amoxicillin is the antibiotic of choice in situations where prophylactic antibiotics are necessary and the surgery involves a breach of the oral or nasal mucosa. Two grams of oral cephalexin is the recommended antibiotic for surgical sites involving glabrous skin. For patients who are penicillin-allergic, 600 mg of oral clindamycin can be substituted for amoxicillin or cephalexin [20] (VI/C).

In late 2008, Wright et al. published an advisory statement in the Journal of the American Academy of Dermatology with recommendations for implementing antibiotic prophylaxis in dermatologic surgery. The authors based their recommendations not on evidence from large-scale prospective trials, but rather loosely followed the guidelines set forth by the American Heart Association, the American Dental Association, and the American Academy of Orthopedic Surgeons. They then adjusted the recommendations from these groups to make it more pertinent to the field of dermatologic surgery. The statement advised the practice of pretreating patients with systemic antibiotics in three major instances. First, if the dermatologic procedure will involve infected skin or the oral mucosa and

**Table 10.5** High-risk cardiac conditions for which antibiotic prophylaxis is indicated for patients undergoing dermatologic surgery on infected skin or that involves breach of oral mucosa

| |
| --- |
| Prosthetic cardiac valve |
| Previous infective endocarditis |
| Congenital heart disease (CHD) |
| – Unrepaired cyanotic CHD, including palliative shunts and conduits |
| – Completely repaired CHD with prosthetic material or device, whether placed by a surgical or catheter intervention, during the first 6 months after procedure |
| – Repaired CHD with residual defects at site or adjacent to the site of prosthetic patch or prosthetic device (which inhibits endothelialization) |
| Cardiac transplantation recipients who develop cardiac valvulopathy |

From Wright et al. [4], VI/C

**Table 10.6** Patients at potential increased risk of prosthetic joint infection

| |
| --- |
| First 2 years following joint placement |
| Previous prosthetic joint infections |
| Immunocompromised/immunosuppressed patients |
| – Inflammatory arthropathies (e.g., RA, SLE) |
| – Drug- or radiation-induced immunosuppression |
| Insulin-dependent (type 1) diabetes |
| HIV infection |
| Malignancy |
| Malnourishment |
| Hemophilia |

From Wright et al. [4], VI/C

the patient is at high risk for infective endocarditis (Table 10.5). Second, they recommend prophylactic antibiotics when the procedure will involve infected skin or the oral mucosa and the patient is at high risk for hematogenous total joint infection (HTJI) (Table 10.6). Finally, antibiotic prophylaxis is recommended for procedures that put patients at a high risk for surgical site infections (Table 10.7). They recommended similar dosages and choices of antibiotic medications as Maragh et al. [20], and also recommended that oral antibiotics should be administered 30–60 min prior to the start of the procedure [4] (VI/C).

In 1995, AHA guidelines were reviewed and a survey of how dermatologists were prescribing prophylactic antibiotics was taken. It was determined

**Table 10.7** Procedure location and surgical techniques at increased risk for surgical site infection

| |
| --- |
| Lower extremity, especially leg |
| Groin |
| Wedge excision of lip or ear |
| Skin flaps on nose |
| Skin grafting |
| Extensive inflammatory skin disease |

From Wright et al. [4], VI/C

that "the most common indications for prophylaxis were manipulation of infected tissue in patients undergoing any procedure, and any procedure in a patient with a prosthetic heart valve." The most common antibiotics used by dermatologists at the time were cephalosporins and erythromycin, given orally, before and after the surgery. The authors conclude that antibiotic prophylaxis should be used in two situations: "(1) surgical procedures on infected tissue in patients with a high risk cardiac lesion; and (2) any surgical procedure in a patient with a prosthetic heart valve." The authors stress the importance of obtaining pertinent medical history to determine whether or not prophylaxis is necessary [21] (VI/C).

Messingham and Arpey conducted a literature review in 2005 to evaluate findings pertaining to the use of antibiotics in cutaneous surgery. They recommended that for most routine skin procedures, antibiotic use is unwarranted for preventing surgical wound infection, endocarditis, and late prosthetic joint infections. In some situations the use of antibiotics is unclear and decisions should be made on a case-by-case basis; these include prolonged Mohs procedures, delayed repairs, grafts, takedowns of interpolation flaps, and procedures that breach a mucosal surface. In addition, they suggested that systemic prophylactic antibiotics for laser resurfacing and liposuction appear not to be routinely necessary, although patients with known prior herpes infection likely should receive antiviral prophylaxis. Antibiotic use is recommended in high-risk patients, in anatomic locations that are known to have a higher risk of infection, and in situations where overt infections have developed [9] (VI/C).

In January 2003, "leadership of the Medicare National Surgical Infection Prevention Project hosted the Surgical Infection Prevention Guideline Writers Workgroup meeting." In a consensus paper, the workshop noted their thoughts regarding currently published guidelines for antimicrobial prophylaxis. They agreed that "infusion of the first antimicrobial dose should begin within 60 min before surgical incision and that prophylactic antimicrobial agents should be discontinued within 24 h of the end of surgery." This advisory statement provides an overview of other issues related to antimicrobial prophylaxis including specific suggestions regarding "antimicrobial selection" [22] (VI/C).

In a publication entitled "Surgical site infection: Prevention and treatment of surgical site infection," commissioned by Great Britain's National Institute for Health and Clinical Excellence (hereafter referred to as NICE), the authors recommend that systemic antibiotics be given as prophylaxis before clean surgery involving the placement of a prosthesis or implant, clean-contaminated surgery, contaminated surgery, and surgery in which a tourniquet is used. They define clean-contaminated surgery as "An incision through which the respiratory, alimentary or genitourinary tract is entered under controlled conditions but with no contamination encountered." They recommend against the routine use of antibiotic prophylaxis for clean nonprosthetic uncomplicated surgery. They recommended that the appropriate timing of antibiotic prophylaxis is intravenous administration at the onset of anesthesia. They did not comment on the timing or dose of oral antibiotic prophylaxis during outpatient surgery under local anesthesia. They emphasized the importance of following local antibiotic formulary guidelines and considering the potential adverse effects when choosing specific antibiotics for prophylaxis [5] (VI/C).

## Prophylactic Systemic Antibiotics: Case Series and Cohort Studies

Rogues et al. conducted a prospective study that examined all consecutive cutaneous surgeries performed, excluding sebaceous cyst and pyoderma excisions, during a 3-month time frame by a group of 73 French dermatologic surgeons. The study's purpose was to determine patient risk factors and reported safety practices amongst the physicians and to correlate these with wound infection rates. Three thousand four hundred and ninety-one surgical cases were included, and all patients were followed-up just to the date of suture removal, with 1.9% of patients contracting a postoperative infection. The vast majority of the infectious complications detected (94%) were limited to superficial suppuration, with the remaining infections identified as abscesses. Infections were more likely in procedures of longer duration, in surgeries performed on the nose, and in excisions requiring a reconstructive procedure other than primary closure. The authors caution that "excisions with a reconstructive procedure, or certain anatomical sites such as the nose, may require stricter infection control precautions." However, exactly which precautions they believe surgeons should take is unclear. They also acknowledge that infections arising after suture removal may have been missed in the study. Of note, no relationship was established between the use of antibiotic prophylaxis and infection control, and the authors assert that "further investigation appears to be necessary before a definitive recommendation can be made for or against antibiotic administration in this context" [6] (V/B).

In a prospective study of 5,091 excisions of nonmelanoma skin cancers, Dixon et al. evaluated the incidence of infection at different body sites when patients received no antibiotic prophylaxis. The overall infection incidence was found to be 1.47%. Individual procedures had the following infection incidence: curettage 0.73% (3/412); skin flap repairs 2.94% (47/1,601); simple excision and closure 0.54% (16/2,974); skin grafts 8.70% (6/69); and wedge excision 8.57% (3/35). Some regions of the body had a higher risk of infection (>5%): surgery below the knee ($n = 448$) had an infection incidence of 6.92% (31/448); groin excisional surgery had an infection incidence of 10% (1/10). Procedures on the face demonstrated an infection incidence of 0.81% (18/2,209). Diabetic patients, those on warfarin and/or aspirin, and smokers showed no difference in infection incidence. Based on these findings, they recommended that oral antibiotics should be considered in the following cutaneous oncologic procedures: "all procedures below the knee, wedge excisions of lip and ear, all skin grafts, and lesions in the groin." While other circumstances, such as "surgery to the nose, ear, fingers, lips, skin flap surgery, and surgery on diabetics, smokers, and those on anticoagulants have previously been considered for wound infection prophylaxis," the authors find based on their data that antibiotic prophylaxis is not necessary [23] (V/B).

Walia and Alster reported findings of a retrospective study of 133 patients undergoing fullface carbon dioxide laser resurfacing to address whether prophylactic antibiotics given intra and postoperatively prevented bacterial infections. They found that all infections (total of 20) occurred in the 119 patients who received prophylactic antibiotics, while none of the 14 patients receiving no antibiotics had an infection. Their antibiotic regimen consisted of either 1 g of IV cephalexin intraoperatively followed by 1.5 g oral azithromycin over 5 days, 1 g IV cephalexin intraoperatively alone, or 1.5 g oral azithromycin alone over 5 days. The most common organisms isolated from subsequent infections were gramnegative bacilli (enterobacter and pseudomonas species). They concluded that intraoperative and postoperative systemic antibiotics are not effective in preventing bacterial infection after fullface resurfacing. They recommend strict aseptic surgical technique [24] (V/B).

In a prospective study of 356 patients undergoing $CO_2$ laser resurfacing, Manuskiatti et al. investigated the efficacy of various systemic and topical antimicrobial regimens: oral ciprofloxacin, topical antibiotics (intranasal mupirocin ointment and otic solution), oral ketoconazole, and oral fluconazole. Twenty-seven patients had infections (7.6%). Patients who had the prophylactic ciprofloxacin had a lesser chance of developing bacterial infections than those without antibiotic prophylaxis (4.3% compared to 8.2%, statistical significant not provided). Furthermore, those infections usually occurred after ciprofloxacin was discontinued. The authors also discovered that *Staphylococcus aureus* infections occurred exclusively in patients who were randomly assigned to receive mupirocin intranasally, suggesting that

prophylactic intranasal mupirocin is ineffective in preventing *S. aureus* infections in laser resurfacing patients. Yeast infections occurred in 6 patients (1.7%) who had not undergone antifungal prophylaxis, but no patients who had received ketoconazole or flucanazole developed yeast infections. Thus the authors concluded that ciprofloxacin can effectively prevent both gram-positive and gram-negative bacterial infections, while oral ketoconazole and fluconazole can be used to prevent yeast infections [25] (IV/B).

In a retrospective evaluation of 181 pts receiving a chemical peel or dermabrasion of the perioral area, Perkins and associates found that HSV reactivation occurred in 50% of patients (6/12) with a known history who were not on prophylaxis. However, of the patients who received standard prophylaxis (600 mg/day acyclovir), only 8.3% had a recurrence and those receiving a higher dosage of prophylaxis (2,400 mg/day acyclovir) had a 0% chance of recurrence, demonstrating that pretreatment with a high dosage of acyclovir may be especially important in clinically minimizing HSV in patients undergoing perioral chemical peel or dermabrasion. The statistical significance of the differences between groups was not stated. They administered acyclovir starting 2 days prior to the procedure to 14 days afterwards. It is important to note that 6.6% of patients (8/121) who had reported no history oral herpes developed a postoperative herpetic outbreak with an onset between days 5 and 12. Based on their findings, the authors recommend acyclovir prophylaxis in all patients undergoing chemical peel or dermabrasion, as HSV can occur even in patients with no recorded prior history. Based on previous reports of HSV infections after chemical peels and dermabrasion [26, 27], the authors believe that prophylactic acyclovir dosages should be administered in dosages larger than 400 mg/day and active infection treatment should be dosages larger than 1,000 mg/day. They believe that the lower dosages recommended in the past are not adequate in preventing herpetic outbreaks [28] (V/B).

Alster and Nanni evaluated 99 consecutive patients undergoing perioral or full-face $CO_2$ laser resurfacing to compare the efficacy of two different famciclovir dosing strategies in preventing HSV outbreaks. Sixty patients received famciclovir 250 mg twice daily starting 24 h prior to laser resurfacing and continuing for 10 days postoperatively. Thirty-nine patients received 500 mg twice daily over the same period. The overall rate of HSV outbreaks was 10.1%; however, it was not different in each group. Approximately, one-third of patients in each group with a prior history of herpes labialis had a recurrence compared to 5% of those without a history. They concluded that 250 mg of famciclovir twice daily is as effective as 500 mg twice daily in preventing HSV recurrence. Their rate of reactivation in each group was around 33%, which is higher all other quoted rates of HSV reactivation in which antiviral prophylaxis is used. They attribute this to their lower threshold and looser diagnostic criteria for diagnosing a case of HSV reactivation compared with other studies [18] (IV/B).

In a retrospective review of 961 cases where patients received nonablative fractional laser resurfacing, Graber, Tanzi, and Alster found that there were 17 HSV outbreaks (1.77%). Of the 295 patients who had a prior history of oral HSV, 86 patients received antiviral prophylaxis and 173 did not. Six of the 86 patients (7%) receiving antiviral prophylaxis had an HSV outbreak, while 8 of the 173 (4.6%) patients who did not receive antiviral prophylaxis had an outbreak. They did not provide the dosage or antiviral agent used. Less than 1% of patients with no prior history of HSV (7/702) had an HSV outbreak. The authors do not recommend prophylaxis for all patients as no scarring or dissemination occurred [29] (V/B).

In a retrospective analysis of 1,000 nonablative fractional resurfacing treatments by Setyadi et al., only two cases with infectious complications were found. The first case was a presumed HSV infection; however, no tzanck, DFA, or biopsy was performed. The other infection was impetigo diagnosed clinically without a culture. Both infections resolved with treatment and without sequellae. After the first case of HSV infection, they instituted a protocol of valacyclovir prophylaxis for all patients, and subsequently there were zero HSV infections in the subsequent 700 patients treated. In this two-subject case report, the authors suggest that HSV prophylaxis is only necessary in patients with a history of facial HSV infection [30] (V/C).

## Prophylactic Systemic Antibiotics: Randomized Controlled Trials and Meta-Analyses

Baran et al. evaluated 1,400 patients undergoing plastic surgery for reconstruction or cosmetic surgery procedures. Half of patients receive 2 g of a sulbactam–ampicillin combination during the induction of anesthesia, and the other half received a placebo (saline) solution. Wounds were observed daily in the postoperative period, were graded, and were cultured as needed if infection was suspected. They found no statistically significant difference in the infection rates between the two groups. Based on their findings, the authors recommended that phrophylactic antibiotics should not be used routinely in plastic and reconstructive surgery, except in patients who have high risk for infection [31] (II/A).

A study by John Burke published in 1961 has guided the current surgical practice of administering antibiotics prior to the start of surgical procedures. He administered antibiotic agents (Penicillin G, chloramphenicol, erythromycin, and achromycin) to guinea pigs at different time periods in relation to the time an incision was made and an aliquot of S. aureus was placed in the incision. He demonstrated that when the antibiotics were administered 1 h prior to the incision and contamination that the bacterial infection was completely controlled. If the antibiotics were administered at the same time as the incision the response was slightly decreased, and if the antibiotics were administered 3 h after the contamination the clinical outcome was no different as the control guinea pigs which received no antibiotic therapy. Burke concluded that, "There is a definite short period when the developing staphylococcal dermal or incisional infection may be suppressed by antibiotics. This effective period begins the moment bacteria gain access to the tissue and is over in 3 h… Antibiotics cause maximum suppression of infection if given before bacteria gain access to tissue" [32] (II/A).

Surgeons may sometimes prescribe oral fluo-roquinolines after auricular procedures to prevent postoperative infections, especially those caused by *Pseudomonas aeruginosa*. Mailler-Savage et al. conducted a prospective, randomized trial of 82 patients who were randomly assigned to local wound care alone or 500 mg of levofloxacin daily. While 12.2% of patients developed inflammatory chondritis, the infection rate overall was only 2.4%. There was no statistical difference in the infection rates between the two groups. No infections with *P. aeruginosa* occurred in any of the patients. They determined that "levofloxacin is not necessary to prevent postoperative infections of auricular second intention wounds after Mohs surgery," and that local wound care alone is enough [33] (II/A).

Gilbert and McBurney sought to address the proper timing of antiviral prophylaxis before laser resurfacing procedures. In a randomized, prospective study of 84 patients undergoing chemical peel, dermabrasion/dermasanding, or Er/YAG laser resurfacing, patients were randomized to receive 500 mg of valacyclovir twice daily starting either the morning of the procedure or the morning before the procedure. Both groups continued the medication for 14 days. None of the patients had HSV recurrence. They concluded that 500 mg of oral valacyclovir twice daily is effective in preventing HSV reactivation after resurfacing procedures, regardless of whether it is started the day before or the day of surgery [34] (II/A).

A prospective, randomized study of 120 patients undergoing full face or perioral $CO_2$ laser resurfacing by Beeson and Rachel sought to address the duration of antiviral prophylaxis necessary to prevent HSV reactivation. All patient started valacyclovir 500 mg twice daily 1 day preoperatively. They were then randomized to continue therapy for either 10 or 14 days. A Tzank prep was performed on day of the procedure and then weekly for 3 weeks. None of the subjects had a reactivation of HSV, despite 47% of the patients having had a prior clinical history of HSV infection. The authors concluded that the 14-day course of valacyclovir does not confer any additional benefit than the 10-day course. Another interesting point of the study was that 70% of the

patients who reported having no clinical history of prior HSV infection had positive evidence of HSV on serology. This may provide support for the rationale to treat all patients with laser resurfacing with antiviral prophylaxis [14] (II/A).

No randomized controlled trials exist which compare different antiviral medications in their efficacy in preventing HSV infection after laser resurfacing or other resurfacing procedures.

## Prophylactic Systemic Antibiotics: Conclusions

The evidence suggests that prophylactic antibiotic administration should be reserve for instances in which the risk of infection is high (Tables 10.1, 10.2, and 10.7) or in appropriate situations when the consequences of infection are disastrous (such as hematogenous joint infection or infective endocarditis) (VI/C). Procedures that have the highest risk of infection, and therefore would warrant antibiotic prophylaxis include those where the oral or nasal mucosa is encountered, prolonged procedures, skin flaps on the nose, skin grafts, and procedures on the lower legs (V/B). For antibiotic prophylaxis to be the most effective, the medication should be administered 30–60 min prior to the start of surgery (II/A). The antibiotic of choice should be appropriate to cover the pathogenic organisms that most commonly colonize and subsequently infect the surgical site. For dermatologic procedures in most locations on the skin, the pathogenic organism responsible for most infections is *S. aureus*, and cephalexin is the recommended antibiotic of choice (VI/C). However, in surgeries which breach the oral mucosa, amocicillin is the antibiotic of choice to cover *Streptococcus* species (VI/C). In geographic areas where the incidence of *MRSA* skin infection is high, an antibiotic which covers MRSA may be an appropriate choice for antibiotic prophylaxis (VI/C). There is no evidence that antibiotic treatment antibiotics in the days following surgery is effective in preventing surgical wound infection.

Antiviral prophylaxis at appropriate dosing should be administered to all patients undergoing fractional ablative and fully-ablative facial resurfacing (II/A); however, the evidence does not clearly demonstrate that systemic antibiotics are effective at preventing bacterial infections (V/B). The evidence does not support the use of antiviral prophylaxis is necessary in nonablative fractional laser resurfacing (V/B).

## Preoperative Preparation of Patient

Since microbial flora residing on patients' skin or mucous membranes can be a source of wound infections, methods to reduce or eliminate these organisms prior to surgery have been sought. There may be a difference between *transient* microorganisms which are transferred to the skin by touch and which are easily removed with antiseptics, and the *resident* flora which reside in hair follicles and other appendages and are less effectively removed with soaps or antiseptic washes [5]. The most standard practice for reducing flora is cleansing, or "prepping" the area of surgery immediately prior to surgery with a variety of antiseptic solutions. Other interventions include instructing patients to bathe with antibacterial soaps or solutions in the days leading up to surgery or to apply intranasal antibacterial ointment to decrease colonization of S. aureus. These interventions have the goal of decreasing the number of potentially infecting organisms which might contaminate the wound during surgery. As body hair can make a surgical procedure more difficult (hair becoming caught in sutures or otherwise obstructing the surgery) or represent a source of wound contamination, surgeons have sought answers to the questions of whether hair removal lowers infection rates and which method of hair removal results in the lowest infection rate.

### Preoperative Preparation of Patient: Consensus Documents

In a review article entitled "Acute surgical complications: Cause, prevention, and treatment," Stuart Salasche recommends 4% chlorhexidine gluconate in a detergent base as a safe, effective, nontoxic way of killing gram-positive and gram-negative bacteria [35] (VI/C).

NICE recommends that patients should shower or have a bath with regular soap either the day before or the day of surgery. The authors discourage the use of hair removal routinely to reduce the risk of surgical site infection. They stress that if the hair has to be removed, that it be removed on the day of surgery with electric clippers with a single use head. Razors should not be used for hair removal, as they increase the risk of surgical infection. The authors also recommend that the skin at the surgical site be prepared immediately before incision using either an aqueous or alcohol-based antiseptic preparation of chlorhexidine or povidone-iodine. They do not recommend one specific antiseptic solution over another [5] (VI/C).

Mangram et al., in a review published as a CDC guideline, give recommendations similar to NICE regarding bathing, hair removal, and preoperative skin preparation. In addition, they stress the importance of pre and postoperative serum glucose control in patients who are diabetic and the encouragement of smoking cessation [8] (VI/C).

### Preoperative Preparation of Patient: Case Series and Cohort Studies

Dzubow et al. compared the efficacy of three antiseptic protocols in reducing aerobic bacterial levels on the faces of 14 subjects. They found that a 10-s wipe of 70% isopropyl alcohol was as effective as a 60-s alcohol wipe or a 60-s chlorhexidine or povidone-iodine solution application in reducing bacterial levels at the 5-min postoperative period. In addition, they found that povidone-iodine maintained higher efficacy at 60 min after the application than the 10 or 60-s alcohol wipe. They also reported that none of the preparations significantly reduced the anaerobic flora present on the highly sebaceous regions of the face [36] (III/B).

In the prospective study of 356 $CO_2$ laser resurfacing patients mentioned above, Manuskiatti et al. investigated the efficacy of various systemic and topical antimicrobial regimens in preventing postoperative infections. One of the interventions used was preoperative intranasal mupirocin ointment and otic solution. They found that S. aureus infections occurred exclusively in patients who were randomly assigned to

**Table 10.8** Summary of skin and nail preparation methods evaluated in Becerro et al. [39] (II/A)

| Method 1 | 7.5% Povidone-iodine scrub for 5 min + 10% povidone-iodine paint |
|---|---|
| Method 2 | Prewash with 70% isopropyl alcohol for 3 min + 7.5% povidone-iodine scrub for 5 min + 10% povidone-iodine paint |
| Method 3 | 4% Chlorhexidine gluconate scrub for 5 min + 70% isopropyl alcohol paint |
| Method 4 | Immersion of foot in 5 L of water and 250 mL of 4% chlorhexidine gluconate + prewash with 70% isopropyl alcohol for 3 min + 7.5% povidone-iodine scrub for 5 min + 10% povidone-iodine paint |

receive mupirocin intranasally, suggesting that prophylactic intranasal mupirocin is ineffective in preventing postoperative staph infections in laser resurfacing patients [25] (IV/B).

## Preoperative Preparation of Patient: Randomized Controlled Trials and Meta-Analyses

Randall et al. conducted a randomized, controlled trial of 64 patients comparing showering with 4% chlorhexidine against no showering, and found no difference in the surgical site infection rate [37] (II/A).

Wihlborg compared showering with 4% chlorhexidine to no washing in a randomized, controlled trial of 978 general surgery patients. There was a statistically significant decreased rate of infection (9/541, 1.7%) in the chlorhexidine group compared to the group that did not bathe (20/437, 4.6%) [38] (II/A).

A prospective, randomized study by Becerro et al. published in the JAAD in 2009 compared four protocols of skin and nail preparation of the foot (Table 10.8). Each scrub was tested on 28 different feet, and efficacy was measured by comparing differences in total bacterial load before and after the skin preparation. They demonstrated a significantly increased efficacy when a combination of isopropyl alcohol and povidone-iodine solution scrubs are incorporated into the preparatory regimen when compared with other protocols. The authors acknowledged that they did not measure clinically relevant infections, and that the results may not correlate with decreased infection rates postoperatively. This study quantitatively tested different antiseptic scrubs in the area of the feet and toes. It is unclear whether the results can be applied to other surgical sites [39] (II/A).

In a Cochrane Review, Webster and Osborne analyzed six randomized controlled trials in a meta-analysis which included over 10,000 patients undergoing surgery in the traditional operating room setting, to evaluate the efficacy of preoperative full-body bathing or showering with antiseptics in reducing wound infections after surgery. The collective evidence did not support the use of 4% chlorhexidine gluconate as a preventative measure in infection control; there was no significant difference in the infection rates of patients using the scrub vs. those showering with a placebo or nothing. The authors conclude that "efforts to reduce the incidence of nosocomial surgical site infection should focus on interventions where effects have been demonstrated." In addition, the review found no evidence of the benefit of clorhexidine gluconate scrub vs. other products [40] (I/A).

In a meta-analysis by Tanner et al. of 11 randomized controlled trials involving 5,031 patients, the effect of preoperative hair removal at the surgical site on the occurrence of treatment-related infections was evaluated. The cumulative evidence demonstrated no significant differences between the infection rates in patients who had undergone hair removal and those who had not. Significantly, they did find that shaving the hair preoperatively results in more wound infections that using a depilatory cream or clipping the hair. Based on their findings, the authors recommend that if hair removal is necessary, "clipping and depilatory cream result in fewer surgical site infections than shaving with a razor." The timing of hair removal proved unimportant; no differences in the rate of infectious complications existed between patients who had hair clipped on the day of surgery vs. those who had had hair clipped 1 day preoperatively [41] (I/A).

In a meta-analysis of seven randomized controlled trials in the traditional surgery literature, Edwards et al. found that there was insufficient evidence to demonstrate that the use of one preoperative antiseptic solution was advantageous over another. One study resulted in fewer surgical site infections when chlorhexidine scrubs were used compared to iodine, but multiple other studies demonstrated no difference between the two. Four trials showed that "there is no evidence that iodophor impregnated incise drapes reduce infections when compared to using no incise drape. Patients' skin at the operation site is routinely cleaned with antiseptic solutions before surgery." The authors concluded that further research to determine the effects of preoperative skin antiseptics on postoperative surgical wounds is needed before any conclusions can be drawn [42] (I/A).

A randomized, double-blind, placebo-controlled study of 4,030 patients undergoing general, gynecologic, neurologic, or cardiothoracic surgery received intranasal mupirocin or a placebo ointment in a preoperative protocol. Overall, the rate of postoperative infection with *S. aureus* was not different between the two groups (2.3% in the mupirocin group and 2.4% in the placebo group). However, of the 891 patients who had *S. aureus* cultured in their nares prior to their study, there were significantly lower rates of nosocomial infections in those receiving mupirocin compared to those receiving placebo (4.0% compared to 7.7%, odds ratio for infection 0.49; 95% confidence interval 0.25–0.92, $P=0.02$). They concluded that "Prophylactic intranasal application of mupirocin did not significantly reduce the rate of *S. aureus* surgical-site infections overall, but it did significantly decrease the rate of all nosocomial *S. aureus* infections among the patients who were *S. aureus* carriers" [43] (II/A).

### Preoperative Preparation of Patient: Conclusions

Preoperative patient skin preparation with antiseptic solutions is universally accepted as a procedure to minimize the risk of wound contamination with bacterial organisms that reside on the patient's skin. The most extensively studied antiseptic solutions are chlorhexidine gluconate and povidone iodine; however, there is no conclusive evidence that one of these solutions is superior to the other (I/A). The time duration of the scrub (some scrubs in studies are as short as 10 s, while other are as long as, 8 min),

extent of coverage around the treated area, or the method of administration of applying the solution (a brush, sponge, gauze, or other tool) have not been studied sufficiently to provide recommendations. Studies have not demonstrated a benefit of instructing patients to bathe preoperatively with antiseptic soaps; however, one concensus guideline recommends preoperative showering with regular soap as close as possible before surgery [5] (VI/C). Removing hair prior to surgery has not proven to lower the infection rate; however, if the decision is made to remove the hair then using a depilatory cream or clipping with a single use disposable head is recommended over shaving, which has a higher risk of infection (I/A). The timing of hair removal is also not important, as infection rates are the same when hair is removed on the day of surgery as when it is removed 1 day preoperatively (I/A). Serum glucose control and smoking cessation may also reduce the risk of wound infection (VI/C).

Patient use of preoperative topical antibiotic ointments and creams has been suggested as a way to prevent postoperative infection; however, studies have not demonstrated a benefit in lowering infection rates with this method. In addition, intranasal mupirocin ointment with the goal of decreasing *S. aureus* colonization has not been shown to decrease the wound infection rate. In fact, Manuskiatti et al. found postoperative *S. aureus* infections in $CO_2$ resurfacing patient occurred only in patients who had used preoperative intranasal mupirocin ointment [25] (IV/B); however, this is the only study to date with this finding.

### Attire Worn/Protocol of Surgical Team

Sterile protective attire worn by the surgical team is thought to decrease the risk of wound contamination. Aseptic operating technique has long been a focus of dermatologic surgeons; however, there is debate over the level of sterility required for skin surgery in the outpatient setting [44, 45]. In the traditional surgical literature, an area of extensive study has been the comparison of different hand-washing protocols and the infect they have on bacterial counts and surgical site infections. However, it is not a common practice among dermatologic surgeons to undertake lengthy handwashing protocols. Other interventions which have been studied include the wearing of facemasks and the comparison of the use of sterile vs. nonsterile gloves when performing dermatologic surgical procedures.

## Attire Worn/Protocol of Surgical Team: Consensus Documents

NICE recommends that the operating team remove hand jewelry, artificial nails, and nail polish prior to procedures. They recommend that sterile gowns be worn in the operating room, that two pairs of sterile gloves be worn when the risk of glove perforation is high and the consequences of contamination are serious [5] (VI/C).

In his review article on the prevention and treatment of acute surgical complications, Salasche recommends the wearing of sterile gloves and masks. Depending on the surgical setting and the extent of the procedure, sterile caps and gowns may provide additional benefit. While difficult in the outpatient setting, air filtration, multiple use-rooms, and limiting personnel traffic during the procedure may provide additional preventive benefit. He also discusses the importance of proper aseptic technique and gentle tissue handling to avoid causing devitalized tissue that may have decreased local resistance. The proper use of toothed forceps and skin hooks can avoid crushing the tissue. In addition, sutures tied too tightly could compromise host defenses [35] (VI/C).

## Attire Worn/Protocol of Surgical Team: Case Series and Cohort Studies

The findings of Rogues et al., who published the results of a prospective multicenter study evaluating a variety of safety interventions in 3,471 dermatologic surgical cases, were addressed more in detail in the preceding section on prophylactic antibiotics. The authors found that the only safety practice which significantly correlated with lower infection rates was the wearing of sterile gloves over nonsterile gloves when performing surgical excisions which required a flap

or graft reconstruction. In the case of excision with primary closure, there was no difference in the infection rates when comparing use of nonsterile and sterile gloves [6] (V/B).

A retrospective, chart review study conducted by Rhinehart et al. found that "the use of sterile vs. nonsterile gloves in the tumor extirpation phase of MMS" does not affect infection rates. "Statistically significant infection rates were discovered for patients with cartilage fenestration with secondary healing and malignant melanoma diagnosis only. There was no statistical difference in infection rates with all other measured variables to include the use of sterile or clean, nonsterile gloves." Thus clean, nonsterile gloves are safe and effective in MMS [46] (V/B).

An orthopedic surgery study attempted to demonstrate whether surgical team decolonization would reduce the risk of surgical site infections. Surgical team members had cultures taken of nasal swabs. Carriers of *S. aureus* were treated with intranasal mupirocin. In the 1,000 cases prior to the intervention, there were six surgical site infections. After initiation of the protocol, there were no infections in the subsequent 300 cases. The authors acknowledge that "more data need to be collected," but suggest that this intervention might be a useful intervention to reduce the rate of surgical infections. The applicability of this intervention to dermatologic surgery is unknown [47] (V/C).

## Attire Worn/Protocol of Surgical Team: Randomized Controlled Trials and Meta-Analyses

In a Cochrane Review, Lipp and associates evaluated the use of disposable surgical facemasks on the prevention of postoperative wound infections in a meta-analysis of two randomized controlled studies in the traditional surgery literature. The authors concluded that it was "unclear whether the wearing of surgical masks by the surgical team results in any harm or benefit for the patient." Because this analysis focuses exclusively on "clean" surgeries in the operating room setting, its application to the field of dermatology is extremely limited, and the results cannot be extrapolated to other categories of surgery. Despite the limited applicability of this analysis to dermatologic surgery, it is the routine practice of many dermatologic surgeons to wear disposable face-masks while operating, and this review does abate the concern that facemasks may be contributors to surgical wound infection [48] (I/A).

Arrowsmith et al. found that nail polish and finger rings had no effect on postoperative wound infection rates. It was previously hypothesized that nail polish (varnish) and rings hide bacteria and lead hand scrubbing to be less effective in reducing the number of bacteria on the hands of operating theater staff, but "the review [of one RCT] found no evidence from trials about the effect of staff wearing rings. One small trial suggests that there might be differences between varnished and unvarnished nails, but there is not enough evidence to be certain." They concluded that removing nail polish and finger rings to prevent surgical infection is unnecessary [49] (I/A).

Tanner et al. performed a meta-analysis, which was published as a Cochrane Review in 2008 to address whether or not preoperative hand antisepsis of the surgical team decreased surgical site infection rates or lowered the number of bacterial colony forming units present on the hands of the surgical team. They also sought to address whether one method of preoperative washing was superior over others. One of the ten randomized control trials analyzed evaluated the primary outcome measure of postoperative infection, finding that alcohol rubs with additional active ingredients were as effective as aqueous preparations in preventing surgical site infections. The authors were hesitant to make a recommendation based on these findings because they had not been replicated. However, when assessing colony forming units, the evidence supports the use of either an alcohol rub or an aqueous scrub to reduce the microflora present on the hands of the surgical team. The authors stated that they could not draw firm conclusions to recommend one antiseptic agent over another because "results of studies comparing alcohol rubs with aqueous scrubs are mixed." None of the studies assessed compared different types of alcohol rubs, but four studies demonstrated the superiority of chlorhexidine gluconate-based aqueous scrubs over povidone iodine-based

aqueous scrubs. The authors tentatively suggest "that aqueous scrub solutions of chlorhexidine gluconate should be [chosen] for surgical hand antisepsis." Although the studies examined in this analysis were limited to those examining surgeries performed in operating theaters under sterile conditions, hand-washing with anti-microbial agents is certainly a precaution against infection that can be applied in the field of dermatologic surgery [50] (I/A).

## Attire Worn/Protocol of Surgical Team: Conclusions

Handwashing prior to performing dermatologic surgery is a common practice which is thought to reduce the risk of infection (VI/C). The traditional surgery literature has demonstrated that alcohol based scrubs are as effective as aqueous scrubs in reducing bacterial colony counts (I/A) and that among aqueous scrubs that chlorhexidine is more effective than iodine-based scrubs at decreasing colony counts (I/A). There is no clear evidence that one surgical hand scrub is more effective than another at decreasing surgical site infection rates (I/A). The evidence does not support the removal of rings or nail polish by the surgical team as an intervention to prevent wound infections (I/A). During the tumor extirpation of Mohs surgery clean, nonsterile gloves can be worn (IV/B); however, sterile gloves should be worn during surgical repairs, especially flap and graft procedures (IV/B). The decolonization of the surgical team with intranasal mupirocin or other methods has not been shown to decrease the risk of surgical infection. It is also unclear whether the wearing of facemasks or preoperative hand antisepsis of the operating team lowers the infection rate in dermatologic surgery; however, both of these practices are widely used.

## Postoperative Wound Care

In addition to prophylactic antibiotics, patient preparation, and the attire and protocol of the surgical team, postoperative wound care has an area of focus in preventing procedure-associated infection. Interventions include cleansing the wound with specific solutions or protocols, using different dressing materials and protocols, and applying topical antibiotics or other preparations. An area of debate has been the most effective postoperative care after full face laser resurfacing. Occlusive dressings after full face laser resurfacing generally speed up healing and decrease pain intensity, but it has also been suggested that occlusive dressings left on for more than 3–5 days may increase the risk of infection [51] (VI/C).

## Postoperative Wound Care: Consensus Documents

Mangram et al. recommend that a postoperative wound be protected with a sterile dressing for 24–48 h postoperatively for a wound that has been closed primarily. Hands should be washed before and after dressing changes or any other contact with the surgical site, and a sterile technique should be used for dressing changes. The authors also recommend educating the patient and family regarding the proper care of the incision, the symptoms of infection, and the importance of reporting these symptoms. They do not give a recommendation on the need to cover an incision closed primarily beyond 48 h, nor on the length of time to wait showering or bath with an uncovered incision [8] (VI/C).

A literature review by Messingham and Arpey addressed topical antibiotic use in dermatologic surgery. They recommend topical antibiotics in contaminated or infected wounds (Class III or IV), but recommend that in class I or II wounds that white petrolatum be used due to its low cost, lower rate of contact dermatitis, and comparable associated infection rates. The authors also state that while topical antibiotics may be overused, "silver sulfadiazine may have an undeserved negative reputation among dermatologists." Silver sulfadiazine is a mainstay of treatment in burn units and among burn surgeons. They note that while silver sulfadiazine can induce bone marrow suppression, cause local and systemic argyria, and induce contact sensitivity, the rates of these occurring in patients who are not burn patients is low, and silver sulfadiazine has far fewer case reports of contact sensitivity, anaphylaxis, and other adverse events with the use of silver sulfadiazine when compared with bacitracin and other topical antibiotics that dermatologists use frequently [9] (VI/C).

In their guidelines for preventing surgical site infections, NICE recommends that the surgical incision be covered with an appropriate interactive dressing immediately at the end of the procedure. For wound cleansing the authors recommend sterile saline for the first 48 h and tap water thereafter, including if the wound is healing by second intention or if the wound has separated or been opened to drain pus. They recommend against the use of topical antibiotics on surgical wounds that are healing by primary intention. For wounds that heal by second intention, the authors recommend that a tissue viability nurse or other healthcare professional with tissue viability expertise be consulted for advice on appropriate dressings and wound management [5] (VI/C).

## Postoperative Wound Care: Case Series and Cohort Studies

In a retrospective study of 354 patients who underwent full-face $CO_2$ laser resurfacing, Christian et al. treated their patients with polyurethane foam occlusive dressings and empiric oral cephalexin postoperatively. Of the 354 patients there were four cases of culture-proven infection (1.13% overall), and 3 out of the 4 occurred 3–5 weeks after the procedure. The organisms cultured were. S. Aureus, P. aeruginosa, Staphylococcus epidermidis, Escherichia coli, Klebsiella, and Hafnia Alvei. The authors suggested an exogenous source of infection in these cases, as most infections after laser resurfacing occur between postoperative days 2 and 10. Based on their findings, the authors claimed that occlusive dressings do not increase the risk of infections. They stressed that patients should be educated about how to properly maintain the area in which they were treated and to avoid "double dipping of wound care products until wounds are completely healed," as infection can occur weeks after the procedure [52] (V/B).

In a retrospective study of 395 patients undergoing $CO_2$ laser resurfacing, Sriprachya et al. identified the most common infections. There were 17 cases of "culture-proven infection" for a total incidence of 4.3%, with symptoms arising 2–10 days postoperation. Most of the infections (11/17) occurred when occlusive dressings were used without systemic antibiotics. Several patients had multiple infections with different microorganisms. Among the most common agents were *P. aeruginosa* (41% of all infected cases), *S. aureus* (35%), *S. epidermidis* (35%), and Candida species (24%). In addition, "multiple drug-resistant, gram-negative bacteria were found in four cases, implicating the possibility of hospital-acquired infections. Almost all isolates of gram-positive bacteria were resistant to both erythromycin and penicillin, but not oxacillin." The authors suggest that infections occur more often in patients who undergo full face resurfacing and those using a bio-occlusive dressing postoperatively [53] (V/B).

## Postoperative Wound Care: Randomized Controlled Trials and Meta-Analyses

In a randomized, controlled, double-blind study of 1,249 wounds in 922 dermatologic surgery patients published in *JAMA*, Smack et al. compared petroleum ointment to bacitracin ointment for wound care. The overall infection rate was 2%, and they found no difference in postoperative infection rates or healing times. Of the infections developing in the petroleum group, 90% were methicillin-sensitive *S. aureus*, which can easily be treated with systemic antibiotics. The most common organisms cultured in the bacitracin-treated group were ciprofloxacin-sensitive gram-negative organisms. The authors concluded that infection rates are comparable between petrolatum and bacitracin. They also commented that the bacitracin group was 4 times more expensive to treat because of the higher cost of treating gram-negative infections, the 0.9% rate of contact allergy due to bacitracin, and the higher cost of bacitracin over petrolatum [54] (I/A).

A Cochrane Review by Fernandez et al. published in 2007 sought to evaluate the data from randomized controlled trials comparing different solutions and protocols for wound cleansing. They found seven trials which compared infection rates between wound cleansed with water

and with normal saline. Tap water was more effective than saline in preventing infection in acute wounds in adults (RR 0.65, 95% CI 0.40–0.99), however. Three trials compared cleansing with saline to no cleansing, and a meta-analysis of these trials showed no difference infection rates [55] (I/A).

In a prospective randomized placebo controlled double blind multicenter trial in Australia, 972 patients undergoing minor dermatological surgery were given either a single topical dose of chloramphenicol or a placebo paraffin ointment, to determine the efficacy of chloramphenicol in preventing wound infection. Chloramphenicol is known to have "a broad spectrum of activity against Gram positive and Gram negative bacteria, Rickettsias, and Chlamydia," and the authors wished to determine how effective it was in preventing infection after patients had minor skin excisions. The incidence of infection in patients who had chloramphenicol treatment was 6.6%, while those in the control group had an 11% incidence (relative risk of wound infection of 1.7). The authors determined that the application of a single dose of chloramphenicol to "high risk sutured wounds after minor surgery produces a moderate absolute reduction in infection rate that is statistically but not clinically significant." The authors acknowledge that it is uncertain whether the placebo had pro-infective or anti-infective properties [56] (II/A).

## Postoperative Wound Care: Conclusions

Wounds should be dressed with sterile dressings immediately after the procedure (VI/C). The dressing material should be adequate to absorb drainage from the wound without producing maceration or become too dry (VI/C). White petrolatum is suggested over topical bacitration or combination antibiotic ointments in Class I or II surgical wounds because of its similar efficacy, lower cost, and lower rate of allergic contact dermatitis (I/A). Topical silver sulfadiazine may also have a role, as may topical cloramphenicol. However, topical chloramphenicol is not widely available for use in many areas of the world. Wounds can be cleansed with tap water (I/A). Occlusive dressings after completely ablative facial resurfacing procedures speeds healing and provides comfort; however, the evidence about their ability to prevent infection is conflicting, with some studies suggesting that they increase the rate of infection and others showing that they do not affect the infection rate.

## Treatment of Wound Infections

Most of current practice in diagnosing and treating wound infections is based on clinical practice and convention and not from the results of well-designed studies. Difficulty in interpreting treatment recommendations for wound infections in dermatologic surgery arises because of (1) differences in definition of wound infections (lumping them together instead of dividing them into superficial, deep, and organ cavity), and (2) the large number of papers addressing general surgery wound infections and not directly dermatologic surgery.

### Treatment of Wound Infections: Consensus Documents

Salache, in a review article entitled "Acute surgical complications: Cause, prevention, and treatment," stresses that it is important to recognize wound infections early and to distinguish them from contact dermatitis or reactions to suture material. He stresses that pain, tenderness, and purulent drainage are the most important diagnostic clues, but warmth, edema, erythema are also signs of wound infection (Fig. 10.2). He recommends establishing adequate drainage when a wound infection is diagnosed. A Gram's stain and culture should be performed, and the most appropriate emperic antibiotic should be started until the laboratory results are available. In most cases, emperic coverage for *S. aureus* is important, but if *Pseudomonas* or other gram-negative organisms are suspected then acetic acid compresses and appropriate antibiotic coverage should be initiated. Sutures should be removed if there is substantial exudate evident or if there is fluctuance or substantial edema under the suture line. In these cases the wound should be opened, irrigated with saline and packed lightly with

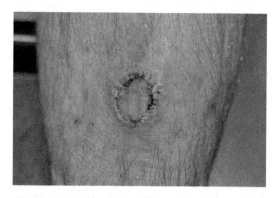

**Fig. 10.2** Infected postoperative wound showing signs of edema, warmth, erythema, and minor dehiscence. A culture of the discharge revealed *Staphylococcus aureus*

iodoform gause strips. Dressing changes and antibiotics should be continued until secondary intention healing is well underway. Scar revision can be undertaken at a later time when healing is complete [35] (VI/C).

May et al. recommend vigilant postoperative monitoring and diagnosis of superficial incisional wound infections, looking for the following signs: Purulent drainage from the incision, organisms cultured from fluid or tissue from the incision, pain, tenderness, redness, heat, or localized swelling. They recommend monitoring for a deeper soft tissue infection (suggested by a temperature >38°C, a spontaneous dehiscence, or purulent drainage from the wound) or severe infections such as necrotizing faciitis. Emperic systemic antibiotic therapy should be initiated (Table 10.9, likely pathogens), and agents directed at community-acquired MRSA should be considered in most settings. If a gram-negative or polymicrobial infection is suspected based on the location of surgery or the history and physical examination, broad-spectrum antibiotics may be indicated. The antibiotic medication should be changed based on the results of microbiological tests. If an abscess is suspected, an I&D should be performed with care to remove all loculations, if present [1] (VI/C).

NICE [5] stress vigilant monitoring in the postoperative period for signs of superficial wound infection (heat, redness, tenderness, drainage of pus). The presence of these signs is more important than results of microbiological cultures at the

**Table 10.9** Rank order of bacterial pathogens producing skin and soft tissue infections in North America, 1998–2004

| Rank | Pathogen | No. of isolates (% of total) |
|------|----------|------------------------------|
| 1 | *Staphylococcus aureus* | 2,602 (44.6) |
| 2 | *Pseudomonas aeruginosa* | 648 (11.1) |
| 3 | *Enterococcus* spp. | 542 (9.3) |
| 4 | *Escherichia coli* | 422 (7.2) |
| 5 | *Enterobacter* spp. | 282 (4.8) |
| 6 | *Klebsiella* spp. | 248 (4.2) |
| 7 | *B-hemolytic Streptococcus* | 237 (4.1) |
| 8 | *Proteus mirabilis* | 166 (2.8) |
| 9 | Coagulase-neg *Staphylococcus* | 161 (2.8) |
| 10 | *Serratia* spp. | 125 (2.1) |

Data obtained by the SENTRY Program [57]

**Table 10.10** Criteria for defining a superficial incisional surgical site infection [8] (VI/C)

| |
|---|
| Infection occurs within 30 days after the operation |
| *and* |
| Infection involves only skin or subcutaneous tissue of the incision |
| *and* at least *one* of the following |
| 1. Purulent drainage, with or without laboratory confirmation, from the superficial incision |
| 2. Organisms isolated from an aseptically obtained culture of fluid or tissue from the superficial incision |
| 3. At least one of the following signs or symptoms of infection: pain or tenderness, localized swelling, redness, or heat *and* superficial incision is deliberately opened by surgeon, *unless* incision is culture-negative |
| 4. Diagnosis of superficial incisional SSI by the surgeon or attending physician |

*Note*: Do *not* report a stitch abscess (minimal inflammation and discharge confined to the points of suture penetration) as a surgical site infection

wound edge, as multiple organisms normally colonize the skin. They recommend removal of sutures in an infected wound and the drainage of any purulent fluid (VI/C). They stress that drainage of fluid from a wound is often not due to infection but rather due to normal tissue exudation or an early failure of the wound to heal, which may be more common in patients with a high body mass index. In these situations the open wound edges can be closed with a delayed primary closure with sutures or adhesive strips rather than by treatment with systemic antibiotics. In situations where wound infection is suspected, treatment with the appropriate antibiotic to cover the most likely infectious organism should be initiated. The choice of antibiotic should be based on local resistant patterns and the results of microbiologic test results. The authors discuss the management of large open wounds from general surgery, and they stress the importance of the use of a multidisciplinary team approach, with involvement of specialists in wound care, tissue viability, and infection disease. The applicability of this team approach to dermatologic surgery wound management is limited, as wounds in dermatologic surgery are usually small and superficial and managed on an outpatient basis [5] (VI/C).

Mangram et al., in a review published as a CDC guideline, recommend criteria for the diagnosis of superficial wound infections [8] (Table 10.10).

A review paper by Bowler et al. addressing wound microbiology and approaches to wound infection management stresses that with the exception of clean surgeries, surgical wound infections have a polymicrobial etiology which involves both aerobic and anaerobic microorganisms. While prophylactic antibiotics immediately prior to surgery are the most effective, if they are used imperically to treat an active postoperative infection, broad spectrum antibiotics should be used, including coverage of facultative and aneorobic bacteria. The authors do not distinguish treatment for superficial wound infections and deeper wound infections, including intraabdominal infections. If necrotic material is present, it should be debrided to reduce the bacterial burden and to provide a wound margin that is more favorable for epithelial migration [58] (VI/C).

Garman and Orengo explain that "dermatologic procedures disrupt skin integrity, [altering] the body's protective barrier and predispose individuals to cutaneous infection." The authors note that "unusual infections have been reported to complicate excisions, biopsies, skin grafts, chemical peels, dermabrasion, laser resurfacing, liposuction, blepharoplasty, and injections (e.g., with anesthetic solutions or botulinum toxin)." For this reason, they strongly advise obtaining a thorough patient history (especially pertaining to prior HSV infections or immuno-compromising factors). In addition, patients and physicians should be vigilant for any possible wound infection for "several months postoperatively." They note that antimicrobial prophylaxis for reducing the infection risk in some cases, but recommend that clinicians become "familiar with the causes and clinical manifestations of unusual dermatologic postoperative wound infections. Following the recognition of an infectious process, appropriate diagnostic procedures allow for pathogen identification and the prompt institution of indicated therapy" [2] (VI/C).

## Treatment of Wound Infections: Case Series and Cohort Studies

No case series or cohort studies exist addressing the treatment of surgical wound infections in dermatologic surgery.

Rogues et al. mention that in their study hemorrhagic complications which occurred with an excision and primary repair had a sixfold increase in the risk of infection. They defined hemorrhagic complication as uncontrolled bleeding during or immediately after the procedure or a subsequent hematoma. This provides evidence to support the clinical practice of evacuating a hematoma as an intervention to treat or prevent an infection [6] (V/B).

## Treatment of Wound Infections: Randomized Controlled Trials and Meta-Analyses

No Randomized Controlled Trials or Meta-analyses exist addressing the treatment of surgical wound infections in dermatologic surgery.

## Treatment of Wound Infections: Conclusions

Most interventions used to treat wound infections are based on tradition and clinical experience rather than on rigorous scientific study. When an infection is encountered, the patient should be evaluated and monitored for more severe sequelae such as sepsis, toxic shock syndrome, and necrotizing fasciitis, as these complications have been reported after excisional skin surgery [59, 60] (VI/C). Any hematoma or abscess should be drained, and devitalized material should be surgically debrided (VI/C). Appropriate diagnostic tests for suspected organisms should be performed such as a gram stain and culture for bacteria and a Tzanck smear, viral culture, or direct fluorescent antibody test for viruses (VI/C). Emperic treatment with systemic antibiotics is indicated, with coverage for MRSA in locations where the incidence of MRSA is high. If gram-negative or anaerobic organisms are suspected then appropriate medications which cover these organisms should be considered. The treatment should then be guided by the results of biologic test results (VI/C).

| **Evidence-Based Summary** | |
|---|---|
| Findings | Evidence level |
| Procedures that have the highest risk of infection include those where the oral or nasal mucosa is encountered, prolonged procedures, skin flaps on the nose, skin grafts, and procedures on the lower legs (V/B) | (V/B) |
| Prophylactic antibiotics should be administered when the risk of surgical site infection is high or in appropriate situations where the risk of hematogenous joint infection or infective endocarditis is substantial (see Tables 10.5–10.7) (VI/C) | (VI/C) |
| Antibiotic prophylaxis is most effective when administered 30–60 min prior to surgery (II/A). Cephalexin or other antibiotics which cover *S. aureus* are the agents of choice except in cases where the oral mucosa is breached (VI/C) | (II/A); (VI/C) |
| Antiviral prophylaxis should be given to all patients undergoing fractional ablative and fully-ablative facial resurfacing (II/A); however, the evidence does not demonstrate that systemic antibiotics are effective at preventing bacterial infections (V/B) | (II/A); (V/B) |

**Evidence-Based Summary** (continued)

| Findings | Evidence level |
|---|---|
| Antiviral prophylaxis is not necessary in nonablative fractional laser resurfacing (V/B) | (V/B) |
| Neither chlorhexidine gluconate nor povidone iodine superior the other in preventing wound infections when used to cleanse the surgical site (I/A) | (I/A) |
| Removing hair prior to surgery does not lower the infection rate; however, if the decision is made to remove the hair then using a depilatory cream or clipping with a single use disposable head is recommended over shaving, which has a higher risk of infection (I/A) | (I/A) |
| The use of intranasal mupirocin by patients or the surgical team with the goal of decreasing *S. aureus* has not been shown to decrease the postoperative infection rate | |
| Alcohol-based hand washing scrubs are as effective as aqueous scrubs in reducing bacterial colony counts (I/A). Among aqueous surgical hand chlorhexidine is more effective than iodine-based scrubs at decreasing colony counts (I/A); however, no evidence suggests that one scrub is more effective than another at decreasing infection rates (I/A) | (I/A); (I/A); (I/A) |
| The evidence does not support the removal of rings or nail polish by the surgical team as an intervention to prevent wound infections (I/A) | (I/A) |
| During the tumor extirpation of Mohs surgery clean, nonsterile gloves can be worn (IV/B), however sterile gloves should be worn during surgical repairs, especially flap and graft procedures (IV/B) | (IV/B); (IV/B) |
| Wounds can be cleansed with tap water after 24 h (I/A) | (I/A) |
| White petrolatum is suggested over topical bacitracin or combination antibiotic ointments for Class I or II surgical wounds because of similar efficacy, lower cost, and lower rate of allergic contact dermatitis (I/A) | (I/A) |
| Treatment of wound infection involves evaluating for systemic complications; removing hematoma, purulence, or necrotic material; performing appropriate microbiologic tests; and beginning empiric antibiotic treatment (VI/C) | (VI/C) |

# References

1. May AK, Stafford RE, Bulger EM, Heffernan D, Guillamondegui O, Gochicchio G, et al. Treatment of complicated skin and soft tissue infections. Surg Infect. 2009;10(5):467–99.
2. Garman ME, Orengo I. Unusual infectious complications of dermatologic procedures. Dermatol Clin. 2003;21(2):321–35.
3. Haas AF, Grekin RC. Antibiotic prophylaxis in dermatologic surgery. J Am Acad Dermatol. 1995;32(2):155–76.
4. Wright TI, Baddour LM, Berbari EF, Roenigk RK, Phillips PK, Jacobs MA, et al. Antibiotic prophylaxis in dermatologic surgery: advisory statement 2008. J Am Acad Dermatol. 2008;59(3):464–73.
5. National Institute for Health and Clinical Excellence. Surgical site infection. 2008 (Clinical guideline 74). www.nice.org.uk/CG74. Accessed March 2009.
6. Rogues AM, Lasheras A, Amici JM, Guillot P, Beylot C, Taïeb A, et al. Infection control practices and infectious complications in dermatological surgery. J Hosp Infect. 2007;65(3):258–63.
7. Rubin RH. Surgical wound infection: epidemiology, pathogenesis, diagnosis, and management. BMC Infect Dis. 2006;6:171.
8. Mangram AJ, Horan TC, Pearson ML, Silver LC, Jarvis WR. Guideline for prevention of surgical site infection. Hospital Infection Control Practices Advisory Committee. Infect Control Hosp Epidemiol. 1999;20(4):250–78; quiz 279–80.
9. Messingham MJ, Arpey CJ. Update on the use of antibiotics in cutaneous surgery. Dermatol Surg. 2005;31 (8 Pt 2):1068–78.
10. Cook JL, Perone JB. A prospective evaluation of the incidence of complications associated with Mohs micrographic surgery. Arch Dermatol. 2003;139(2):143–52.
11. Kimyai-Asadi A, Goldberg LH, Peterson SR, Silapint S, Jih MH. The incidence of major complications from Mohs micrographic surgery performed in office-based and hospital-based settings. J Am Acad Dermatol. 2005;53(4):628–34.
12. Maragh SL, Brown MD. Prospective evaluation of surgical site infection rate among patients with Mohs micrographic surgery without the use of prophylactic antibiotics. J Am Acad Dermatol. 2008;59(2):275–8.

13. Amici JM, Rogues AM, Lasheras A, Gachie JP, Guillot P, Beylot C, et al. A prospective study of the incidence of complications associated with dermatological surgery. Br J Dermatol. 2005;153(5):967–71.
14. Beeson WH, Rachel JD. Valacyclovir prophylaxis for herpes simples virus infection or infection recurrence following laser skin resurfacing. Dermatol Surg. 2002;30(4):331–6.
15. Apfelberg DB. Perioperative considerations in laser resurfacing. Int J Aesthet Restor Surg. 1997;5:21.
16. Monheit GD. Facial resurfacing may trigger the herpes simplex virus. Cosmet Derm. 1995;8:9–16.
17. Wall SH, Ramey SJ, Wall FP, et al. Anti-viral prophylaxis in laser resurfacing procedures [abstract SE.21]. In: 1998 global summit on aesthetic surgery. Los Angeles, 1–6 May 1998.
18. Alster TS, Nanni CA. Famciclovir prophylaxis of herpex simplex virus reactivation after laser skin resurfacing. Dermatol Surg. 1999;25(3):242–6.
19. Rapaport MJ, Kamer F. Exacerbation of facial herpes simplex after phenolic peels. J Dermatol Surg Oncol. 1984;10(1):57–8.
20. Maragh SL, Otley CC, Roenigk RK, Phillips PK. Antibiotic prophylaxis in dermatologic surgery: updated guidelines. Dermatol Surg. 2005;31(1):91–3.
21. Rabb DC, Lesher Jr JL. Antibiotic prophylaxis in cutaneous surgery. Dermatol Surg. 1995;21(6):550–4.
22. Bratzler DW, Houck PM, Surgical Infection Prevention Guideline Writers Workgroup. Antimicrobial prophylaxis for surgery: an advisory statement from the National Surgical Infection Prevention Project. Am J Surg. 2005;189(4):395–404.
23. Dixon AJ, Dixon MP, Askew DA, Wilkinson D. Prospective study of wound infections in dermatologic surgery in the absence of prophylactic antibiotics. Dermatol Surg. 2006;32(6):819–26; discussion 826–7.
24. Walia S, Alster TS. Cutaneous $CO_2$ laser resurfacing infection rate with and without prophylactic antibiotics. Dermatol Surg. 1999;25(11):857–61.
25. Manuskiatti W, Fitzpatrick RE, Goldman MP, Krejci-Papa N. Prophylactic antibiotics in patients undergoing laser resurfacing of the skin. J Am Acad Dermatol. 1999;40(1):77–84.
26. Brody HJ. Complications of chemical peeling. J Dermatol Surg Oncol. 1989;15:1010.
27. Collins PS. The chemical peel. Clin Dermatol. 1987;5:57.
28. Perkins, SW, Sklarew EC. Prevention of facial herpetic infections after chemical peel and dermabrasion: new treatment strategies in the prophylaxis of patients undergoing procedures of the perioral area. Plast Reconstr Surg. 1996;98(3):427–33; discussion 434–5.
29. Graber EM, Tanzi EL, Alster TS. Side effects and complications of fractional laser photothermolysis: experience with 961 treatments. Dermatol Surg. 2008;34(3):301–7.
30. Setyadi HG, Jacobs AA, Markus RF. Infectious complications after nonablative fractional resurfacing treatment. Dermatol Surg. 2008;34(11):1595–8.
31. Baran CN, Sensöz O, Ulusoy MG. Prophylactic antibiotics in plastic and reconstructive surgery. Plast Reconstr Surg. 1999;103(6):1561–6.
32. Burke JF. The effective period of preventive antibiotic action in experimental incisions and dermal lesions. Surgery. 1961;30(1):161–8.
33. Mailler-Savage EA, Neal Jr KW, Godsey T, Adams BB, Gloster Jr HM. Is levofloxacin necessary to prevent postoperative infections of auricular second intention wounds? Dermatol Surg. 2008;34(1): 26–30.
34. Gilbert S, McBurney E. Use of valacyclovir for herpes simplex virus-1 (HSV-1) prophylaxis after facial resurfacing: a randomized clinical trial of dosing regimens. Dermatol Surg. 2000;26(1):50–4.
35. Salasche SJ. Acute surgical complications: cause, prevention, and treatment. J Am Acad Dermatol. 1986; 15(6):1163–85.
36. Dzubow LM, Halpern AC, Leyden JJ, Grossman D, McGinley KJ. Comparison of preoperative skin preparations for the face. J Am Acad Dermatol. 1988;19(4):737–41.
37. Randall PE, Ganguli L, Marcuson RW. Wound infection following vasectomy. Br J Urol. 1983;55(5):564–7.
38. Wihlborg O. The effect of washing with chlorhexidine soap on wound infection rate in general surgery. A controlled clinical study. Ann Chir Gynaecol. 1987;76(5):263–5.
39. Becerro de Bengoa Vallejo R, Inglesias MEL, Cervera LA, Fernandez DS, Priety JP. Preoperative skin and nail preparation of the foot: comparison of the efficacy of 4 different methods in reducing bacterial load. J Am Acad Dermatol. 2009;61(6):986–92.
40. Webster J, Osborne S. Preoperative bathing or showering with skin antiseptics to prevent surgical site infection. Cochrane Database Syst Rev. 2007;(2):CD004985. DOI:10.1002/14651858.CD004895.
41. Tanner J, Woodings D, Moncaster K. Preoperative hair removal to reduce surgical site infection. Cochrane Database Syst Rev. 2006;(3):CD004122. DOI:10.1002/14651858.CD004122.pub3.
42. Edwards P, Lipp A, Holmes A. Preoperative skin antiseptics for preventing surgical wound infections after clean surgery. Cochrane Database Syst Rev. 2004;(3):CD003949. DOI:10.1002/14651858. CD003949.pub2.
43. Perl TM, Cullen JJ, Wenzel RP, Zimmerman MB, Pfaller MA, Sheppard D, et al. Intranasal mupirocin to prevent postoperative *Staphylococcus aureus* infections. N Engl J Med. 2002;346(24):1871–7.
44. Finn L, Crook S. Minor surgery in general practice – setting the standards. J Public Health Med. 1998; 20:169–74.
45. Naimer SA, Trattner A. Are sterile conditions essential for all forms of cutaneous surgery? The case of

ritual neonatal circumcision. J Cutan Med Surg. 2000;4:177–80.

46. Rhinehart MB, Murphy MM, Farley MF, Albertini JG. Sterile versus nonsterile gloves during Mohs micrographic surgery: infection rate is not affected. Dermatol Surg. 2006;32(2):170–6.

47. Portigliatti BM, Mognetti B, Pecoraro S, Picco W, Veglio V. Decolonization of orthopedic surgical team *S. aureus* carriers: impact on surgical-site infections. J Orthop Traumatol. 2010;11(1):47–9.

48. Lipp A, Edwards P. Disposable surgical face masks for preventing surgical wound infection in clean surgery. Cochrane Database Syst Rev. 2002;(1): CD002929. DOI:10.1002/14651858.CD002929. Updated 3 Feb 2008.

49. Arrowsmith VA, Maunder JA, Sargent RJ, Taylor R. Removal of nail polish and finger rings to prevent surgical infection. Cochrane Database Syst Rev. 2001;(4): CD003325.

50. Tanner J, Swarbrook S, Stuart J. Surgical hand antisepsis to reduce surgical site infection. Cochrane Database Syst Rev. 2008;(1):CD004288. DOI:10. 1002/14651858.CD004288.pub2.

51. Rosenberg GJ, Gregory Chernoff W, Apfelberg DB, Seckel BR. Treatment of postlaser resurfacing complications. Aesthet Surg J. 1997;17(2):119–23.

52. Christian MM, Behroozan DS, Moy RL. Delayed infections following full-face $CO_2$ laser resurfacing and occlusive dressing use. Dermatol Surg. 2000; 26(1):32–6.

53. Sriprachya-Anunt S, Fitzpatrick RE, Goldman MP, Smith SR. Infections complicating pulsed carbon dioxide laser resurfacing, for photo-aged facial skin. Dermatol Surg. 1997;23:527–35.

54. Smack DP et al. Infection and allergy incidence in ambulatory surgery patients using white petrolatum vs. bacitracin ointment. A randomized controlled trial. JAMA. 1996;276(12):972–7.

55. Fernandez R, Griffiths R, Ussia C. Water for wound cleansing. Cochrane Database Syst Rev. 2008;(1): DC003861. DOI:10.1002/14651858.CD003861.pub2.

56. Heal CF et al. Does single application of topical chloramphenicol to high risk sutured wounds reduce incidence of wound infection after minor surgery? Prospective randomised placebo controlled double blind trial. BMJ. 2009;338:a2812.

57. Moet GJ, Jones RN, Biedenbach DJ, et al. Contemporary causes of skin and soft tissue infections in North America, Latin America, and Europe: report from the SENTRY Antimicrobial Surveillance Program (1998–2004). Diagn Microbiol Infect Dis. 2007;57:7–13.

58. Bowler PG, Duerden BI, Armstrong DG. Wound microbiology and associated approaches to wound management. Clin Microbiol Rev. 2001;14(2):244–69.

59. Moiemen NS, Frame JD. Toxic shock syndrome after minor dermatological surgery. Br Med J. 1993;306:386–7.

60. Gibbon KL, Bewley AP. Acquired streptococcal necrotizing fasciitis following excision of malignant melanoma. Br J Dermatol. 1999;141:717–9.

## Self-Assessment

1. Antibiotic prophylaxis is most effective when initiated immediately after surgery and continuing for at least 5 days postoperatively.
   (a) True
   (b) False

2. A patient who had a knee replacement surgery 6 months ago is undergoing Mohs surgery on the nasal ala, and you suspect the nasal mucosa will be breached. What is the most appropriate management?
   (a) 2 g of oral cephalexin should be administered 30–60 min prior to the procedure.
   (b) 2 g of oral amoxicillin should be administered 30–60 min prior to the procedure.
   (c) Antibiotic prophylaxis is not necessary.

3. Which preoperative antiseptic agent is most effective in preventing postoperative wound infections?
   (a) Povidone-iodine
   (b) Chlorhexidine gluconate
   (c) Providone-iodine and chlorhexidine gluconate are equally effective.

4. If hair needs to be removed in the surgical site prior to surgery, which of the following protocols is suggested in minimize the risk of infection
   (a) The area should be shaved on the day of surgery immediately prior to the procedure
   (b) The area should be shaved with a razor 1 day prior to surgery
   (c) The hair should be removed with clippers or a depilatory cream either on the day or surgery or 1 day prior to surgery

5. Which topical ointment is recommended for placing on class I or II wounds?
   (a) Bacitracin
   (b) White petrolatum
   (c) Mupirocin
   (d) Bacitracin/polymyxin B

## Answers

1. b: Antibiotic prophylaxis is most effective when given 30–60 min preoperatively.

2. a: Antibiotic prophylaxis is recommended to prevent hematogenous joint infection in patients with a joint replacement surgery within the past 2 years if the procedure breaches the oral or nasal mucosa or has a high risk for infection. The most common organism in the nasal mucosa is S. aureus, which will be covered by cephalexin.

3. c: No evidence indicates that either povidone-Iodine and chlorhexidine gluconate is superior to the other in preventing infection.

4. c: Hair removal has not proven to prevent surgical site infections. If the hair needs to be removed, then it is best removed with clippers with a disposable head or with a depilatory cream. The timing of hair removal is not important.

5. b: White petrolatum. The evidence does not demonstrate that topical antibiotic ointments are more effective in preventing infections than white petrolatum. In addition to the increased cost of antibiotic ointment, there is also a higher rate of contact dermatitis with these agents.

# Prevention and Treatment of Bleeding Complications in Dermatologic Surgery

**11**

Murray A. Cotter, Siegrid S. Yu, and Isaac M. Neuhaus

## Introduction

In general, the rate of complications in dermatologic surgery is extremely low. A single-center prospective analysis of 1,343 cases of Mohs micrographic surgery reported an overall complication rate of 1.6% (22/1,343), including wound infection, postoperative hemorrhage, hematoma, wound dehiscence, and flap or graft necrosis [1] (IV/B). This chapter reviews the available evidence regarding the prevention and management of bleeding complications of cutaneous surgery. Although much of the data will be generated from the collective dermatologic experience with Mohs micrographic surgery, the conclusions drawn will be applicable to standard excisional surgery, as well other common procedures of the dermatologist and dermatologic surgeon. Not only is peri-operative bleeding the most common complication associated with cutaneous surgery, but it is also the subject for which the most robust evidence exists. It is additionally important to note that complications involving dehiscence, necrosis, poor wound healing, and infection often occur after difficulties with hemostasis.

## Consensus Documents

A review of the websites of the American Academy of Dermatology (AAD), the American Society of Dermatologic Surgery (ASDS), the American College of Mohs Surgeons (ACMS), and the Association of Professors in Dermatology (APD) reveals no published consensus documents regarding complications in Dermatologic Surgery. Similarly there are no relevant documents published by Cochrane.

## Bleeding

The first step in the prevention of bleeding complications occurs through preoperative assessment of an individual patient's risk. A complete and directed preoperative history is the first step in assessing potential risk for bleeding in a patient undergoing a dermatologic surgery procedure. Common medical problems such as hypertension and anxiety can contribute significantly to bleeding, especially intra-operatively, and every effort should be made to adequately manage these medical problems in the pre- and peri-operative periods. History taking should also include medical conditions that can contribute to altered platelet

M.A. Cotter
Dermatologic Surgery and Laser Center,
University of California, 1701 Divisadero Street,
San Francisco, CA 94115, USA

Dermatology Associates of Northern Michigan,
Petoskey, MI 49770, USA

S.S. Yu • I.M. Neuhaus (✉)
Dermatologic Surgery and Laser Center,
University of California, 1701 Divisadero Street,
San Francisco, CA 94115, USA
e-mail: neuhausi@derm.ucsf.edu

M. Alam (ed.), *Evidence-Based Procedural Dermatology*,
DOI 10.1007/978-0-387-09424-3_11, © Springer Science+Business Media, LLC 2012

function and coagulation. This includes, but is not limited to, liver disease, renal dysfunction, and both hematologic and solid malignancies. A recent paper reports a case of disseminated intravascular coagulation in a patient with metastatic prostate cancer unmasked by Mohs micrographic surgery for a relatively small basal cell carcinoma on the forehead [2] (V/B). Poor nutritional status must also be considered a risk factor for excessive bleeding. This is especially relevant in the elderly population, the most common group of patients undergoing surgery for cutaneous malignancy. Clinicians should specifically assess for any prior history of significant bleeding during low-risk surgical procedures (i.e., dental extractions). Though a patient's description of prior operative bleeding is often very subjective, a previous history of excessive bleeding in this setting may indicate an inherited bleeding disorder such as hemophilia or von Willebrand disease, the most common hereditary bleeding disorder. Peterson and Joseph have provided an excellent review on inherited bleeding disorders in dermatologic surgery patients [3] (V/B). They emphasize the importance of working in conjunction with an experienced hematologist when dealing with this patient population.

Much more common than inherited bleeding disorders are acquired abnormalities in coagulation or platelet function secondary to medications and ingested products. It is well-known that ethanol consumption contributes to bleeding via decreased vasoconstriction and impaired platelet and coagulation function [4] (VI/C). Though this effect is difficult to quantify, patients who routinely consume alcoholic beverages may be advised to abstain for several days before and after cutaneous surgery. The use of alternative medicines and therapies has dramatically increased in recent years. Reports demonstrate that 22% of presurgical patients take various herbs and 51% consume vitamin supplements [5] (V/B). Vitamins and herbal supplements were often overlooked in the preoperative history. Patients often do not readily reveal their alternative medications to their physicians and physicians frequently do not specifically ask patients. One report found that over 35% of patients on alternative therapies did not inform their doctor during the medical history [6] (V/B). As further evidence, an anesthesiology study found that 89% of patients consuming herbal plant products did not consider them to be a medication, and that 91% would not have told an anesthesiologist about them on routine interview [7] (V/B). Dinehart and Henry recently published an excellent comprehensive review on dietary supplements and altered bleeding and coagulation [8] (I/A). They report that many dietary supplements can alter coagulation and platelet function, with many effects on platelets being irreversible. Therefore, the recommendation is for patients to stay off all vitamins and supplements for 7–10 days prior to surgery. The exceptions are vitamin E and ginkgo, which can be discontinued several days prior to surgery [8] (IV/B). Nonetheless, for the sake of simplicity, the authors typically advise patients to discontinue all of their supplements and herbals for the full 7–10 days.

While most patients can easily discontinue their alternative therapies or alcohol consumption in the peri-operative period, discontinuation of nonsteroidal anti-inflammatory drugs (NSAIDs) or anticoagulant and antiplatelet medications such as warfarin and aspirin is a much more complex issue that continues to be debated among dermatologic and other surgeons. A large percentage of patients are on NSAIDs for musculoskeletal aches and pains as well as other chronic inflammatory conditions. A significant proportion of the U.S. population takes aspirin for primary prevention of cardiac and cerebrovascular events, with primary prevention being defined as treatment aimed at preventing vascular events in patients who currently have no evidence of vascular disease. Furthermore, a variety of anticoagulants and blood thinning agents are currently utilized in patients as secondary prevention for thromboembolic events. Secondary preventative efforts focus on identifying and treating those with established disease, or those at very high risk for developing thromboembolic disease. Common indications for secondary prevention include patients with artificial heart valves or

**Table 11.1** Blood thinning agents and their mechanisms of action

| Class | Subclass/mechanism | Chemical (brand) name |
|---|---|---|
| Antiplatelet | Block formation of thromboxane A2 via inhibition of cyclooxygenase | Aspirin<br>Ticlopidine hydrochloride (Ticlid) |
| | Inhibitors of ADP-induced activation of platelets | Clopidogrel (Plavix) |
| | Glycoprotein IIb/IIIa inhibitors | Abciximab (Reopro) |
| | (block platelet adhesion) | Eptifibatide (Integrilin)<br>Tirofiban hydrochloride (Aggrastat) |
| Antithrombin | Unfractionated heparin (binds antithrombin III and rapidly inactivates coagulation enzymes) | Heparin<br>Hirudin (Refludan) |
| | Direct thrombin inhibitors | Agatroban (Novastan) |
| | Low molecular weight heparins | Enoxaparin sodium (Lovenox) |
| | (similar mechanism to unfractionated heparin) | Warfarin (Coumadin) |
| | Coumarins (antagonists of vitamin K which decrease vitamin K dependent clotting factors II, VII, IX, X, and protein C and S) | |
| Thrombolytic | Plasminogen activators (activate plasminogen and hence cause fibrinolysis) | Streptokinase (Streptase)<br>Alteplase (tPA) |

Adapted from Alam and Goldberg [28]

valvular heart disease, history of stroke or myocardial infarction, atrial fibrillation, underlying coagulopathies, and a history of pulmonary embolism and/or deep venous thrombosis (DVT) [9] (V/B). Table 11.1 summarizes the currently utilized anti-platelet and anti-thrombotic agents, with brief explanations of their mechanisms of action [9]. It is important to note that the various anticoagulants act at different levels in the process of coagulation and are therefore theoretically predicted to result in problems at different times in the peri-operative period. Antiplatelet agents such as aspirin interfere with primary hemostasis: platelet aggregation and activation at the site of blood vessel injury. These agents are therefore predicted to cause more difficulty in the initiation of hemostasis intraoperatively. This is distinct from that which might be expected from warfarin which interferes with secondary hemostasis; the enzymatic activity of coagulation factors that leads to the formation of a fibrin clot. These agents might therefore be expected to cause more problems postoperatively since they handicap the terminal portion of the coagulation process.

The decision of whether or not to discontinue anticoagulant therapy in patients with significant thromboembolic risk has been subject to significant study and debate in dermatologic surgery and other fields. The deliberations center around balancing the possible increased risk of bleeding and hemorrhage with the low, but potentially life-threatening, risk of a thrombotic event if anticoagulant therapy is temporarily discontinued. The vast majority of published literature involves the use of warfarin and aspirin. The effects of peri-operative discontinuation of other blood thinning agents are not well studied.

In order to provide guidelines regarding anticoagulant use in dermatologic surgery, several factors need to be taken into consideration:

- What is the overall rate of hemorrhagic complications in dermatologic surgery?
- Is the risk of hemorrhagic complications in patients taking blood thinning agents higher than this overall risk?
- Does temporary peri-operative discontinuation of blood thinning agents significantly decrease the risk of hemorrhagic complications?
- Are there objectively measurable adverse operative effects of warfarin and aspirin?
- What is the risk of thromboembolic events following temporary peri-operative discontinuation of blood thinning agents?
- What is the relative magnitude of bleeding vs. thrombotic complications?

**Table 11.2** Summary of studies examining the incidence of dermatologic surgical complications in patients on blood thinners

| Drug and study | No. of patients | Controlled study | Increased severe complications[a] | Evidence level |
|---|---|---|---|---|
| *Aspirin and NSAIDs* | | | | |
| Otley et al. [11] | 286 | Yes, retrospective | No | IV/B |
| Billingsley and Maloney [12] | 97 | Yes, prospective | No | III/B |
| Lawrence et al. [24] | 61 | Yes, prospective | No | IV/B |
| Bartlett [19] | 52 | Yes, prospective | No | V/B |
| Shalom and Wong [18] | 41 | Yes, prospective | No | III/B |
| Kargi et al. [20] | 37 | Yes, prospective | No | III/B |
| *Warfarin/multiple agents* | | | | |
| Otley et al. [11] | 26 | Yes, retrospective | No | IV/B |
| Billingsley and Maloney [12] | 12 | Yes, prospective | No | III/B |
| Lam et al. [15] | 13 | Yes | No | IV/B |
| Alcalay and Alkalay [13] and Alcalay [14] | 16 | Yes, prospective | No | III/B, V/B |
| Kargi et al. [20] | 21 | Yes, prospective | Yes | III/B |
| Syed et al. [16] | 47 | Yes, prospective | No | IV/B |
| Lewis and DuFresne [21] | 1,373 | Meta-analysis | Yes | IV/B |
| Shimizu et al. [23] | 760 | Yes, retrospective | Yes | III/B |

[a]Excessive bleeding (>1 h despite pressure), hematoma, flap/graft necrosis, wound dehiscence, or infection

As previously mentioned, there is a very low baseline risk of hemorrhagic complications in dermatologic surgery. One prospective study investigating immediate and delayed dermatologic surgery complications demonstrated an overall complication rate of 1.64%. The majority of these complications (postoperative hemorrhage, hematoma formation, flap or graft necrosis, wound dehiscence, and infection) were either directly or indirectly related to problems with hemostasis [10] (IV/B). In this series, none of the patients required hospitalization or the assistance of another specialist. This demonstrated 1.64% rate of complications is comparable to two additional reports estimating 2% rates of significant hemorrhage or hematoma in control patients undergoing dermatologic surgical procedures in the absence of blood thinning agents [11, 12] (III/B). While there are no randomized controlled studies on the subject, the question of continuing or discontinuing anticoagulants lends itself to a study design where rates of hemorrhagic complications are compared between patients who underwent surgery on anticoagulants vs. those who underwent surgery without. While the study of this kind cannot control for the possible contribution of the underlying indication for anticoagulation to a patient's risk of bleeding, the data are relatively consistent across studies and therefore lend themselves to making confident recommendations. Numerous studies have compared the rate of hemorrhagic complications in patients on vs. off of blood thinning agents. A review of these published reports reveals the near unanimous conclusion that there is no increased risk of severe hemorrhagic complications in anticoagulated patients. Furthermore, the literature suggests that perioperative discontinuation of anticoagulants does not decrease the risk of bleeding complications [24]. Several of these studies even focused specifically on Mohs surgical procedures, during which difficulties with hemostasis would have been expected to be tested by increased defect size, extensive undermining, and relatively more complex repair methods. Sufficient data exist to support that blood thinning agents may be safely continued in dermatologic surgery without exposing the patient to a significant increase in risk for bleeding complications (see Table 11.2).

The largest prospective study regarding anticoagulant use in dermatologic surgery was published by Billingsley and Maloney [12]. The authors reported no significant increase in severe adverse events in Mohs micrographic surgery patients on blood thinning agents (12 patients on warfarin and 97 on either aspirin or NSAID) compared with controls. There was also no significant difference between these groups in the complexity of repair performed. Thirty-three percent of the aspirin/NSAID group and 8% in the warfarin group underwent flaps or grafts, compared with 34% in the control group. The only statistically significant finding noted was that 5/12 (42%) of warfarin patients had "excessive intra-operative bleeding," defined as excessive if the time required to achieve hemostasis at the time of closure was greater than 3 min [12].

Otley et al. published a large retrospective study of warfarin, aspirin, and NSAID use in cutaneous surgery patients [11]. In this study, incidence of severe complications was reported for 653 patients undergoing Mohs surgical and excisional surgical procedures. Severe complications were defined as significant intraoperative or postoperative hemorrhage, wound bleeding greater than 1 h and not stopped with pressure, acute hematoma, necrosis of flap or graft, or dehiscence greater than 2 mm. Of the 26 patients who continued warfarin, one experienced a severe complication compared with one severe event in the 101 patients in whom warfarin was held. Similarly, four severe events were reported in the 286 patients continuing aspirin or NSAID compared to three out of the 240 patients who discontinued these medications peri-operatively. Based on these results, Otley et al. concluded that continuation of warfarin or platelet inhibitors is associated with a very low risk of severe complications, and that the rate of complications is not statistically significantly increased compared to patients in whom the same medications are discontinued. It is worth noting that only 54 (8%) of the 653 patients underwent flap or graft repairs, with 2 out of the 5 severe events in patients on warfarin or blood thinners occurring in these more complex repairs [11].

Other smaller prospective studies have also supported the safety of blood thinning agents in cutaneous surgical procedures. Alcalay and Alkalay reported no significant adverse events in 68 consecutive patients undergoing Mohs micrographic surgery while on warfarin [13, 14] (IV/B).

Similarly, Lam et al. found no difference in adverse events in a small group of dermatologic surgery patients continuing warfarin therapy during the procedure as compared to those patients who had their warfarin stopped and were treated with peri-operative heparin [15] (IV/B). The most recently published study addressing warfarin alone was by Syed et al. [16] (IV/B). Syed et al. published a prospective study of 47 patients on warfarin undergoing cutaneous surgery. In this report, nine patients experienced minor bleeding without any major adverse events, three of whom had an intra-operative international normalized ratio (INR) of 3.5 or greater. Of note, only 5 out of 47 patients had intra-operative INRs of 3.5 or greater, with 60% of those experiencing the minor bleeding episodes [16] (IV/B). This was the first study to directly address INR values and attempt to correlate with bleeding complications in cutaneous surgery patients taking warfarin. A more recent study has prospectively addressed the potential correlation between INR values and bleeding complications in patients undergoing excisional surgery while anticoagulated on warfarin. While very few patients were noted to have INR values greater than 3, no correlation was found between increased INR value and intraoperative or postoperative bleeding [17] (III/B). One can conclude that peri-operative INRs may only serve to identify the small subset of patients with supratherapeutic values who may be at particular risk for bleeding complications, postoperative, or otherwise.

Shalom and Wong recently reported a statistically increased incidence of intra-operative suture ligation for hemostasis in 41 patients on aspirin compared with 212 controls undergoing excisions of cutaneous and subcutaneous lesions [18] (V/B). However, the authors did not find any increased risk of significant bleeding events in those patients taking aspirin. Finally, Barlett reported no increased incidence of minor, severe, or overall bleeding complications in 52 patients undergoing minor dermatologic surgery while on aspirin compared with 119 patients who were not taking aspirin [19] (III/B). Only one group has published data suggesting significantly increased major bleeding complications in patient undergoing minor cutaneous surgery while on warfarin [20] (IV/B). Of 21 patients on warfarin, 5 (24%) experienced a major bleeding complication, which was defined as persistent bleeding, wound hematoma, loss of skin graft, or wound infection. This number was significantly higher than that in the 37 patients on aspirin and the 44 controls. This study did not report on INR values or monitoring in the warfarin-treated patients. No significant difference between the aspirin and control groups with regard to bleeding complications was observed [20].

A recent meta-analysis increases the power of many of the aforementioned small studies [21] (I/A). Somewhat surprisingly, there was a statistically significant increase in bleeding complications for patients taking warfarin vs. controls. A similar but much less robust trend was observed for patients taking aspirin; however, this distinction failed to meet statistical significance. The reliability of this meta-analysis is somewhat compromised by virtue of summing data from several small heterogeneous studies. It is also important to note that additional medical comorbidities were not controlled for in any of the aforementioned anticoagulation studies. It is likely true that anticoagulated patients tend to be older and have greater number and severity of medical problems. If the risk of bleeding complications is somewhat higher in anticoagulated patients, the question of acceptable risk persists. As pointed out by Alcalay, the observed complications have never been reported as life-threatening, while there are numerous reported cases of life-threatening complications potentially attributable to the discontinuation of anticoagulants perioperatively [13] (V/B).

While multiple studies in the dermatologic surgery literature have addressed NSAID, aspirin, and warfarin use, there are currently no published reports addressing bleeding complications in patient on clopidogrel (Plavix®, Bristol-Myers Squibb) as a single agent. Clopidogrel is a selective inhibitor of platelet adhesion to fibrinogen and aggregation via inhibition of ADP-induced platelet activation. Its use continues to increase as a component of secondary prevention among cardiac and cerebrovascular patients, and it is

often used in combination with aspirin. The only published study regarding clopidogrel and bleeding complications is in the pulmonary literature. A 2006 prospective cohort report found that clopidogrel significantly increased the bleeding risk in patients undergoing transbronchial biopsy, with the effect exacerbated by concomitant aspirin use [22] (III/B). As this agent continues to be utilized in more patients, studies regarding its effects on dermatologic surgery complications will be beneficial.

An increasingly relevant subject for which there is little published has to do with patients on multiple anticoagulants. There are many frequent combinations of both prescription and nonprescription agents that may or may not act synergistically in terms of enhancing risk of bleeding, especially when there are agents interfering with both primary and secondary hemostases as described above. This subject is difficult to study since the number of patients on any particular combination is much less than the total number of dermatologic surgery patients on any one particular agent. Nonetheless one recent report addresses the subject retrospectively through a chart review [23] (V/B). There were no significant bleeding complications in 227 patients undergoing Mohs surgery on one anticoagulant (ASA, warfarin, clopidogrel, dipyridamol/ASA, vitamin E, or fish oil). There were three cases of significant bleeding in 58 total patients on two or more agents. While the authors did show statistical significance for these findings, they are somewhat limited by the very low number of adverse events. Furthermore, none of the patients exhibited any significant morbidity associated with their bleeding complications. This is consistent with the absence in the literature of any life-threatening or lethal bleeding complications after cutaneous surgery. The subject deserves more study with larger numbers to better quantify the increased risk potentially associated with multiple agents. Regardless, it seems difficult to justify modifying a patient's multiple anticoagulant regimen on the basis of this study alone.

Despite the belief by many surgeons that they can predict anticoagulant or blood thinner status intra-operatively, a recent dermatologic surgery study demonstrated that physicians at all levels of training were equally unable to assess blood thinner status based on visual inspection of intra-operative oozing [25] (V/B). This is similar to findings reported in coronary artery bypass patients, in which surgeons' impressions of aspirin status were unreliable [26] (II/A).

There are now documented reports of serious thromboembolic events occurring in patients who discontinued warfarin or aspirin therapy for dermatologic surgery.

Kovich recently reported data from a survey of 504 members of the American College of Mohs Micrographic Surgery and Cutaneous Oncology [27] (VI/C). One hundred and sixty-eight respondents reported 46 patients who experienced thrombotic events. These were all serious events and included 24 strokes, three cerebral emboli, five myocardial infarctions, eight transient ischemic attacks, three deep venous thromboses, two pulmonary emboli, one retinal artery occlusion leading to blindness. Three deaths were reported. Of the 46 patients who experienced thrombotic events, 54% had an event when warfarin was held, 39% occurred when aspirin was held, and 4% of events happened when both medications were held [27]. There are other documented case reports in the dermatologic surgery literature of stroke, pulmonary embolus, and clotted prosthetic valve occurring in patients in whom anticoagulation or antiplatelet medications were discontinued peri-operatively [28, 29] (V/B). A review in the New England Journal of Medicine highlights the potential gravity of thromboembolic complications. A patient who experiences a recurrent episode of venous thromboembolism has a 6% mortality risk, and 2% risk for serious permanent disability. Arterial thromboembolism morbidity and mortality rates are higher, with 20% of events being fatal and 40% resulting in serious permanent disability [30] (I/A). The risk of these grave complications varies somewhat depending upon the circumstance and indication for anticoagulation. Patients with older mechanical cardiac valves or a mechanical mitral valve are at higher risk than those with newer or aortic mechanical valves. Patients with DVT are at much greater risk if the DVT was diagnosed

within 1 month of the peri-operative period. In addition, patients with stable, lone atrial fibrillation who have no history of stroke or other risk factor for stroke are at much lower risk than those atrial fibrillation patients who do have such a history [31] (V/B).

For two of the common indications for warfarin (atrial fibrillation and artificial heart valve replacement), the estimated risks of thromboembolism are 1–20% per year and 8–22% per year, respectively [31] (IV/B). For the third most common indication, DVT, the estimated clotting risk is 1% per day for patients who have had a DVT within 1 month, and 0.2 and 0.04% for patients with DVTs within 2–3 months and over 3 months, respectively. Using these numbers, the estimated 2-day risk of a thrombotic event in a patient taken off warfarin for a dermatologic procedure is 0.01–0.3% in the setting of atrial fibrillation and 0.08–0.4% for a patient with an artificial heart valve replacement. For DVT patients, the 2-day risk is 4–6% in those less than 1 month after a DVT, 0.8–1.2% in those 2–3 months after DVT, and 0.16–0.24% in those more than 3 months after DVT [31].

These data lend themselves to the clinical recommendations summarized below with their accompanying evidence levels. While it is generally clear that patients should be maintained on anticoagulants for secondary prevention, some cases inevitably merit further discussion. It is important to remember that these guidelines have not necessarily been adopted by other surgical fields who often extrapolate data from more invasive surgeries in considering the risk of continuing an anticoagulant during surgery. Therefore communication with our colleagues in the other surgical disciplines is critical if, for example, the dermatologic surgeon anticipates referral to a plastic or head and neck surgeon for repair of a Mohs surgery defect in an anticoagulated patient. Our consulting colleagues may wish to hold anticoagulants for large defects, defects involving the scalp or eyelids or any reconstruction that is expected to require extensive and/or deep undermining. Though the data in the dermatologic surgery literature is quite clear, it is important to remember that the decision to withhold anticoagulants preoperatively depends upon numerous clinical factors and assessment of risk must be conducted on a case-by-case basis. This decision depends not only upon a critical appraisal of the relevant literature but also on the clinical acumen of the surgeon performing the procedure. Furthermore, while it seems common to consult with a patient's cardiologist or primary care physician regarding peri-operative anticoagulants, the value of this practice is limited by these physicians' lack of familiarity with the above reviewed literature and dermatologic surgery procedures in general.

Cutaneous surgery is performed commonly on patients taking medically necessary blood thinning medications such as warfarin and aspirin. Available data suggests that the risk of severe hemorrhagic complications is not increased if these medications are continued. Importantly, brief peri-operative discontinuation does NOT lower this already minimal hemorrhagic risk. Life-threatening thromboembolic complications have been related temporally to peri-operative discontinuation of both warfarin and aspirin. In general, the risks of stopping anticoagulants far outweigh the risks of continuing them for most dermatologic surgery procedures. As the use of these agents increases, the onus is on the dermatologic surgeon to help prevent bleeding complications through careful preoperative assessment, meticulous intraoperative hemostasis, effective use of pressure dressings, and excellent postoperative care and follow-up.

## Evidence-Based Summary

| Recommendations regarding peri-operative use of blood thinning agents | Evidence level |
|---|---|
| All vitamin supplements and herbal medications should be discontinued 7–10 days preoperatively, and resumed 1 week following surgery. For practical purposes, and since many supplements and over-the-counter vitamins can affect bleeding, we do not distinguish between various agents with regard to recommending patient discontinuation | IV/C |
| Nonsteroidal anti-inflammatory medications (NSAIDs) should be stopped 3 days prior to surgery, with recommended resumption 1 week following the procedure. Because of their reversible effect on platelet aggregation via cyclooxygenase inhibition and the relatively short drug half-life, 3 days of preoperative discontinuation is sufficient for resumption of platelet function, and we find that most patients can tolerate being off NSAIDs for that period of time | V/B |
| Primary preventative aspirin, which irreversibly inhibits platelet function, should be discontinued 10–14 days prior to surgery, and re-started 1 week after the procedure | III/B |
| Medically necessary warfarin and aspirin should be continued, with an INR value recommended within at least 1 week of surgery. Care must be taken to assess in the preoperative history whether or not the warfarin doses and INR measurements are stable. In addition, a careful medication history assessing for new medication additions that may affect warfarin levels is crucial | I/A |
| We currently recommend that patients continue clopidogrel in the peri-operative period, although further studies regarding this medication and complications are warranted | III/B |

# References

1. Cook JL, Perone JB. A prospective evaluation of the incidence of complications associated with Mohs micrographic surgery. Arch Dermatol. 2003;139: 143–52.
2. Guldbakke KK, Schanbacher CF. Disseminated intravascular coagulation unmasked by Mohs micrographic surgery. Dermatol Surg. 2006;32:760–4.
3. Peterson SR, Joseph AK. Inherited bleeding disorders in dermatologic surgery. Dermatol Surg. 2001;27: 885–9.
4. Wolfort FG, Pan D, Gee J. Alcohol and preoperative management. Plast Reconstr Surg. 1996;98(7): 1306–9.
5. Tsen LC, Segal S, Pothier M, et al. Alternative medicine use in presurgical patients. Anesthesiology. 2000;35:226–7.
6. Barraco D, Valencia G, Riba AL, et al. Complementary and alternative medicine (CAM) use patterns and disclosure to physicians in acute coronary syndromes patients. Complement Ther Med. 2005;13:34–40.
7. Valencia Orgaz O, Orts Castro A, Castells Armenter MV, et al. Assessing preoperative use of medicinal plants during preanesthetic interviews. Rev Esp Anesthesiol Reanim. 2005;52:453–8.
8. Dinehart SM, Henry L. Dietary supplements: altered coagulation and effects on bruising. Dermatol Surg. 2005;31:819–26.
9. Schanbacher CF. Anticoagulants and blood thinners during cutaneous surgery: always, sometimes or never? Skin Therapy Lett. 2004;9:5–8.
10. Goldsmith SM, Leshin B, Owen J. Management of patients taking anticoagulants and platelet inhibitors prior to dermatologic surgery. J Dermatol Surg Oncol. 1993;19:578–81.
11. Otley CC, Fewkes JL, Frank W, et al. Complications of cutaneous surgery in patients who are taking warfarin, aspirin, or nonsteroidal anti-inflammatory drugs. Arch Dermatol. 1996;132:161–6.
12. Billingsley EM, Maloney ME. Intraoperative and postoperative bleeding problems in patients taking warfarin, aspirin, and nonsteroidal anti-inflammatory agents. Dermatol Surg. 1997;23:381–5.
13. Alcalay J, Alkalay R. Controversies in perioperative management of blood thinners in dermatologic surgery: continue or discontinue? Dermatol Surg. 2004;30:1091–4.
14. Alcalay J. Cutaneous surgery in patients receiving warfarin therapy. Dermatol Surg. 2001;27:756–8.
15. Lam J, Lim J, Clark J, et al. Warfarin and cutaneous surgery: a preliminary prospective study. Br J Plast Surg. 2001;52:372–3.
16. Syed S, Adams BB, Liao W, et al. A prospective assessment of bleeding and international normalized ratio in warfarin-anticoagulated patients having cutaneous surgery. J Am Acad Dermatol. 2004;51:955–7.
17. Blasdale C, Lawrence CM. Perioperative international normalized ratio level is a poor predictor of postoperative bleeding complications in dermatological surgery patients taking warfarin. Br J Dermatol. 2008;158:522–6.
18. Shalom A, Wong L. Outcome of aspirin use during excision of cutaneous lesions. Ann Plast Surg. 2003;50:296–8.
19. Bartlett GR. Does aspirin affect the outcome of minor cutaneous surgery? Br J Plast Surg. 1999;52:214–6.
20. Kargi E, Babuccu O, Hosnuter M, et al. Complications of minor cutaneous surgery in patients under anticoagulant treatment. Aesthetic Plast Surg. 2002;26: 483–5.
21. Lewis KL, DuFresne RG. Meta-analysis of complications attributed to anticoagulation among patients following cutaneous surgery. Dermatol Surg. 2008;34: 160–5.
22. Ernst A, Eberhardt R, Wahidi M, et al. Effect of routine clopidogrel use on bleeding complications after transbronchial biopsy in humans. Chest. 2006;129: 734–7.
23. Shimizu I, Jellinek N, Dufresne D, et al. Multiple antithrombotic agents increase the risk of postoperative hemorrhage in dermatologic surgery. J Am Acad Dermatol. 2008;58:810–6.
24. Lawrence C, Sakuntabhai A, Tiling-Grosse S. Effect of aspirin and nonsteroidal anti-inflammatory drug therapy on bleeding complications in dermatologic surgical patients. J Am Acad Dermatol. 1994;31: 988–92.
25. West SW, Otely CC, Nguyen TH, et al. Cutaneous surgeons cannot predict blood-thinner status by intraoperative visual inspection. Plast Reconstr Surg. 2002;110:98–103.
26. Kallis P, Tooze JA, Talbot S, et al. Pre-operative aspirin decreases platelet aggregation and increases postoperative blood loss: a prospective, randomized, placebo controlled, double-blind clinical trial in 100 patients with chronic stable angina. Eur J Cardiothorac Surg. 1994;8:404–9.
27. Kovich O, Oltey CC. Thrombotic complications related to discontinuation of warfarin and aspirin therapy perioperatively for cutaneous operation. J Am Acad Dermatol. 2003;48:233–7.
28. Alam M, Goldberg LH. Serious adverse vascular events associated with perioperative interruption of antiplatelet and anticoagulant therapy. Dermatol Surg. 2002;28:992–8.
29. Schanbacher CF, Bennett RG. Postoperative stroke after stopping warfarin for cutaneous surgery. Dermatol Surg. 2000;26:785–9.
30. Kearon C, Hirsh J. Management of anticoagulation before and after elective surgery. N Engl J Med. 1997;336:1506–11.
31. Spandorfer J. The management of anticoagulation before and after procedures. Med Clin North Am. 2001;85:1109–16.

## Self-Assessment

1. Clopidogrel is an anticoagulant that acts in inhibiting secondary hemostasis
   True or False

2. Cessation of anticoagulants prior to dermatologic surgery has resulted in severe thromboembolic complications
   True or False

3. In most studies there does not appear to be an increased rate of hemorrhagic complications in anti-coagulated patients undergoing cutaneous surgery
   True or False

4. Dermatologic surgeons are generally able to predict whether a patient is anticoagulated or not based on intraoperative bleeding.
   True or False

5. The overall rate of complications associated with Mohs surgery is approximately:
   0.16%, 1.6%, 4.8%, 16%

## Answers

1. False
2. True
3. True
4. False
5. 1.6%

# Vascular Lasers and Lights

## Nicole E. Rogers and Marc R. Avram

## Introduction

Vascular lasers and lights have evolved considerably over the last 30 years since Anderson and Parrish published their landmark paper on selective photothermolysis [1]. Previously, continuous wave (argon and copper vapor) lasers were used to treat vascular lesions, but resulted in significant side effects such as scarring or pigmentary changes. With the understanding that laser energy can be modified for preferential absorption by the intended target, or chromophore, heat could be delivered in a more controlled manner that did not result in destruction of surrounding tissues. The laser wavelength could be matched to the absorption spectra of the targeted chromophore. By the 1990s, the pulsed dye laser (PDL) was established as the gold standard for vascular lesions [2]. Its wavelengths of 577–595 nm match the spectrum for oxyhemoglobin, which is in blood vessels. Figure 12.1 demonstrates the absorption spectra of hemoglobin. The 532 nm wavelength has also been explored for its strong absorption by hemoglobin.

N.E. Rogers (✉)
Department of Dermatology, Tulane University School of Medicine, Old Metairie Dermatology, 701 Metairie Road, Suite 2A-205, Metairie, LA, USA
e-mail: nicolerogers11@gmail.com

M.R. Avram
Department of Dermatology,
New York Presbyterian Hospital,
Weill Cornell Medical College, New York, NY, USA

Using the PDL, longer wavelengths can be used to target deeper structures. Likewise, longer pulse durations are used to sufficiently heat larger vessels. This is based on the principle of thermal relaxation time (TRT). The pulse duration (also called pulse width) should approximate the vessel TRT, defined as the time required for the affected tissue to lose half the heat it gained from the laser. The TRT of a vessel is proportional to the square of its diameter. Pulses which are too short will result in insufficient heating of the vessel, and pulses which are too long can result in excess heat diffusion, which can adversely affect surrounding structures.

## Childhood Hemangiomas and Port-Wine Stains

The earliest application of these lasers has been in the treatment of childhood hemangiomas and port-wine stains (PWS). Both conditions can result in serious psychological effects for the affected child and should be treated as soon as possible. Although hemangiomas of infancy can often involute, PWS continue to grow in thickness and usually darken in color. In this chapter, we focus on the evidence supporting the use of different lasers (and parameters) to treat simple, refractory, and hypertrophic vascular anomalies. A discussion of the use of lasers in treating leg veins will also be included.

While the 1990s saw a shift from argon and copper based technologies to the PDL, the first

M. Alam (ed.), *Evidence-Based Procedural Dermatology*,
DOI 10.1007/978-0-387-09424-3_12, © Springer Science+Business Media, LLC 2012

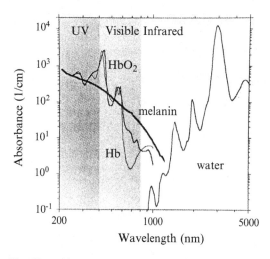

**Fig. 12.1** Absorption spectra of hemoglobin

**Table 12.1** Vascular wavelengths

| 532 nm | KTP |
|---|---|
| 532 nm | Nd:YAG, frequency doubled |
| 577–585 nm | Conventional PDL with pulse duration = 0.45 ms |
| 595 nm | Long-pulsed dye laser, pulse duration = 1.5 ms |
| 500–1,200 nm | Noncoherent intense pulsed light (IPL) |
| 755 nm | Alexandrite |
| 800, 810 nm | Diode |
| 1,064 nm | Long-pulsed Nd:Yag |

decade of the twenty-first century showed an exploration of second-generation PDLs with slightly longer wavelengths, higher fluence, and longer pulse duration, in order to treat recalcitrant PWS and hemangiomas. The use of cryogen spray and contact cooling not only increases patient comfort but also protects the epidermis from thermal injury as the laser penetrates the skin. Other modalities such as intense pulsed light (IPL) sources, long pulsed alexandrite, and infrared lasers have been tried for refractory lesions, these and other vascular lasers have been developed to comprise a broad range of wavelengths (Table 12.1). The use of lasers in darker skin types has also been investigated. Newer techniques have involved combining injectable photosensitizers with PDL to create photodynamic therapy (PDT) for vascular lesions. Topical agents like imiquimod and rapamycin have also been investigated. The following studies will

summarize our present knowledge and practices for each of these modalities.

## Consensus Documents and Guidelines

A limited Medline search was conducted using the following terms: (vascular) laser, PWS, hemangioma, and leg vein. Two recent sets of guidelines were identified. Most of these documents include protocols for diagnosis and imaging as well as treatment. For the sake of limiting this discussion to vascular lasers, we will focus on their recommendations for laser treatments specifically.

The European Society for Laser Dermatology published guidelines for care using vascular lasers and IPL sources in 2007 [3]. These guidelines were assembled by members of the dermatology departments in Sweden, Switzerland, Germany, and Slovenia. They begin by stressing the importance of properly diagnosing vascular lesions, emphasizing that arterial malformations should never be treated with laser or IPL. Careful attention should be paid to the lesion being treated, the skin type, and the anatomic location so that the correct parameters are chosen. Test treatments are advised. Their treatment principles include the following: (1) smaller vessels need shorter pulses; larger vessels need longer pulses; (2) the deeper the blood vessel is located in the dermis, the larger the spot size, the longer the wavelength, and the longer the pulse duration should be, combined with cooling to protect the epidermis; and (3) darker skin types need longer pulses and longer pulse intervals.

The authors provide guidelines for treating a variety of congenital and acquired vascular lesions. Most benefit from treatments every 4–6 weeks and patients should avoid sun exposure prior to and after laser treatment. Areas prone to scarring, such as the anterior chest or neck, or where skin is fragile such as periorbita should be treated with a 10–20% reduction in fluence. Table 12.2 outlines the laser recommendations for a variety of different conditions, including conditions such as telangiectasias, rosacea, venous lakes, leg veins, PWS, and hemangiomas of infancy.

**Table 12.2**  Guidelines for care from the European Society for Laser Dermatology (2007)

| Vascular lesion | Recommended laser | Notes |
|---|---|---|
| Facial telangiectasias | First choice: FPDL, KTP (532), IPL<br>Second choice: APDL, argon,<br>copper vapor (with great care) | Contact cooling or topical anesthetic<br>recommended |
| Rosacea | First choice: FPDL, KTP (532), IPL<br>Second choice: APDL, argon,<br>copper vapor (with great care) | The erythema (first stage of rosacea)<br>can only be treated with FPDL, KTP,<br>or IPL |
| Hemangiomas<br>of infancy | First choice: FPDL, IPL, Nd:Yag, KTP | Patients older than a year can be<br>treated with topical anesthetic<br>or nerve blocks |
| Port wine stain (PWS) | First choice: FPDL, IPLS, Nd:Yag, KTP<br>(large spot) | |
| Spider angiomas | First choice: KTP, FPDL, IPLS, Nd:Yag<br>Second choice: argon, copper vapor | Occurs in 15% of normal individuals.<br>More common in children, pregnancy,<br>liver dz |
| Poikiloderma of civatte | First choice: FPDL, IPL<br>Second choice: KTP (caution to avoid<br>scarring depending on area) | Reduce the fluence when treating<br>scar-prone areas such as chest<br>and neck, with larger spot sizes |
| Venous lakes | First choice: KTP, Nd:Yag, FPDL, IPL | Dilated venules without the<br>proliferation of vascular tissue |
| Cherry angioma | First choice: KTP, Nd:Yag, IPL, FPDL | Disappear in extreme old age |
| Leg veins and<br>telangiectasias | First choice: Nd:Yag (1,064)<br>Second choice: for small diameter<br>(<1 mm) can use KTP, FPDL<br>(long pulse), IPL<br>Second choice: for large diameter can<br>also use Nd:Yag, alexandrite, diode, IPL | Overall, lasers are second choice after<br>sclerotherapy |

For hemangiomas of infancy, which can have long-lasting psychosocial effects, they recommend treating all hemangiomas with laser as early as possible (Fig. 12.2a, b). This helps prevent the proliferative phase and its associated complications such as ulceration, bleeding, or infection. The authors remind readers that laser treatment will only affect the superficial component of the hemangioma and that it is often difficult predicting whether there will be a deep component.

PWS are vascular malformations which continue to increase in size throughout life. Unlike hemangiomas, they do not involute. Some remain as pale, erythematous macules, or patches while others grow rapidly during adolescence. The authors recommend starting laser treatment as soon as the PWS turns darker or thicker. This is because smaller PWS (less than 20 cm²) clear better than larger ones, irrespective of age. However, pink PWS, especially in children, are more difficult to lighten than mature red PWS. Thus clinical experience must be used to establish starting time. Deep purple and nodular PWS

respond least well to laser treatment; longer wavelengths (755, 800–900, and 1,064 nm) are more suitable. Other guidelines mention that PWS on the distal extremities are more difficult to clear than on proximal extremities, centrofacial lesions (and those in the V2 distribution) are less responsive to laser therapy than PWS located more laterally on the face, and PWS on the head and neck respond better to laser treatment than lesions elsewhere on the body (Fig. 12.3a, b).

For treatment of leg veins, lasers are less successful due to increased hydrostatic pressure, thicker surrounding adventitial tissue, greater depth in the dermis, and more energy required to target vessels (with greater resultant damage to overlying epidermis). Because of the need for longer wavelength, the neodymium:yttrium-aluminum-garnet (Nd:Yag) (1,064 nm) has emerged as the laser of choice for leg veins. The authors recommend that lasers be considered prior to sclerotherapy only in patients with needle phobia, who fail or do not tolerate sclerotherapy, or who are prone to telangiectatic matting. Fair skinned individuals whose

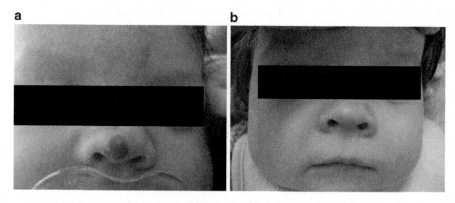

**Fig. 12.2** (**a**) Hemangioma of infancy on the nose, prior to treatment, (**b**) same lesion 4 months later after three treatments of 595 nm PDL (courtesy of Jeffrey Poole, MD)

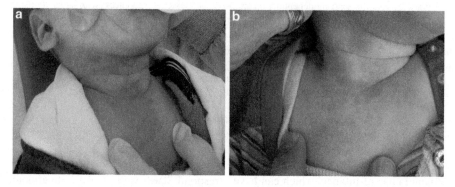

**Fig. 12.3** (**a**) Port wine stain (capillary malformation) of the chest, before treatment with PDL, (**b**) same lesion following treatment with 595 nm PDL (courtesy of Jeffrey Poole, MD)

feet and ankles have numerous vessels <2 mm may also be treated with laser.

Another set of guidelines was published in 2008 by the German Society of Dermatology together with the German Societies for Pediatric Surgery and Pediatric Medicine [4]. This focused specifically on the treatment for hemangiomas of infancy and childhood, and included recommendations for nonlaser therapies as well. They based their recommendations for treatment on the phase of hemangioma growth. Rapidly proliferating hemangiomas, and especially those located in problematic areas such as near the eye or anogenital region, should be treated promptly. Likewise, lesions which may ulcerate should be treated promptly (Fig. 12.4a, b). However, hemangiomas in the quiescent or regression phase may take a "wait and see" approach.

The authors describe laser therapy as the best approach for flat hemangiomas. Specifically, flashlamp-pumped pulse dye laser (FPDL) or IPL with resultant purpura can help resolve the lesions. Scars are reported to occur in 1% of cases. No specific recommendations for laser settings or treatment intervals are provided. They discuss the Nd:Yag as helpful for greater penetration of subcutaneous hemangiomas. It can be used with topical cooling or intralesionally via quartz fibers. Such treatment may help reduce the volume of very large hemangiomas before a planned surgical procedure. The authors also discuss cryotherapy for flat lesions, stating that the results are comparable to those of laser therapy. Systemic corticosteroids or cytotoxic agents can be used in cases of very rapidly proliferating (Fig. 12.5a–c) or life-threatening hemangiomas.

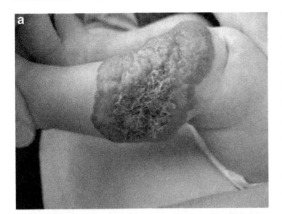

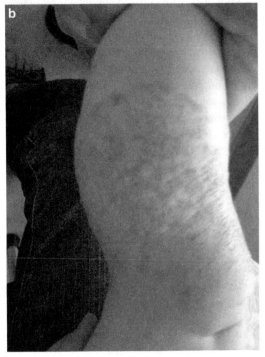

**Fig. 12.4** (**a**) Segmental superficial ulcerating hemangioma of infancy on the leg, tender and painful prior to treatment, (**b**) same lesion 10 months later after six treatments with 595 nm PDL (courtesy of Jeffrey Poole, MD)

Less recent guidelines are available from the American Academy of Dermatology, which were written in 1997 [5]. They recommend the use of FPDLs but urge caution in lasers such as the argon which may result in hypopigmentation or scarring. These guidelines will presumably be updated soon to reflect the enormous advances in laser technology since they were written.

## Case Series and Cohort Studies

Several large studies dating back 10 years have established the role of the FPDL in treating PWS and hemangiomas. A case series of 617 cases of mostly superficial childhood hemangiomas using the 585 nm PDL with 0.45 ms pulse duration reported the cessation of further growth in 96.6% of patients [6]. However, side effects included blister formation, crusts, and pigment changes in 7% of patients as well as 4% with small atrophic scars, likely due to the fact that contact cooling had not yet been introduced. Another study showed that the deeper component of mixed hemangiomas responded less well to the 585 nm, due to the limited penetration of the PDL (0.8–1.0 mm) [7]. The subcutaneous components were recalcitrant to treatment and even continued to proliferate in most cases. The benefits had to be weighed with the side effects of pigmentary and textural changes.

Darker skin types also faced a dilemma in that, their epidermal pigmentation provided a barrier to laser penetration. They risked blister formation or scarring where the laser energy was absorbed. In a 2002 study of 107 Chinese patients who were randomized to treatment with the 585 nm PDL, the 532 nm potassium titanyl phosphate (KTP),

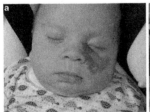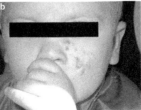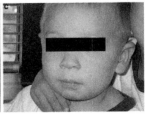

**Fig. 12.5** (**a**) Proliferating superficial hemangioma of infancy, untreated, (**b**) same lesion 10 months later after four treatments of 595 nm PDL, (**c**) proliferating superfi-cial HOI, after 21 months and five treatments of 595 nm PDL (courtesy of Jeffrey Poole, MD)

or both, the authors found that they were less responsive to laser treatment, required more treatments, and had a higher complication rate [8].

Another interesting problem with the lasers was that these deeper, incompletely treated lesions could re-emerge years later. Redarkening of PWS 10 years after PDL treatment was reported in 18 of 51 patients (35%) [9]. They were still lighter than they had been prior to treatment, but darker than after the treatments were finished. Another larger study found that 15 of 110 (13.4%) patients treated with 585 nm laser for PWS found their lesions to re-emerge [10]. These areas reemerged an average of 31.3 months after discontinuing treatment. Spider nevi can also recur, and a 2-year study found that 50 out of 139 patients (36%) questioned 27–51 months after finishing treatment reported a recurrence [11]. The most common time for return was between 6 and 18 months.

The challenge, therefore, was to find ways to reduce side effects, increase penetration, and reduce recurrence of these lesions. These techniques included the introduction of contact cooling, which allowed for higher fluences to be used. Increasing the wavelength allowed for the delivery of energy to the deeper vessels, and increasing the pulse duration allowed for the treatment of larger vessels.

## Contact Cooling

In 2000, Geronemus used a modified PDL with a tetrafluoroethane spray prior to and just after each laser pulse, to treat 16 infants with facial PWS

[12]. In this same group, he increased the pulse duration to 1.5 ms and increased the energy fluence to 11–12 J/cm². Sixty-three percent had a greater than 75% clearing after an average of 4 treatments. Although it was only a pilot study, the multiple modifications made set the stage for investigating many different parameters [12].

Asian patients were found to benefit from the use of cryogen spray cooling, in that their darker skin was protected from the effects of the laser. One prospective, split-area study from 2003 compared the use of the 585 nm PDL alone vs. the 585 nm laser with cryogen spray cooling to treat PWS in 35 Chinese patients [13]. It is found that patients treated with cryogen spray achieved greater clearance, probably because significantly higher fluences could be used. Pain scores were higher and blistering more common in the PDL-alone-treated group. Overall, patients preferred the cryogen spray for its increased comfort and greater clearance.

By 2007, a retrospective report described 49 facial PWS in newborns, which had all improved with the 595 nm wavelength at 1.5 ms and at fluences of 7.75–9.5 J/cm² and the use of cryogen cooling [14]. The clearance for the V1 distribution was highest (93.8%), followed by V2 (91.1%), and V3 (84.3%). No cases of atrophy or scarring resulted and the authors remarked that this was an excellent option for patients 6 months of age or younger (Fig. 12.6a, b). Since then, a 2009 retrospective chart review of 90 patients with 105 hemangiomas reported excellent clearing with the 595 nm long PDL with dynamic epidermal cooling at 2–8 week intervals [15].

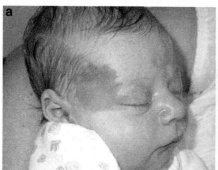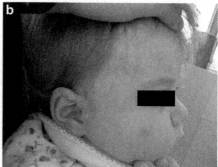

**Fig. 12.6** (a) Port wine stain of the V2 distribution, (b) same lesion following nine treatments with the 595 nm PDL. Lesion was mostly resolved after four treatments (courtesy of Jeffrey Poole, MD)

Near-complete or complete clearance in color
was achieved for 85 (81%) of lesions and in
thickness for 67 (64%) of hemangiomas. No
instances of scarring or atrophy occurred, but
hyper- and hypopigmentation occurred in 4 and
14% of hemangiomas respectively.

## Changing Wavelength

In 2001, a study of 62 patients with untreated
PWS compared the traditional 585 nm, 45 ms
PDL with a longer-tunable dye laser (585–
600 nm) which demonstrated just as optimal fading and no side effects so long as the epidermis
was additionally cooled with a spray cooling
device [16].

The use of the 595 nm wavelengths in darker
skin types has also proven to be helpful. A 2006
case series of 239 Korean patients (Fitzpatrick
skin types III–V) were treated with the 595 nm
PDL, 1.5 ms pulse duration for nevus flammeus,
telangiectasias, or hemangiomas [17]. Over half
(51.9%) of the patients had either good (51–75%)
or excellent (76–100%) clearance. As with the
Caucasian populations, lesions on the head and
neck responded more favorably, and superficial
hemangiomas showed a better clinical response
than deep hemangiomas. Hyper- and hypopigmentation was noted in 10 (27.2%) and 2 (5.4%)
of patients. Another study published the same
year showed that of 66 Japanese patients treated
with the 595 nm for PWS, 67% had a good or
excellent response [18].

Prior to this, the KTP 532 nm laser was used
to treat vascular lesions. A Polish case series published in 2005 found that 81% of 155 patients had
fair (23%), good (27%), or excellent (31%)
improvement [19]. There were no reports of scarring or persistent pigmentary changes in the epidermis. The laser worked best on lesions localized
to the face and neck; lesions on the trunk and
extremities were quite resistant. A prospective
cohort of 30 patients in the UK treated for PDL-
resistant PWS found that 16 patients (53%) had a
>25% response and 5 patients (17%) had a >50%
response [20]. Patients preferred the KTP, citing
less discomfort and minimal purpura. Six patients
had side effects, including scarring in 2 (7%),

hyperpigmentation in 3 (10%) and prolonged
healing phase over 4 weeks in 1 (3%).

The frequency doubled Nd:YAG 532 nm laser
was also investigated for treatment of vascular
lesions. A Turkish case series of 89 patients
treated for PWS found that results were excellent
(>95% improvement) for 13% of patients, good
(75–94% improvement) in 38% of patients, moderate (50–74% improvement) in 44% of patients,
and mild (25–50% improvement) in 5% [21].
Side effects included hyperpigmentation in two
patients (2.25%), hypopigmentation in one patient
(1.12%) and atrophic scarring in one patient
(1.12%). When the frequency doubled Nd:YAG
(532 nm) laser was compared with the 585 nm
laser in a retrospective trial of 50 infants with 62
superficial hemangiomas, a cessation of growth
was achieved in 93 and 70% of the PDL and
Nd:YAG treated lesions, respectively [22].
Complete regression was seen in 41% of the PDL
treated lesions and 30% of Nd:YAG treated
lesions. Because the PDL was more effective, the
authors concluded that PDL was still the preferred therapy for hemangiomas.

The frequency-doubled Nd:YAG 532 nm laser
was tried in the treatment of PWS in Chinese
patients, but a retrospective review of the 22
treated patients demonstrated just 33% of patients
with more than 50% clearing and 62% of patients
with more than 25% clearing [23]. Pigmentary
and texture changes were noted in 11–33% of
patients, and very high fluences were required to
achieve clearing. The authors concluded that
Nd:YAG was only partially effective for the treatment of PWS in Chinese patients and that, while
contact cooling helps protect the epidermis, textural changes could still occur.

## Increased Fluence

A prospective case series reported using a high-
energy device that delivered 9.5 J/cm$^2$ at 595 nm
with a 1.5 ms pulse duration and 10 mm circular
spot [24]. Twenty patients with PWS who had
become refractory to the conventional 585 nm
laser were included in the study and had an average
improvement of 76% following an average of 3.1
treatments.

The tradeoff with increased fluence is the appearance of greater purpura postoperatively. This appearance of bruising can limit patient acceptance but has been shown to increase clearing. A prospective, randomized controlled trial of 11 patients with facial telangiectasias demonstrated a greater improvement in areas treated 0.5 J/cm$^2$ above the purpura threshold than patients treated 1 J/cm$^2$ less than the threshold [25].

Another suggestion has been the use of pulse stacking (repetitive treatments at a lower fluence) to improve results without causing the same degree of purpura. In a randomized study, 25 patients underwent a single 595 nm pulse on one cheek and 3–4 pulses on the opposite cheek [26]. Both sides used the sub-purpuric fluence of 7.5 J/cm$^2$ and greater clearance was noticed on the pulse-stacked side. This remains an option for patients who do not want to have postoperative purpura. One case of edema was noted in the pulse-stacked group.

## Increased Pulse Duration

In 2005, a longer pulse duration of 1.5 ms was also found to increase the efficacy of the 585 nm laser for treating PWS, in a study of 95 patients with 104 areas of involvement by PWS. Twenty-one of these patients had failed previous treatment using a conventional 0.45 ms device, but showed improvement with the longer pulse duration [27]. A comparative study of 18 patients, examining the use of the 595 nm laser with the 585 nm lasers at the same pulse duration of 1.5 ms demonstrated little difference between the two settings, and found that the use of even longer pulse durations (6 ms) yielded no significant advantage [28].

Another prospective study compared the use of two wavelengths (585 and 595 nm) as well as two pulse durations (0.5 and 20 ms) in 15 patients with PWS [29]. They found that increasing the pulse duration all the way to 20 ms with the 595 nm laser (and increasing the fluence to 13 J/cm$^2$) conferred no additional advantage over simply using the 585 nm wavelength with the 0.5 ms pulse duration at 5.5 J. A uniform spot size of 7 mm was used for all treatment groups. Overall,

they found that purple PWS responded better than lesions which were red or pink.

## Noncoherent Light Sources

Several studies have investigated the use of IPL systems, which included a broad range of noncoherent wavelengths, to treat vascular lesions. The largest of these tested a 515–1,200 nm IPL for rosacea in 60 patients, treating a total of 508 sites with an average of 4.1 treatments per site [30]. The patients had a mean clearance rate of 77.8% over 3 years, recurrence was noted in only 4 of 508 treated sites. Four other, smaller studies examined the use of IPL for PWS. Their results are summarized in Table 12.3 [31–34].

As indicated in Table 12.3, the IPL technology does not provide more than a moderate improvement in either previously treated or untreated PWS. Direct randomized controlled trials of PDL with IPL are described in the next section of randomized controlled trials, and indicate that PDL is still the best technology for treating vascular lesions.

## Infrared Light Sources

A 2009 case series of 20 patients describes the use of the 755 nm alexandrite laser for treatment of hypertrophic and resistant PWS. They found that these lesions showed significant lightening after treatment with a 755 nm laser in combination with PDL, but not all were successful. Side effects included pain, edema, bullae, crusting, and rare scarring. Although the results were promising, the authors urged their colleagues to be cautious choosing a fluence at or near the threshold for clinical response. The deeply penetrating nature of this laser could result in serious sequelae [35].

A pilot open-label clinical study of 17 patients with PWS compared using three sessions each with the 595 nm PDL (1.5 ms and dynamic cooling) and with the 1,064 nm Nd:YAG laser [36]. Fluences 1.0, 0.8, and 0.6 times the minimum purpura dose were applied for the Nd:YAG group and both groups had similar clearing, but the Nd:YAG caused greater perivascular and

**Table 12.3** Summary of studies using intense pulsed laser for port wine stains

| References | No. of patients | Study design | Outcome |
|---|---|---|---|
| Ozdemir et al. [31] | 12 Turkish patients with untreated facial and/or neck PWS | Patients received 3–6 treatments every 4–6 weeks | Moderate improvement (50–75% clearing) was seen in 47% of patients Complete clearing in only one patient (8.3%) |
| Reynolds et al. [32] | 12 British patients with untreated PWS on the body (less visible areas) | Treated with IPL cutoff filters of 550–1,100 nm for 2–9 treatments, case-controlled within-patient | 8/12 had some degree of fading 4/12 had no response (and all had pink PWS) Darker, more caudal lesions had a better response |
| Ho et al. [33] | 22 Chinese patients with untreated PWS | Treated 5–7 times at 3–4 week intervals | 9% achieve complete clearing Majority (50%) had only 25–50% clearing |
| Bjerring et al. [34] | 15 Danish patients with PDL resistant PWS | Treated four times with second generation IPL system and evaluated 2 months after last treatment | 46.7% of patients responded to IPL (had more than 50% clearance; 87% of these had 75–100% clearance) 53.3% did not respond to IPL (had less than 25% clearance) V2 area did not respond to treatments |

epidermal injury. Again, the authors warn that Nd:Yag can be as effective but can cause scarring at higher fluences.

Perhaps the most interesting of recent studies has combined the use of the 595 nm PDL with the 1,064 nm laser for treatment of recalcitrant and hypertrophic PWS in adults and children. Twenty-five patients who had incomplete clearance despite ten previous treatments with PDL were treated by Alster and Tanzi using a novel device that delivers sequential pulses of 595 and 1,064 nm wavelengths [37]. Additional clinical improvement was noted in all patients, although none had complete clearance. It was found to be slightly more uncomfortable by adult patients, but none had pigmentary alterations or scarring.

In describing their 20 years of experience in treating the pediatric population, Burns and Navarro describe how they use the 1,064 nm Nd:Yag laser only on patients whose hemangiomas have begun to involute [38]. Otherwise, they noticed higher rates of skin ulceration and necrosis. They theorize that the proliferative lesions are already at higher risk for ulceration, and the laser heating can place an increased metabolic demand that hastens or even causes ulceration. Similar results are suggested by a 2006 publication reporting 12 patients who had

complications following PDL for hemangiomas of infancy [39]. Eight developed ulcerations and four had permanent atrophic scarring. All were treated between the ages of 5 days and 4 months, when the hemangiomas were likely to have still been in the proliferative phase. However, 11 of the 12 were treated without any dynamic cooling to the surface, which may have resulted in more epidermal injury.

A direct comparison of the 755 nm alexandrite, 1,064 nm Nd:YAG, 550–1,100 nm IPL, and 532 nm KTP lasers with the PDL as control was performed in 18 patients with capillary malformations [40]. All 18 had received at least five treatments with a PDL 585 nm, for 0.45 ms to lesions on their head or neck, and received test treatments of all five different systems. The alexandrite laser showed the most improvement using Munsell color charts, improving ten patients, while the KTP and Nd:YAG lasers were least effective, with fading seen in just two patients. Six patients improved with the IPL. Five had further fading with the PDL. The tradeoff was a higher rate of side effects seen in the alexandrite laser. Hyperpigmentation and scarring developed in four patients, likely due to the deeper penetration and lower specificity for oxyhemoglobin-carrying vessels.

# Photodynamic Therapy

One relatively new area of study is the use of an intravenous photosensitizer prior to treatment with a laser. In 2007, 1,949 cases of PWS in 1,385 patients received IV hematophorphyrin derivative or hematoporphyrin monomethyl ether (HMME) prior to undergoing laser irradiation with different wavelengths (488–578 nm) at varying fluences [41]. Among the treated lesions, 6.6% achieved 100% clearance, 38.3% achieved >75% clearance, and 47.4% achieved 50–75% clearance. Darker stains required two sessions or more, while pink PWS had better response with only one session. The authors reported almost no risk of scarring.

In 2009, 75 patients in China with PWS were injected with photosensitizer (Photocarcinorin, PsD-007) and exposed to copper vapor laser [42]. Complete clinical remission was observed in 57.3% of patients and some improvement was seen in 94% of patients after no more than four courses of treatment. Twenty percent of the complete responders required only two courses or less.

# Adjunctive Topical Treatments

Imiquimod is a topical immune-response modifier which has been FDA approved for treatment of genital warts, actinic keratoses, and basal cell carcinoma. Its use in a variety of other skin conditions has been explored, and in 2008 a pilot study examined its use in treating PWS birthmarks, alone and in conjunction with 585 nm PDL (1.5 ms) for a group of 20 Asian patients [43]. In each patient, three test areas were identified for treatment: PDL alone, imiquimod alone, and PDL + imiquimod. PDL test sites received a single laser treatment of spot size 7 mm using 10 J/cm$^2$ and cryogen spray cooling. For the imiquimod sites, the patients applied the agent once daily for 1 month after PDL exposure. They were followed at 1, 3, 6, and 12 months after the initial laser exposure, and a blanching response was evaluated using a dermospectrophotometer. They found that over time, the group treated with PDL and imiquimod had the best response ($P < 0.05$) with superior blanching over the other two treatment

groups. No hypopigmentation or scarring was seen, and any hyperpigmentation resolved within 6 months.

Rapamycin is an anti-angiogenic agent, which has been shown to inhibit growth of blood vessels. It was investigated in conjunction with laser pulses in golden Syrian hamsters to see whether it could inhibit reperfusion of photocoagulated blood vessels in an animal model [44]. Two treatment groups were established: one treated with laser only, and one treated with laser and then topical rapamycin daily for 14 days after laser exposure. In the laser only group, they found that 23 of the 24 photocoagulated blood vessels reperfused within 5–14 days. The combination treated group had 36% less reperfusion than the laser-only group. There was no correlation with the concentration of rapamycin used and the reperfusion rate, but the results suggest that topical anti-angiogenic therapy may help improve results with laser therapy.

# Conclusions

– PDL remains the gold standard for treating vascular lesions. Side effects include purpura (transient) and ulceration in highly proliferative lesions.
– The 1,064 Nd:YAG can also be used for PWS but should be used with caution due to the possibility of scarring at high fluences [36]. The combination of 595 + 1,064 is especially promising [37].
– The 532 nm wavelength can provide adjunctive therapy, but has risk of pigmentary changes and scarring [20–23], especially in darker skin types [23].
– Epidermal cooling is essential to help mitigate textural and pigmentation changes [14, 15].
– IPL laser therapy can help lighten vascular lesions but is not a panacea [31–34].
– The deeper components (>1 mm) of HOI remain difficult to treat.
– Increasing the wavelength to 1.5 ms with either the 585 or 595 PDL can improve results for refractory lesions [27].
– Increasing the energy to 9.5 J/cm$^2$ with the 595 PDL can improve results for refractory PWS [24].

- The 595 nm PDL with 1.5 ms pulse duration is presently the standard of care for PWS and HOI.
- Longer wavelengths (>6 ms) confer no additional advantage in clearing the lesions [28, 29].
- Pulse stacking can provide comparable clearing without the purpura that results from using higher fluences [26].
- PDT using photosensitizers prior to laser treatment can improve PWS [41, 42, 50].
- Patients born with PWS should undergo treatment as early as possible and as many times are necessary to avoid hypertrophy and nodularity, which are more difficult to treat.

## Randomized Controlled Trials and Meta-Analyses

A search of the Pubmed English literature for the terms "port-wine stain," "hemangioma," and "telangiectasias" was conducted to identify all existing randomized controlled trials and meta-analyses for the last 10 years. The following includes a description of the findings. Many randomized controlled trials were identified, but there were no meta-analyses. As with most of the previous studies, these involved improving upon existing treatments for PWS and hemangiomas, including those which are hypertrophic or resistant to therapy.

In 2002, a randomized controlled study of early PDL treatment for 121 infants with uncomplicated hemangiomas demonstrated no significant difference in the rate of clearing between treated and untreated groups [45]. The side effects of skin atrophy (seen in 28% of treated patients) and hypopigmentation (45% of treated patients) made the treatment not worthwhile. This study used traditional 585 PDL wavelength with a 0.45 μs pulse duration but with no epidermal cooling. We know from subsequent studies that the epidermal cooling is crucial to minimizing side effects.

In 2005, a randomized, blinded controlled study demonstrated a higher proportion of clearance when the pulse duration was near to or higher than the TRT [46]. This was achieved by varying different pulse durations in patients treated with the KTP

532 nm laser for telangiectatic facial vessels. A 2006 prospective, randomized controlled trial enrolling 52 Japanese infants compared the clearance of hemangiomas treated with traditional PDL (585 nm, with pulse duration = 0.45 ms) with long-pulsed (595 nm, pulse duration 10–20 ms) using cryogen spray cooling to protect the epidermis [47]. It found that the PDL group had 54% had complete clearance while the LPDL group had 65% clearance. Although this result was not statistically significant, the degree of side effects (hyperpigmentation, hypopigmentation, and textural changes) was significantly lower in the long pulsed PDL group. Likewise, the LPDL group had a significantly shorter time period of proliferation by the hemangiomas (177 days for PDL vs. 106 days for LPDL).

PWS can be quite refractory to laser treatment, even with longer wavelengths and increased pulse durations. The use of higher fluences, along with cooling of the epidermis was investigated in one randomized controlled trial in 2007. This study treated 11 patients with PWS, who were partitioned into three groups [48]. All three groups were treated with 585 nm PDL, (1) 6 J/cm$^2$ with no cold air cooling, (2) 6 J/cm$^2$ with cold air cooling, and (3) 9 J/cm$^2$ with cold air cooling. The third treatment group demonstrated a slightly but not significantly higher rate of clearance (59 vs. 57%) than the first group. Because pain was also lowered, the authors recommended in favor of using contact cooling.

Another suggestion for improving results was to increase the frequency of treatments. In 2006, a British group enrolled 15 patients with PWS to compare treatments at 2- and 6-week intervals [49]. On their first visit, the entire lesion was treated with a 595 PDL. Then, half the lesion was randomly allocated to be treated again after 2 weeks and the other half to be treated at 6 weeks. Both areas were examined by independent observers after 12 weeks and the endpoint was the degree of lightening as measured with a reflectance spectrophotometer. In 11 of the 13 patients who completed the trial, the 2 week treatment interval resulted in a significantly greater reduction in reflectance than the 6-week interval ($P = 0.003$). No adverse reactions were reported and the results suggest that shorter treatment intervals are more effective.

A randomized internally controlled trial of eight patients with PWS combined the use of a photosensitizer (5-aminolevulinic acid) with a 585 nm PDL to see if patients would achieve better clearance than in areas treated with PDL alone [50]. Five-ALA is a porphyrin derivative, which is converted in vascular endothelial cells to the active photosensitizer PpIX. One of the peaks in its absorption spectrum is 576 nm which has been utilized for the treatment of actinic keratoses. The researchers found no significant benefit from combining PDT with PDL. However, the authors suggest that further research in using longer pulse durations, higher fluences, or larger doses of 5-ALA may demonstrate better results.

Three randomized controlled trials investigated whether IPL sources could offer better treatment of vascular lesions than PDLs. In the first study, 20 patients in Denmark with PWS were allocated to receive side by side treatments of 595 nm PDL treatment and IPL [51]. Treatment outcomes were evaluated by blinded observers and skin reflectance measurements. They found that the PDL treated group has significantly better clearance rates (75 vs. 30%) as well as better lightening on skin reflectance (33 vs. 12%) than the IPL treated spots. Eighteen of the 20 patients preferred to continue treatments with PDL rather than IPL. No adverse events were reported in either group.

In a second study containing 20 patients, individuals with photodamaged skin were randomly assigned to receive LPDL (595 nm, with dynamic cooling and a 3–20 ms pulse duration depending on the size of the vessels being treated) to one half-face and IPL (without cooling) on the other half of their face [52]. The patients received a series of three treatments at 3 week intervals, and were evaluated at end point for telangiectasias, pain, and adverse effects. Superior vessel clearance was observed via blinded clinical evaluations as well as patient self-assessments for the LPDL treated sides. Likewise, patients preferred the LPDL treatments over the IPL because it was less painful. Results of a third smaller but nearly identical split-lesion study comparing LPDL with IPL for telangiectasia after radiotherapy for breast cancer showed a significant improvement in vessel clearance with LPDL (90%)

over IPL (50%) [53]. Lower pain score and higher patient satisfaction were reported in among 11 of the 13 patients who enrolled in the trial.

One randomized controlled trial from 2009 compared nonpurpuragenic PDL settings (595 nm, 6 ms pulse duration) with IPL settings using 560 nm cutoff filter and chilled crystal tip to treat erythemotelangiectatic rosacea [54]. The fluence of the PDL was adjusted up or down to achieve transient purpura. Three monthly treatment sessions were performed in this single-blind split face trial of 29 patients. Both systems resulted in significant reduction of erythema, telangiectasia, and patient reported symptoms, with no difference noted between the two treatments.

Other modifications for improving response over the PDL included changing the wavelength to 532 nm with the KTP laser (Fig. 12.7a, b). Fifteen patients with facial telangiectasias were treated in a split-face, single-blind, controlled comparison study using the 595 nm PDL on one cheek and the 532 nm KTP laser on the opposite cheek [55]. They underwent three treatments, every 3 weeks, and were evaluated 3 weeks after the last treatment. The KTP laser achieved 62% clearing after the first treatment and 85% clearing at final evaluation, while the PDL achieved just 49 and 75% clearing for the same time intervals. However, the areas treated with the 532 nm laser noted 58% erythema while PDL treated areas had only 8%. This study suggests that the KTP laser is more effective for facial telangiectasias but causes more swelling and erythema.

Another randomized controlled trial published in 2010 investigated the use of PDL (595 nm), KTP (532 nm) and electrodessication for treating cherry angiomata [56]. Fifteen volunteers had three areas on the trunk demarcated with four lesions each. Each area was randomly assigned to undergo one of the three treatments, two times and spaced 2 weeks apart. The areas were analyzed for color and texture on visual analog scales. Lesions treated with electrodessication were significantly less improved than those treated with PDL ($P = 0.001$) and KTP ($P = 0.003$). No difference in textural change was noted between the KTP and PDL lasers. However, there was more textural change associated with electrodessication than with laser.

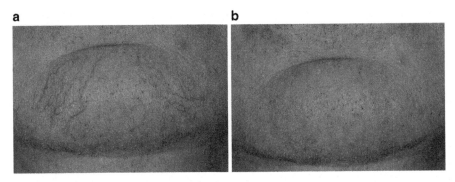

**Fig. 12.7** (**a**) Facial telangiectasias of the chin, untreated, (**b**) same facial telangiectasias after a single KTP 532 nm treatment (courtesy of Patricia Farris, MD)

In 2008, researchers tested the combination of PDL (595 nm) and Nd:YAG (1,064 nm) with PDL or Nd:YAG alone using a dual wavelength laser system for treatment of facial telangiectasias [57]. Twenty patients underwent the sequential delivery of PDL and Nd:YAG on one cheek, and were randomized to receive either PDL or Nd:YAG on the opposite cheek. Results were evaluated 4 weeks later by blinded assessment of before and after photographs. They found no statistical difference in efficacy between the single wavelength treated sides, but there was a significant improvement ($P < 0.05$) seen in the dual-wavelength group.

## Conclusions

– The PDL is still the best treatment option over the IPL for PWS and hemangiomas.
– Combined wavelengths of 595 with 1,064 may allow improved penetration of deeper vessels.
– The 532 nm KTP laser may be helpful in treating very superficial facial telangiectasias.

## Lasers and Lights for the Leg Telangiectasias

The treatment of leg veins with vascular lasers is slightly more challenging. This has been attributed to several factors: (1) lower content of oxygenated blood returning from the lower extremities to the heart (2) thick surrounding interstitial tissue and fibrosis surrounding the vessel walls, and (3) increased hydrostatic pressure in the lower extremities [3]. As a result, the most promising lasers have been in the near-infrared range, targeting 750–1,100 nm.

Initial studies investigated the use of the 532 nm wavelength for treatment of leg veins. One randomized, controlled trial used the KTP lasers for spider leg veins in 70 female volunteers [58]. Three treatment sessions were provided each for vessels less than or equal to 0.6 mm in diameter, and for vessels 0.7–1.0 mm in diameter. They found that the smaller size vessels showed complete resolution in 33%, a decrease in vessel diameter in 40%, and no change in appearance for 27%. The larger size vessels were all still visible after three sessions. Hyperpigmentation occurred in 13 of the 56 patients who completed the study. Another study investigated the long-pulsed Nd:YAG laser at 532 nm with a chilled sapphire tip and found that it could treat leg veins of 0.5–1.0 mm diameter with greater than 50% clearance at 44% of sites with a single treatment [59]. Higher fluences of 16 J/cm$^2$ improved the clearance rate, but also had greater adverse effects, including atrophic scarring for up to a year.

The alexandrite (755 nm) laser has also been tried for leg veins. A 2002 trial involved treating 20 female volunteers (skin types 1–3) with 0.3–1.3 mm leg telangiectasias with test spots of increasing fluence (40–90 J/cm$^2$) and a spray cooling system [60]. They found that 15 out of 20 subjects had a clearance rate between 26 and 75%. Hyperpigmentation was observed in 15 patients, and hypopigmentation occurred in two patients. No edema, purpura, scarring, or blistering was seen. Another alexandrite study from 2009 enrolled 15 patients with 0.2–1.0 mm vessels (and skin types I–III) with varying pulse durations of 3–100 ms [61]. Optimal settings were identified though blinded evaluation of pre and post treatment photographs. The average fluence required for vessel closure was 89 J/cm$^2$ and the optimal pulse duration was 60 ms for most patients. These parameters provided a clearance approaching 65%, 12 weeks after a single treatment. Four patients did experience transient hyperpigmentation, but the study concluded that a longer pulse width reduced purpura and improved the side effect profile.

Investigation of the Nd:YAG 1,064 nm laser has provided the most promising results for the treatment of leg telangiectasias. A 2002 side-by-side comparative study of the 1,064 nm Nd:YAG, 810 nm diode, and 755 nm alexandrite lasers was performed in 30 female volunteers, skin types I–V, for 0.3–3 mm leg veins [62]. In the 22 patients who completed the study, 36 sites were treated with the Nd:YAG laser, 18 sites were treated with the diode laser, and 12 vein sites were treated with the alexandrite. Greater than 75% improvement was seen in 88% of the Nd:YAG treated sites, 29% of the diode treated sites, and 33% of the alexandrite treated sites. Greater than 50% improvement was seen in 94% of Nd:YAG treated sites, 33% of diode treated sites, and 58% of alexandrite treated sites. Less than 25% improvement was seen in 6% of the Nd:YAG treated sites, 39% of the diode treated sites, and 33% of the alexandrite treated sites. Post-treatment purpura and telangiectatic matting was seen with the alexandrite laser. Overall the authors concluded that the Nd:YAG provided the best treatment with least side effects.

Optimal pulse durations for the Nd:YAG laser have since been identified as 40–60 ms. A 2006 study of 18 patients with leg veins found that this provided clearance of 71% of vessels with a single laser treatment, and minimal post inflammatory pigmentation [63]. Shorter pulse durations (<20 ms) increased tendency for purpura and postinflammatory pigmentation. One comparative

study suggested that the Nd:YAG 1,064 long pulse laser could yield results similar to policodanol 0.5% sclerotherapy in the treatment of small leg veins [64]. It involved treating four sites on each of 14 patients with 0.4–2 mm veins: sclerotherapy alone, laser alone, sclerotherapy then laser, and laser then sclerotherapy. The best clinical results were seen with sclerotherapy followed by laser, but this improvement was not statistically significant over either modality alone.

Nonetheless, most dermatologists still use injectable sclerotherapy as their gold standard for leg vein treatment. A 2002 study comparing the long-pulsed Nd:YAG with sodium tetradecyl sulfate (STS) sclerotherapy in 20 patients with size-matched superficial leg telangiectasias found that the veins responded best to sclerotherapy, in fewer treatment sessions, than to long-pulsed 1,064 laser therapy [65]. Other sclerosing agents include glycerin, which has been showed to provide a better, more rapid clearance of previously treated telangiectasias [66], and liquid polidocanol, which offers comparable results as STS [67], but is not yet approved for use in the United States. Hypertonic saline is used by many doctors in the U.S. and has been found comparable to polidocanol in efficacy and patient satisfaction [68].

## Conclusions

- Sclerotherapy continues to be the gold standard for treatment of leg veins.
- The best laser for treatment of leg veins appears to be the long-pulsed Nd:YAG (1,064 nm).
- Lasers can be helpful for patients with needle phobia, sclerosant allergy, or who are prone to telangiectatic matting.

## Conclusion

Most of the studies performed in the last decade have focused on how to improve the resolution of vascular lesions that are resistant to traditional PDL settings. These include efforts to investigate

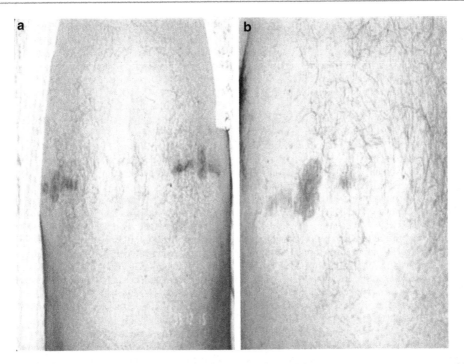

**Fig. 12.8** (**a**) Surgical scar following male breast reduction, untreated, (**b**) same scar after four treatments with PDL 595 nm, 1.5 ms at 5.5 J/cm² with 7 mm spot size (courtesy of Marc Avram, MD)

changes in wavelength, pulse duration, and fluency. Also more work has been done to investigate the IPL for use in refractory PWS and hemangiomas. PDT, alone or in conjunction with PDL has also been investigated. Also, the use of adjunctive topical agents, such as imiquimod and rapamycin, offers interesting areas for further investigation.

Vascular lasers are playing an increasingly valuable role in the treatment of other conditions, such as psoriasis, warts, surgical scars (Fig. 12.8a, b), striae, rhinophyma, acne, and Poikiloderma of Civatte or photodamaged skin. As more lasers are tried for various applications we will have more experience to report.

## References

1. Anderson RR, Parrish JA. Selective photothermolysis: precise microsurgery by selective absorption of pulsed radiation. Science. 1983;220:524–7.
2. Alster TS, Wilson F. Treatment of port-wine stains with the flash lamp-pumped pulsed dye laser: extended clinical experience in children and adults. Ann Plast Surg. 1994;32:478–84.
3. Adamic M, Troilius A, Adatto M, Drosner M, Dahmane R. Vascular lasers and IPLs: guidelines for care from the European Society for Laser Dermatology (ESLD). J Cosmet Laser Ther. 2007;9:113–24.
4. Grantzow R, Schmittenbecher P, Cremer H, Hoger P, Rossler J, Hamm H, et al. Hemangiomas in infancy and childhood. S 2k guideline of the German Society of Dermatology with the working group Pediatric Dermatology together with the German Society for Pediatric Surgery and the German Society for Pediatric Medicine. J Dtsch Dermatol Ges. 2008;6:324–9.
5. Frieden IJ, Eichenfield LF, Esterly NB, Geronemus R, Mallory SB. Guidelines of care for hemangiomas of infancy. American Academy of Dermatology Guidelines/Outcomes Committee. J Am Acad Dermatol. 1997;37:631–7.
6. Hohenleutner S, Badur-Ganter E, Landthaler M, Hohenleutner U. Long-term results in the treatment of childhood hemangioma with the flashlamp-pumped pulsed dye laser: an evaluation of 617 cases. Lasers Surg Med. 2001;28:273–7.
7. Poetke M, Philipp C, Berlien HP. Flashlamp-pumped pulsed dye laser for hemangiomas in infancy: treatment of superficial vs mixed hemangiomas. Arch Dermatol. 2000;136:628–32.
8. Ho WS, Chan HH, Ying SY, Chan PC. Laser treatment of congenital facial port-wine stains: long-term efficacy and complication in Chinese patients. Lasers Surg Med. 2002;30:44–7.

9. Huikeshoven M, Koster P, de Borgie C, Beek JF, Gemert M, van der Horst C. Redarkening of port-wine stains 10 years after pulsed-dye laser treatment. N Engl J Med. 2007;356:1235–40.

10. Soueid A, Waters R. Re-emergence of port wine stains following treatment with flashlamp-pumped dye laser 585 nm. Ann Plast Surg. 2006;57:260–3.

11. Sivarajan V, Al Aissami M, Maclaren W, Mackay IR. Recurrence of spider naevi following treatment with 585 nm pulsed dye laser. J Plast Reconstr Aesthet Surg. 2007;60:668–71.

12. Geronemus RG, Quintana AT, Lou WW, Kauvar A. High-fluence modified pulsed dye laser photocoagulation with dynamic cooling of port-wine stains in infancy. Arch Dermatol. 2000;136:942–4.

13. Chiu CH, Chan HH, Ho WS, Yeung CK, Nelson JS. Prospective study of pulsed dye laser in conjunction with cryogen spray cooling for treatment of port wine stains in Chinese patients. Dermatol Surg. 2003;29:909–15.

14. Chapas AM, Eickhorst K, Geronemus RG. Efficacy of early treatment of facial port wine stains in newborns: a review of 49 cases. Lasers Surg Med. 2007;39:563–8.

15. Rizzo C, Brightman L, Chapas AM, Hale EK, Cantatore-Francis JL, Bernstein LJ, et al. Outcomes of childhood hemangiomas treated with the pulsed-dye laser with dynamic cooling: a retrospective chart analysis. Dermatol Surg. 2009;35:1947–54.

16. Scherer K, Lorenz S, Wimmershoff M, Landthaler M, Hohenleutner U. Both the flashlamp-pumped dye laser and the long-pulsed tunable dye laser can improve results in port-wine stain therapy. Br J Dermatol. 2001;145:79–84.

17. Woo SH, Ahn HH, Kim SN, Kye YC. Treatment of vascular skin lesions with the variable-pulse 595 nm pulsed dye laser. Dermatol Surg. 2006;32:41–8.

18. Asahina A, Watanabe T, Kishi A, Hattori N, Shirai A, Kagami S, et al. Evaluation of the treatment of port-wine stains with the 595 nm long pulsed dye laser: a large prospective study in adult Japanese patients. J Am Acad Dermatol. 2006;54:487–93.

19. Latkowski IT, Wysocki MS, Siewiera IP. Own clinical experience in treatment of port-wine stain with KTP 532 nm laser [article in Polish]. Wiad Lek. 2005;58:391–6.

20. Chowdhury MM, Harris S, Lanigan SW. Potassium titanyl phosphate laser treatment of resistant port-wine stains. Br J Dermatol. 2001;144:814–7.

21. Pence B, Aybey B, Ergenekon G. Outcomes of 532 nm frequency-doubled Nd:YAG laser use in the treatment of port-wine stains. Dermatol Surg. 2005;31:509–17.

22. Raulin C, Greve B. Retrospective clinical comparison of hemangioma treatment by flashlamp-pumped (585 nm) and frequency-doubled Nd:YAG (532 nm) lasers. Lasers Surg Med. 2001;28:40–3.

23. Chan HH, Chan E, Kono T, Ying SY, Wai-Sun H. The use of variable pulse width frequency doubled Nd:YAG 532 nm laser in the treatment of port-wine stain in Chinese patients. Dermatol Surg. 2000;26:657–61.

24. Bernstein EF. High-energy 595 nm pulsed dye laser improves refractory port-wine stains. Dermatol Surg. 2006;32:26–33.

25. Alam M, Dover JS, Arndt KA. Treatment of facial telangiectasia with variable-pulse high-fluence pulsed-dye laser: comparison of efficacy with fluences immediately above and below the purpura threshold. Dermatol Surg. 2003;29:681–4.

26. Rohrer TE, Chatrath V, Iyengar V. Does pulse stacking improve the results of treatment with variable-pulse pulsed-dye lasers? Dermatol Surg. 2004;30 (2 Pt 1):163–7.

27. Bernstein EF, Brown DB. Efficacy of the 1.5 millisecond pulse-duration, 585 nm, pulsed-dye laser for treating port-wine stains. Lasers Surg Med. 2005;36:341–6.

28. Yung A, Sheehan-Dare R. A comparative study of a 595-nm with a 585-nm pulsed dye laser in refractory port wine stains. Br J Dermatol. 2005;153:601–6.

29. Greve B, Raulin C. Prospective study of port wine stain treatment with dye laser: comparison of two wavelengths (585 nm vs. 595 nm) and two pulse durations (0.5 milliseconds vs. 20 milliseconds). Lasers Surg Med. 2004;34:168–73.

30. Schroeter CA, Haaf-von Below S, Neumann HA. Effective treatment of rosacea using intense pulsed light systems. Dermatol Surg. 2005;31:1285–9.

31. Ozdemir M, Engin B, Mevlitoglu I. Treatment of facial port-wine stains with intense pulsed light: a prospective study. J Cosmet Dermatol. 2008;7:127–31.

32. Reynolds N, Exley J, Hills S, Falder S, Duff C, Kenealy J. The role of the lumina intense pulsed light system in the treatment of port wine stains – a case controlled study. Br J Plast Surg. 2005;58:968–80.

33. Ho WS, Ying SY, Chan PC, Chan HH. Treatment of port wine stains with intense pulsed light: a prospective study. Dermatol Surg. 2004;30:887–90.

34. Bjerring P, Christiansen K, Troilius A. Intense pulsed light source for the treatment of dye laser resistant port-wine stains. J Cosmet Laser Ther. 2003;5:7–13.

35. Izikson L, Nelson JS, Anderson RR. Treatment of hypertrophic and resistant port wine stains with a 755 nm laser: a case series of 20 patients. Lasers Surg Med. 2009;41:427–32.

36. Yang MU, Yaroslavsky AN, Farinelli WA, Flotte TJ, Rius-Diaz F, Tsao SS, et al. Long-pulsed neodymium:yttrium-aluminum-garnet laser treatment for port-wine stains. J Am Acad Dermatol. 2005;52 (3 Pt 1):480–90.

37. Alster TS, Tanzi EL. Combined 595-nm and 1,064-nm laser irradiation of recalcitrant and hypertrophic port-wine stains in children and adults. Dermatol Surg. 2009;35:914–8.

38. Burns AJ, Navarro JA. Role of laser therapy in pediatric patients. Plast Reconstr Surg. 2009;124(Suppl):82e–92.

39. Witman PM, Wagner AM, Scherer K, Waner M, Frieden IJ. Complications following pulsed dye laser treatment of superficial hemangiomas. Lasers Surg Med. 2006;38:116–23.

40. McGill DJ, MacLaren W, Mackay IR. A direct comparison of pulsed dye, alexandrite, KTP, and Nd:YAG lasers and IPL in patients with previously treated capillary malformations. Lasers Surg Med. 2008;40:390–8.

41. Gu Y, Huang NY, Liang J, Pan YM, Liu FG. Clinical study of 1949 cases of port wine stains treated with vascular photodynamic therapy (Gu's PDT) [article in French]. Ann Dermatol Venereol. 2007;134(3 Pt 1): 241–4.

42. Lu YG, Wu JJ, Yang YD, He Y. Photodynamic therapy of port-wine stains. J Dermatolog Treat. 2010;21:240–4.

43. Chang CJ, Hsiao YC, Mihm Jr MC, Nelson JS. Pilot study examining the combined use of pulsed dye laser and topical imiquimod versus laser alone for treatment of port wine stain birthmarks. Lasers Surg Med. 2008;40:605–10.

44. Jia W, Sun V, Tran N, Choi B, Liu SW, Mihm Jr MC, et al. Long-term blood vessel removal with combined laser and topical rapamycin antiangiogenic therapy: implication for effective port wine stain treatment. Lasers Surg Med. 2010;42:105–12.

45. Batta K, Goodyear HM, Moss C, Williams HC, Hiller L, Waters R. Randomized controlled study of early pulsed dye laser treatment of uncomplicated childhood hemangiomas: results of a 1-year analysis. Lancet. 2002;360:521–7.

46. Cameron H, Ibbotson SH, Ferguson J, Dawe RS, Moseley H. A randomized, blinded, controlled study of the clinical relevance of matching pulse duration to thermal relaxation time when treating facial telangiectasia. Lasers Med Sci. 2005;20:117–21.

47. Kono T, Sakurai H, Groff WF, Chan HH, Takeuchi M, Yamaki T, et al. Comparison study of a traditional pulsed dye laser versus a long-pulsed dye laser in the treatment of early childhood hemangiomas. Lasers Surg Med. 2006;38:112–5.

48. Hammes S, Roos S, Raulin C, Ockenfels HM, Greve B. Does dye laser treatment with higher fluences in combination with cold air cooling improve the results of port-wine stains? J Eur Acad Dermatol Venereol. 2007;21:1129–33.

49. Tomson N, Lim SP, Abdullah A, Lanigan SW. The treatment of port-wine stains with the pulsed-dye laser at 2-week and 6-week intervals: a comparative study. Br J Dermatol. 2006;154:676–9.

50. Evans AV, Robson A, Barlow RJ, Kurwa HA. Treatment of port wine stains with photodynamic therapy, using pulsed dye laser as a light source, compared with pulsed dye laser alone: a pilot study. Lasers Surg Med. 2005;36:266–9.

51. Faurschou A, Togsverd-Bo K, Zachariae C, Haedersdal M. Pulsed dye laser vs. intense pulsed light for port-wine stains: a randomized side-by-side trial with blinded response evaluation. Br J Dermatol. 2009;160:359–64.

52. Jorgensen GF, Hedelund L, Haedersdal M. Long-pulsed dye laser versus intense pulsed light for photodamaged skin: a randomized split-face trial with blinded response evaluation. Lasers Surg Med. 2008;40:293–9.

53. Nymann P, Hedelund L, Haedersdal M. Intense pulsed light vs. long-pulsed dye laser treatment of telangiectasia after radiotherapy for breast cancer: a randomized split-lesion trial of two different treatments. Br J Dermatol. 2009;160:1237–41.

54. Neuhaus IM, Zane LT, Tope WD. Comparative efficacy of nonpurpuragenic pulsed dye laser and intense pulsed light for erythematotelangiectatic rosacea. Dermatol Surg. 2009;35:920–8.

55. Uebelhoer NS, Bogle MA, Stewart B, Arndt KA, Dover JS. A split-face comparison study of pulsed 532-nm KTP laser and 595-nm pulsed dye laser in the treatment of facial telangiectasias and diffuse telangiectatic facial erythema. Dermatol Surg. 2007;33:441–8.

56. Collyer J, Boone SL, White LE, Rademaker A, West DP, Anderson K, et al. Comparison of treatment of cherry angiomata with pulsed-dye laser, potassium titanyl phosphate laser, and electrodessication: a randomized controlled trial. Arch Dermatol. 2010;146:33–7.

57. Karsai S, Roos S, Raulin C. Treatment of facial telangiectasia using a dual-wavelength laser system (595 and 1,064 nm): a randomized controlled trial with blinded response evaluation. Dermatol Surg. 2008;34:702–8.

58. Spendel S, Prandl EC, Schintler MV, Siegl A, Wittgruber G, Hellborn B, et al. Treatment of spider leg veins with the KTP (532 nm) laser – a prospective study. Lasers Surg Med. 2002;31:194–201.

59. McMeekin TO. Treatment of spider veins of the leg using a long-pulsed Nd:YAG laser (Versapulse) at 532 nm. J Cutan Laser Ther. 1999;1:179–80.

60. Brunnberg S, Lorenz S, Landthaler M, Hohenleutner U. Evaluation of the long pulsed high fluence alexandrite laser therapy of leg telangiectasia. Lasers Surg Med. 2002;31:359–62.

61. Ross EV, Meehan KJ, Gilbert S, Domankevitz Y. Optimal pulse durations for the treatment of leg telangiectasias with an alexandrite laser. Lasers Surg Med. 2009;41:104–9.

62. Eremia S, Li C, Umar SH. A side-by-side comparative study of 1064 nm Nd:YAG, 810 nm diode and 755 nm alexandrite lasers for treatment of 0.3–3 mm leg veins. Dermatol Surg. 2002;28:224–30.

63. Parlette EC, Groff WF, Kinshella MJ, Domankevitz Y, O'Neill J, Ross EV. Optimal pulse durations for the treatment of leg telangiectasias with a neodymium YAG laser. Lasers Surg Med. 2006;38:98–105.

64. Levy JL, Elbahr C, Jouve E, Mordon S. Comparison and sequential study of long pulsed Nd:YAG 1,064 nm laser and sclerotherapy in leg telangiectasias treatment. Lasers Surg Med. 2004;34:273–6.

65. Lupton JR, Alster TS, Romero P. Clinical comparison of sclerotherapy versus long-pulsed Nd:YAG laser treatment for lower extremity telangiectasias. Dermatol Surg. 2002;28:694–7.

66. Leach BC, Goldman MP. Comparative trial between sodium tetradecyl sulfate and glycerin in the treatment of telangiectatic leg veins. Dermatol Surg. 2003;29:612–4.

67. Rao J, Wildemore JK, Goldman MP. Double-blind prospective comparative trial between foamed and liquid polidocanol and sodium tetradecyl sulfate in the treatment of varicose and telangiectatic leg veins. Dermatol Surg. 2005;31:631–5.

68. McCoy S, Evans A, Spurrier N. Sclerotherapy for leg telangiectasia – a blinded comparative trial of polidocanol and hypertonic saline. Dermatol Surg. 1999;25: 381–5.

## Self-Assessment

1. Which phrase *does not* characterize a childhood hemangioma?
   (a) Vascular growth that appears at birth or shortly afterward
   (b) Undergoes a process of growth followed by involution
   (c) Must be treated as soon as possible
   (d) Prompt treatment is recommended in areas of anatomic importance or ulceration

2. Which phrase *does not* characterize a PWS?
   (a) Remains flat throughout life
   (b) Light pink lesions can resist laser therapy
   (c) Can increase in thickness and develop nodularity over time
   (d) Peripheral lesions can be more resistant to laser therapy than truncal/facial lesions

3. What is the gold standard laser treatment for vascular malformations?
   (a) Nd:Yag (1,064 nm)
   (b) KTP (532 nm)
   (c) PDL (585 and 595 nm)
   (d) Alexandrite (755 nm)

4. Which modality is the best for treatment for leg telangiectasias (spider veins)?
   (a) Nd:Yag laser (1,064 nm)
   (b) Sclerosing agents such as hypertonic saline, STS, or polidocanol injected directly into the veins
   (c) Alexandrite (755 nm)
   (d) PDL (585 or 595 nm)

5. Several conditions make it wise to treat hemangiomas of infancy as soon as possible with laser therapy. Which of these *are not* reasons to treat early on?
   (a) Ulcerating lesions
   (b) Lesion on or near the eye
   (c) Lesion on or near the arm
   (d) Lesion in the anogenital region

6. What special adjustments should be used for laser treatment of darker skin types?
   (a) Longer wavelengths
   (b) Shorter wavelengths
   (c) Epidermal cooling
   (d) Both a and c

7. What medication(s) can assist in the clearing of vascular lesions?
   (a) Imiquimod
   (b) Triamcinolone (intralesional)
   (c) Rapamycin
   (d) All of the above

## Answers

1. c: Must be treated as soon as possible
2. a: Remains flat throughout life
3. c: PDL (585 or 595 nm)
4. b: Sclerosing agents such as hypertonic saline, STS, or polidocanol injected directly into the veins.
5. c: Lesion on or near the arm
6. d: Both a and c
7. d: All of the above

# Pigment Lasers and Lights

# 13

Voraphol Vejjabhinanta,
Mohamed L. ElSaie, Su Luo, Nidhi Avashia,
Rawat Charoensawad, and Keyvan Nouri

## Introduction

The versatility of lasers has truly manifested itself in various medical and cosmetic procedures. Patients consider a number of benign pigmented cutaneous lesions objectionable because of their color, size, number, or location. These lesions include lentigines, café-au-lait macules, ephelides, junctional nevi, seborrheic keratoses, dermal melanosis, and tattoos [1]. Removal of these lesions involves destroying the epidermis to remove the unwanted lesion. For superficial lesions, physicians can treat these lesions with multiple modalities. In addition, almost all epidermal injuries heal without scarring. For deep dermal pigmented lesion, however, selective damaging to the lesions usually is performed by using the Q-switched laser systems.

V. Vejjabhinanta
Department of Dermatology, Siriraj Hospital,
Bangkoknoi, Bangkok, Thailand

M.L. ElSaie • S. Luo (✉) • N. Avashia • K. Nouri
Department of Dermatology and Cutaneous Surgery,
University of Miami Miller School of Medicine,
Miami, FL, USA
e-mail: sluo@med.miami.edu

R. Charoensawad
Department of Dermatology, Suphannahong
Dermatology Institute, Prathmuwan, Lumpinee, Thailand

## Principle of Selective Photothermolysis

The theory of selective photothermolysis is the science behind the process of laser hair removal and treatment of vascular and pigmented skin lesions. Melanin is the main chromophore and most concentrated in the basal cell layer of the epidermis. It has a broad absorption spectrum, being most intense in the ultraviolet range, and then dropping off through the visible to the near-infrared spectra. Melanin's absorption spectrum ranges from 250 to 1,200 nm. Melanin is densely packed within melanosomes, which are located in melanocytes and keratinocytes. Melanosomes, the primary sites of injury during laser therapy of epidermal pigmented lesions, are selectively injured with high-intensity pulsed light and are at various wavelengths across the spectrum. Shorter wavelengths require less energy to damage pigment cells, whereas greater energy is required for longer wavelengths because the absorption coefficient for melanin decreases as the wavelength increases. Longer wavelengths penetrate more deeply and more effectively target pigmented cells that are at greater depths in the epidermis. In addition to the wavelength, the pulse duration also determines the extent of injury to the melanosomes.

M. Alam (ed.), *Evidence-Based Procedural Dermatology*,
DOI 10.1007/978-0-387-09424-3_13, © Springer Science+Business Media, LLC 2012

## Basic Principles of Pigmented Lasers and Light-Based Devices

The term "laser" is an acronym that stands for "light amplification by stimulated emission of radiation." Stimulated emission is a process through which an already excited electron absorbs a photon of equal energy and then reverts to the resting orbit. During this process, two photons of light are released, both with the wavelength, phase, and direction of the absorbed photons. The energy is provided by an external power source. Lasers are named after the constituents of the medium and the pulse characteristics of the beam. This medium can be a gas, liquid, or solid. The beam may be continuous, pulsed, or quality switched [2]. Continuing advances in technology have expanded the dermatologist's armamentarium for treatment of solar lentigines and other skin lesions. The Q-switched ruby, the Q-switched alexandrite, the Q-switched Nd:YAG, the long-pulse duration-pulsed dye laser, and the long-pulse duration alexandrite lasers are often used.

## Q-Switched Laser

Q-switching is a technique that produces nanosecond laser pulses by suddenly releasing all of the excited-state energy from a laser medium. Nanosecond pulsed lasers such as the Q-switched ruby, alexandrite, and Nd:YAG cause melanosome cavitation and selective death of pigment-containing cells (photoacoustic reaction). This causes the whitening reaction seen upon exposure to this laser (Fig. 13.1). The Q-switched ruby laser (QSRL) (694 nm) has been used successfully in the removal of tattoos and a variety of cutaneous pigmented lesions. The frequency-doubled Q-switched neodymium:yttrium-aluminum-garnet laser (QSNd: YAG) (1,064 and 532 nm) has also been shown to be effective in the treatment of pigmented lesions. Tse et al. reported a study that compared the efficacy and side effect profile of the QSRL and the frequency-doubled QSNd:YAG lasers in the removal of cutaneous pigmented lesions, including lentigines, café-au-lait macules, nevus of Ota,

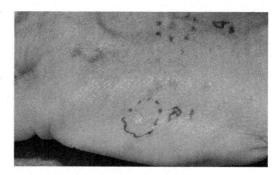

**Fig. 13.1** Immediate whitening reaction of a freckle on the left hand after Q-switched 532-nm laser

Becker's nevus, postinflammatory hyperpigmentation (PIH), and melasma. Results showed that a minimum of 30% lightening was achieved in all patients after only one treatment with either the QSRL or the frequency-doubled QSNd:YAG laser. The QSRL seems to provide a slightly better treatment response than the QSNd:YAG laser. Neither laser caused scarring or textural change of the skin. Most patients found the QSRL to be more painful during treatment, but the QSNd:YAG laser caused more postoperative discomfort [3] (IIA). The Q-switched lasers' high energy and short pulse widths permit less heat diffusion from the target melanosomes [4]. The 1,064-nm Nd:YAG has the longest wavelength and deepest penetration among the aforementioned laser systems available. It is not very well absorbed by melanin, but is sufficient in achieving selective photothermolysis and has superior penetration. This laser is able to penetrate the skin 5–7 mm, a depth at which most of the target structures lay. Furthermore, the combination of a low melanin absorption and deep penetration leads to less collateral damage to the melanin-containing epidermis. These features make this particular laser the safest method to treat all skin types especially tanned or darker skin patients. Although the Q-switched alexandrite laser is effective for discrete solar lentigines, the "violent" destruction of the melanosomes can be associated with significant postinflammatory pigmentation [5] in darker patients [6, 7]. The QSRL with its wavelength of 694 nm and a pulse duration of around 40 ns is an effective modality for the removal of tattoos and cutaneous pigmented lesions. Based on the principle of selective photothermolysis, selective damage to cutaneous pigment or pigmented cells is possible, allowing the scar-free elimination of endogenous or exogenous pigment in the skin. Main indications for the treatment with the QSRL are tattoos (amateur, professional, accidental, or cosmetic) and lentigines but the QSRL can also be used for lightening or even removing other pigmented lesions such as nevus spilus or café au lait macules. Furthermore, pigmented lesions of mucous membranes can be removed easily [8]. Thus, the Q-switched 694, 755, and 1,064/532-nm lasers are the key laser devices for pigmented lesions.

## Long-Pulsed Laser

### The Long-Pulsed Dye Laser

The 595-nm long-pulsed dye laser (LPDL) has been used for the treatment of vascular lesions and although it is well absorbed by oxyhemoglobin, it is also absorbed by melanin. In a study by Kono et al. the QSRL was compared with the LPDL using a flat glass lens to the tip of the laser's handpiece, allowing compression of the skin during treatment for lentigines in Asians. In doing so, the absorption by oxyhemoglobin was eliminated. Results showed that the degree of clearing achieved with the two lasers was 70.3 and 83.3% for QSRL and LPDL, respectively. All QSRL-treated areas developed erythema whereas only 4 of 18 LPDL-treated areas developed erythema. Hyperpigmentation was seen in four patients after QSRL, but not after LPDL. There was no scarring or hypopigmentation [9] (IIA). Subsequently, in another study by Kono et al., LPDL delivered with compression for treatment of facial lentigines was evaluated. Results showed that LPDL delivered with the compression method is effective in the treatment of facial lentigines in Asian patients, and the side effect profile is minimal. The compression technique allows the traditional "vascular" LPDL to be used for treating a variety of pigmented lesions [10] (IIA).

## The Long-Pulsed Alexandrite Laser

The long-pulsed alexandrite laser has a wavelength of 755 nm. This longer wavelength allows deeper penetration into the dermis with less absorption by epidermal melanin. This causes less adverse side effects such as pigmentation in darker skin patients. This laser is still typically used for patients with lighter skin types, but can also be used in those with darker skin. The adverse effects of this laser, when used on patients with darker skin types, can include blistering, crusting, and alterations of pigment, even when skin cooling devices are used. In patients classified as having the darkest skin, residual hypo- or hyperpigmentation is the rule with the alexandrite laser.

Although the alexandrite 755-nm-wavelength laser is effective in the treatment of unwanted hair, its use in treating pigmented skin lesions has not been well documented. A recent study by Trafeli et al. reported that a long-pulsed alexandrite laser is effective in clearing solar lentigines because patients with darker lentigines had greater lesion clearance than those patients with lighter-colored lentigines. Shorter pulse widths and treatment without cryogen cooling both, independently, lowered the fluence threshold for lentigo clearance [4] (IIA).

## Intense Pulsed Light

The intense pulsed light (IPL) system is not a laser, but emits broad-wavelength pulses of divergent light that cannot be tightly focused [11]. The most powerful IPLs deliver about 1,000 W of optical power per square centimeter. It has been used for virtually all of the same indications as laser systems. IPL systems utilize a xenon bulb as a light source, which produces polychromatic light with wavelengths from 515 to 1,200 nm. This is in contrast to laser light sources, which produce monochromatic light of a specific wavelength. Light emitted by the bulb passes through a filter that excludes shorter wavelengths that may severely damage skin. The ability to "tune" the wavelength of light emitted by these systems gives IPL systems the advantage of versatility. Using different filters, a pulsed light system could mimic any number of laser systems, allowing the operator to treat many different conditions amenable to light therapy. In an open study by Kawada et al., IPL's efficacy was tested after 3–5 treatments. Forty-eight percent of patients had more than 50% improvement and 20% had more than 75% improvement. In the group of solar lentigines, 40% of patients showed more than 50% improvement and 16% had more than 75% improvement. Patients with small plaques of solar lentigines responded well, whereas patients with small to large and large plaques showed poor response. Patients with solar lentigines + ephelides and ephelides responded remarkably with 75 and 71% of patients, respectively, having more than 50% improvement [12] (III B). In a study by Jorgensen et al., LPDL was compared to IPL for photodamaged skin and treatment of telangiectasias. Telangiectasias improved from LPDL and IPL treatments with superior vessel clearance from LPDL treatments. Irregular pigmentation and skin texture improved from both treatments with no significant side-to-side differences [13] (II A). Comparing with laser therapy, IPL has been known to have weaker intensity and no down time. Recently, a new second generation IPL source with stronger irradiation and various filters has been developed. In a study by Konishi et al., this new second generation IPL system was tested as to the efficacy on facial pigmentary lesions such as solar lentigines and ephelides [14].

### Summary of Lasers for Superficial Pigmented Lesions

Solar lentigines, ephelides, and seborrheic keratoses can be treated with many types of lasers, but good results have been reported with the Q-switched 532-nm Nd:YAG, 694-nm Q-switched ruby, and 755-nm Q-switched alexandrite lasers. IPLs have also been shown to be of benefit in treating these superficial lesions. Patients should be forewarned that a temporary effect after treatment with any of these devices is a "dirty" look for 5–10 days [9]. As stated above, Q-switched lasers have been used for the treatment of lentigines but PIH can be an issue especially in darker skin individuals.

## Lasers for Dermal Pigmented Lesions and Tattoos

The types of lasers used in treatment of pigmented dermal lesions and removal of tattoos are often the same. Therefore, this section will cover the two topics together. The basic requirements of selective photothermolysis theory of Anderson and Parrish (appropriate wavelength, pulse duration, and energy setting) reveal why the quality-switch mode is optimal for pigmented dermal lesion and tattoo removal. In both cases, the targeted chromophore is located deeper in the dermis, requiring a longer wavelength to provide deeper penetration. Consideration of the short thermal relaxation time (TRT) of the small-sized melanin and ink particles indicates need for even shorter pulses of light in order to minimize thermal diffusion injury to surrounding structures. The pulses of light must deliver enough energy to achieve a therapeutic effect. There are three commonly used quality-switched (QS) lasers for deep pigmented lesions and tattoos, the QSRL delivering a 694-nm wavelength, the QS Alexandrite (QS Alex) delivering 755 wavelength, and the QS Neodymium:yttrium-aluminum-garnet (QS Nd:YAG) which can deliver a 1,064-nm wavelength. In addition, using a KTP crystal, the QS Nd:YAG laser can deliver a doubled-frequency 532-nm wavelength for treatment of superficial lesions and red tattoo pigment (Table 13.1).

**Table 13.1** Lasers types and parameters

| Laser (Q-switched) | Abbreviations | Wavelength (nm) | QS Pulse width (ns) |
| --- | --- | --- | --- |
| Ruby | QSRL | 694 | 28–40 |
| Alexandrite | QS Alex | 755 | 50–100 |
| Neodymium: yttrium-aluminum-garnet | QS Nd:YAG | 1,065 | 10–20 |
|  |  | 532 | 10–20 |

Adapted from Kuperman-Beade et al. [52]

## Lasers for Dermal Pigmented Lesions

Many patients seek removal of various dermal pigmented lesions due to their unappealing size, color, or location. We will include a discussion of lasers' role in lightening of such lesions, including nevus of Ota, Hori's nevus, melanocytic nevi, and drug-induced hyperpigmentation.

### Nevus of Ota

The nevus of Ota, or oculodermal melanocytosis, appears as a light brown/black to blue/gray macule-patch confined to the first and second trigeminal dermatomes, usually unilaterally. Ocular involvement as well as other extracutaneous disease can be present. The nevus of Ota is most often seen in black and Asian females and is associated with low malignant potential in these populations. Cosmetic removal is frequently sought due to its facial distribution and permanent quality. However, the nevus of Ota in the white population has been shown to portend a greater risk for malignant transformation. Therefore, laser-assisted removal is controversial as sublethal laser damage may promote residual melanocyte growth and play a yet unestablished role in malignant transformation. Reports of benign recurrence after successful laser treatment convey this uncertainty [15] (V/C). Assessment for removal must be made with clinical judgment in each individual case.

Numerous studies on all three QS lasers have showed them to be efficacious and safe for treatment of nevus of Ota (Table 13.2). There are differing reports on effective fluence, number of treatment sessions, and intervals, perhaps due to the variability of each lesion. The earliest studies reported therapeutic success with QSRL [16] (V/C) [17] (V/C). Yang studied the response to QSRL therapy of 81 Korean patients with nevus of Ota, and found it effective in achieving over 50% removal of nevus pigment when patients were assessed at 2 years. Transient hyperpigmentation was seen in about a third of patients and hypopigmentation in only three patients [18] (III/B). The efficacy of QSRL was reconfirmed in a study of 114 patients with nevus of Ota that demonstrated significant lightening after three or

more treatments, and the only side effect seen was transient hyperpigmentation after the first treatment [19] (III/B). Pediatric populations also respond favorably to QSRL therapy. In fact, earlier vs. later laser therapy may anticipate fewer side effects and recurrences [20] (III/B). However, few studies have explored the long-term complications of QSRL in treatment of nevus of Ota. One retrospective study described that although recurrence was rare, hypopigmentation was relatively common and could be permanent [21] (V/C). The other QS lasers are effective in eliminating nevus of Ota as well. Several studies demonstrated histological evidence of QS Alex laser-induced dermal melanocyte destruction and subsequent pigment clearing. These changes were associated with minimal transient pigmentary side effects and no scarring [22–24] (III/B). A recent retrospective study in China analyzing 602 cases of nevus of Ota treated with QS Alex and reaffirmed the safety and efficacy of this laser therapy application [25] (V/B). Chan conducted a series of studies comparing QS Alex with 1,064-nm QS Nd:YAG for nevus of Ota removal. Greater lightening was subjectively reported in the lesion half treated with QS Nd:YAG, although statistical significance was only determined in one case [26] (III/B). QS Alex treatment was better tolerated long-term than QS Nd:YAG, although it was associated with more immediate pain during treatment sessions. This pain was reducible with pre- and postoperative skin cooling methods [27, 28] (III/B). Comparisons of the side effect profiles between QS Alex, QS Nd:YAG, and combination therapy showed common hypopigmentation, less frequent hyperpigmentation, and scarring, but increased incidence of all side effects when both lasers were used [29] (V/B). Most recently, a case report described complete clearance of a nevus of Ota using fractionated photothermolysis with a 1,440-nm Nd:YAG laser [30] (V/C). More pilot studies are required to explore the application of this novel treatment modality for nevus of Ota therapy.

### Hori's Nevus

Hori's nevus is also known by several other names including acquired bilateral nevus-of-Ota-like

**Table 13.2** Laser treatment of nevus of Ota

| References | Design | QSRL 694 nm Laser | QS Alex 755 nm | QS Nd:YAG 1,065 nm | Fluence (J/cm$^2$) Settings | Spot size (mm) | Pulse width (ns) | Interval (months) |
|---|---|---|---|---|---|---|---|---|
| Kono et al. [20] | Trial: 46 children and 107 adults | ✓ | | | 5–7 | 4 | 30 | 3–4 |
| Kono et al. [21] | Retrospective: 101 patients | ✓ | | | 5–7 | 4 | 30 | – |
| Yang et al. [18] | 81 patients | ✓ | | | 6–8.5 | 4–6 | 40 | 1–4 |
| Watanabe and Takahashi [19] | 114 patients | ✓ | | | 6 | 4 | 30 | 3–4 |
| Chan et al. [26] | Trial: 40 patients. Each half of lesion was tx with either QS Alex or QS Nd:YAG | | ✓ | ✓ | A: 6–9, Y: 7–9 | 2 | A: 75, Y: 6 | 3–9 |
| Chan et al. [29] | Retrospective: 171 patients. Tx with QSAlex (A), QS Nd:YAG (Y) or both (B) | | ✓ | ✓ | A: 5–11, Y: 4–11 | 2–3 | A: 75, Y: 6 | – |
| Suh et al. [23] | Trial: 87 patients | | ✓ | | 6–7.75 | 3 | 100 | 1–2 |
| Wang et al. [25] | Trial: 602 patients | | ✓ | | 7.2±10 | – | – | 2–3 |
| Alster and Williams [22] | Trial: 7 patients | | ✓ | | 4.75–7 | – | 100 | 2–3 |
| Kang et al. [24] | Trial: 55 patients | | ✓ | | 7.5 | 3 | 100 | 3 |

| No. of treatments (mean) | % clearing | Hypopig-mentation (%) | Hyperpig-mentation (%) | Textural Δ (%) | Scarring (%) | Recur-rence (%) | Not reported |
|---|---|---|---|---|---|---|---|
| Results | | Side effects | | | | | Conclusions |
| 3.5*5.9 | 100*100 | 0*14 | 2*7 | 0*2 | 0*1 | 0*1 | Early QSRL treatment of nevus of Ota in children results in fewer required sessions and complications, but recurrence is still a concern Children |
| 5.5 | 75 | 16.8 | 5.9 | 3 | 1 | 1 | Most common QSRL treatment side effects are pigmentary changes; mainly hypopigmentation that may be permanent. Recurrence is rare but important in childhood cases |
| 5 | ≥50 | 3.7 | 40 | 0 | 0 | – | QSRL treatment is efficacious and safe, without scarring. However, transient pigmentary changes, especially hyperpig-mentation, are common |
| 4–5 3 2 1 | 70 40–69 10–39 9 | 0 | 7 | 0 | 0 | – | Multiple treatment sessions with QSRL increases response rate, and transient hyperpigmentation is the main side effect |
| 3–6 | A: 10–26, Y: 35–62 | A: 2.5, Y: 2.5 | A: 2.5, Y: 2.5 | A: 2.5, Y: 2.5 | A: 2.5, Y: 0 | – | QS Nd:YAG is superior to QS Alex in subjective assessments of lightening, but no statistical difference in efficacy was determined |
| Varied | Varied | A: 6, Y: 8, B: 18 | A: 2, V: 3, B: 1 | A: 2, V: 2, B: 2 | A: 1, V: 0, B: 1 | 18 | The most common side effect of QS Alex or QS Nd:YAG treat-ment is hypopigmentation, especially when both lasers are used. Recurrence is an important issue with special consideration to children |
| 1–15 | Varied: 7 7% pt with improve-ment | 9 | 16 | 0 | 0 | – | QS Alex is safe and effective, with better results after repeated treatments. Histologic evidence of laser-induced thermal damage of melanocytes demonstrated |
| 1–9 | Varied | 1.2 | 0.8 | – | 0 | – | QS Alex treatment is safe and effective with few cases of transient hypopigmentation as the main side effect. Increased treatment sessions yielded better results |
| 5 2 | 100 50 | 0 | 0 | 0 | 0 | – | QS Alex treatment is efficacious and can be without side effects. Histologic evidence demonstrates laser-induced elimination of upper dermal pigmenta-tion without epidermal disruption |
| 3 | ≥75 | 0 | 55 | 0 | 0 | – | QS Alex treatment is safe and effective but limited by hyperpig-mentation in darker skin types, delay in therapeutic effect, and lack of complete clearing. Histologic evidence of laser-induced selective destruction of melanocytes is demonstrated |

macules (ABNOM) and nevus fuscoceruleus zygomaticus (NFZ). It is a symmetrically distributed, blue or grayish-brown dermal melanocytosis that almost always involves the malar region. Onset is late, around age 20, with prevalence in Asian females.

Unlike nevus of Ota, this lesion is notorious for being difficult to remove by laser, as recurrence and PIH are frequent. Histological examination reveals more dermal melanocytes located in clusters and perivascularly than nevus of Ota, suggesting that laser-induced vascular damage may play a role in the increased PIH [31] (III/B). ABNOM can resemble melasma, and like melasma, also has significant epidermal pigmentation in addition to the dermal component. Thus, clearance of the epidermal pigmentation prior to laser treatment has shown to increase the efficacy of laser therapy. Newer therapeutic options of combining laser with other treatment modalities have shown great promise.

QSRL has been explored in combination with various other treatments for efficacy in removing ABNOM. One of the latest studies examined the combined use of IPL and QSRL in treating patients with complex dyspigmentation involving lesions such as ABNOM. They found this treatment modality to be effective in producing a 76–100% improvement in at least 60% of the patients with minimal side effects of transient hypo- and hyperpigmentation observed [32] (III/B). One study used a combination of QSRL and a topical bleaching protocol (0.1–0.4% tretinoin gel and 5% hydroquinone) given in repeated sessions and was able to achieve successful clinical results with less PIH than with QSRL therapy alone [33] (III/B). Another study utilizing topical bleaching pretreatment of ABNOM with QSRL showed similar results [34] (III/B). Manuskiatti conducted a split-face experiment using scanning $CO_2$ laser pretreatment on one side prior to QSRL and sole QSRL treatment on the other. Response was measured as decrease in melanin index and supported that epidermal ablation with $CO_2$ laser prior to QSRL produced significantly greater response and fewer cases of hypopigmentation [35] (II/A).

The other QS lasers have also been explored in treatment of ABNOM. The QS Alex laser showed promise in achieving at least 50% clearing in the majority of patients, however associated also with frequent erythema, hypo-, and hyperpigmentation [36] (III/B). QS Nd:YAG proved effective with repeated treatment sessions, achieving good-to-excellent clearing in half of the patients after three or more treatments. Still, the results were inferior to those seen with nevus of Ota [37] (III/B). A split-face study assessing the use of double-frequency 532-nm QS Nd:YAG before 1,065-nm QS Nd:YAG showed improved pigment clearance than 1,065-nm treatment alone [38] (III/B).

## Drug-Induced Hyperpigmentation

Drug-induced hyperpigmentation results when drug complexes precipitate in the dermis. These complexes are chromophores and give an unnatural hue to the overlying skin. One example includes the amiodarone-induced blue–gray or purple discoloration seen in a photosensitive distribution. QS lasers have been reported as an effective treatment option [39] (V/C).

Minocycline-induced hyperpigmentation (MIH) occurs not only in skin, but also in mucosal surfaces, nails, and teeth, leading to much patient distress. QS Alex has been described to effectively clear MIH with side effects limited to transient purpura and mild desquamation [40] (V/C). A 2002 review described varied results from use of the three QS lasers. It claimed that only one QS Nd:YAG study was successful in clearing MIH by employing up to eight treatment sessions. Other studies with QS Nd:YAG were not successful when fewer sessions were delivered. The QSRL demonstrated significant lightening of leg and facial hyperpigmentation, and both the 532-nm QS Nd:YAG and QS Alex were efficacious in the treatment of MIH. The reviewers then described their own findings of effective QSRL treatment of lingual MIH [41] (I/B).

## Melanocytic Nevi

Congenital melanocytic nevi can cause much social stigmatism due to their visible location or large size. Often, the anatomical position of the nevus makes surgical excision impossible to achieve for an aesthetically and functionally satisfactory result. A combination of using epithelial abrasion with $CO_2$ laser followed by QS Alex treatment showed efficacy and was associated with less pain, quicker recovery, and few required treatment sessions [42] (IV/B).

Giant congenital melanocytic nevi (GCMN) are rare and can be hugely disfiguring in addition to harboring malignant potential. Thus, treatment is focused on excision and lasers are only used when the surgical option is not feasible. Michel conducted an excellent review of the clinical studies that examined laser treatment of melanocytic nevi. He described that long-pulse ruby laser therapy actually showed enhanced penetration and fewer recurrences than QSRL. However, normal mode is still the most used pulse modality, demonstrating effective clearance without repigmentation after 6 weeks. There is histological evidence of laser-induced nevomelanocyte destruction, theoretically reducing the chance of malignant transformation [43] (I/B). However, some argue that laser treatment should be avoided as it is inadequate to remove malignant potential and only achieves mediocre clinical results [44] (V/C). Er:YAG laser resurfacing is another treatment option for inoperable medium-sized GCMN [45, 46] (III/B).

## Lasers and Tattoos

Tattooing is a sociocultural phenomenon that has arisen independently across various isolated civilizations throughout early human history [47] (I/B). Archeological evidence traces the most primitive tattoos to the Stone Age, approximately 12,000 bc. These crude patterns were created during acts of bereavement by rubbing ash into self-inflicted wounds [48]. Tattoo images appeared subsequently, around 400 bc, with the earliest known image portraying the Egyptian god, Bes. Considering our fickle human nature, it is not surprising that tattoo removal attempts arose early as well. The first record described salabrasion and was authored by the Greek physician Aetius in 543 ad. Abrasive techniques, such as salabrasion, involved mechanical induction of epidermal injury and inflammation in order to facilitate transdermal migration of pigment through the denuded surface. Other destructive modalities using caustic chemicals, infrared coagulation, electrocautery, or cryotherapy were also tried, but most often resulted in significant scarring with residual pigmentation. Surgical excision did not always achieve cosmetically pleasing results either. Unfortunately, these crude methods were the only option until the 1960s, when laser techniques in tattoo removal were introduced [47] (I/B).

In 1963, Goldman documented the first laser application in tattoos, using the normal mode ruby laser [49] (V/C). He closely followed this with a series of studies including reports of successful pigment clearance with the Nd:YAG and QSRL lasers [50, 51] (V/B). These results were largely overlooked at the time. Ironically, the scientific community remained focused on the familiar concept of tissue destruction; now using novel laser modalities of the $CO_2$ (10,600 nm) and argon lasers (488 and 514 nm) [48] (I/B). While these lasers offered more precise and uniform epidermal ablation [47] (I/B), their non-selective wavelengths and the continuous energy delivery caused significant collateral thermal injury. Similar to other abrasive techniques, hypertrophic scarring, textural and pigmentary alterations were frequent [52] (I/B). Two decades passed before the more selective QS delivery mode was revisited. This remains the mainstay of laser-assisted tattoo removal.

## Tattoo Types and Ink Substances

Various reasons motivate tattooing including self- or group-identity, cosmetic coverage, and most often, simple decoration. Tattoos are also acquired involuntarily; by medical need to demarcate a radiation treatment field, or by traumatic embedment of foreign, pigmented matter in explosions and other accidents. This results in a wide range of tattoo types (Table 13.3) [47] (I/B). The most important classification in regard to laser removal is the method of placement, either

**Table 13.3** Types of tattoos

| Type | Examples | Ink characteristics | Laser response | Side effects |
|---|---|---|---|---|
| Amateur | Cultural, tribal, or gang identification | Most often black India Ink, but also various other organic substances [48] | Excellent: complete clearance can be achieved with few treatment sessions | Few |
| Professional | Most common type | Diverse pigments, often inorganic metal salts [48] | Difficult: pigment densely and deeply placed. Various vibrant colors poorly targeted by available wavelengths [59] | Pigmentary changes and residual ink frequently seen. Allergic reactions possible [53] |
| Cosmetic | Scar coverage, eye or lip liner, enhanced eyebrows, lips, or rosy cheeks | Often brown, white or flesh-tones enhanced with iron or titanium | Difficult: flesh-tone pigments poorly target table by available wavelengths [59] | Risk of paradoxical darkening [60] |
| Medicinal | Radiation field markings | Most often blue–black India ink | Easily removed in 1–2 sessions | Few |
| Iatrogenic | Amalgam tattoos | Metallic | Good response to QSAlex and QSRL | Few |
| Traumatic | Following abrasions, explosions | Pigment from gunpowder, tar, and other particulate matter | Varies | Special care with combustible pigments [81] |

Adapted from Kuperman-Beade et al. [52] with additional data from Buchner [89] professional or amateur. The creation of amateur tattoos with uneven, but superficially placed, monochromatic ink allows excellent laser response with few complications. By contrast, professional tattoos involve a wider variety of pigments that are placed deeply and densely into the dermis. This creates challenges in selecting the appropriate laser and achieving complete clearance.

Each tattoo type achieves pigmentation with use of different substances as ink. Traumatic tattoos require special consideration as the responsible pigment may react dangerously with laser therapy [53] (V/C). Amateur tattoos most often employ black India ink, but concoctions of organic substances such as burnt wood, cotton, and paper, as well as vegetable matter have also been used [48] (I/B). Professional tattoos are notorious for their wide range undocumented chemical compositions and will continue to pose therapeutic challenges if government regulations are not implemented. Inorganic substances such as metal salts have been used in professional pigments, like chromium green, cobalt blue, or cadmium yellow. These chemicals are known to cause adverse cutaneous reactions [54] (V/C) and are already banned in Germany. Newly developed, quality-ensured organic pigments may show greater promise in accommodating laser removal. These include mono- and di-azo dyes, polycyclic pigments of phthalocyanine, and the pigment classes of dioxazine and quinacridone [55] (I/B). Very recently developed Freedom-2 ink technology uses microencapsulated polymer beads of biodegradable ink to allow complete clearance with just one laser treatment [56]. Current studies surrounding this controversial ink are lacking. The history of a tattoo should therefore be accurately assessed as certain characteristics of ink, laser treatment response, and side effects can be associated with each type [52] (I/B).

## Color-Based Laser Selection

Tattoo ink is an exogenous chromophore in the skin. Each pigment is maximally absorptive at specific wavelengths. In principle, elucidating this information allows a more targeted selection of laser device that produces the wavelength most similar to pigment's absorption spectra. However, the frequently undocumented chemical makeup of the tattoo pigments and further mixing of pigment in use make it very difficult to follow this principle. Previous in vitro and in vivo studies have revealed that some pure pigments are maximally absorptive at their complementary color wavelength [57] (IV/B) [58] (V/C). Beute et al. expanded on this finding with in vitro spectral analysis [59] (V/C). They used QS wavelengths of 532 and 752 nm to irradiate agar plates mixed with 28 various tattoo pigments and recorded their reaction. Consistent with previous trials, black and India ink had wide absorption spectra, thus responding well to both laser treatments. Red and green were best targeted at their complementary colors, by use of QS Nd:YAG 532 nm and QSRL, respectively. Yellow, orange, and flesh-toned shades poorly absorbed over the available QS treatment wavelengths, explaining why cosmetic tattoo removal is so challenging. They also made note of the paradoxical darkening of these pigments, first noted by Anderson et al. [60] (V/B), as they often contain iron and titanium that are oxidized by the laser (Table 13.4).

## Treatment Procedure

Prior to laser treatment, the patient should be interviewed regarding his/her tattoo as well as patient's medical history to anticipate possible complications (Table 13.5) [52] (I/B).

Other preoperative considerations include pain control. If needed, either a 1–2% lidocaine injection or anesthetic cream placed under occlusive dressing can be used prior to treatment to reduce pain. Recently, a compressive technique known as pneumatic skin-flattening has been shown to decrease perception of pain using the gate theory of pain transmission [61] (V/C). Posttreatment wound care with antibacterial ointments is argued, but most do recommend occlusive dressing with a moisturizing creams and avoidance of sun exposure.

**Table 13.4** Color-based laser selection

| Color | Max absorption (nm)*/spectrum | QS Nd:YAG 532 nm | QSRL 694 nm | QS Alex 755 nm | QS Nd:YAG 1,064 nm | Pulsed dye laser |
|---|---|---|---|---|---|---|
| | | Laser (fluence and no. of sessions – if reported) | | | | |
| Black | 600–800 | Ø | ✓✓† | ✓✓✓‡§ | ✓✓✓†‡ | |
| | Orange, red and near IR | | | (4–8, 8.9)§ | | |
| India ink | 600–800 | | | ✓† | | |
| | Orange, red and near IR | | | | | |
| Brown | 410–550 | | | | ✓‡ | |
| | Violet, blue, green | | | | | |
| Blue | 656–808 | Ø | | ✓✓✓‡§ | ✓✓✓ | |
| | Red and near IR | | | (4.8, 8.9)§ | | |
| Green | 570–800 | | ✓† | ✓✓‡‖ | Ø/✓ | |
| | Yellow, orange, red | | | (5.8, 9)‖ | | |
| Yellow | 470–485 | | | Ø | | |
| | Blue | | | | | |
| Orange | 420–540 | ✓ | | Ø | Ø/✓‡ | |
| | Violet, blue green | | | | | |
| Red | 500–570 | ✓/✓✓✓†‡ | | Ø/✓‖ | Ø/✓† | ✓¶ |
| | Green | (2–4)† | | (6.1, 9.7)‖ | (5–6)† | (3, 2)¶ |
| Purple | – | | ✓‡ | ✓‖ | | |
| | | | | (6.2, 10)‖ | | |
| Flesh | None | Darker | | Darker | | |
| | None | | | | | |
| White | 790 | Darker | | Ø | | |
| | Near IR | | | | | |

✓ minimal response; ✓✓ good response; ✓✓✓ excellent response; Ø no response
*Beute et al. [59] (in vitro data, QSRL wavelength equivalent of 752 nm was used)
†Levine and Geronemus [66]
‡Zelickson et al. [90]
§Fitzpatrick and Goldman [68]
‖Stafford et al. [91]
¶Alster [70]

**Table 13.5** Questions prior to laser tattoo removal

| Questions to ask prior to laser tattoo removal |
|---|
| Regarding tattoo |
|   What type of tattoo? |
|   When was it applied? |
|   How was it applied? |
|   Any allergic cutaneous reactions after application? |
| Regarding patient |
|   History of keloid formation? |
|   Allergies to antibacterial ointment? |
|   History of gold ingestion? |

## Selective Laser Systems

The QS laser systems remain the treatment of choice for tattoo removal, as recently emphasized by many reviews and studies (Table 13.6). While more than one laser type may be required for multicolored tattoos, appropriate device selection can achieve clearance with few incidence of scarring or permanent pigmentary alterations [47, 52, 55, 62] (I/B). The QSRL was the first of the QS laser systems to be explored in tattoo removal. Studies agree that black and dark blue pigments respond excellently to QSRL treatment [63] (II/A) [64] (III/B). Studies of newer QSRLs support good clearance of green pigment as well [65, 66] (V/B). In general, professional tattoos were harder to remove, requiring 6–10 or up to 20 treatment sessions. More recently placed tattoos with deeply located pigment on a distal site were also harder to remove due to less lymphatic involvement in removing residual ink particles [55] (I/B). These patterns were observed with other QS laser systems as well. A recent comparison study showed QSRL treatment resulted in greatest clearance rate of blue–black tattoos. However, it was also associated with the highest incidence of transient hypopigmentation [67] (III/B).

Like the other QS laser systems, QS Alex also effectively treats black and blue pigments [52] (I/B), but is better than others in removal of green pigment [47] (I/B). Fitzpatrick and Goldman demonstrated 95% clearance of black pigment after 8.9 average treatment sessions [68] (III/B). They followed up with an animal model demonstrating good removal of green as well but poor clearance of red [69] (III/B). Alster used a 510-nm pulsed dye laser to target residual red pigments after QS Alex therapy, and achieved clearance of amateur and professional tattoos in 4.6 and 8.5 treatment sessions, respectively. This study demonstrated no long-term pigmentary alterations, in contrast to the 50% incidence of hypopigmentation seen in the Fitzpatrick study [70] (III/B).

The QS Nd:YAG serves several particular uses. The 1,064-nm device is the laser of choice for removal of blue–black pigments in darker skin types. Its longer wavelength is less competitively absorbed by melanin and thus fewer pigmentary alterations result [65] (III/B). One study achieved 75–95% clearance of tattoo in Fitzpatrick type VI skin, without textural change or scarring and only two cases of hypopigmentation [71] (III/B). The frequency-doubled QS Nd:YAG with 532 nm facilitates clearance of red pigments after an average of three treatments [72] (II/A) [73] (III/B).

## Complications

The three leading complications following laser tattoo removal are pigmentary alterations, textural changes, and scarring. Risks of these adverse effects increase at higher fluences, which are often used when ink becomes refractory to a given laser [47, 52] (I/B). Instead, more than one laser system should be incorporated to utilize their different selectivities and prevent need to increase fluence.

Transient hypopigmentation is most frequent, typically lasting 2–6 months [55] (I/B). Due to wavelength parameters, a higher incidence of hypopigmentation is seen with QSRL and QS Alex compared to 1,064-nm QS Nd:YAG, making the latter a more suitable selection for darker skin [67] (III/B). Lower fluences can prevent hypopigmentation, along with pretreatment efforts to lighten darker skin like sunscreen use and bleaching with hydroquinone [47] (I/B). Hyperpigmentation can follow treatment with QS Nd:YAG, with incidence varying between 9 and 77%, and most cases transient [73] (III/B) [74] (II/A). It can be improved with hydroquinone and sun avoidance, and possibly also fractional photodermolysis [55] (I/B).

Textural changes occur infrequently with QS Nd:YAG, but can occur up to 12% following QS Alex treatment [52] (I/B). Improvement of textural change may be achieved after treatment with Erbium:YAG laser, $CO_2$ laser, or fractional photodermolysis [55] (I/B). Scarring is typically rare with appropriate laser treatment. Further reduction in incidence of scarring after QS Nd:YAG treatment has been shown with use of adjunctive measures such as Contractubex gel, a combination of onion extract, heparin, and allantoin gel [74] (II/A).

Cosmetic tattoos pose a special challenge, as they can darken immediately following laser treatment [60] (V/C). These tattoos contain various hues of red, white, and flesh-toned pigments created by iron, zinc, and titanium oxide content. Darkening of these pigments has been observed following treatment with the QS laser systems and other lasers [47] (I/B). This phenomenon may be partially explained by the oxidation of the ferrous oxide to the black-colored ferric oxide at the high temperatures induced by laser. Extensively repeated QS laser treatments can remove some of these darkened tattoos, although others may require ablative techniques with $CO_2$ laser that can result in scarring [75, 76] (V/C). Allergic reactions following laser treatment are serious but rare complications. Due to their

**Table 13.6** Laser treatment of tattoos

| Study | Design | Grade | QS Nd:YAG 532 nm Laser | QSRL 694 nm | QS Alex 755 nm | QS Nd:YAG 1,065 nm | Fluence (J/cm²) Settings | Spot size (mm) | Pulse width (ns) | Interval (months) |
|---|---|---|---|---|---|---|---|---|---|---|
| Ricotti et al. [88] | RCT: 20 patients given laser therapy with 5% imiquimod or placebo cream | II/A | ✓ | | ✓ | ✓ | – | – | – | 1–1.5 |
| Kilmer et al. [72] | RCT: 25 patients with 39 blue–black or multicolored tattoos | II/A | | | | ✓ | 6–12 | – | 10 | 0.75–1 |
| Taylor et al. [63] | RCT: 35 amateur and 22 professional blue–black tattoos | II/A | | ✓ | | | 1.5–8 | – | 40–80 | 0.8 |
| Ross et al. [85] | Trial: 16 tattoos each treated in designated area with pico- and nanosecond pulses | III/B | | | | ✓ | 0.6 | 1 | 35 ps 10 ns | 1 |
| Alster [70] | Trial: 24 multicolored professional (P) and 18 blue–black amateur (A) tattoos | III/B | | | ✓ | | P: 5.5–8 A: 4.75–8 | 3 | ## | 2 |
| Ferguson and August [73] | Trial: 221 amateur and 27 professional tattoos | III/B | ✓ | | | ✓ | 5–7 10–14 | 2 | 5–10 | – – |
| Ho et al. [74] | RCT: 144 professional tattoos | II/A | | | | ✓ | 3.6–4.8 | 3 | 6 | 2–2.5 |
| Fitzpatrick and Goldman [68] | Trial: 17 professional and 8 amateur tattoos | III/B | | | ✓ | | 4–8 | 3 | ## | – |
| Leuenberger et al. [67] | Comparative trial: 42 blue–black tattoos. Simultaneous treatment with QSRL, QS Alex, and QS Nd:YAG | III/B | | ✓ | ✓ | ✓ | 4–10 6–8 5–10 | 5 3 3 | 25–40 50–100 10–20 | 1.5–1.75 |

| Average no. of treatments | Results | Hypopig-mentation (%) | Hyperpig-mentation (%) | Textural Δ (%) | Scarring (%) | −: not reported |
|---|---|---|---|---|---|---|
| Results | | Side effects | | | | Conclusions |
| 6 | Mean clearance of around 51–75% seen in both groups | – – – | – – – | – – – | – – – | Imiquimod is an ineffective adjunct to laser tattoo removal. No statistical difference in clearance or treatment sessions was noted compared to placebo. More frequent side effects including pruritis, erythema, scale, burning, erosions and urticaria occurred in test group |
| 4 | >75% ink clearance in black tattoos; >95% black pigment clearance in multicolored tattoos | 0 | 0 | 0 | 0 | QS Nd:YAG effective for black tattoo ink removal, while bright colors were less responsive. Higher fluences yielded better results with good tolerance. No significant side effects observed |
| 5 | Complete clearance in 78% amateur and 23% professional | 0 | 0 | 0 | 1.8 | QSRL treatment is effective. Greater clearance seen at higher fluences with optimal fluence between 4 and 8 J/cm² |
| 4 | 12 of 16 tattoos showed greater lightening in picosecond-treated areas | # 0 | 0 0 | 0 0 | 0 12 | Picosecond pulses are more effective than nanosecond pulses in removal of black pigment. Histological evidence shows laser-induced changes in optical properties of ink are responsible for tattoo lightening |
| P: 8.5 A: 4.6 | 100 % clearance | 8 0 | 0 0 | 0 0 | 0 0 | QS Alex achieves comparable results to other lasers but with fewer incidence of pigmentary change, avoidance of tissue splatter, and minimal pain |
| 1–5 A:2, P:6.3 | 75% clearance in red 75% clearance | 2 | 77 | 0 | 1 | QS Nd:YAG effective in treating black pigment at 1,065 nm, and red at 532 nm. No response seen for yellow, orange blue, and green. Significant incidence of transient hyperpigmentation seen |
| 5.3 5.4 | Contractubex: 82% clearance Control: 80% clearance | # # | # 9 | – – | 11 24 | Contractubex is effective in reducing incidence of scar compared to control after QS Nd:YAG treatment. Hypopigmentation observed was permanent while hyperpigmentation was transient |
| 8.9 | 95% clearance | 50 | 0 | 12 | 0 | QS Alex is effective for removal of black tattoo pigment. Moderate effectiveness observed for blue and green, and only minimal effectiveness for red. Clinical and histologic consensus proved no scarring |
| 4–6 | >95% clearance in 38% of QSRL, 31% of QSAlex, and 23% of QS Nd:YAG sites | 38 2 0 | 0 0 7 | – – – | – – – | QSRL achieved the greatest clearance rate of blue–black tattoos with improved results after more treatment sessions. However, it was associated with the highest incidence of hypopigmentation, 38% |

potentially fatal consequences, a special mention of this complication follows.

Cutaneous allergic reaction to certain tattoo pigments is well known. Various pigments like chromium green, cobalt blue, or cadmium yellow contain metal salts that can trigger localized edema, erythema, or pruritis at the site of the tattoo. Red pigment has been notorious for causing the most tattoo-related allergic reactions. In the past, the suspected culprit was cinnabar (mercuric sulfide), but now additional immunogenic chemicals such as aromatic azo compounds have been identified in the red pigments [77] (V/C). Many individuals may asymptomatic at tattoo application but manifest a delayed reaction weeks after. Several studies report success in selectively removing the inflammatory lesions in red tattoo reactions with the $CO_2$ laser [78, 79], (V/C) and QS Erbium:YAG laser [80] (V/C).

Paradoxically, injury to the tattoo site, such as laceration and even laser application, may provoke allergic reaction in otherwise asymptomatic individuals. It is important to note that individuals who do exhibit cutaneous allergic reactions within a tattoo should be careful when seeking laser tattoo removal, as they are at greater risk for a systemic reaction from the procedure. There are no extensive reviews focusing on this complication of laser therapy but many case reports do exist.

The only known case of immediate cutaneous hypersensitivity reaction to QS Nd:YAG laser tattoo removal was published by England in 2002 [81] (V/C). The individual of study underwent laser treatment of two tattoos. Treatment of the first tattoo was without incident, but treatment of the second resulted in localized urticaria and induration within 30 min. No other immediate hypersensitivity reactions to laser tattoo removal have been reported but cases of delayed hypersensitivity reactions are well documented. They describe generalized urticaria developing days to weeks after QSRL and QS Nd:YAG treatments, as well as eczematous reaction presenting several weeks after $CO_2$ laser treatment [54, 82] (V/C).

A report was published this year describing two cases of noncutaneous immunoreactivity after laser removal of professional tattoos. They were attributed to laser-induced release or modification of pigment chemicals that manifested as regional lymphadenopathy, which eventually spontaneously resolved [83] (V/C).

The mechanism through which immunologic reaction occurs is unclear. Microscopic analysis studies of tattoo reaction to laser therapy has shown that laser application rapidly disrupts the membrane of pigment-laden cells and causes explosive vacuolization, leading to the extravasation of pigment particles into extracellular space [84] (V/C). No longer sequestered, the foreign particles may interact with immunologic cells and lead to the development of allergic reaction.

## Future Direction

The QS laser systems operate on the concept that shorter pulses allow great temperature increase with minimal collateral damage. Based on this, picosecond range pulses should be superior in delivering thermally confined damage and achieving greater tattoo clearance. Ross et al. tested this hypothesis and demonstrated that QS Nd:YAG treatment delivered in 35 ps pulses accomplished greater lightening than nanosecond-treated areas [85] (III/B). Similarly, use of the new, picosecond pulsed titanium-sapphire laser (795 nm) showed greater clearance than traditional QS alexandrite in a guinea pig model [86] (III/B). These studies suggest great promise in clinical use of picosecond pulses but more in vivo investigations are required.

Various modalities have been applied in attempts to enhance laser-assisted tattoo removal. One animal model used topical immunomodulator, Imiquimod, to achieve clinical and histological clearance of acute-phase tattoos [87] (III/B). A recent study applied this evidence to laser tattoo removal, but demonstrated Imiquimod an ineffective adjunct. Compared to laser and placebo cream, no statistical difference in clearance or treatment sessions and significantly greater side effects occurred [88] (II/A).

**Evidence-Based Summary**

| Findings | Evidence level |
|---|---|
| Pulsed dye laser delivered with compression for treatment of facial lentigines in Asians showed that LPDL delivered with the compression method is effective with a minimal side effect profile | II/A |
| QSRL provides a better treatment potential for superficial pigmented lesions than the frequency-doubled Q-switched neodymium:yttrium-aluminum-garnet laser (QSNd:YAG). Both showed no textural changes of the skin, yet QSRL is more painful and discomfortable than the frequency-doubled Nd:YAG | II/A |
| Shorter pulse widths of long-pulsed alexandrite laser in the treatment of solar lentigines as well as treatment without cryogen cooling both, independently, lowers the fluence threshold for lentigo clearance | II/A |
| Comparing with laser therapy, IPL has been shown to have weaker intensity and no down time when treating superficial pigmentation | III/B |
| Complete clearance of a nevus of Ota using fractionated photothermolysis with a 1,440-nm Nd:YAG laser had been described lately and with minimal side effects or adverse events | V/C |
| For melanocytic nevi, a combination of using epithelial abrasion with $CO_2$ laser followed by QS Alex treatment showed efficacy and was associated with less pain, quicker recovery, and few required treatment sessions | IV/B |
| Imiquimod proved to be an ineffective adjunct in laser tattoo removal | II/B |

# References

1. Kilmer SL, Goldman MP, Fitzpatrick RE. Treatment of benign pigmented cutaneous lesions. In: Goldman MP, Fitzpatrick RE, editors. Cutaneous laser surgery: the art and science of selective photodermolysis. 2nd ed. St. Louis: Mosby; 1999. p. 179–211.

2. Goldberg DJ. Procedures in cosmetic dermatology series: lasers and lights, vol. 1. New York: Saunders; 2005.

3. Tse Y, Levine VJ, McClain SA, Ashinoff R. The removal of cutaneous pigmented lesions with the Q-switched ruby laser and the Q-switched neodymium: yttrium-aluminum-garnet laser. A comparative study. J Dermatol Surg Oncol. 1994;20(12):795–800.

4. Trafeli JP, Kwan JM, Meehan KJ, et al. Use of a long-pulse alexandrite laser in the treatment of superficial pigmented lesions. Dermatol Surg. 2007;33(12): 1477–82.

5. Wang CC, Sue YM, Yang CH, Chen CK. A comparison of Q-switched alexandrite laser and intense pulsed light for the treatment of freckles and lentigines in Asian persons: a randomized, physician-blinded, split-face comparative trial. J Am Acad Dermatol. 2006;54(5):804–10.

6. Halder RM, Nootheti PK. Ethnic skin disorders overview. J Am Acad Dermatol. 2003;48(6 Suppl): S143–8.

7. Tanzi EL, Alster TS. Cutaneous laser surgery in darker skin phototypes. Cutis. 2004;73(1):21–4, 7–30.

8. Michel S, Hohenleutner U, Baumler W, Landthaler M. Q-switched ruby laser in dermatologic therapy. Use and indications. Hautarzt. 1997;48(7):462–70.

9. Kono T, Manstein D, Chan HH, Nozaki M, Anderson RR. Q-switched ruby versus long-pulsed dye laser delivered with compression for treatment of facial lentigines in Asians. Lasers Surg Med. 2006;38(2):94–7.

10. Kono T, Chan HH, Groff WF, et al. Long-pulse pulsed dye laser delivered with compression for treatment of facial lentigines. Dermatol Surg. 2007;33(8):945–50.

11. Sakamoto FH, Wall T, Avram MM, et al. Lasers and flashlamps in dermatology. In: Wolff K, Goldsmith LA, Katz SI, et al., editors. Fitzpatrick's dermatology in general medicine. New York: McGraw-Hill; 2008.

12. Kawada A, Shiraishi H, Asai M, et al. Clinical improvement of solar lentigines and ephelides with an intense pulsed light source. Dermatol Surg. 2002;28(6):504–8.

13. Jorgensen GF, Hedelund L, Haedersdal M. Long-pulsed dye laser versus intense pulsed light for photodamaged skin: a randomized split-face trial with blinded response evaluation. Lasers Surg Med. 2008;40(5):293–9.

14. Konishi N, Kawada A, Kawara S, et al. Clinical effectiveness of a novel intense pulsed light source on facial pigmentary lesions. Arch Dermatol Res. 2008;300 Suppl 1:S65–7.

15. Chan HH, Leung RS, Ying SY, Lai CF, Chua J, Kono T. Recurrence of nevus of Ota after successful treatment with Q-switched lasers. Arch Dermatol. 2000;136(9):1175–6.

16. Goldberg DJ, Nychay SG. Q-switched ruby laser treatment of nevus of Ota. J Dermatol Surg Oncol. 1992;18(9):817–21.

17. Geronemus RG. Q-switched ruby laser therapy of nevus of Ota. Arch Dermatol. 1992;128(12): 1618–22.

18. Yang HY, Lee CW, Ro YS, Yu HJ, Kim YT, Kim JH. Q-switched ruby laser in the treatment of nevus of Ota. J Korean Med Sci. 1996;11(2):165–70.

19. Watanabe S, Takahashi H. Treatment of nevus of Ota with the Q-switched ruby laser. N Engl J Med. 1994;331(26):1745–50.

20. Kono T, Chan HH, Ercocen AR, et al. Use of Q-switched ruby laser in the treatment of nevus of Ota in different age groups. Lasers Surg Med. 2003; 32(5):391–5.

21. Kono T, Nozaki M, Chan HH, Mikashima Y. A retrospective study looking at the long-term complications of Q-switched ruby laser in the treatment of nevus of Ota. Lasers Surg Med. 2001;29(2):156–9.

22. Alster TS, Williams CM. Treatment of nevus of Ota by the Q-switched alexandrite laser. Dermatol Surg. 1995;21(7):592–6.

23. Suh DH, Hwang JH, Lee HS, Youn JI, Kim PM. Clinical features of Ota's naevus in Koreans and its treatment with Q-switched alexandrite laser. Clin Exp Dermatol. 2000;25(4):269–73.

24. Kang W, Lee E, Choi GS. Treatment of Ota's nevus by Q-switched alexandrite laser: therapeutic outcome in relation to clinical and histopathological findings. Eur J Dermatol. 1999;9(8):639–43.

25. Wang HW, Liu YH, Zhang GK, et al. Analysis of 602 Chinese cases of nevus of Ota and the treatment results treated by Q-switched alexandrite laser. Dermatol Surg. 2007;33(4):455–60.

26. Chan HH, Ying SY, Ho WS, Kono T, King WW. An in vivo trial comparing the clinical efficacy and complications of Q-switched 755 nm alexandrite and Q-switched 1064 nm Nd:YAG lasers in the treatment of nevus of Ota. Dermatol Surg. 2000;26(10): 919–22.

27. Chan HH, King WW, Chan ES, et al. In vivo trial comparing patients' tolerance of Q-switched Alexandrite (QS Alex) and Q-switched neodymium:yttrium-aluminum-garnet (QS Nd:YAG) lasers in the treatment of nevus of Ota. Lasers Surg Med. 1999;24(1): 24–8.

28. Chan HH, Lam LK, Wong DS, Wei WI. Role of skin cooling in improving patient tolerability of Q-switched Alexandrite (QS Alex) laser in nevus of Ota treatment. Lasers Surg Med. 2003;32(2):148–51.

29. Chan HH, Leung RS, Ying SY, et al. A retrospective analysis of complications in the treatment of nevus of Ota with the Q-switched alexandrite and Q-switched Nd:YAG lasers. Dermatol Surg. 2000;26(11): 1000–6.

30. Kouba DJ, Fincher EF, Moy RL. Nevus of Ota successfully treated by fractional photothermolysis using a fractionated 1440-nm Nd:YAG laser. Arch Dermatol. 2008;144(2):156–8.

31. Lee B, Kim YC, Kang WH, Lee ES. Comparison of characteristics of acquired bilateral nevus of Ota-like macules and nevus of Ota according to therapeutic outcome. J Korean Med Sci. 2004;19(4):554–9.

32. Park JM, Tsao H, Tsao S. Combined use of intense pulsed light and Q-switched ruby laser for complex dyspigmentation among Asian patients. Lasers Surg Med. 2008;40(2):128–33.

33. Yoshimura K, Sato K, Aiba-Kojima E, et al. Repeated treatment protocols for melasma and acquired dermal melanocytosis. Dermatol Surg. 2006;32(3):365–71.

34. Momosawa A, Yoshimura K, Uchida G, et al. Combined therapy using Q-switched ruby laser and bleaching treatment with tretinoin and hydroquinone for acquired dermal melanocytosis. Dermatol Surg. 2003;29(10):1001–7.

35. Manuskiatti W, Sivayathorn A, Leelaudomlipi P, Fitzpatrick RE. Treatment of acquired bilateral nevus of Ota-like macules (Hori's nevus) using a combination of scanned carbon dioxide laser followed by Q-switched ruby laser. J Am Acad Dermatol. 2003;48(4):584–91.

36. Lam AY, Wong DS, Lam LK, Ho WS, Chan HH. A retrospective study on the efficacy and complications of Q-switched alexandrite laser in the treatment of acquired bilateral nevus of Ota-like macules. Dermatol Surg. 2001;27(11):937–41; discussion 41–2.

37. Polnikorn N, Tanrattanakorn S, Goldberg DJ. Treatment of Hori's nevus with the Q-switched Nd:YAG laser. Dermatol Surg. 2000;26(5):477–80.

38. Ee HL, Goh CL, Khoo LS, Chan ES, Ang P. Treatment of acquired bilateral nevus of Ota-like macules (Hori's nevus) with a combination of the 532 nm Q-Switched Nd:YAG laser followed by the 1,064 nm Q-switched Nd:YAG is more effective: prospective study. Dermatol Surg. 2006;32(1):34–40.

39. Wiper A, Roberts DH, Schmitt M. Amiodarone-induced skin pigmentation: Q-switched laser therapy, an effective treatment option. Heart. 2007; 93(1):15.

40. Alster TS, Gupta SN. Minocycline-induced hyperpigmentation treated with a 755-nm Q-switched alexandrite laser. Dermatol Surg. 2004;30(9):1201–4.

41. Friedman IS, Shelton RM, Phelps RG. Minocycline-induced hyperpigmentation of the tongue: successful treatment with the Q-switched ruby laser. Dermatol Surg. 2002;28(3):205–9.

42. Chong SJ, Jeong E, Park HJ, Lee JY, Cho BK. Treatment of congenital nevomelanocytic nevi with the $CO_2$ and Q-switched alexandrite lasers. Dermatol Surg. 2005;31(5):518–21.

43. Michel JL. Laser therapy of giant congenital melanocytic nevi. Eur J Dermatol. 2003;13(1):57–64.

44. Helsing P, Mork G, Sveen B. Ruby laser treatment of congenital melanocytic naevi – a pessimistic view. Acta Derm Venereol. 2006;86(3):235–7.

45. Rajpar SF, Abdullah A, Lanigan SW. Er:YAG laser resurfacing for inoperable medium-sized facial congenital melanocytic naevi in children. Clin Exp Dermatol. 2007;32(2):159–61.

46. Ostertag JU, Quaedvlieg PJ, Kerckhoffs FE, et al. Congenital naevi treated with erbium:YAG laser (Derma K) resurfacing in neonates: clinical results and review of the literature. Br J Dermatol. 2006;154(5):889–95.

47. Bernstein EF. Laser treatment of tattoos. Clin Dermatol. 2006;24(1):43–55.

48. Kilmer SL, Goldman MP, Fitzpatrick RE. Treatment of tattoos. In: Goldman MP, Fitzpatrick RE, editors. Cutaneous laser surgery: the art and science of selective photodermolysis. 2nd ed. St. Louis: Mosby; 1999. p. 213–57.

49. Goldman L, Blaney DJ, Kindel Jr DJ, Franke EK. Effect of the laser beam on the skin. Preliminary report. J Invest Dermatol. 1963;40:121–2.

50. Goldman L, Wilson RG, Hornby P, Meyer RG. Radiation from a Q-switched ruby laser. Effect of repeated impacts of power output of 10 megawatts on a tattoo of man. J Invest Dermatol. 1965;44:69–71.

51. Goldman L, Rockwell RJ, Meyer R, Otten R, Wilson RG, Kitzmiller KW. Laser treatment of tattoos. A preliminary survey of three year's clinical experience. JAMA. 1967;201(11):841–4.

52. Kuperman-Beade M, Levine VJ, Ashinoff R. Laser removal of tattoos. Am J Clin Dermatol. 2001;2(1): 21–5.

53. Fusade T, Toubel G, Grognard C, Mazer JM. Treatment of gunpowder traumatic tattoo by Q-switched Nd:YAG laser: an unusual adverse effect. Dermatol Surg. 2000;26(11):1057–9.

54. Ashinoff R, Levine VJ, Soter NA. Allergic reactions to tattoo pigment after laser treatment. Dermatol Surg. 1995;21(4):291–4.

55. Pfirrmann G, Karsai S, Roos S, Hammes S, Raulin C. Tattoo removal – state of the art. J Dtsch Dermatol Ges. 2007;5(10):889–97.

56. Freedom-2, LLC to Offer the First Permanent but Removable Tattoo Ink. Business Wire. 18 Oct 2006. http://www.allbusiness.com/services/business-services/3944154-1.html. Accessed 10 Nov 2008.

57. Haedersdal M, Bech-Thomsen N, Wulf HC. Skin reflectance-guided laser selections for treatment of decorative tattoos. Arch Dermatol. 1996;132(4):403–7.

58. Baumler W, Landthaler M. Laser therapy for tattoos. MMW Fortschr Med. 2006;148(41):37, 9–40.

59. Beute TC, Miller CH, Timko AL, Ross EV. In vitro spectral analysis of tattoo pigments. Dermatol Surg. 2008;34(4):508–15; discussion 15–6.

60. Anderson RR, Geronemus R, Kilmer SL, Farinelli W, Fitzpatrick RE. Cosmetic tattoo ink darkening. A complication of Q-switched and pulsed-laser treatment. Arch Dermatol. 1993;129(8):1010–4.

61. Lapidoth M, Akerman L. Pain inhibition in Q-switched laser tattoo removal with pneumatic skin flattening (PSF): a pilot study. J Cosmet Laser Ther. 2007;9(3):164–6.

62. Burris K, Kim K. Tattoo removal. Clin Dermatol. 2007;25(4):388–92.

63. Taylor CR, Gange RW, Dover JS, et al. Treatment of tattoos by Q-switched ruby laser. A dose-response study. Arch Dermatol. 1990;126(7):893–9.

64. Scheibner A, Kenny G, White W, Wheeland RG. A superior method of tattoo removal using the Q-switched ruby laser. J Dermatol Surg Oncol. 1990;16(12):1091–8.

65. Kilmer SL, Anderson RR. Clinical use of the Q-switched ruby and the Q-switched Nd:YAG (1064 nm and 532 nm) lasers for treatment of tattoos. J Dermatol Surg Oncol. 1993;19(4):330–8.

66. Levine VJ, Geronemus RG. Tattoo removal with the Q-switched ruby laser and the Q-switched Nd:YAGlaser: a comparative study. Cutis. 1995;55(5): 291–6.

67. Leuenberger ML, Mulas MW, Hata TR, Goldman MP, Fitzpatrick RE, Grevelink JM. Comparison of the Q-switched alexandrite, Nd:YAG, and ruby lasers in treating blue-black tattoos. Dermatol Surg. 1999;25(1): 10–4.

68. Fitzpatrick RE, Goldman MP. Tattoo removal using the alexandrite laser. Arch Dermatol. 1994;130(12): 1508–14.

69. Fitzpatrick RE, Goldman MP, Ruiz-Esparza J. Use of the alexandrite laser (755 nm, 100 nsec) for tattoo pigment removal in an animal model. J Am Acad Dermatol. 1993;28(5 Pt 1):745–50.

70. Alster TS. Q-switched alexandrite laser treatment (755 nm) of professional and amateur tattoos. J Am Acad Dermatol. 1995;33(1):69–73.

71. Jones A, Roddey P, Orengo I, Rosen T. The Q-switched ND:YAG laser effectively treats tattoos in darkly pigmented skin. Dermatol Surg. 1996;22(12):999–1001.

72. Kilmer SL, Lee MS, Grevelink JM, Flotte TJ, Anderson RR. The Q-switched Nd:YAG laser effectively treats tattoos. A controlled, dose-response study. Arch Dermatol. 1993;129(8):971–8.

73. Ferguson JE, August PJ. Evaluation of the Nd/YAG laser for treatment of amateur and professional tattoos. Br J Dermatol. 1996;135(4):586–91.

74. Ho WS, Ying SY, Chan PC, Chan HH. Use of onion extract, heparin, allantoin gel in prevention of scarring in Chinese patients having laser removal of tattoos: a prospective randomized controlled trial. Dermatol Surg. 2006;32(7):891–6.

75. Herbich GJ. Ultrapulse carbon dioxide laser treatment of an iron oxide flesh-colored tattoo. Dermatol Surg. 1997;23(1):60–1.

76. Fitzpatrick RE, Lupton JR. Successful treatment of treatment-resistant laser-induced pigment darkening of a cosmetic tattoo. Lasers Surg Med. 2000;27(4): 358–61.

77. Bendsoe N, Hansson C, Sterner O. Inflammatory reactions from organic pigments in red tattoos. Acta Derm Venereol. 1991;71(1):70–3.

78. Kyanko ME, Pontasch MJ, Brodell RT. Red tattoo reactions: treatment with the carbon dioxide laser. J Dermatol Surg Oncol. 1989;15(6):652–6.

79. Bhardwaj SS, Brodell RT, Taylor JS. Red tattoo reactions. Contact Dermatitis. 2003;48(4):236–7.

80. De Argila D, Chaves A, Moreno JC. Erbium:Yag laser therapy of lichenoid red tattoo reaction. J Eur Acad Dermatol Venereol. 2004;18(3):332–3.

81. England RW, Vogel P, Hagan L. Immediate cutaneous hypersensitivity after treatment of tattoo with Nd:YAG laser: a case report and review of the literature. Ann Allergy Asthma Immunol. 2002;89(2):215–7.

82. Zemtsov A, Wilson L. $CO_2$ laser treatment causes local tattoo allergic reaction to become generalized. Acta Derm Venereol. 1997;77(6):497.

83. Izikson L, Avram M, Anderson RR. Transient immunoreactivity after laser tattoo removal: report of two cases. Lasers Surg Med. 2008;40(4):231–2.

84. Taylor CR, Anderson RR, Gange RW, Michaud NA, Flotte TJ. Light and electron microscopic analysis of tattoos treated by Q-switched ruby laser. J Invest Dermatol. 1991;97(1):131–6.

85. Ross V, Naseef G, Lin G, et al. Comparison of responses of tattoos to picosecond and nanosecond Q-switched neodymium: YAG lasers. Arch Dermatol. 1998;134(2):167–71.

86. Herd RM, Alora MB, Smoller B, Arndt KA, Dover JS. A clinical and histologic prospective controlled comparative study of the picosecond titanium:sapphire (795 nm) laser versus the Q-switched alexandrite (752 nm) laser for removing tattoo pigment. J Am Acad Dermatol. 1999;40(4):603–6.

87. Solis RR, Diven DG, Colome-Grimmer MI, Snyder NT, Wagner RF Jr. Experimental nonsurgical tattoo removal in a guinea pig model with topical imiquimod and tretinoin. Dermatol Surg. 2002;28(1):83–6; discussion 6–7.

88. Ricotti CA, Colaco SM, Shamma HN, Trevino J, Palmer G, Heaphy Jr MR. Laser-assisted tattoo removal with topical 5% imiquimod cream. Dermatol Surg. 2007;33(9):1082–91.

89. Buchner A. Amalgam tattoo ( amalgam pigmentation) of the oral mucosa: clinical manifestations, diagnosis, and treatment. Refuat Hapeh Vehashinayim. 2004; 21(3):25–8, 92.

90. Zelickson BD, Mehregan DA, Zarrin AA, Coles C, Hartwig P, Olson S, Leaf-Davis J. Clinical, histologic, and ultrastructural evaluation of tattoos treated with 3 laser systems. Lasers Surg Med. 1994; 15(4):364–72.

91. Stafford TJ, Lizek R, Tan OT. Role of the Alexandrite laser for removal of tattoos. Lasers Surg Med. 1995; 17(1):32–8.

## Self-Assessment

1. Visible (400–760 nm) wavelength lasers produce light which is well absorbed by the:
   (a) Cornea
   (b) Retina
   (c) Iris
   (d) Sclera

2. An advantage of using an Nd:YAG 1,064-nm laser includes:
   (a) Decreased absorption by epidermal melanin
   (b) Decreased discomfort during treatments
   (c) Increased efficacy when compared to similar devices
   (d) Increased absorption by epidermal melanin

3. Multicolored tattoos are most effectively treated with a combination of the following lasers:
   (a) Q-switched Nd:YAG (1,064 nm) and frequency-doubled Q-switched Nd:YAG (532 nm)
   (b) Pulsed dye(585 nm) and Q-switched Nd:YAG (1,064 nm)
   (c) Pulsed Er:YAG (2,940) and Q-switched Alexandrite (755 nm)
   (d) Frequency-doubled Q-switched Nd:YAG (532 nm) and continuous $CO_2$ (10,600 nm)

4. The following pigmented lesion(s) respond(s) best to the least number of laser treatments:
   (a) Lentigines
   (b) Nevus of Ota
   (c) Melasma
   (d) Café au lait macules

5. The proposed mechanism(s) of action for laser tattoo removal includes:
   (a) Lymphatic elimination of micronized pigment particles
   (b) Phagocytosis of pigment particles
   (c) Elimination of pigment particles via an epidermal wound
   (d) All of the above

6. Nd:YAG 532 nm and QSRL(ruby) best target which tattoo colors
   (a) Black
   (b) Red
   (c) Green
   (d) (b) and (c)
   (e) All

7. The laser of choice for removal of blue–black pigments in darker skin types is:
   (a) 1,064
   (b) 532
   (c) Both (a) and (b)
   (d) 585
   (e) 595

## Answers

1. 1.b: Retina
2. 2.a: Decreased absorption by epidermal melanin
3. 3.a: Q-switched Nd:YAG (1,064 nm) and frequency-doubled Q-switched Nd:YAG (532 nm)
4. 4.a: Lentigines
5. 5.c: Elimination of pigment particles via an epidermal wound
6. 6.d: (b) and (c)
7. 7.a: 1,064

# Ablative Resurfacing: Laser, Chemical Peels, and Dermabrasion

Ali Jabbari and Vicki J. Levine

## Introduction and Procedure Overview

Improving the appearance of facial rhytides and scars can be addressed by ablative resurfacing techniques. The goal of these methods is to eliminate the epidermis and at least a portion of the underlying dermis in a controlled fashion to allow for healing to a more cosmetically acceptable endpoint. Ablative resurfacing techniques include mechanical disruption, chemical disruption, or photothermolysis, achieved by dermabrasion, chemical peels, and laser-based modalities, respectively.

Dermabrasion is a technique used to mechanically disrupt the skin to improve rhytides or revise scars. The types of tools used include the motor-driven rotating diamond fraise (see Fig. 14.1) or wire brush as well as manual dermasanding instruments. Dermabrasion is more commonly used to correct the appearance of scars and for the improvement of local facial rhytides, as opposed to more widespread facial resurfacing. In addition to appropriate patient selection, the successful use of dermabrasion is thought to highly depend on user experience.

Chemical peeling is the use of a chemical exfoliant to improve facial rhytides and photodamaged skin [1]. Peels are classified as superficial, medium, or deep-based on the depth of tissue ablation; superficial peels affect only the epidermis, medium-depth peels affect the epidermis and papillary dermis, and deep peels go beyond the papillary dermis into the reticular dermis. Superficial peels are not thought to be sufficient for resurfacing purposes, as they leave the dermis largely unaffected.

Medium depth chemical peels cause necrotic changes of the epidermis and papillary dermis [2]. Trichloroacetic acid (TCA), at concentrations ranging from 35 to 50%, is the agent most often used in medium-depth peel preparations. When used alone, concentrations of TCA at the higher end of this range are often needed to achieve a favorable cosmetic outcome; however, these higher concentrations have a higher rate of side effects including pigmentary and topographic irregularities. Combination peels have been developed in which lower concentrations of TCA are used that achieve adequate absorption while limiting morbidity. The most commonly used preparations used for medium-depth chemical peels include the sequential use of either Jessner's solution (see Table 14.1) [3] or 70% glycolic acid [4] prior to the application of 35% TCA.

Deep chemical peels may be used for patients with deep facial rhytides or more pronounced facial photoaging. Virtually, the only preparation in use for deep chemical peels is the Baker Gordon formula, in which phenol is the active component [5]. Precautions such as the incremental application of the formula to successive cosmetic units and intravenous fluid administration are taken to

A. Jabbari • V.J. Levine (✉)
Ronald O. Perelman Department of Dermatology,
NYU Medical Center, New York, NY 10016, USA
e-mail: vickilevine1@gmail.com

M. Alam (ed.), *Evidence-Based Procedural Dermatology*,
DOI 10.1007/978-0-387-09424-3_14, © Springer Science+Business Media, LLC 2012

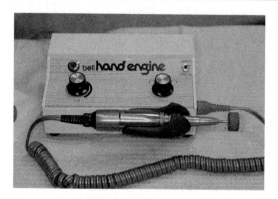

**Fig. 14.1** Motor-driven dermabrasion unit

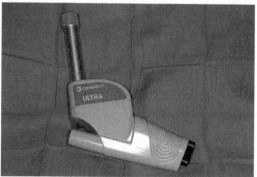

**Fig. 14.2** Handpiece for scanning $CO_2$ laser

**Table 14.1** Preparation used for medium-depth chemical peels

| Component | Amount |
| --- | --- |
| Lactic acid | 14 mL |
| Resorcinol | 14 g |
| Salicylic acid | 14 g |
| Ethanol (95%) | QSAD 100 mL |

limit systemic absorption and toxicity during the procedure. Perioperative cardiac monitoring and oxygen supplementation are also required. These precautions, as well as the procedure's time-consuming nature and higher rate of side effects, limit its use.

Laser-based resurfacing is the newest ablative modality for treatment of facial rhytides and photoaging. The carbon dioxide ($CO_2$) and the erbium:yttrium-aluminum-garnet (Er:YAG) lasers emit photons at wavelengths absorbed by water, resulting in vaporization of the cutaneous skin. Besides the wavelength of emitted photons, the depth of tissue injury is also dependent on the fluence and spot size of the laser.

The first lasers used for ablative resurfacing were $CO_2$ lasers (see Fig. 14.2). The two most commonly used models are a pulsed $CO_2$ laser and a scanning $CO_2$ laser (in which the laser beam is focused and scanned in a spiral pattern to limit dwell time) [6]. These lasers emit photons at a wavelength of 10,600 nm, causing immediate tissue vaporization as well as a minimal amount of residual thermal damage. The residual thermal damage is thought to be important in immediate collagen shrinkage and skin tightening [7]. The $CO_2$

lasers have the advantage of causing coagulative hemostasis, resulting in minimal bleeding.

Er:YAG lasers emit photons at a wavelength of 2,940 nm, resulting in 12–18 fold greater absorption by water when compared with the $CO_2$ lasers [8]. In comparison to the $CO_2$ lasers, the Er:YAG produces less residual thermal damage and therefore less immediate collagen shrinkage and skin tightening. Ablation of the epidermis usually requires more passes with the Er:YAG than with the $CO_2$ laser at standard fluences. Additionally, the Er:YAG does not cause the same degree of hemostasis as the $CO_2$ lasers, leading to relatively more intraoperative bleeding.

Fractional laser systems will be discussed in other chapters.

## Consensus Statements

Guidelines for dermabrasion were last published in the *Journal of the American Academy of Dermatology* in 1994. This document outlines the indications, physician qualifications, preoperative diagnostic criteria, intraoperative recommendations, and postoperative care as it pertains to the dermabrasion procedure.

There are no published guidelines for chemical peels. A useful review with practical information is cited below [2].

There are no published guidelines specifically for ablative resurfacing using lasers. However, the American Society for Laser Medicine and Surgery is a professional society that has devised standards and guidelines for laser therapeutics in all fields of medicine. This organization has released a set of documents under the heading of "standards of practice" that is accessible on the Internet (http://www.aslms.org/public/standards.shtml). Relevant documents, as it pertains to the practicing dermatologist using laser technology for ablative resurfacing purposes, include guidelines for office-based laser procedures and standards of training for dermatologists.

## Evidence

Listed below are what we deemed were the highest quality studies addressing the questions listed. No meta-analyses were encountered in our review of the literature. For the purposes of rating the level of evidence of each study, we considered prospective, split-face, and split-scar models in which each hemiface or half-scar received a randomly assigned treatment to be considered a rating of II.

## How Effective Is Manual Dermabrasion at Reducing Scars?

Poulos et al. examined the use of dermasanding in treating facial scars formed following a surgical excision [9] (II/A). Fifteen patients who had undergone a surgical procedure on the face within 8 weeks prior to enrollment with scars at least 2 cm in length that were not largely asymmetric were enrolled in this prospective study. Dermasanding using sterile sandpaper was performed on a randomly assigned half of the facial scar, and the other half was not manipulated. Photographs were taken at 1, 3, and 6 months following the procedure, and the appearance of the halves was compared to each other by two blinded reviewers. At 1 and 3 months after dermasanding, the dermasanded side was thought to have a better overall appearance only 57% (8 of 14 scars) and 54% (6 of 11) of the time, respectively, with the untreated side having equal or better overall appearance the remaining percentages of the time. At 6 months following the procedure, however, the side that was treated with dermasanding was assessed to

have a better overall appearance in 12 of 15 (80%) scars. Three of 15 (20%) scars were graded to have a better clinical appearance on the untreated side; the authors state that this may be due to minor asymmetry in the scars, as all three scars involved the "the lower aspect of the nose in areas with inherent asymmetry." In total, though, the authors conclude that dermasanding is an effective treatment for scars.

## How Does Manual Dermasanding Compare with Motorized Dermabrasion with a Diamond Fraise in the Treatment of Facial Scars?

Gillard et al. compared dermasanding with a hand-held motorized diamond fraise to manual dermasanding in the treatment of postsurgical facial scars [10] (II/A). Twenty-one patients with facial scars, made up of 14 patients who had undergone reconstruction following Mohs excisions 6–12 weeks prior and seven patients who had wounds left to heal by secondary intention 4–32 weeks prior, were enrolled in this prospective study. Scars were divided in half and each side was randomly assigned to treatment by either motorized dermabrasion with a diamond fraise or dermasanding with a medium-grade drywall-plaster sanding screen. A blinded reviewer judged each scar, comparing the two halves to each other based on a specific list of variables depending on the time after the procedure. No significant differences were observed in terms of erythema, contour correction, hypertrophic scarring, scar line visibility, or pigmentary changes at any time point up to 6 months following the procedures; additionally no changes were observed in the first 4 weeks in terms of re-epithelialization, number of milia, infection, or patient's pain, the only time points where these variables were assessed. Interestingly, no patient exhibited any perceived difference in correction of contour at any time point between the two treated halves. The authors conclude from this study that manual dermasanding and motorized dermabrasion are equally effective in the treatment of facial scars.

## How Does Dermabrasion Compare with Laser Resurfacing at Reducing Facial Rhytides?

Kitzmiller et al. compared an electric rotary dermabrader to a pulsed $CO_2$ laser in the treatment of perioral rhytides [11] (II/A). Twenty female patients were subjected to dermabrasion to a randomly assigned half of the perioral area and 2–4 passes of pulsed $CO_2$ treatment (300 mJ) to the opposite half of the perioral area. Photographs were taken at 1 week, 1 month, and 6 months following the procedures, and a blinded panel of ten plastic surgeons graded the improvement of the perioral rhytides in the photographs. The authors reported a small but statistically significant greater improvement of the perioral rhytides on the side treated with the pulsed $CO_2$ laser at 1 month and at 6 months; both treatments reduced the facial rhytides by about 50%. An increased amount of erythema was also reported for the pulsed $CO_2$ laser-treated area when compared to the dermabrasion-treated area at 1 month, however. Also included in the study was a patient-reported survey taken 6 months after treatment. The patients' overall impression was that the laser gave a better result, but was also associated with worse intraoperative pain and postoperative drainage. Interestingly, patients reported that they would recommend both procedures equally to a friend. The authors concluded that the pulsed $CO_2$ laser is slightly more effective at improving perioral rhytides than dermabrasion, although they acknowledged that this change may not have been observed if they were more aggressive with their dermabrasion technique and recommend weighing the operator's experience with each technique before determining which modality would be optimal for a specific patient.

Holmvist and Rogers compared a pulsed, scanning $CO_2$ laser with dermabrasion treatments in the treatment of perioral rhytides in a similar split-face manner [12] (II/A). Fifteen patients received $CO_2$ laser treatment (4.24 $J/cm^2$) to a randomly assigned half of the perioral area and dermabrasion with either a motor-driven diamond fraise or manual dermasanding with a medium-grade drywall sanding screen. The choice of dermabrasion technique was randomly determined. All patients were treated with tretinoin and hydroquinone for 2 weeks prior to the procedures. At different time points up to 4 months following the procedure, two blinded lab technicians examined the patients and together decided on a score based on a graded scale. No statistically significant differences were found for improvement in rhytides between the laser-treated side and aggregate dermabrasion-treated side at 4 months, although it was observed that the laser-treated side exhibited delayed re-epithelialization and a longer duration of erythema. When the patients were surveyed as to which side exhibited the superior outcome, most stated either the laser-treated side (7 of 14 patients) or no difference between the two sides (6 of 14 patients), with only one respondent endorsing the dermabrasion treatment. The blinded observers conducted a similar exercise and their preferences largely reflected that of the patients (with 6 of 14 judging the laser-treated side to have a superior outcome, 7 of 14 stating no difference, and 1 of 14 preferring the dermabrasion-treated side). The authors concluded that both methodologies were effective in the improvement of perioral rhytides, although the $CO_2$ laser treatment was associated with prolonged side effects.

Gin et al. used a similar approach to evaluate and compare the efficacies of a scanning $CO_2$ laser with motorized dermabrasion with either a pear-shaped or a dome-shaped diamond fraise in the treatment of perioral rhytides (II/A) [13]. The perioral area was divided into halves, and one half was randomly selected to be treated with the motor-driven diamond fraise and the other half with the $CO_2$ laser. Rhytides were evaluated on a graded scale preoperatively and at different time points following the procedure out to 26 weeks; it is unclear from the article who did the evaluating. Of the 19 patients who completed the study, the mean rhytide score for the laser-treated and dermabrasion-treated side went from $4.4 \pm 0.2$ and $4.3 \pm 0.2$ (out of 5), respectively, to $1.8 \pm 0.3$ and $1.5 \pm 0.3$; the difference between the laser treatment and the dermabrasion treatment was not statistically significant. Major differences were not observed for postoperative erythema between the two techniques. These authors concluded that these techniques are equally effective in the treatment of perioral rhytides.

## How Does Chemical Peeling Compare to Laser Resurfacing in Reducing Facial Rhytides?

Reed et al. compared a medium depth, Jessner/35% TCA peel to scanning $CO_2$ laser treatment in the improvement of periorbital rhytides [14]. Treatments were compared within the same patient such that one hemiface was treated with the chemical peel and the other hemiface was treated with the $CO_2$ laser. A single blinded reviewer graded the degree of periorbital rhytides preoperatively and at 6 months postoperatively on a 5-point graded scale. The laser-treated side exhibited a statistically significantly higher degree of improvement than the chemical peel treatment (mean wrinkle score of 4.00 preoperatively to 1.75 postoperatively compared to 4.13 preoperatively to 3.29 postoperatively, respectively). However, the laser-treated side also exhibited a protracted healing course with delayed crust resolution (ranging 10–14 days as compared to 5–10 days for the chemical peel-treated side) as well as prolonged erythema (average 4.5 months compared to 2.5 months for the chemical peel-treated side). The authors concluded that the scanning $CO_2$ laser treatment was more effective than the medium depth chemical peel at improving facial rhytides, but was also associated with more side effects.

Chew et al. compared deep chemical peels to $CO_2$ laser in the treatment of perioral rhytides [15] (II/A). Twenty females were treated with 3 passes of a scanning $CO_2$ lasers to the upper lip area on a randomly assigned one half of the face and a Baker's phenol peel to the upper lip area on the other half. An independent, blinded investigator assigned wrinkle severity scores on a 5-point scale prior to treatment and at 6 months postoperatively. Whereas the pretreatment wrinkle severity scores were similar for both halves, the chemical peel-treated side showed statistically significantly greater improvement of perioral rhytides at 6 months (mean wrinkle severity score of 4.3 pretreatment, 0.47 at 6 months) when compared to the $CO_2$ laser-treated side (mean wrinkle severity score of 4.2 pretreatment, 1.11 at 6 months). In this study, the amount of improvement for the $CO_2$ laser-treated side was much greater than that observed for most other studies. With regard to the observed greater improvement in perioral rhytides after the deep peel treatment, the authors point out that additional phenol treatments were done to the deeper scars on the chemical peel-treated side, whereas no additional treatments were done for the $CO_2$-treated side. The chemical peel-treated side did have a higher rate of complications, with greater erythema/amount of coagulum than the $CO_2$ laser-treated side (30% with greater erythema/amount of coagulum on the deep peel treatment side vs. 10% with greater erythema/amount of coagulum on the $CO_2$ laser-treated side). The authors conclude that deep chemical peels are more effective than $CO_2$ laser treatment in the improvement of perioral rhytides.

## How Does the Scanning $CO_2$ Laser Compare with the Pulsed $CO_2$ Laser in the Improvement of Facial Rhytides?

Ross et al. compared a pulsed $CO_2$ laser to a scanning $CO_2$ laser in the treatment of facial rhytides [16] (II/A). Twenty-eight patients were randomized to receive 1–3 passes with either a pulsed $CO_2$ laser (fluences of 3.5–7 J/cm$^2$) or a scanning $CO_2$ laser (fluences of 15–18 J/cm$^2$). A panel of five dermatologists graded facial rhytides as seen on photographs of patients taken preoperatively and at 2 and 12 months postoperatively. There was no statistical difference in rhytide improvement between the two lasers, with the scanned laser showing a reduction of the wrinkle score from 5.6±1.4 (scale maximum of 9) to 3.3±1.2 at 1 year and the pulsed $CO_2$ laser reducing the wrinkle score from 5.8±1.4 to 3.8±1.5 at 1 year. These lasers were also compared in five patients in a side-by-side scheme as in other studies, in which each side was subjected to a different treatment; two patients were treated in the perioral areas, two patients were treated in the periorbital areas, and one patient was treated on the forehead. The authors state no statistically significant differences were found in rhytide improvement when the lasers were compared, although they do state that slightly better improvement was appreciated on the scanning laser side of 3 of the 5 patients.

Optical profilometry, a method in which dental impression material was used to create negative replicas of the patients' faces and the topography of these was graded when tangential light was cast across the replicas, was used to compare the improvement of facial rhytides after laser treatment in the same study. The five "hemiface" patients and two representative patients each from the pulsed laser and scanned laser groups were used for this analysis. This analysis also did not show a statistically significant difference in improvement of facial rhytides at 1 year following laser treatment.

Lastly, histologic analyses of punch biopsies from seven patients, including 4 of the 5 "hemiface" patients, assessed the immediate thermal damage immediately postoperatively and the depth of fibroplasias at 1 year postoperatively. The scanning laser exhibited a greater mean depth of thermal damage immediately postoperatively as well as a greater depth of fibroplasias at 1 year, indicating more aggressive tissue destruction as well as a deeper zone of healing; statistical analyses of these data, however, was not reported. This is consistent with another study that qualitatively reported histological analyses of punch biopsies done postoperatively showing delayed reformation of the epidermal layer as well as prolonged edema and inflammation after scanning laser treatment when compared to pulsed laser treatment [17].

In total, the authors conclude that both lasers were equally efficacious in the treatment of facial rhytides. The scanning $CO_2$ laser, however, may induce more of the histological changes thought to be consistent with a favorable cosmetic result.

## How Do the $CO_2$ Lasers Compare with the Er:YAG Laser in the Improvement of Facial Rhytides?

Robert Adrian compared the efficacy of the Er:YAG laser to the pulsed $CO_2$ laser in the treatment of facial rhytids [18] (III/B). Twenty patients with perioral ($n = 12$) or periocular ($n = 8$) rhytides underwent treatment with the Er:YAG to involved

areas on half of the face and the $CO_2$ to the contralateral half; the authors did not state whether the treatment was randomized. The periorbital areas were treated with either 5–10 passes of the Er:YAG laser (1.0 J/cm²) or 2–3 passes with the $CO_2$ laser (300 mJ). Upper lips were treated with 12–15 passes of the Er:YAG laser (5.0 J/cm²) or 2–3 passes with the $CO_2$ laser (300 mJ). Blinded observers rated the degree of improvement after treatment in photographs at time points ranging from 1 day postoperatively to 3 months. The author reports that 12 of 12 perioral areas treated with the $CO_2$ laser improved 75–100%, whereas only 5 of 12 perioral areas treated with the Er:YAG laser improved to the same degree. In the periocular area, the $CO_2$ laser treatment resulted in 5 of 8 improving 75–100% and 3 of 8 improving 50–75%, whereas only 2 of 8 Er:YAG-treated periocular areas improved by 75–100%, 4 of 8 improved 50–75%, and 2 of 8 improved 25–50%. No statistical analyses were reported. However, the Er:YAG-treated areas showed slightly earlier re-epithelialization and a shorter duration of periocular erythema postoperatively, although postoperative pain and postoperative perioral erythema were deemed to be the same. The author concluded that the $CO_2$ laser was more efficacious at improving facial rhytides than the Er:YAG laser.

Ross et al. compared single pass pulsed $CO_2$ laser treatment to multipass Er:YAG laser treatment in the improvement of facial rhytides [19] (II/A). The rationale behind this comparison stemmed from studies done in live porcine models showing relatively equivalent depths of fibroplasia 60 days after treatment with either a single pass of the pulsed $CO_2$ laser or 5 passes of the Er:YAG laser [20]. Approximately 13 patients were treated with either a single pass of the pulsed $CO_2$ laser (10 J/cm²) or 4 passes of the Er:YAG laser (5 J/cm²) in the perioral, periorbital, or both perioral and periorbital areas. The assignment of right and left sides was randomized. Photographs were taken preoperatively and at various time points up to 6 months postoperatively. The photographs were assessed for wrinkle reduction, erythema, hyperpigmentation, and scarring by a panel of nine physicians not involved in the study. The authors reported no statistical differences in wrinkle reduction (approximate reduction from mean wrinkle score 4.2 out of 5 preoperatively to approximately 3.0 for both groups at 6 months postoperatively) or hyperpigmentation between the two treatments. Further, they describe postoperative erythema was slightly greater in the Er:YAG-treated areas at 2 weeks, but no statistically significant differences were found at any of the later time points. The authors conclude that a single pass with the $CO_2$ laser can approximate the results in facial rhytide improvement as multiple passes with the Er:YAG.

Khatri et al. compared the Er:YAG and pulsed $CO_2$ lasers in the treatment of facial rhytides [21] (II/A). Of the total 21 patients, 12 patients were treated for perioral rhytides and 9 patients were treated for periorbital rhytides. One half of each patient's face was treated with the $CO_2$ laser and the other half with the Er:YAG laser; the lasers were alternated to each side with successive patients to prevent selection bias. The $CO_2$ laser-treated sides received 2 or 3 passes (approximately 5–6.5 J/cm$^2$ for the initial pass and 3.5 J/cm$^2$ for subsequent passes), and the Er:YAG-treated sides received 2–3 passes with the initial set of patients (between 1 and 1.5 J/cm$^2$ per pass). After the study had begun, the investigators increased the number of passes with the Er:YAG laser as it was not generating as marked of an effect as the $CO_2$ laser treatment. Wrinkle improvement was graded on a qualitative scale by a blinded panel of dermatologists. The authors reported the mode score of each set of patients; they state that the most common grade reported by the blinded panel was "excellent improvement" by the $CO_2$-treated sides as well as the Er:YAG-treated sides in which at least 5 passes were performed, and "fair" improvement was the most common grade reported when less than 5 passes were performed with the Er:YAG laser. When an aggregate score was determined that was made up of the scores given by the blinded reviewers, the investigators, and the patients, the authors state that the $CO_2$ laser-treated sides exhibited a statistically significant greater degree of improvement when compared to all Er:YAG-treated areas. They do state, however, that this was not the case when the $CO_2$ laser-treated sides were compared to the sides treated with at least 5 passes of the Er:YAG laser. In these statistical analyses, the grades were not actually reported.

In terms of side effects, the $CO_2$ laser-treated sides exhibited statistically significantly greater incidence of erythema at 2 and 8 weeks postoperatively (following $CO_2$ laser treatment, 95% erythema at 2 weeks and 62% at 8 weeks, as compared to following Er:YAG laser treatment which exhibited 67% at 2 weeks and 24% at 8 weeks). No statistically significant differences were found in the incidence edema or hyperpigmentation. Further, the $CO_2$ laser-treated sides exhibited a statistically significant higher incidence of a visible line of dermarcation at 6 months (43%) when compared with the Er:YAG-treated areas (5%).

## How Do the $CO_2$ Lasers Compare with the Long/Variable-Pulse Er:YAG Laser in the Improvement of Facial Rhytides?

Robert Andrian compared the pulsed $CO_2$ laser to the long-pulse Er:YAG laser in the treatment of facial rhytides [22] (II/A). Twelve patients received treatments to the perioral areas and 2 of these 12 additionally received treatments to the periocular areas. Patients received 3 passes with the pulsed $CO_2$ laser at 300 mJ/pulse to one side of the face and 10–12 pulses at 5 J/cm$^2$ at 10 ms pulse duration with a 5 mm handpiece Er:YAG laser to the contralateral areas. The patient, physician, and two nurses then graded the percent improvement at 4 months; the paper does not state whether or not this assessment was blinded. The authors state that no difference was found between the two treatments. Of the Er:YAG laser-treated perioral areas, 8 of 12 patients exhibited 75–100% improvement, and 4 of 12 patients exhibited 50–75% improvement. Of the $CO_2$ laser-treated areas, 10 of 12 patients exhibited 75–100% improvement and 2 of 12 patients exhibited 50–75% improvement. Additionally, of the two patients treated in the periocular areas, both the Er:YAG and the $CO_2$ lasers improved rhytides 50–75%. No statistical analysis was shown, but the author found both lasers to be equally effective in the treatment of facial rhytides. The text of the paper mentions that there was no difference in patient postoperative discomfort. The author additionally states that less postoperative bleeding was seen with the long-pulse Er:YAG than the conventional Er:YAG laser, although this was an interstudy comparison (no conventional Er:YAG lasers were used in this study). The author suggests that the long-pulse Er:YAG laser can closely reproduce the effects of the $CO_2$ laser at the improvement of facial rhytides.

Rostan et al. compared the resurfacing effects of the pulsed $CO_2$ laser to that of the long/variable-pulsed Er:YAG laser [23] (II/A). Sixteen patients received treatments with the pulsed $CO_2$ laser (2 or 3 passes) to a randomly assigned half of the face and with the Er:YAG laser (passes 1 through 3 at 10–10.5 $J/cm^2$, 10 ms pulse, 5 mm spot size, 4–10 Hz, with the third pass restricted to areas of the greatest photodamage/scarring) to the contralateral face. These treatments were followed by a short-pulsed erbium with a 5–7 mm spot size, 1.5 J, 7.7 $J/cm^2$, 0.5 ms, 10 Hz. Photographs were taken at time points up to 12 weeks following the procedure, and a blinded physician assessed the photographs for evidence photoaging (scale of 1–9), erythema, edema, and pigmentary changes (scale of 0–4). The authors state that the amelioration of photodamage was essentially equal between the two treatments at 2 months, with 1 of 15 patients determined to have greater improvement on the Er:YAG-treated side, and 3 of 15 patients determined to have greater improvement on the $CO_2$-treated side. At 3 months, 3 of 16 patients were judged to exhibit greater improvement on the $CO_2$-treated side, and 2 of 16 patients were judged to exhibit greater improvement on the Er:YAG-treated side. The $CO_2$-treated side more frequently exhibited more severe erythema and edema when compared to the contralateral face than the Er:YAG-treated side; whether or not these differences were statistically significant was not mentioned. However, "faster healing than the contralateral face" was more frequently noted on the Er:YAG-treated side at 1 and 2 weeks following the procedure (12 patients and 10 patients, respectively, as compared with 1 patient and no patients for $CO_2$ laser-treated side). Furthermore, histologic samples were compared after 1 or 2 passes of the $CO_2$ and Er:YAG lasers. After 1 pass with the Er:YAG

laser, thermal damage/residual thermal necrosis was seen at an average depth of 11.0 µm of thermal damage as compared to 29.5 µm after 1 pass with the $CO_2$ laser ($n=4$). After 2 passes, the Er:YAG laser created 36.4 µm of thermal damage, compared to 55.0 µm by the $CO_2$ laser ($n=9$). Additionally, samples from five patients were examined after 3 month postoperatively for depth of new collagen. The Er:YAG laser created $35.4\pm28.2$ µm of new collagen deposition, much less than the $115.4\pm15.12$ by the $CO_2$ laser. No statistical analyses were done for the histologic studies. The authors conclude that the variable-pulse Er:YAG laser can achieve a similar degree of facial rhytide improvement despite inducing decreased thermal tissue effects.

Newman et al. compared the long/variable-pulse Er:YAG laser to the pulsed $CO_2$ laser in the improvement of perioral rhytides [24] (II/A). Twenty-one were randomized to receive treatment to the perioral area of one hemiface by the pulsed $CO_2$ laser (2 passes, 300 mJ, 2.25 mm spot diameter, 7.5 $J/cm^2$) or by the Er:YAG laser (6 total passes made up of 4 passes with a 5 mm handpiece at 1.5 J, 5.2 $J/cm^2$, 500 ms pulse, then 1 pass at 2.6 $J/cm^2$ at 10 ms pulse duration, then 1 pass 1.5 J, 5.2 $J/cm^2$, 500 ms pulse duration), with the other laser used to treat the contralateral hemiface. The $CO_2$ laser treatment resulted in greater improvement in facial rhytides (63% as compared with 54% after Er:YAG laser treatment) at 2 months following the procedure as determined by a blinded panel of reviewers, although no statistical analysis to determine statistical significance was reported. The authors stratified this data based on Fitzpatrick wrinkle class and showed that the difference in improvement was greatest with the Fitzpatrick class III wrinkles (approximately 70% improvement for the $CO_2$ laser as compared with approximately 35% for the Er:YAG laser), with lesser differences identified for class I or II wrinkles. It was not stated whether these differences were statistically significant. However, the patients reported greater time to re-epithelialization after $CO_2$ laser treatment (average 7.8 days as compared with 3.5 days for the Er:YAG laser). The authors observed no adverse events such as dyspigmentation, scarring, infections, or contact dermatitis. They concluded that the $CO_2$ laser is more efficacious in the treatment of facial rhytides, especially in the treatment of the more severe grades of rhytides.

## How Do the $CO_2$ Lasers Compare with Combined Sequential $CO_2$ and Er:YAG Laser in the Improvement of Facial Rhytides?

Goldman and Manuskiatti compared the use of a pulsed $CO_2$ laser alone with the sequential use of a pulsed $CO_2$ laser followed by an Er:YAG laser in the treatment of facial wrinkles [25] (II/A). Ten patients underwent 3 passes with the pulsed $CO_2$ laser to a randomly selected half of the face and 2 passes of the $CO_2$ laser followed by 2 passes with the Er:YAG laser to the other half of the face. Photographs were taken preoperatively and post-operatively at 1 and 4–8 weeks, respectively. Blinded reviewers graded wrinkle improvement and erythema, pigmentation and healing in the photographs. The authors found no differences in wrinkle improvement or edema between the two techniques, although raw data and statistical analyses were not shown. They state that the pulsed $CO_2$ treatment alone resulted in persistent erythema at 8 weeks following treatment, whereas treatment with the pulsed $CO_2$ followed by the Er:YAG showed resolution of erythema by 3 weeks in 7 of 10 patients. Histological analyses were also conducted on punch biopsies taken at 2–3 days, 1 week, and 4–8 weeks postoperatively; some patients had additional biopsies taken at days 4, 5, or 6 postoperatively. The authors describe less inflammation in the $CO_2$/Er:YAG-treated skin at 2–3 days postoperatively and state that re-epithelialization occurred more quickly after this treatment. Only representative sections were shown and quantitative data or statistical analyses were not reported. The authors concluded from this study that the sequential use of the pulsed $CO_2$ laser and the Er:YAG resulted in a similar cosmetic outcome while limiting adverse sequelae.

McDaniel et al. compared pulsed $CO_2$ to pulsed $CO_2$ followed by Er:YAG in the treatment of perioral rhytides [26] (II/A). Twenty patients were treated with 2 passes with the pulsed $CO_2$ laser to the perioral area, and a randomly selected right or left hemiface was additionally treated with 3 passes (10% overlapping) of the Er:YAG laser. Color, black/white, and ultraviolet photographs were taken preoperatively and at set time points up to 4 months following treatment. No difference in rhytide improvement was reported after 4 months postoperatively, as graded by a panel of blinded reviewers. Furthermore, the authors report a reduction in mean duration crusting (6.0 days compared to 7.2 days), swelling (6.0 days compared with 6.3 days), and itching (4.0 days compared to 5.2 days) in the $CO_2$/Er:YAG-treated areas as compared to the $CO_2$ alone-treated areas, although no statistical analyses were reported. They concluded that the additional Er:YAG treatments helped to reduce adverse sequelae without affecting the cosmetic outcome.

## Conclusions

Ablative resurfacing is the use of mechanical, chemical, or photothermal means to create a controlled wound of the skin to allow for healing to a more favorable cosmetic result. Dermabrasion, chemical peels, and laser treatments are modalities to achieve this end. It is important for the dermatologist to identify what these techniques are capable of achieving and in what specific circumstances with these techniques offer the patient the desired outcome.

The reviewed studies above begin to better define the circumstances in which these ablative resurfacing procedures are optimally effective. The preponderance of negative or conflicting results may be due to several factors, including author experience with a given modality, technique used with a given modality (i.e., settings used for a laser, the number of passes with a given laser), and alteration of techniques to suit individual patient characteristics. It is therefore unclear how useful many of these studies will be to the individual clinician in determining what would be the optimal technique for a particular scenario.

**Evidence-Based Summary**

| Findings | Evidence level |
|---|---|
| Manual dermabrasion is effective in postsurgical scar treatment | II/A |
| $CO_2$ laser treatment is more effective than medium depth peeling in treating facial rhytides | II/A |
| Deep chemical peels are more effective in treating facial rhytides than $CO_2$ laser treatment | II/A |
| Negative or conflicting studies | |
| Comparison of manual dermasanding and motorized dermabrasion in the treatment of surgical scars | |
| Comparison of dermabrasion vs. $CO_2$ laser in the treatment of facial rhytides | |
| Comparison of pulsed vs. scanning $CO_2$ laser treatment in the treatment of facial rhytides | |
| Comparison of $CO_2$ laser and Er:YAG laser in the treatment of facial rhytides | |
| Comparison of $CO_2$ laser and long/variable-pulse Er:YAG laser in the treatment of facial rhytides | |

# References

1. Cox SE, Butterwick KJ. Chemical peels. In: Robinson JK, Sengelmann RD, Hanke CW, Siegel DM, editors. Surgery of the skin, procedural dermatology. 1st ed. New York: Elsevier Mosby; 2005. p. 463–82.
2. Monheit GD. Medium-depth chemical peels. Dermatol Clin. 2001;19(3):413–25. vii.
3. Monheit GD. The Jessner's + TCA peel: a medium-depth chemical peel. J Dermatol Surg Oncol. 1989; 15(9):945–50.
4. Coleman III WP, Futrell JM. The glycolic acid trichloroacetic acid peel. J Dermatol Surg Oncol. 1994;20(1): 76–80.
5. Baker TJ. The ablation of rhitides by chemical means. A preliminary report. J Fla Med Assoc. 1961;48:451–4.
6. Hamilton MM. Carbon dioxide laser resurfacing. Facial Plast Surg Clin North Am. 2004;12(3):289–95. v.
7. Airan LE, Hruza G. Current lasers in skin resurfacing. Facial Plast Surg Clin North Am. 2005;13(1):127–39.
8. Alster TS, Lupton JR. Erbium:YAG cutaneous laser resurfacing. Dermatol Clin. 2001;19(3):453–66.
9. Poulos E, Taylor C, Solish N. Effectiveness of dermasanding (manual dermabrasion) on the appearance of surgical scars: a prospective, randomized, blinded study. J Am Acad Dermatol. 2003;48(6):897–900.
10. Gillard M, Wang TS, Boyd CM, Dunn RL, Fader DJ, Johnson TM. Conventional diamond fraise vs manual spot dermabrasion with drywall sanding screen for scars from skin cancer surgery. Arch Dermatol. 2002; 138(8):1035–9.
11. Kitzmiller WJ, Visscher M, Page DA, Wicket RR, Kitzmiller KW, Singer LJ. A controlled evaluation of dermabrasion versus $CO_2$ laser resurfacing for the treatment of perioral wrinkles. Plast Reconstr Surg. 2000;106(6):1366–72. discussion 1364–73.
12. Holmkvist KA, Rogers GS. Treatment of perioral rhytides: a comparison of dermabrasion and super-pulsed carbon dioxide laser. Arch Dermatol. 2000; 136(6):725–31.
13. Gin I, Chew J, Rau KA, Amos DB, Bridenstine JB. Treatment of upper lip wrinkles: a comparison of the 950 microsec dwell time carbon dioxide laser to manual tumescent dermabrasion. Dermatol Surg. 1999;25(6):468–73. discussion 464–73.
14. Reed JT, Joseph AK, Bridenstine JB. Treatment of periorbital wrinkles. A comparison of the SilkTouch carbon dioxide laser with a medium-depth chemical peel. Dermatol Surg. 1997;23(8):643–8.
15. Chew J, Gin I, Rau KA, Amos DB, Bridenstine JB. Treatment of upper lip wrinkles: a comparison of 950 microsec dwell time carbon dioxide laser with unoccluded Baker's phenol chemical peel. Dermatol Surg. 1999;25(4):262–6.
16. Ross EV, Grossman MC, Duke D, Grevelink JM. Long-term results after $CO_2$ laser skin resurfacing: a comparison of scanned and pulsed systems. J Am Acad Dermatol. 1997;37(5 Pt 1):709–18.
17. Trelles MA, Rigau J, Mellor TK, Garcia L. A clinical and histological comparison of flashscanning versus pulsed technology in carbon dioxide laser facial skin resurfacing. Dermatol Surg. 1998;24(1):43–9.
18. Adrian RM. Pulsed carbon dioxide and erbium-YAG laser resurfacing: a comparative clinical and histologic study. J Cutan Laser Ther. 1999;1(1): 29–35.
19. Ross EV, Miller C, Meehan K, et al. One-pass $CO_2$ versus multiple-pass Er:YAG laser resurfacing in the treatment of rhytides: a comparison side-by-side study of pulsed $CO_2$ and Er:YAG lasers. Dermatol Surg. 2001;27(8):709–15.
20. Ross EV, Naseef GS, McKinlay JR, et al. Comparison of carbon dioxide laser, erbium:YAG laser, dermabrasion, and dermatome: a study of thermal damage, wound contraction, and wound healing in a live pig model: implications for skin resurfacing. J Am Acad Dermatol. 2000;42(1 Pt 1):92–105.
21. Khatri KA, Ross V, Grevelink JM, Magro CM, Anderson RR. Comparison of erbium:YAG and carbon dioxide lasers in resurfacing of facial rhytides. Arch Dermatol. 1999;135(4):391–7.

22. Adrian RM. Pulsed carbon dioxide and long pulse 10-ms erbium-YAG laser resurfacing: a comparative clinical and histologic study. J Cutan Laser Ther. 1999;1(4):197–202.

23. Rostan EF, Fitzpatrick RE, Goldman MP. Laser resurfacing with a long pulse erbium:YAG laser compared to the 950 ms pulsed CO(2) laser. Lasers Surg Med. 2001;29(2):136–41.

24. Newman JB, Lord JL, Ash K, McDaniel DH. Variable pulse erbium:YAG laser skin resurfacing of perioral rhytides and side-by-side comparison with carbon dioxide laser. Lasers Surg Med. 2000;26(2): 208–14.

25. Goldman MP, Manuskiatti W. Combined laser resurfacing with the 950-microsec pulsed $CO_2$ + Er:YAG lasers. Dermatol Surg. 1999;25(3):160–3.

26. McDaniel DH, Lord J, Ash K, Newman J. Combined $CO_2$/erbium:YAG laser resurfacing of peri-oral rhytides and side-by-side comparison with carbon dioxide laser alone. Dermatol Surg. 1999;25(4): 285–93.

## Self-Assessment

1. Which ablative resurfacing technique requires intraoperative cardiac monitoring?
   (a) $CO_2$ laser treatment
   (b) Er:YAG laser treatment
   (c) Dermabrasion with a diamond fraise
   (d) Phenol chemical peels

2. T or F; in the treatment of scars, dermabrasion is more often associated with prolonged erythema than $CO_2$ laser treatment.

3. T or F; it is likely that a single pass with the $CO_2$ laser is more effective than a single pass with the conventional Er:YAG laser in the improvement of facial rhytides.

4. T or F; the Er:YAG laser is more effective than the $CO_2$ laser in the treatment of facial rhytides because it exhibits less absorption by water.

5. T or F; there are specific, evidence-based guidelines for the use of chemical peels in the treatment of facial rhytides.

# Answers

1. d: Phenol chemical peels
2. False
3. True
4. False
5. False

# Nonablative and Minimally Ablative Resurfacing

**15**

## Shraddha Desai and Ashish C. Bhatia

## Introduction

Skin damage, resulting from surgery, trauma, acne scarring, or excessive skin exposure, often prompts patients to seek medical advice. Nowadays, even expected signs of aging, such as rhytides and "age spots," can be distressing enough to lead patients to inquire about treatment. Traditional treatment modalities include the use of topical retinoids, bleaching agents, chemical peels, microdermabrasion, and lasers. With the recent advances in technology, lasers and light sources have now become the technique of choice for skin resurfacing. Conventional lasers, like the carbon dioxide ($CO_2$) or erbium:yttrium aluminum garnet (Er:YAG), are ablative and thus remove the entire epidermis and portions of the dermis during treatment. Consequently, results are impressive, but there is a great degree of associated postoperative morbidity. Patients are often advised to expect 1–2 weeks of "downtime" in order to recover from the swelling, oozing, crusting, and discomfort that results from the procedure [1] (V/B). Because of this expected result, newer minimally ablative and nonablative lasers and light sources were created. Minimally ablative lasers are still able to perform precise skin vaporization with less morbidity (3 days of downtime as opposed to 7), while nonablative lasers provide satisfactory clinical results with no postoperative morbidity. Results, as expected, are less dramatic than traditional lasers, but the adverse effect profile is similar to treatment with a light source. Due to these advantages, the use of minimally ablative and nonablative methods for skin resurfacing has greatly increased. See Table 15.1 for a summary of the devices that will be discussed.

## Consensus/Review

The demand for newer methods of skin resurfacing (for acne scarring, pigmentation, and improvement of skin texture and pore size) has made the use of nonablative lasers and light devices a must at the dermatologists' office. These treatment modalities work on deeper skin layers without removing the epidermis, resulting in collagen synthesis and remodeling without protracted healing [2] (V/B). Consequently, nonablative technology has several benefits. It is a safe and effective treatment in all skin types and colors with a minimal amount of required recovery time

S. Desai (✉)
Division of Dermatology, Loyola University - Stritch School of Medicine, 2160 South First Avenue, Maywood, IL 60153, USA
e-mail: shdesai@lumc.edu

A.C. Bhatia
Department of Dermatology, Feinberg School of Medicine, Northwestern University, Chicago, IL, USA

The Dermatology Institute of DuPage Medical Group, 2155 CityGate Lane, Suite 225, Naperville, IL 60563, USA

M. Alam (ed.), *Evidence-Based Procedural Dermatology*,
DOI 10.1007/978-0-387-09424-3_15, © Springer Science+Business Media, LLC 2012

**Table 15.1** Overview of discussed devices

| Name | Type of device | Wavelength | Indication |
|---|---|---|---|
| KTP | Vascular-selective laser | 532 nm | Red/brown pigment<br>Texture |
| PDL | Visible light laser | 585 nm<br>595 nm | Vascular lesions<br>Red pigment<br>Texture |
| IPL | Broadband light source | 500–1,200 nm | Red/brown pigment<br>Fine wrinkling |
| Cool Touch | Mid-IR laser | 1,320 nm | Acne scars<br>Wrinkles |
| Smooth Beam | Diode mid-IR laser | 1,450 nm | Acne scars<br>Wrinkles |
| Aramis | Er:glass mid-IR laser | 1,540 nm | Acne<br>Acne scars<br>Wrinkles |
| Q-switched | Nd:YAG IR laser | 1,064 nm | Skin tone<br>Texture |
| LP | Nd:YAG IR laser | 1,064 nm | Red pigment<br>Vascular lesions |
| Fraxel | Erbium-doped fiber laser | 1,550 nm | Wrinkles<br>Pigmented lesions<br>Melasma<br>Scarring |
| LED | Low intensity light source | Range from UV<br>and visible to IR | Texture<br>Wrinkles |
| Portrait PSR | Plasma-RF | – | Wrinkles<br>Actinic keratoses<br>Viral warts<br>Seborrheic keratoses |

after the procedure and relatively few side effects. Nonablative devices include (1) vascular lasers like the 532 nm pulsed KTP (potassium titanyl phosphate), 585 nm PDL (pulsed dye laser) and long-pulsed (LP) 595 nm PDL, (2) IPL (intense pulse light), (3) IR (infrared) lasers like the Nd:YAG (neodymium-doped yttrium aluminium garnet), (Q-switched [QS] 1,064 nm, LP 1,064 nm, 1,319 nm Nd:YAG, and 1,320 nm), diode lasers (980 and 1,450 nm), (4) LEDs (light-emitting diodes), and (5) RF (radiofrequency) [3] (I/A). The vascular, infrared, and IPL lasers were among the first to be used for nonablative resurfacing and treating hypertrophic scars, striae distensae and acne scars (KTP and PDL), rhytides (PDL and infrared), and dyspigmentation and

vascularity (IPL). As expected, treatment parameters vary greatly among the different laser systems. The vascular lasers are operated at subpurpuric fluences and pulse durations with minimal overlap during passes [3] (I/A). Approximately five treatments are administered every 3–4 weeks. IPL devices vary among systems, but all require cold aqueous gel application prior to treatment. A series of 5–6 sessions is usually necessary with multiple passes during each session [3] (I/A). IR lasers are operated at the highest tolerated energy level to ensure the best results. A cryogen spray is delivered milliseconds before laser pulsing in order to protect the epidermis from thermal injury. Treatments generally occur in a series of 5–6 sessions at 2–4 week intervals [3] (I/A). Depending on the laser used, 1–3 passes with the laser can be made per treatment.

Unlike the nonablative lasers, light-based treatments like the LEDs do not cause gross thermal heating, but instead cause subtle molecular changes in the tissue for clinical improvement. For example, yellow (590 nm) LED irradiation is known to downregulate metalloprotease-1 (collagenase) and stimulate fibroblasts to increase procollagen production, while continuous red (633 nm) LED irradiation stimulates mast cell degranulation and increased fibroblast growth factor production. Several LEDs exist: Gentlewaves (LightBioscience, Virginia Beach, VA), Dermillume (Care Electronics, Boulder, CO), Lumiphase (Opusmed, Montreal, Canada), Omnilux (Photo Therapeutics, Manchester, UK), and the SoliTone (Custom Esthetics, Woburn, MA) [4] (V/B). The pulsed yellow LED (Gentlewaves), when used twice a week for 4 weeks, was shown in two prospective blinded studies (with 183 patients) to mildly improve skin texture, dyspigmentation, erythema, and fine lines in the periorbital region in the majority of patients as assessed by blinded observers, patient reports, digital microscopy, and ultrasound. The recommended treatment course consists of less than 1 min irradiations twice a week for 4 weeks, followed by a monthly booster treatment. Exfoliation with an enzymatic peel or microdermabrasion prior to treatment is also recommended [4] (V/B). There is no discomfort during treatment or an expected recovery period afterwards. Treatment parameters for other LED devices have not yet been determined. Consequently, LED therapy is an effective treatment modality for subtle skin resurfacing, but more studies are necessary.

Although beneficial, the nonablative modalities do not provide the same degree of clinical results as the ablative lasers. So, in order to bridge the gap between nonablative and ablative devices, a new nonablative fractional resurfacing technique was developed. Similar to nonablative lasers, the fractional laser (1,550 nm erbium-doped and 1,540 nm erbium:glass) emits infrared light that is absorbed by water-containing tissue.

This laser procedure, approved for the treatment of facial rhytides, atrophic scarring, pigmentary irregularities, and soft tissue coagulation, works by treating portions of the skin by creating multiple 3-dimensional, deep zones of thermal injury to dermal collagen, while leaving intact skin in between [2, 5] (V/B). Because the stratum corneum is spared, keratinocyte migration and healing occur rapidly with very little wound production. Consequently, nonablative fractional laser therapy provides a good clinical response with only minimal risk and downtime. Only a few contraindications, similar to other laser procedures, exist to this treatment. Patients on chronic systemic corticosteroids or those with serious underlying illnesses should be evaluated by their primary care physician before undergoing this procedure. Additionally, patients who have a history of herpes facialis should be placed on the appropriate antiviral prophylaxis prior to the procedure. Moreover, those with a propensity for excessive scarring, pigmentary changes, and/or keloid formation may be at an increased risk for developing these changes after therapy and should be made aware of these possibilities beforehand. Finally, there are no studies available on the safety and efficacy of treatment of pregnant or lactating women, and thus treatment of these individuals should be avoided [2] (V/B).

The first fractional laser device was the Fraxel SR750 Laser™ (Reliant Technologies, Palo Alto, CA), a 1,550 nm Erbium-doped fiber laser system that could be adjusted to vary both depth and the percent skin surface coverage. This allowed for the safe treatment of various skin types. A later model, the Fraxel SR1500™, was completed in 2006 and was capable of delivering higher energy fluences (up to 40 J/cm$^2$), along with the production of wider and deeper zones of thermal injury (up to 40% surface area coverage, and a depth of 1.114 mm) [5] (V/B). Since then, several companies have produced fractional lasers, like the Mixto SX (Lasering USA, Inc., San Ramon, CA), the Palomar Lux 1540™ (Palomar Medical Technologies, Inc., Burlington, MA), which is an erbium:YAG laser that delivers high precision microbeams, and the Affirm™ Workstation (Cynosure, Inc., Westford, MA),

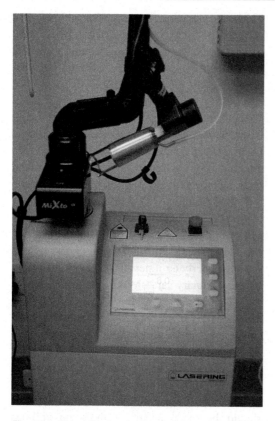

**Fig. 15.1** Example of a microfractional device: Mixto SX laser

a combination device of a 1,440 nm Nd:YAG fractionated laser at a fixed pulse width and a variable-width xenon pulsed light (560–950 nm) [5] (V/B). See Fig. 15.1. Regardless of which fractional laser system is used, the technique and recommendations remain consistent.

Topical anesthesia may be used to provide intraoperative comfort. Additional oral analgesics and regional nerve blocks may be needed depending on the patients' comfort level. Nevertheless, forced cool air and contact cooling have been demonstrated to significantly reduce pain and increase patient comfort during fractional laser treatment. Fraxel treatments require direct skin contact at 90° to the surface area, while the Affirm and Lux 1540 devices do not require this contact. Treatment zones should be overlapped by 50% and be laid down in the same direction. After the area is completely covered, subsequent passes are to be delivered perpendicular to initial treatment zones [6] (V/B). Usually, the procedure requires 3–8 passes and mild erythema and edema is expected to occur immediately postprocedure. This typically resolves within 24–72 h, followed by 1–3 days of fine desquamation. Patients should expect a rough texture and dryness during this time period and often require extra moisturizing. The use of oral corticosteroids posttreatment is still up for debate as there is evidence that they may speed recuperation, but it has also been suggested that they can impede the inflammatory response, thereby negatively impacting collagen synthesis and reorganization. Consequently, when used postoperatively, steroids should only be used for up to 3 days [2] (V/B). For photorejuvenation and treatment of scarring, a total of 3–5 treatments performed at 3–4 week intervals are generally necessary. Single treatments every 6–12 months thereafter are recommended to maintain results. Adverse effects, although rare, consist of acneiform eruptions and herpes simplex reactivation (hence prophylaxis prior to treatment). If an eczematous dermatitis occurs, a low potency topical steroid cream should be applied to the affected areas. Pigmentary changes or the recurrence of melasma are also possible. As a result, lower fluences should be used in darker skin types.

Further technological developments have resulted in the use of the radiofrequency and light devices for skin rejuvenation, particularly for the treatment of skin laxity by heating deeper skin and subcutaneous tissue, causing skin and tissue tightening. These devices will be discussed in greater detail in Chap. 16. However, a new RF tool, the Portrait® plasma skin regeneration (PSR³) device, has been shown to improve skin texture, tone, fine lines, dyschromia, and rhytides [7] (V/B). The plasma is emitted in millisecond pulses to deliver energy to the desired tissue without reliance on a skin chromophore, and energy settings on the device can be varied for different depths. One disadvantage of this technology is that there is about a 1-week period of required downtime [7, 8] (V/B). Since few cohort studies exist, additional investigations will be required to substantiate clinical outcomes from these studies and to determine appropriate treatment parameters for the device.

In spite of what treatment modality is chosen, all of the devices are effective to some degree, and the ideal patient for skin resurfacing remains the same. The best candidates are relatively young (25–65 years of age), have minimal facial skin sagging, and should be made aware that skin texture and fine lines will improve, but will not be eliminated. Furthermore, since the effects of treatment are cumulative, it is important to reiterate that multiple treatments will be more beneficial than a single treatment [9] (II/A). With this in mind, both the patient and physician will be greatly satisfied with results.

## Case Reports/Cohort Studies

### Vascular Laser-PDL

The PDL was first developed to treat vascular lesions, like port wine stains and hemangiomas, due to its ability to selectively target hemoglobin. This resulted in coagulation within a vessel, leading to thrombosis and termination of the vessel. Later, independent studies by Zelickson and Kilmer determined that purpurogenic doses of the PDL to a vessel also induced fibroblast proliferation and the production of the Grenz zone of new collagen in the papillary dermis, beneficial for resurfacing [1, 9] (II/A,V/B). Initial studies with this device showed a good histological response, but with low patient satisfaction scores. In 2004, Trelles et al. compared the effects of the 595 nm PDL to a 1,450 nm diode laser and to a combination treatment with both lasers [6] (V/B). Ten women (group A) received five treatment sessions by the PDL immediately followed by the 1,450 nm diode laser. Two other groups, each consisting of ten demographically similar patients, were treated with the PDL alone (Group B) or the diode laser alone (Group C). Overall better and faster results were seen in Group A with higher patient satisfaction scores. These patients also exhibited good dermal collagen remodeling, and at 6 months, the clinical outcome was best in this group followed by Group C and Group B. It is believed that after the removal of the vascular-associated pigment from the superficial dermis by the PDL, the following pulse with the 1,450 nm diode might have penetrated deeper into the skin, helping to amplify the wound-healing response [10] (V/B). However, individuals in Group A also received twice as many laser pulses as those in the other groups. Therefore, it can be argued that the dual treatment was only better because patients received more pulses in total.

The combination of PDL with other laser systems continued to gain favor, and in 2007, Berlin et al. studied the effects of a combined 595/1,064 nm laser on photoaging [11] (V/B). Fifteen subjects with photodamaged skin received five sequential treatments with the PDL/Nd:YAG (Cynergy, Cynosure Inc., Westford, MA) laser at monthly intervals. The PDL energy level was set at 1 J/cm$^2$ below the purpura threshold and the Nd:YAG varied between 35 and 50 J/cm$^2$, depending on patient comfort. Telangiectasias and diffuse erythema were the most improved, followed by pigment irregularities and lentigines, results which were generally maintained at 3 months. Some subjects also benefited by improved smoothness, radiance, and pore size. Patient satisfaction scores reflected these results. Consequently, it was determined that the Cynergy laser could be used to treat several signs of photoaging with the benefit of using just one laser system. Still, further studies are necessary to determine if this effect is simply additive or synergistic, and whether improvement is maintained for longer than 3 months.

### Broadband Light-IPL

IPL devices emit white light at a spectrum of 515–1,200 nm and affect the three most common signs of photoaging: telangiectasias and erythema, lentigines and other dyspigmentation, and fine wrinkling [12] (V/B). Bitter first proposed that a series of treatments with the IPL (photorejuvenation) would improve these signs [13] (V/B). Forty-nine patients were treated with 4–6 IPL sessions every 3 weeks and evaluated nine categories on a 9-point scale before and after all treatments: severity of fine wrinkles, skin texture,

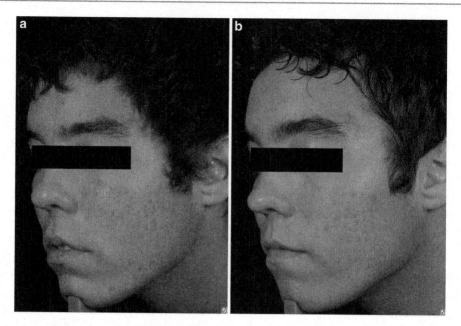

**Fig. 15.2** (**a**) Acne lesions before treatment with IPL. (**b**) Acne lesions after treatment with IPL

skin laxity, irregular pigmentation, pore size, telangiectasias, facial flushing, and facial redness. More than 90% of patients had improvement in all aspects of photoaging: 50% or greater improvement was noted by 46% of patients for fine wrinkles, 72% for skin smoothness, 70% for telangiectasias, 67% for decreased pore size, 59% for facial erythema, and 50% for flushing [12] (V/B). Since then, this regimen has been modified, but several studies confirm the results of serial treatments. See Fig. 15.2a, b.

In a 2004 multicenter study of 93 patients (skin phototypes I–III, Fitzpatrick Wrinkle Classes I–II, and Elastosis Scores 1–6), Sadick et al. administered up to five full-face IPL treatments at monthly intervals with the 560 or 640 nm cutoff filter [14] (V/B). Results showed that the average Wrinkle Class and Elastosis Score improved significantly ($p < 0.001$) at the 4- and 6-month follow-up visits. Consequently, they determined that IPL treatment is an effective noninvasive method for photorejuvenation with only minimal side effects, zero downtime, excellent long-term results, and a very high measure of patient satisfaction. Smaller cohort studies verify this claim [15] (V/B). Furthermore, Negishi et al. demonstrated that, by using longer pulse dura-

tions with a longer cutoff filter at 590 nm, IPL can be safely and effectively used to treat photoaging in skin type IV [1, 16] (V/B). A long-term follow-up study by Weiss et al. suggested that clinical improvement after IPL treatment of the face, neck, and chest is sustained at 4 years [1] (V/B).

## IR Laser-1,064 nm Nd:YAG

The LP and QS 1,064 nm Nd:YAG lasers have been utilized as nonablative resurfacing modalities for years. The LP Nd:YAG laser, like the PDL, is vasculature-selective and works best for treating red pigment and vascular lesions [9] (II/A). On the other hand, the QS laser was initially developed for the treatment of epidermal and dermal pigmentation and tattoos. Recently, its use has extended to the treatment of photodamaged skin, improving dyspigmentation, skin tone, and texture. An early study assessed the efficacy of this laser in comparison with the scanned and pulsed $CO_2$ laser in 11 patients with perioral and periorbital rhytides [17, 18] (V/B). Three patients had similar results to those with the $CO_2$ laser, 6 had some improvement and 2 had no improvement. In an ensuing study, the QS laser was used for the treatment of periocular and perioral rhytides, postacne scars, and melanotic and vascular eyelid pigmentation [19] (V/B). Twenty-two patients with facial wrinkles reported very good results after only two treatments, 28 patients with acne scarring were found to have excellent results, and 16 patients with eyelid pigmentation exhibited good results. In 1999, this laser was also used with a topical carbon suspension and lower fluences in 61 patients with photodamaged skin on the face and hands [17, 20] (V/B). The patients received three treatments at monthly intervals with a fluence of 2.5 J/cm$^2$ and a 7 mm spot size. At 32 weeks, patients reported at least a slight improvement in 71% of class I rhytides and 68% of class II rhytides, while observers reported improvement at 97 and 86%, respectively. Profilometry results showed a significant decrease ($p = 0.01$) in wrinkle depth. As a result, the QS laser is considered a modestly effective treatment for wrinkles, lentigines, and acne scarring.

In 2006, a short-pulsed 1,064 nm Nd:YAG laser was developed for more effective acne scar reduction. In a pilot study, 9 patients with moderate-to-severe facial acne scars received 8 low fluence (14 J/cm$^2$) sequential treatments with this laser [21] (V/B). Acne scarring improved in 100% of the patients. Scar severity scores improved by almost 30%, and 89% of patients reported greater than 10% improvement of their scars. Although the optimal treatment parameters have yet to be determined, the ones used in this study (14 J/cm$^2$, 0.3 ms, 5 mm spot size, 7 Hz pulse rate, 2,000 pulses per side of face) were successful. Future studies should concentrate on determining treatment protocols and address long-term clinical effects of treatment.

## IR Laser-1,320 nm Nd:YAG

The CoolTouch laser (CoolTouch, Roseville, CA) was the first device specifically designed for nonablative resurfacing and improving skin texture. It employs the use of a cooling spray to cool the epidermis in order to protect it from thermal damage. Several studies have demonstrated the

effectiveness of this device with modest improvement in wrinkles and acne scarring [12, 22–24] (V/B). Chan et al. studied this laser's effect on wrinkle reduction and the treatment of acne scarring in 27 Asian females [12] (V/B). The subjects received monthly treatments for 6 months, with 3 passes per session. Overall, the patients' satisfaction was rated as a 4.9 (range 0–9.8) and 4.0 (range 0–10) for wrinkle reduction and improved scarring, respectively. Objectively, only mild improvement or no change was seen in most cases. In 2006, Bhatia et al. performed a study utilizing structured interviews of 34 patients 3 months after undergoing a series of 6 monthly treatments with the CoolTouch laser for the treatment of acne scarring or photodamage [22] (V/B). Patient satisfaction with treatment was rated at 62% (slightly higher for the treatment of acne scarring than photodamage), with textural improvement at 31% at the end of six sessions and 30% at the date of interview. Overall improvement was rated as 5.4 for acne scarring and 3.8 for wrinkling on a 1–10 scale. These studies suggest that although the 1,320 nm Nd:YAG shows a mild-to-moderate benefit for wrinkling and acne scarring, patients are more than satisfied with results. Moreover, longer follow-up investigations may reveal additional positive results.

In a split-face comparison with the Lyra 1,064 nm Nd:YAG laser for the nonablative treatment of acne scars in 12 patients, the CoolTouch laser was found to have no statistical difference based on profilometric studies [24] (V/B). Interestingly, clinical investigators reported the Lyra laser to have a greater response. This may in part be due to the fact that the 1,064 nm wavelength is less absorbed by water and can therefore more effectively penetrate the dermis.

## IR Laser-1,450 nm Diode

Similar to the CoolTouch laser, the 1,450 nm diode (SmoothBeam, Candela, Wayland, MA) uses a cryogen cooling device to protect the epidermis during treatment and delivers energy via a 4- or 6-mm spot. In addition to its thermal effects on the dermis, it also damages sebaceous glands, thereby making it a useful treatment option for acne [12] (V/B). In the first study to prove its efficacy, 16 patients with rhytids underwent four split-face treatments every 3 weeks [25] (V/B). The other side of the face was treated with cryogen cooling alone. Mild-to-moderate improvement was seen in 12 of the 16 patients on the treated side. Further studies confirm this result [10, 26] (V/B). In a study of 25 patients with mild-to-moderate perioral or periorbital wrinkles, Tanzi et al. determined that all of the patients treated with this laser had mild-to-moderate improvement of wrinkles. An increase in dermal collagen was seen at 6 months after the last treatment, and patient satisfaction scores reflected the histological and photographic changes [10] (V/B). Tanzi and Alster later compared this laser to the 1,320 nm Nd:YAG for the treatment of atrophic facial scars in 20 patients receiving three successive treatments with a LP 1,320 nm Nd:YAG laser on one side of the face and with a LP 1,450 nm diode laser on the other side [27] (V/B). Both lasers improved atrophic scarring. However, the 1,450 nm diode laser showed a greater clinical scar response. After the initiation of this study, other investigators suggested that 3 passes with the 1,320 nm Nd:YAG may provide improved results. As a result, it is possible that using the 3 pass protocol with the Nd:YAG laser may yield similar or greater results to the 1,450 nm diode.

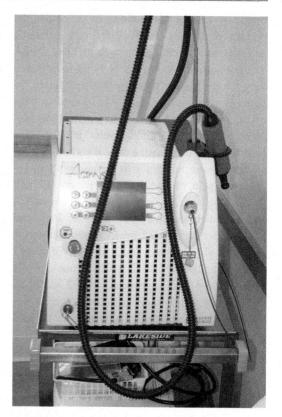

**Fig. 15.3** Aramis laser

the papillary dermis from biopsy specimens. Further studies have indicated that this laser is effective for treating fine-to-moderate wrinkles, acne scarring, and even acne [12, 29] (V/B).

## IR Laser-1,540 nm Erbium:Glass

The 1,540 nm Erbium:glass laser (Aramis, Quantel Medical, Clermont-Ferrand, France), like the SmoothBeam and CoolTouch, also uses contact cooling for epidermal protection. See Fig. 15.3. Unlike these lasers, it has a smaller spot size (4 mm), and therefore treatments are relatively comfortable and require no topical anesthesia [12] (V/B). In a study of 60 patients, Fournier et al. determined that the erbium:glass laser results in progressive improvement of perioral and periorbital rhytids at 6 and 14 months [28] (V/B). New collagen formation was also noted at

## IR Laser-1,550 nm Erbium-Doped Fiber

Manstein et al. performed the first study of the fractional laser by treating 15 subjects with varying densities on the distal forearm [30] (V/B). Biopsies taken from the treated sites at 48 h, 1 week, 1 month, and 3 months were used to help describe the wound-healing process. Results from this study eventually led to FDA approval for the use of the fractional laser for soft tissue coagulation in 2003 [31] (V/B). Since then, the laser has been sanctioned for the following indications: periorbital rhytids, pigmented lesions, melasma, skin resurfacing, and scarring. In 2007, 50 patients underwent three successive treatments with the Fraxel laser at 3–4 week intervals to evaluate safety and efficacy of the laser for the treatment of facial and nonfacial photodamage [32] (V/B). Objective assessments of photos taken at baseline and 3, 6, and 9 months posttreatment revealed a 51–75% improvement in photodamage at 9 months in 73% of facial- and 55% of nonfacial-treated skin. Patient satisfaction scores reflected these results. The lack of pigmentary changes and adverse effects suggested that this laser was an effective and safe treatment for photodamaged skin. See Fig. 15.4a–f. Kono et al. studied the effect of varying laser density and energy in 30 Asian females for skin rejuvenation [33] (V/B). Adverse effects (pain, erythema, edema) occurred when patients were treated with higher densities and fluences. Higher densities also resulted in postinflammatory hyperpigmentation in two patients. Patient satisfaction was greatest with higher fluences. Thus, the ideal treatment parameters seem to be high fluence with low density when treating Asian skin.

## Light-Emitting Diodes

LEDs are small devices that emit electromagnetic radiation at wavelengths in the UV, visible, and IR ranges and are able to modify the biologic activity of keratinocytes and fibroblasts by increasing the metabolic activity of mitochondria. Early studies demonstrated that various LED light sources used at assorted fluences with varying additional parameters could unregulate procollagen synthesis, resulting in significant clinical skin changes [34, 35] (V/B). A 90-subject prospective study by Weiss et al. using a 590 nm nonthermal full-face LED (eight treatments over 4 weeks with a minimum of 48 h between treatments) showed a global improvement of more than 85% and a self-assessment improvement of 84% in patients at 4 months. With digital imaging, there was a 90% reduction in the signs of photoaging: smoother texture, and reduced periorbital wrinkles, erythema, and pigmentation. However, profilometry results only showed a 10% improvement by surface measurements [35] (V/B). In a prospective study using the Omnilux™ LED system, a combination of IR

(633 nm) and near-IR (830 nm) light with fluences of 126 and 66 J/cm$^2$, respectively, 31 patients underwent 9 treatments: 830 nm light on days 1, 3, 5, 15, 22, and 29, and 633 nm light on days 8, 10, and 12 [36] (V/B). Patient satisfaction scores, photos, and profilometry were used to assess improvement at 9 and 12 weeks. A clinically significant reduction in surface roughness, maximum profile peak height, and maximum height of the profile was demonstrated. Fifty-two percent of the subjects had a 25–50% improvement in photoaging scores at 12 weeks, and 81% displayed a significant improvement in periorbital rhytides at the end of the study. Consequently, LED combination therapy is a safe and effective method of skin resurfacing, but in order to optimize treatment parameters, further studies are necessary.

## Plasma Skin Rejuvenation Device: Portrait® PSR$^3$

The Rhytec Portrait® PSR$^3$ System was developed in an attempt to produce rapid and precise treatment of photodamaged skin areas with minimal thermal effects on surrounding tissue [7] (V/B). The device works by using RF to convert nitrogen gas into plasma. As energy from the plasma is given up to the skin, the skin rapidly heats, providing its skin rejuvenation effect. A two-site prospective study of 24 subjects assessed the safety and efficacy of a single-pass of the full face with this device. Patients were separated into three groups at specific starting energy levels that were increased at 0.5 J increments. Clinical and histological effects were evaluated. Textural improvement was consistently high with all energies used, and each cohort showed similar results. Patients with preexisting pigmentary irregularities also had improvement at the 90-day follow-up visit. Histologic evaluation did not reveal any adverse effects in the epidermis and dermis. In a study of 30 skin areas treated with the PSR System at three different energy settings, Alster and Konda demonstrated clinical improvement in the chest (57%), hands (48%), and neck (41%). Significant improvements in wrinkle severity, hyperpigmentation, and skin smoothness were

**Fig. 15.4** (**a**) Rhytides before treatment with the Mixto SX laser (*front*). (**b**) Rhytides 15 days after treatment with the Mixto SX laser (*front*). (**c**) Rhytides before treatment with the Mixto SX laser (*right*). (**d**) Rhytides 15 days after treatment with the Mixto SX laser (*right*). (**e**) Rhytides before treatment with the Mixto SX laser (*left*). (**f**) Rhytides 15 days after treatment with the Mixto SX laser (*left*)

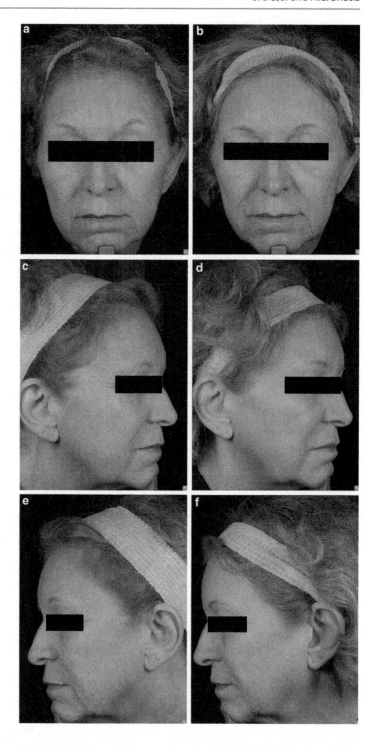

seen [37] (V/B). Bogle et al. further demonstrated that a multiple low-energy treatment technique can successfully treat photodamaged facial skin with minimal downtime [8] (V/B). In addition, histological studies have confirmed continued collagen production, reduction in elastosis, and progressive skin rejuvenation even after more than 1 year posttreatment [38] (V/B). Furthermore, this device has recently received FDA clearance for the treatment of rhytids, superficial skin lesions, actinic keratoses, viral papillomata, and seborrheic keratoses. It can be used to treat photoaging, skin laxity, acne scarring, and dyschromias [38] (V/B). Unfortunately, due to the economy, further development of this product has ceased.

## Randomized Controlled Trials/ Meta-Analyses

Although cohort studies and case series were helpful in determining the safety and efficacy of the above devices, it is the randomized controlled trials and meta-analyses that truly provide the evidence to support the use of these devices for skin resurfacing.

In a randomized controlled split-face trial using IPL, 32 females with skin types I–III and class I or II rhytides received either three IPL treatments at monthly intervals or no treatment to one side of the face [39] (II/A). Patient self-assessments and blinded clinical and photographic evaluations were used to judge improvement. There was a clinically significant improvement in skin texture in 82% of patients ($p < 0.006$) that peaked at 1 month and became nonsignificant at 6 months. Fifty-eight percent of patients self-reported this improvement as mild or moderate. Significant improvements in telangiectasias and irregular pigmentation were seen at all assessments. However, there was no significant difference in rhytides between the treated and untreated sides. Adverse effects included pain related to the treatment as well as scarring to one patient.

In a split-face comparison with IPL and the long-pulsed dye laser (LPDL), 20 females with skin types I–III and class I–II rhytids received a series of three treatments at 3-week intervals of the 595 nm LPDL to one side of the face and IPL to the other [15] (II/A). The LPDL provided greater clearance of telangiectasias at 3 and 6 months per postoperative side-to-side evaluations and patient assessments. Irregular pigmentation and skin texture were improved, but not signifi-

cantly when compared side-to-side. There was no reduction in rhytides with either treatment. Treatment-related pain was lower with LPDL and more patients preferred this device over the IPL. Therefore, it is evident that IPL is effective in treating pigmentary irregularities, although there is pain associated with the procedure, but other methods are more effective for the treatment of rhytides.

In a single-blinded randomized controlled study with the Omnilux Revive LED device, 23 subjects underwent 20 facial treatments 3 times a week at 3-week intervals, with the untreated side acting as a control [40] (II/A). Ninety-one percent of the patients reported visible changes in their skin (fine lines, wrinkles, skin tone, and general appearance), 76% had clinical improvement, and 59% were reported to have a clinical response after evaluation of blinded photos. Cutometer readings failed to demonstrate significant changes in skin hydration or elasticity. This study revealed that LEDs are useful and safe for skin rejuvenation with good patient satisfaction.

## Conclusions

Clinical evaluations of nonablative and minimally ablative therapy generally rely on patient and physician (blinded and nonblinded) assessments of before and after photographs. Additional objective methods of skin texture measurement include profilometry and ultrasound, among others. Differences in before and after results can be subtle, even with the use of digital photography. Still, these therapeutic interventions remain popular among both patients and physicians, suggesting that although differences may not always be clear, results are real.

Determining which patients are suitable for skin resurfacing depends in part on the patients' desires and expectations with treatment. Relatively young individuals (aged 25–65 years) with minimal facial skin sagging are ideal. It is important to emphasize that skin texture and fine lines will be improved, but the latter will not be eradicated. Additionally, since changes occur gradually over time and often require multiple treatments, patients should be aware that immediate results may not be evident. Dark-skinned individuals or those with the tendency to develop hyperpigmentation after skin trauma can be safely treated with nonablative IR lasers as these devices are less prone to causing pigmentary changes. Conversely, non-IR lasers must be used with care in darker-skinned or Asian patients. Although studies suggest that these patients infrequently develop pigment irregularities, they are at a higher risk than lighter-skinned individuals to do so.

Pain with the nonablative lasers for skin resurfacing is variable. Of these devices, IR lasers are likely to cause the most pain, although

it is typically less than minimally ablative and ablative methods. Erythema and edema also occur following treatment. These side effects occurring after IR laser treatment last only for a few hours, but when PDL, IPL, or Nd:YAG devices are used, these tissue effects last longer. Postoperative care focuses mainly on sun protection after the use of any of these devices. It is abundantly clear that lasers and light sources should be used in accordance to the patients' desires. Choosing the most appropriate device, based on individual characteristics, can help provide the best outcome. Moreover, the development of new combination devices will likely further improve results.

**Evidence-Based Summary**

| Findings | Evidence level |
| --- | --- |
| Nonablative and minimally ablative devices are safe and effective alternatives to traditional ablative devices | (V/B) |
| IR lasers are best for improving the appearance of rhytids and acne scarring and have little to no effect on pigment abnormalities | (II/A) |
| IR lasers can be safely used in darker skin types | (V/B) |
| Red pigment is best treated by KTP, IPL, PDL, and LP- and Q-switched Nd:YAG lasers | (V/B) |
| Brown pigment is best treated by KTP, IPL, Nd:YAG, and Q-switched lasers | (V/B) |
| IPL is a multipurpose device that can treat both pigment and textural irregularities | (V/B) |
| Fractional $CO_2$ lasers are a good bridge between nonablative and ablative skin resurfacing modalities | (V/B) |

# References

1. DeHoratius DM, Dover JS. Nonablative tissue remodeling and photorejuvenation. Clin Dermatol. 2007;25: 474–9.
2. Non-ablative/light-based treatment information. http://www.asds.net/NonAblativeLightBasedTreatment Information.aspx. Accessed 22 Sept 2008.
3. Alexiades-Armentakas MR, Dover JS, Arndt KA. The spectrum of laser skin resurfacing: nonablative, fractional, and ablative laser resurfacing. J Am Acad Dermatol. 2008;58(5):719–37.
4. Technology report: LED photorejuvenation. http://www.asds.net/TechnologyReportLEDRejuvenation. aspx. Accessed 22 Sept 2008.
5. Technology report: fractional photothermolysis. http://www.asds.net/fractional_photothermolysis. aspx. Accessed 22 Sept 2008.
6. Trelles MA, Allones I, Levy JL, et al. Combined nonablative skin rejuvenation with the 595- and 1450-nm lasers. Dermatol Surg. 2004;30:1292–8.
7. Kilmer S, Semchyshyn N, Shah G, Fitzpatrick R. A pilot study on the use of a plasma skin regeneration device (Portrait PSR[3]) in the full facial rejuvenation procedures. Lasers Med Sci. 2007;22:101–9.
8. Bogle MA, Arndt KA, Dover JS. Evaluation of plasma skin regeneration technology in low-energy full-facial rejuvenation. Arch Dermatol. 2007;143(2):168–74.
9. Alam M, Dover JS. Nonablative laser and light therapy: an approach to patient and device selection. Skin Therapy Lett. 2003;8(4):4–7.

10. Tanzi EL, Williams CM, Alster TS. Treatment of facial rhytides with a nonablative 1,450-nm diode laser: a controlled clinical and histological study. Dermatol Surg. 2003;29:124–8.

11. Berlin AL, Hussain M, Goldberg DJ. Cutaneous photoaging treated with a combined 595/1064 nm laser. J Cosmet Laser Ther. 2007;9:214–7.

12. Chan HHL, Lam L, Wong DYS, et al. Use of 1,320 nm Nd:YAG laser for wrinkle reduction and the treatment of atrophic acne scarring in Asians. Lasers Surg Med. 2004;34:98–103.

13. Bitter PH. Non-invasive rejuvenation of photodamaged skin using serial, full face intense pulsed light treatments. Dermatol Surg. 2000;26:835–43.

14. Sadick NS, Weiss R, Kilmer S, Bitter P. Photorejuvenation with intense pulsed light: results of a multicenter study. J Drugs Dermatol. 2004;3(1):41–9.

15. Jorgensen GF, Hedelund L, Haedersdal M. Long-pulsed dye laser versus intense pulsed light for photodamaged skin: a randomized split-face trial with blinded response evaluation. Lasers Surg Med. 2008;40:293–9.

16. Negishi K, Kushikata N, Takeuchi K, et al. Photorejuvenation by intense pulsed light with objective measurement of skin color in Japanese patients. Dermatol Surg. 2006;32:1380–7.

17. Ang P, Barlow RJ. Nonablative laser resurfacing: a systematic review of the literature. Clin Exp Dermatol. 2002;27:630–5.

18. Goldberg DJ, Whitworth J. Laser skin resurfacing with the Q-switched Nd:AYG laser. Dermatol Surg. 1997;23:903–7.

19. Cisneros JL, Rio R, Palou J. The Q-switched neodymium (Nd):YAG laser with quadruple frequency. Clinical histological evaluation of facial resurfacing using different wavelengths. Dermatol Surg. 1998;23:345–50.

20. Goldberg DJ, Metzler C. Skin resurfacing utilizing a low fluence Nd:YAG laser. J Cutan Laser Ther. 1999; 1:23–7.

21. Lipper GM, Perez M. Nonablative acne scare reduction after a series of treatments with a short-pulsed 1,064-nm neodymium:YAG laser. Dermatol Surg. 2006;32:998–1006.

22. Bhatia AC, Dover JS, Arndt KA, Stewart B, Alam M. Patient satisfaction and reported long-term therapeutic efficacy associated with 1,320 nm Nd:YAG laser treatment of acne scarring and photoaging. Dermatol Surg. 2006;32:346–52.

23. Levy JL, Trelles M, Lagarde JM, Mordon S. Treatment of wrinkles with the nonablative 1,320-nm Nd:YAG laser. Ann Plast Surg. 2001;47(5):482–8.

24. Yaghmai D, Garden JM, Bakus AD, et al. Comparison of a 1,064 nm laser and a 1,320 nm laser for the nonablative treatment of acne scars. Dermatol Surg. 2005;31:903–9.

25. Ross EV, Sajben FP, Hsia J, et al. Non ablative skin remodeling: selective dermal heating with mid-infrared laser and contact cooling combination. Lasers Surg Med. 2000;26:186–95.

26. Shah G, Kilmer S. Combined nonablative rejuvenation techniques. Dermatol Surg. 2005;31:1206–10.

27. Tanzi EL, Alster TS. Comparison of a 1450-nm diode laser and a 1320-nm Nd:YAG laser in the treatment of atrophic facial scars: a prospective clinical and histologic study. Dermatol Surg. 2004;30: 152–7.

28. Fournier N, Dean S, Barneon G, et al. Non ablative remodeling: clinical, histologic, ultrasound imaging and profilometric evaluation of a 1540 nm Er:glass laser. Dermatol Surg. 2001;27:799–806.

29. Bogle MA, Dover JS, et al. Evaluation of the 1,540-nm erbium:glass laser in the treatment of inflammatory facial acne. Dermatol Surg. 2007;33:810–7.

30. Manstein D, Herron GS, Sink RK, et al. Fractional photothermolysis: a new concept for cutaneous remodeling using microscopic patterns of thermal injury. Lasers Surg Med. 2004;34(5):426–38.

31. Rahman Z, Alam M, Dover JS. Fractional laser treatment for pigmentation and texture improvement. Skin Therapy Lett. 2006;11(9):7–11.

32. Wanner M, Tanzi EL, Alster TS. Fractional photothermolysis: treatment of facial and nonfacial cutaneous photodamage with a 1,550-nm erbium-doped fiber laser. Dermatol Surg. 2007;33:23–8.

33. Kono T, Chan HH, Groff WF, et al. Prospective direct comparison study of fractional resurfacing using different fluences and densities for skin rejuvenation in Asians. Lasers Surg Med. 2007;39:311–4.

34. McDaniel DH, Newman J, Geronemus R, et al. Non-ablative non-thermal LED photomodulation – a multicenter clinical photoaging trial. Lasers Surg Med. 2003;15:22.

35. Weiss RA, McDaniel GH, Geronemus R, Weiss MA. Clinical trial of a novel non-thermal LED array for reversal of photoaging: clinical, histologic, and surface profilometric results. Lasers Surg Med. 2005;36:85–91.

36. Russel BA, Kellet N, Reilley LR. A study to determine the efficacy of combination LED light therapy (633 nm and 830 nm) in facial skin rejuvenation. J Cosmet Laser Ther. 2005;7:196–200.

37. Alster TS, Konda S. Plasma skin resurfacing for regeneration of neck, chest and hands: investigation of a novel device. Dermatol Surg. 2007;33(11):1315–21.

38. Foster KW, Moy RL, Fincher EF. Advances in plasma skin rejuvenation. J Cosmet Dermatol. 2008;7(3):169–79.

39. Hedelund L, Due E, Bjerring P, et al. Skin rejuvenation using intense pulsed light: a randomized controlled split-face trial with blinded response evaluation. Arch Dermatol. 2006;142:985–90.

40. Bhat J, Birch J, Whitehurst C, et al. A single-blinded randomized controlled study to determine the efficacy of Omnilux Revive facial treatment in skin rejuvenation. Lasers Med Sci. 2005;20:6–10.

## Self-Assessment

1. Nonablative devices show similar clinical improvement to ablative devices in skin resurfacing.

2. IR lasers are best for treating pigment abnormalities.

3. Patients with skin phototypes IV–VI are not at an increased risk for hyperpigmentation after treatment with the IR lasers.

4. There are no adverse effects with the nonablative and minimally ablative devices.

5. Patients older than 60 are the best candidates for nonablative and minimally ablative skin resurfacing.

## Answers

1. False
2. False
3. True
4. True
5. False

# Nonsurgical Lifting and Tightening

16

Shraddha Desai

## Introduction

Attempts at counteracting the signs of aging, such as redundant facial and neck skin, have become increasingly popular. Traditionally, surgery was the sole treatment for skin laxity. However, with the recent advances in technology, conditions that once required major surgical intervention no longer do so. Devices like nonablative lasers (long pulse 1,064 nm Nd:YAG), have been initiated instead. Primarily created for skin resurfacing with a reduced posttreatment recovery time, these devices also exhibited improvement in skin laxity. Unfortunately, this benefit was modest at best, and thus radiofrequency (RF), infrared, and ultrasound devices were introduced for nonablative tissue tightening via volumetric heating of the deep dermis.

RF energy works to tighten and lift tissue by delivering heat to dermal structures without adversely affecting the epidermis, thus making it an ideal choice for the nonsurgical face-lift [1–3] (V/B). This energy is produced by an electric current that does not diminish by tissue scattering or absorption by a chromophore. Light-based treatments such as lasers and infrared devices, rely on chromophores to produce antiaging effects.

Infrared devices used for tissue tightening emit infrared light at wavelengths of 1,100–1,800 nm and target water as a chromophore. In order to obtain uniform tissue heating, the light is filtered at wavelengths of 1,400–1,500 nm to slow the rate of energy absorption [4] (V/B). Nonablative lasers work in a similar fashion, but emit light of different wavelengths and target melanin instead.

Ultrasound waves induce molecules in deep tissue to vibrate, resulting in tissue heating. Like RF energy, the ultrasound waves spare the epidermis and cause selective heating of the deeper tissues. The advantage of ultrasound devices is the ability to image the area of interest prior to delivering a therapeutic dose of energy [5] (IV/B).

Regardless of the treatment method employed for aging skin, the appropriate use of these devices and selection of patients is crucial to obtaining worthwhile results. Furthermore, because these procedures are still evolving, there is no FDA-approved measurement for skin tightening [3] (V/B).

## Consensus Documents

### Radiofrequency

Therapeutic use of RF technology was first introduced by Bovie and Gushing in the 1920s with the advent of electrocautery. Since then, it has been used for a variety of medical purposes, like joint capsular tightening, corneal curvature

S. Desai (✉)
Division of Dermatology, Loyola University - Stritch School of Medicine, 2160 South First Avenue, Maywood, IL 60153, USA
e-mail: shdesai@lumc.edu

M. Alam (ed.), *Evidence-Based Procedural Dermatology*,
DOI 10.1007/978-0-387-09424-3_16, © Springer Science+Business Media, LLC 2012

**Table 16.1** Overview of discussed devices

| Device type | Mechanism of tissue heating | Frequency or wavelength range | Cooling type |
|---|---|---|---|
| ThermaCool TC | Monopolar RF | 6 MHz | Cryogen |
| Accent | Bipolar RF and unipolar RF | 40.68 MHz | Contact |
| Titan | IR | 1,100–1,800 nm, filtered to 1,400–1,500 nm | Contact |
| Lux-IR | Fractional IR | 850–1,350 nm | Contact |
| Refirme ST | IR and bipolar RF | 700–2,000 nm and 70–120 $J/cm^3$ | Contact |
| Polaris WR | Monopolar RF and diode laser (910 nm) | 10–100 $J/cm^3$ and 10–50 $J/cm^3$ | Contact |
| GentleYAG | Long-pulse Nd:YAG | 1,064 nm | Dynamic cooling |

alteration, incompetent saphenous vein closure, cardiac ablation for arrhythmias, and the removal of prostate and liver neoplasms [6] (V/B). The discovery that this energy could penetrate deep into the dermis and fibrous septae that support underlying structures via the emission of high-frequency radio waves suggested that this technology could also be used to lift and tighten aging skin. Several RF devices (monopolar and combined unipolar and bipolar), infrared light sources, and combination devices have been created for this purpose. All are capable of evenly dispersing large amounts of energy that become transformed into heat by tissue water, over a three-dimensional volume. Consequently, the depth of tissue penetration can be controlled. Concurrently, the epidermis is cooled for the protection of superficial skin layers. See Table 16.1 for a summary of these devices.

In 1999, The ThermaCool TC™ System (Thermage, Inc., Hayward, CA) was the first monopolar radiofrequency (MRF) device developed specifically to tighten dermal structures without epidermal involvement. It was the first nonsurgical treatment of periorbital skin laxity and rhytids approved by the FDA and has since become a common technique for treating aging skin (mid-face, cheeks, jaw line, neck, brows, abdomen, legs, and thighs). It accomplishes its tissue tightening effects via a unique scheme that utilizes MRF energy at a wavelength of 6 MHz. The energy is applied to the skin via a handpiece that contains a single-use electrode tip. A thin capacitive membrane located on the electrode couples RF to the skin by distributing RF energy (in the form of an electrical current) over a volume of tissue under the surface membrane. A return electrode is placed at a distant site on the body, usually on the back, and an electromagnetic field is created that rapidly alternates from positive to negative charge. As charged molecules pass through the electrical field, heat is generated by the resistance of dermal and subcutaneous tissues to the passage of the electric energy. The device's energy output is calculated using the following formula:

$$\text{Energy (J)} = I^2 \times z \times t,$$

where $I$ is current, $z$ is impedance, and $t$ is time in seconds. Energy (J) is created by the impedance ($z$) to electron movement relative to the amount of current ($I$) applied and the total time ($t$) that current is delivered to the tissue. The generated heat is at the appropriate temperature range (65–75°C) to cause collagen damage and to induce an inflammatory response, thereby resulting in skin lifting and tightening [7] (V/B). Quantifiable changes have been seen in brow and superior palpebral crease elevation as well as in the peak angle of the eyebrow and jowl surface area [8] (III/B). A cryogen cooling system is simultaneously applied to the skin surface via a cooling tip for epidermal protection. Treatment parameters vary across clinics and study groups, but in general the previous higher energy, fewer pass practice has now shifted to lower energy and higher pass protocols in order to increase efficiency, tolerability, and safety [9–11] (V/B). Recently, variously sized tips have been produced. The size of the treatment tips depends mostly on the anatomical area being treated, as larger tips cover a larger area of skin. For example, a 1.5 cm² tip should be sufficient for the treatment of the face and neck. Before treatment is initiated, coupling fluid should be applied generously to the area. Then, following the low energy, high pass protocol, RF energy should be applied. In 2005, Fisher et al. routinely treated the face with two passes at 107 J, followed by three or more passes at 83 J. Extra care is given to the neck region, so only 3 or 4 total passes are made at an energy level of 83 J [9] (V/B). Moreover, it was noted that multiple treatments yield significantly better results than a single treatment of the nasolabial folds [12] (V/B). It is important to continuously assess the patient for signs of discomfort, swelling, and skin tightening during the procedure. According to several authors, a good clinical response remains the most useful cut-off guide for treatment [6, 9, 13] (V/B). Initially, it is helpful for the practitioner to make use of the company-supplied grid that is applied to the skin prior to treatment. The grid shows exactly where the handpiece tip should be placed for adequate treatment. As an additional fail-safe, the tip must be in complete contact with the skin or an error message will be displayed. This ensures that the cooling tip will prevent epidermal disruption.

All RF devices should be handled in a similar fashion. The Accent system (Alma Lasers, Ltd., Caesarea, Israel) is a new RF system that uses two different RF handpiece configurations on a single device: unipolar, which permits deep, volumetric tissue heating, and bipolar, which delivers superficial heating of a known depth without requiring aggressive cooling or local anesthesia. This device emits energy at a frequency of 40.68 MHz and heats the tissue in two ways: (1) unipolar RF causes rotational movement of water molecules on the skin in the alternating electromagnetic fields and (2) Bipolar RF increases resistance to the RF-conductive current [14] (V/B). When applied to the skin, the handpieces are moved in continuous sweeping motions starting with horizontal strokes and alternating with vertical strokes until the set time is over [14] (V/B). For the ease of handpiece movement, a

light coating of oil (mineral or baby oil) is applied to the skin just before treatment. Therapeutic power output settings and handpiece selections are generally done based on the anatomic location being treated.

Regardless of whether the ThermaCool or Accent system is chosen for skin tightening, it is clear that RF devices work best for the treatment of mild-to-moderate skin laxity and have only a negligible benefit for patients who have extreme skin redundancy. RF skin tightening would therefore not be advantageous to the elderly and obese. The most appropriate candidate is instead a patient in the mid-thirties to mid-sixties with some sagging of the jowls, but without the need for a surgical lifting procedure [7] (V/B). RF is safe for the use on patients who have had prior cosmetic procedures like laser treatment, botulinum toxin injection, rhytidectomy, etc. It is, however, valuable to advise these patients to wait approximately 3 months before undergoing any additional skin tightening procedures, as the effects of RF therapy continue to work for months after treatment. Use of this device in patients with pacemakers is contraindicated. Relative contraindications include collagen vascular disorders (morphea, scleroderma) [3] (V/B). Additionally, treatment should be avoided in areas of metal implants, hardware, or braces. Of note, monopolar RF is safe and effective in all skin types, and since there is no evidence of damage to hair follicles, men can be treated without risk of facial hair loss [9] (V/B).

## Infrared Light

Infrared light is an alternative source for tissue tightening of aging skin. Titan (Cutera, Brisbane, CA) is a selectively filtered infrared light device that emits light energy in a spectrum of 1,100–1,800 nm, 1,400–1,500 nm when filtered and targets water as a chromophore. This allows for a penetration depth of about 1–2 mm, which is ideal for targeting the reticular dermis [15] (V/B). Light is emitted rapidly in multisecond cycles, so the deep dermal tissue is heated within seconds. A temperature-regulated crystal window provides cooling to the surface skin before, during, and after the procedure for epidermal protection. A device that uses IR technology as a stepping point is the Lux-IR Fractional™ system (Palomar Medical, Inc.), a near infrared halogen lamp device similar to fractional carbon dioxide lasers in that it produces multiple precise thermal lesions in the dermis and hypodermis while sparing the epidermis [15] (V/B). It has a filtered emission spectrum that ranges from 850 to 1,350 nm and has a contact sensor that ensures that IR light is delivered only when the sapphire cooling tip is in complete contact with the skin. Pilot study reports suggest effective tightening of abdominal skin laxity [16] (V/B). Controlled clinical trials will be required in order to acquire more information. Both of these devices are used in a similar way. After the patients wash their faces, protective goggles are worn by the patient and medical staff. Two initial treatment passes are performed over the area of interest, with additional passes given over areas of concern, like the jowls, lower cheeks, forehead, and temples (for eyebrow elevation). Although cooling is supplied during treatment, if a patient complains of an immediate burning sensation after a pulse, ice should be applied to the area right away to prevent further tissue damage. This may suggest that the cooling sapphire crystal was not in complete contact with the skin surface at the time of the pulse. Patients can usually resume normal activities after treatment, but they may expect some mild erythema or edema that resolves within 24 h. If a superficial burn occurs, patients should be treated with standard wound care methods.

## Ultrasound

Since the early 1920s, high intensity focused ultrasound (HIFU) has been studied by medical researchers. First the biological effects were reported, which were then followed by its medical applications in the 1970s [17] (IV/B). These applications have since included ablation of solid organ tumors such as hepatocellular, prostate, and breast, palliation for chronic pain due to malignancy, hemostasis, and more recently tissue tightening and lifting [17–21] (IV/B, III/B, III/B, IV/B, and

IV/B, respectively). Ultrasound causes tissue damage in two ways: by converting mechanical energy into heat and by cavitation. Ultrasound causes tissue vibration and the molecular structures undergo both compression and rarefaction [17] (IV/B). Gas that is released as bubbles during rarefaction oscillates and causes mechanical stress and heat production (See Fig. 16.1). Cavitation depends on ultrasound parameters like pulse length, frequency, and intensity and is used for ablation, whereas heat production from ultrasound creates thermal injury zones (TIZs) that tighten and lift tissues [17–21] (IV/B, III/B, III/B, IV/B, and IV/B, respectively).

Ulthera Inc. is the first company to produce the ultrasound device specifically for esthetic purposes. The UltraSite GT (Ulthera Inc, Mesa, AZ) is an early model, and like the newer version (Ulthera System [Ulthera Inc, Mesa, AZ]), consists of a central power unit, a computer, and a delivery handpiece [18, 19] (III/B). In both devices, parameters such as power output (0.5–1.2 J), exposure time, length of exposure line, distance between exposure zones, and time delay after each exposure can all be controlled [18, 21] (III/B, IV/B). Additionally, the handpiece images the target area for evaluation of underlying layers and structures and delivers energy pulses for a tightening and lifting effect [18, 19] (III/B). More specifically, the Ulthera System is configured to create approximately 1 mm$^3$ TIZs [18] (III/B). In the treatment mode, the handpiece and transducer are moved in a straight line to deliver precise pulses along a linear path.

## Combination Devices

Recently, devices combining RF and light systems were introduced in an attempt to treat both skin laxity and rhytides. These include the ReFirme ST and the Polaris WR systems. ReFirme ST combines broadband IR (700–2,000 nm) and bipolar RF energies (70–120 J/cm$^3$), while the Polaris WR™ system (Syneron Medical Ltd, Israel) combines RF and 900 nm diode laser energies, known as electro-optical synergy or ELOS™ [22, 23] (V/B). The optical energy component is used to selectively heat the target tissue [3] (V/B).

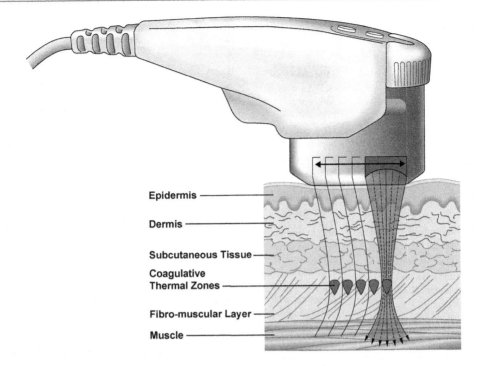

**Fig. 16.1** Dermal heating by radiofrequency devices

The Polaris device is primarily indicated for the treatment of wrinkles, but a variable degree of tissue tightening has been noted. Even so, the IR light source in the ReFirme ST system results in clinical improvement of skin laxity at a lower optical energy than the Polaris WR [23] (V/B). Both devices remain in the early stages of comparative studies. Larger studies are still necessary to obtain further information on these devices.

Despite which treatment method is employed, complications do rarely occur. However, with better patient selection and treatment parameters, the incidence of these adverse events has been reduced [3] (V/B).

## Case Series and Cohort Studies

### Radiofrequency: ThermaCool

Several small prospective and retrospective studies have helped solidify these conclusions. In the largest multicenter study by Fitzpatrick et al., 86 subjects received a single treatment with the ThermaCool TC™ System and were evaluated for up to 6 months after treatment. Subjects of all skin types between the ages of 35 and 70 years with periorbital wrinkles or skin laxity were enrolled [24] (V/B). Of the participants, less than a third were male, most were between the ages of 41–60, and the most common Fitzpatrick skin type was II. The average number of RF treatment applications per subject and energy setting was 68 and 16, respectively. As a standard among all the studies, photographs were used to document the subjects' response to treatment, so photos at 6 months posttreatment were compared to pretreatment photos and evaluated by blinded reviewers using the Fitzpatrick Wrinkle Classification Scale (FWCS). See Table 16.2. About 83% of treated periorbital areas showed a baseline-to-6-month improvement in wrinkle scores. Additionally, 66.4% of left or right eyebrows had an average lift that was greater than or equal to 0.5 mm (the minimum threshold for tissue tightening). This study clearly demonstrated that the ThermaCool System not only worked to improve skin laxity, but also resulted in lifted brows.

**Table 16.2** The Fitzpatrick Wrinkle Classification System (FWCS) [15] (V/B)

| Class | Wrinkling | Score | Degree of elastosis |
|-------|-----------|-------|---------------------|
| I | Fine wrinkles | 1–3 | Mild (fine textural changes with subtly accentuated skin lines) |
| II | Fine-to-moderate depth wrinkles Moderate number of lines | 4–6 | Moderate (distinct popular elastosis [individual papules with yellow translucency under direct lighting] and dyschromia) |
| III | Fine-to-deep wrinkles Numerous lines With or without redundant skin folds | 7–9 | Severe (multipapular and confluent elastosis [thickened yellow and pallid] approaching or consistent with cutis rhomboidalis) |

**Table 16.3** The Leal Laxity Classification System [5] (V/B)

| Laxity type | Description |
|-------------|-------------|
| A | Superficial laxity limited to the skin |
| B | Structural laxity involving subcutaneous tissue |
| AB | Combined superficial and structural laxity |

In another prospective cohort study, Alster and Tanzi studied the effect of neck and cheek laxity after treatment with the ThermaCool Device [25] (V/B). Fifty patients with skin phototypes I to IV, with mild-to-moderate cheek or neck laxity received one treatment with the RF device (fluences ranged from 97 to 144 J/cm$^2$ for the cheeks and 74–134 J/cm$^2$ on the neck). Clinical improvement of the areas was independently determined by three blinded evaluations of baseline, immediately posttreatment, 1 week posttreatment, and 1, 3, and 6-month posttreatment photos using a quartile grading scale: 0 = less than 25% improvement, 1 = 25–50% improvement, 2 = 51–75% improvement, 3 = greater than 75% improvement [25] (V/B). Significant improvement in cheek and neck laxity was observed in 28/30 patients. Patient satisfaction scores also reflected these observations. As with the Fitzpatrick study, side effects were limited to transient erythema, edema, and rare dysethesia. Consequently, noninvasive RF heating of the skin results in safe and effective tissue tightening of the cheeks and neck.

Kushikata et al. studied the effect of this device on Asian skin [26] (V/B). Eighty five Japanese females with skin types III and IV were enrolled for the treatment of the nasolabial folds, marionette lines, and jowls with doses ranging from 74 to 124 J/cm$^2$, and an average of 68 shots per cheek. At 3 and 6 months posttreatment, subjects were evaluated for (1) overall improvement of jowl appearance, (2) depth of marionette lines and nasolabial folds, and (3) improvement in other facial wrinkles. The overall objective improvement rates (50% or more) at 6 months posttreatment for the jowls, marionette lines and nasolabial folds, and other facial wrinkles were 89.0, 89.0, and 83.8%, respectively [26] (V/B). Complications arose in only seven subjects: edema, burn and blister, and secondary hyperpigmentation likely from skin healing effects of mild burns. All cases resolved completely without scarring or prolonged pigmentary change. However, these adverse effects suggest that there might be some race-related differences in the treatment parameters utilized.

Initially, earlier studies used higher treatment energy levels for the treatment of skin laxity with the hypothesis that higher levels would correlate with an improved clinical response. Bogle et al. performed a multicenter study using the ThermaCool device to evaluate the multiple pass, lower fluence treatment algorithm for lower face laxity [27] (V/B). Sixty-six subjects with moderate skin laxity were treated with a maximum of 5 passes over the lower face and neck. The treated areas were then evaluated via photos and the Leal Laxity Classification System. See Table 16.3. The average energy level was 83 J/cm$^2$ with 556 pulses per treatment, and at 6 months, 92% of patients had a measurable improvement in overall appearance, with 84% improvement noted upon photographic review. Compared with the Alster study, the percentage of measurable improvement is similar; however, the degree of improvement is greater with the multiple pass, lower energy setting: one third of patients achieved significantly more improvement at a lower average setting per treatment. These results have been corroborated by other small cohort studies [27, 28] (V/B).

In 2006, Biesman et al. studied the effects of the ThermaCool RF device for eyelid rejuvenation [29] (V/B). Seventy-two patients underwent a single treatment of the eyelids and lateral canthi at a mean energy level of 12 J, using the multiple pass technique, and were then followed for up to 6 months. Upper eyelid tightening and reduction of hooding was noted in 88 and 86% of the subjects, respectively. Lower eyelid tightening was noted in 71–74% of subjects. There was no correlation between the amount of energy applied to the eyelids and the clinical outcome. Regardless, it was determined that RF could be safely and effectively used for eyelid rejuvenation.

## Radiofrequency: Accent

In 2007, Friedman and Gilead studied the efficacy and safety of the Accent RF system in 16 females (skin phototypes II to IV) aged 29–66 [14] (V/B). They received a total of 2–6 treatments within 2–3 weeks and were evaluated by photos taken at 1 month after the last treatment. The treated areas included the chin, forehead, cheeks, jowls, periorbital region, marionette lines, and nasolabial folds. The mean energy level was 120 and 60 W for the unipolar and bipolar handpieces, respectively. Posttreatment patient evaluation of treatment and photographic analysis of laxity and wrinkling were used to assess the outcome. A total of 11 patients (69%) scored their results between satisfied and excellent and, the photo analysis reiterated this improvement. Interestingly, when divided into two age groups (25–45 and 46–66), the younger group reported statistically significant ($p < 0.01$) higher satisfaction scores when compared to the older group. This suggests that although the Accent system is effective in the treatment of wrinkles and lax skin, younger individuals may see a greater benefit from their results. This can in part be contributed to the replacement of heat-labile collagen bonds by irreducible multivalent cross-links as

patients age, making older skin less susceptible to heat-induced tissue tightening [14] (V/B).

In a 2008 randomized, blinded, split-face study, Alexiades-Armenakas et al. compared unipolar and bipolar RF for the treatment of rhytides and skin laxity [30] (V/B). Ten subjects aged 18–75 with rhytides and facial skin laxity received four treatments at 1-week intervals (with four passes per treatment) with random assignment of unipolar RF to one side and bipolar RF to the other. Photographic assessment by two blinded investigators using a 4-point grading scale at baseline, 1 month, and 3 month follow-up visits was done to evaluate clinical improvement. The scale took into consideration the following categories: rhytides, laxity, elastosis, dyschromia, erythema, telangiectasias, keratoses, and skin texture. Grade 0 = none of the above were present. Grade 4 = severe forms of the above were present. Grades 1–3.5 made up the mild-to-advanced forms. Unfortunately, the degree of improvement for both handpieces approached, but did not achieve statistical significance ($p = 0.5599$ unipolar vs. 0.1108 bipolar) [30] (V/B). However, there was a trend towards improvement. As a result, a larger patient population may be required to achieve statistically significant results. As an aside, this treatment was found to be painless and side effects such as erythema resolved completely within 1–3 h of treatment.

## Infrared Light: Titan

In 2007, Goldberg et al. studied the effectiveness of the Titan IR device in 13 US females, for the treatment of soft tissue ptosis of the lower face and neck [31] (V/B). The subjects received two treatment sessions at monthly intervals and were asked to follow up 1, 3, and 6 months after the second treatment for photo evaluation. Changes were dramatic for individuals whose skin envelope appeared to drape separately from deeper soft tissue and included: improved mandibular definition, increased angularity of the cervicomental region, decreased neck skin redundancy, and slimming of the neck contour. In the subjects whose sagging skin remained largely intact with the subcutaneous tissue, only mild-to-moderate improvement was seen [31] (V/B). As a result, the Titan device is likely more beneficial to patients with excess skin and can even induce tightening in older patients.

In a prospective noncomparative open study, Chua et al. treated 21 Asian patients (aged 43–60, skin types IV and V, with facial and/or neck laxity) with the Titan IR device [8] (V/B). The patients received a total of three treatment sessions (with energy levels of 32–40 J/cm$^2$ over soft tissue areas and 28–32 J/cm$^2$ over bony areas) spaced 4 weeks apart. Nineteen percent of the subjects reported mild improvement, 38% reported moderate improvement, and 43% reported good improvement. The physicians reported an observable lifting of sagging skin folds in 86% of patients. Of these, 28% were significant-mild, 38% significant-moderate, and 19% significant-excellent [32] (V/B). The treatments were associated with minimal pain and edema. However, the main adverse effect was superficial blistering in 7 of 63 treatments, which resolved completely. It is likely that the blistering effect was caused by incomplete contact of the cooling tip with the skin during the treatment. As long as contact is made, the Titan IR device can be used safely and effectively in darker skin.

Chan et al. also examined the effects of the Titan system in Asians [33] (III/B). In 2008, a prospective, split-face, single-blinded study of 13 Chinese women was initiated to evaluate the efficacy and complications of this device. One side of the face was treated twice with a 4-week interval between treatments, while the other side remained untreated and served as a control. A subjective assessment via a questionnaire and two independent viewer evaluations of photos taken at 1 and 3 months after the last treatment served as indicators of clinical response. At 3 months after their last visit, 23% of subjects reported mild improvement, 15% moderate improvement, and 54% significant improvement. Objectively, 41% of subjects showed some degree of improvement. Compared to the untreated side, however, the improvement was significant ($p=0.031$) at 1 and 3 months after the second treatment [33] (III/B). As with the Chua study,

blistering occurred and was likely due to poor skin contact with the cooling tip. It is easy to see that the Titan IR device can be a safe and effective treatment modality for skin tightening in all ages and skin types as long as it is used properly.

## ELOS: ReFirme ST

After the introduction of the combination IR and bipolar RF device, ReFirme ST, Yu et al. evaluated its safety and efficacy in Asians [23] (V/B). A prospective cohort study of 19 Chinese subjects of skin types III–V was performed for the treatment of periorbital rhytides and facial laxity. The subjects received three treatments at 3-week intervals (IR energy 700–2,000 nm and RF energy 70–120 J/cm$^3$) and photos were taken at baseline and serially for 3 months to assess improvement of skin laxity. At 3 months, 89.5% of patients reported a moderate-to-significant improvement in skin laxity of the cheek, jowl, periorbital area, and upper neck [23] (V/B). Unfortunately, blinded observers noted only mild improvement over the mid and lower face. Thus, the ReFirme ST system produces only mild improvement of facial laxity in Asians without serious adverse effects, but still meets high patient expectations. More enduring studies are necessary to determine the long-term tissue tightening effects of this device.

## ELOS: Polaris WR

Doshi and Alster treated 20 patients (skin phototypes I–III) with mild-to-moderate rhytides and skin laxity with the Polaris WR combination RF and diode laser device [22] (V/B). Subjects received three treatments at 3-week intervals (RF energy 50–85 J/cm$^3$ and diode laser energy 32–40 J/cm$^2$) and were evaluated via independent photo review, patient satisfaction surveys, and a quartile grading scale. Objectively, only modest improvement of facial rhytides was observed in the majority of patients. Subjective patient satisfaction surveys reflected the observed improvements. Side effects were mild and limited to transient erythema and edema.

No scarring or pigmentary changes were noted. Therefore, the Polaris WR system is a safe, easily tolerable, and effective device for the treatment of mild-to-moderate skin laxity. More long-term studies are necessary to optimize the treatment parameters and energy levels for the most beneficial results.

## Ultrasound

White et al. first studied the IUS device (Ulthera Inc, Mesa, AZ) in porcine tissues. Increasing power settings and varying exposure times (ranging from 1 to 7.6 J) were used to determine the specific source settings required to produce TIZs at given depths using three IUS handpieces: (1) 7.5 MHz/3 mm – superficial, (2) 7.5 MHz/4.5 mm – deep, (3) 4.4 MHz/4.5 mm – deep [5] (IV/B). Prior to treatment, the target area was tattooed with India Ink in a grid-like pattern, and ultrasound still images were taken and stored. Pulses were then delivered along a 25 mm straight line, resulting in select areas of ablation 0.5–5.0 mm apart. Immediately thereafter, the exposure line was marked with Wite-Out® Correction Fluid, and after completing all IUS exposures, the treated region was excised for hematoxylin and eosin staining and nitro blue tetrazolium chloride (NBTC) evaluation. In porcine skin, the 7.5 MHz/4.5 mm probe produced more shallow TIZs as compared to the 4.4 MHz/4.5 mm probe [5] (IV/B). Consequently, handpieces with lower frequency exposures produce TIZs that penetrate deeper into the tissue than those with higher frequency exposures [5] (IV/B).

White et al. furthered their research by studying the effect of IUS on the facial superficial musculoaponeurotic system (SMAS) of human cadaveric specimens [21] (IV/B). Using two IUS handpieces, 202 exposure lines were delivered in multiple facial regions, including the cheek, preauricular area, temple, frontal area, and neck with varying power levels and exposure times. Once again the treatment area was microtattooed with India Ink in lines spaced 10 mm apart to form a grid. Pulses were delivered in one of two ways: (1) up to seven horizontal rows of exposures along the grids with varying energy levels,

or (2) multiple (15–20) parallel line exposures were placed at a fixed energy level 2–3 mm apart. The treated tissue was marked with Wite-Out®, excised, and examined with the NBTC stain to assess for thermal injury. A dose–response relationship was seen with energy level and TIZ depth and size in all treated areas [21] (IV/B). Additionally, reproducible TIZs (contraction of collagen) were seen in the SMAS up to 7.8 mm deep, with sparing of the surrounding epidermis. In general, higher energy levels resulted in a greater percentage of contraction. However, when multiple exposure lines were delivered at a low energy level (1.3 J), tissue shrinkage increased dramatically. This is most likely due to a greater number of TIZs in a given volume of tissue [21] (IV/B).

Based on both of these studies, White et al. determined that tissue shrinkage from IUS is similar to that of lasers, RF, and combination devices. The main benefit of IUS is the ability to sharply focus the energy pulses, without involvement of the surrounding skin [5, 21] (IV/B).

Laubach et al. also studied the effect of IUS on human cadaveric tissue (skin types II–V) using the Ulthera Inc. device. A range of pulses were delivered (50–200 ms) and emitted up to 45 W at 7.5 MHz with a focal distance of 4.2 mm from the transducer membrane. At exposure durations greater than 175 ms, the entire dermis and overlying dermis were affected. Exposure durations up to 125 ms were not clinically detected, but did produce well-defined lesions with loss of NBTC staining within the dermis, whereas durations of 150–174 ms were seen histologically and palpable. Thermal lesions were noted to have an inverted cone shape and produced damage up to a depth of 4 mm within the dermis, while sparing the epidermis [20] (IV/B). By using lower exposure durations and a small amount of energy (less than 15 J), damage to the papillary dermis was avoided and TIZs were created without simultaneous skin cooling [20] (IV/B). Moreover, after evaluating the effect of IUS on multiple skin types, the authors determined that US energy absorption is independent of skin melanin content, and instead depends on the mechanical properties of the tissue [20] (IV/B). Consequently, unlike light-based or laser treatments for skin tightening and lifting, IUS is independent of skin color and chromophores [20] (IV/B).

Gliklich et al. conducted the first clinical IUS study (open-label, phase 1) on 15 patients scheduled to undergo immediate (surgery within 24 h; 7 subjects) or delayed (surgery 4–12 weeks after IUS treatment; 8 subjects) rhytidectomy [19] (III/B). Using up to three of the previously mentioned handpieces, IUS treatments were applied as a series of linear exposures 1.5–2.0 mm apart with different focal depths after ultrasound gel was applied to the treatment area. Histological evaluation of treated tissue with NBTC stain, digital photos, and subject pain ratings was used to evaluate the system. Pathology showed isolated dermal TIZs (as areas of denatured collagen) at exposure levels greater than 0.5 J. Most of the subjects in both immediate and delayed groups had mild, transient erythema immediately after treatment [19] (III/B). Erythema usually resolved in 10 min in patients treated with the superficial probes, while those treated with the deeper focal probes had a milder inflammatory response. Most of the patients rated the pain from 0 (no sensation) to 3 (hot, with moderate transient pain) immediately after treatment, and at 10 min all patients reported no sensation. None of the patients in the delayed treatment groups reported persistent pain at 48 h after treatment, and no delayed adverse effects were seen in any patient. The epidermis was spared [19] (III/B).

In a rater-blinded prospective cohort study by Alam et al., the effect of ultrasound on facial and neck skin tightening for brow-lift was examined [18] (III/B). All subjects were treated with the focused intense ultrasound tightening device (Ulthera System, Ulthera Inc., Mesa, AZ) to the forehead, temples, cheeks, submental region, and side of neck using the (1) 4 MHz, 4.5 mm focal depth, (2) 7 MHz, 4.5 mm focal depth, and (3) 7 MHz, 3 mm focal depth probes. Ultrasound gel was applied to the treatment area, which was then imaged and given a 2-s pulse delivery. The probe was then moved 3–5 mm laterally, parallel to the initial treatment line, and another pulse was delivered. This process was repeated until 110 exposure lines were placed on the face and neck, which took between 15 and 25 min [18] (III/B).

Three masked expert physicians (cosmetic and laser dermatologists and plastic surgeons)-assessed standardized photographs of front and side views were obtained at 2, 7, 28, 60, and 90 days. Pain was rated on a visual analog scale from 0 to 10, with 0 being no pain and 10 being the worst pain imaginable. Adverse events, such as edema, erythema, ulceration/erosion, hypopigmentation, and hyperpigmentation, were graded by the investigator on a scale from 0 to 4 (0 = absent, 1 = trace, 2 = slight, 3 = moderate, 4 = prominent) [18] (III/B). Patient satisfaction was also rated by the use of questionnaires. Of 36 subjects, 35 completed the study. All of the subjects developed at least trace erythema and edema immediately after treatment. Two had moderate erythema and edema, but all had resolution of their erythema by day 7. Pigmentary changes were not seen in any of the patients. The majority of pain scores on the day of treatment were 3–4/10, although five patients who had never before undergone laser, intense light, RF, or chemical peel treatments reported scores greater than 7. All subjects were able to complete treatment. No pain was reported at any of the follow-up visits. Of note, two subjects developed linear white striations on the neck with the 3.0 mm probe [18] (III/B). These areas were treated with high potency steroids and resolved without sequelae within 1 week. Thereafter, only the 7 MHz, 4.5 mm probe was used to treat the neck. The two primary outcome measures of the study were improvement in the comparison of pretreatment and day 90 photos, and objective brow elevation as measured using fixed landmarks. The secondary outcome measure was patient satisfaction [18] (III/B). Thirty subjects (86%) showed clinically significant brow-lift 90 days posttreatment as assessed by the masked raters ($p = 0.00001$). The average change in measured brow height from day 90 photos was 1.7 mm, with the maximum change of 1.9 mm. This improvement was stable at 3 months after treatment [18] (III/B).

According to the author, a limitation of this study was the use of conservative fluences since the treated skin was not to be excised as in previous studies. Therefore, efficacy may not have been as high. Additionally, because there are no fixed landmarks in the lower face, it was difficult to systematically evaluate tightening of this area [18] (III/B). Future studies should attempt to focus the ultrasound energy deeper into the tissue for greater tightening effect.

## Long-Pulsed Nd:YAG

Although lasers have shown skin tightening effects, the clinical improvement remains similar to RF devices while adverse effects are greater. In 2006, Taylor and Prokopenko performed a single-treatment comparison of RF vs. the long-pulsed 1,064 nm Nd:YAG laser [34] (V/B). Six blinded observers noted that clinical improvement was greater for wrinkles and laxity (30% median) on the laser-treated side and essentially the same with both modalities (15% median) for texture, pores, and pigmentation. This improvement was maintained for approximately 2–6 months on both sides without adverse effects [34] (V/B). In 2007, Key confirmed these results in another single-treatment split-face trial. Overall improvement was significantly greater on the laser-treated side of the face (47.5% improvement vs. 29.8%) [35] (V/B). Adverse events, like edema and erythema, last slightly longer on the laser-treated sides in both studies. Further split-face or nonself controlled studies are required to determine the effectiveness of these devices,

especially with multiple treatments. However, for those patients looking for textural and tightening effects, the laser is the better choice.

## Conclusions

For patients who desire a noninvasive approach to skin tightening as well as brow and eyelid lifting, RF, IR light, combination devices, and ultrasound offer a practical alternative for those who are willing to accept modest clinical improvement in exchange for less aggressive treatment and preferred side effect profiles. Treatments are generally delivered at 3–4 week intervals (not yet established for ultrasound) with the expectation that final results will take several months to achieve. At this time, there remains a lack of an FDA-approved method for measuring skin tightening. Consequently, before and after photos are essential in documenting clinical improvement of skin laxity. Although results are not comparable to surgical intervention, the benefit is enough to ensure patient satisfaction even if objective measurements of photos do not mirror this improvement. Large-scale randomized controlled trials are still necessary to determine optimal treatment parameters for these devices and others. With continued research efforts, it is likely that these treatment modalities will soon become commonplace in the dermatologists' repertoire.

| Evidence-Based Summary | |
| --- | --- |
| Findings | Evidence level |
| RF and IR are safe and effective in all Fitzpatrick skin types | (V/B) |
| RF can be safely used in all areas of the face and neck, including the eyelids | (V/B) |
| Excessive skin redundancy leads to negligible results from RF treatment | (V/B) |
| Use of RF in patients with pacemakers is contraindicated | (V/B) |
| Low energy with multiple passes with RF is most effective | (V/B) |
| Complete skin contact with the cooling tip is essential in avoiding burns or blistering with IR devices | (V/B) |
| IR works best for individuals with excess skin that is separate from underlying subcutaneous tissue | (V/B) |
| IR is effective in older individuals | (V/B) |
| IUS produces well-defined TIZs in the dermis while sparing the epidermis | (IVB) |
| IUS images and treats the given target area | (IVB) |
| Photographs are essential to documenting treatment for skin laxity | (V/B) |

# References

1. Koch RJ. Radiofrequency nonablative tissue tightening. Facial Plast Surg Clin North. 2004;12(3):339–46. vi.
2. Technology report: monopolar radiofrequency. http://www.asds.net/TechnologyReportMonopolarRadiofrequency.aspx. Accessed 1 Nov 2008.
3. Technology report: tissue tightening. http://www.asds.net/TechnologyReportTissueTightening.aspx. Accessed 1 Nov 2008.
4. Carniol PJ, Dzopa N, Fernandes N, Carniol ET, Renzi AS. Facial skin tightening with an 1100–1800 nm infrared device. J Cosmet Laser Ther. 2008;10(2):67–71.
5. White M, Makin I, Slayton M, Barthe P, Gliklich R. Selective transcutaneous delivery of energy to porcine soft tissues using intense ultrasound (IUS). Lasers Surg Med. 2008;40:67–75.
6. Alster TS, Lupton JR. Nonablative cutaneous remodeling using radiofrequency devices. Clin Dermatol. 2007;25:487–91.
7. Sukal SA, Geronemus RG. Thermage: the nonablative radiofrequency for rejuvenation. Clin Dermatol. 2008;26:602–7.
8. Nahm WK, Su TT, Rotunda AM, Moy RL. Objective changes in brow position, superior palpebral crease, peak angle of the eyebrow, and jowl surface area after volumetric radiofrequency treatments to half of the face. Dermatol Surg. 2004;30(6):922–8.
9. Fisher GH, Jacobsen LG, Bernstein LJ, et al. Nonablative radiofrequency treatment of facial laxity. Dermatol Surg. 2005;31:1237–41.
10. Narins DJ, Narins RS. Non-surgical radiofrequency facelift. J Drugs Dermatol. 2003;2(5):495–500.
11. Ruiz-Esparza J, Gomez JB. The medical face lift: a noninvasive, nonsurgical approach to tissue tightening in facial skin using nonablative radiofrequency. Dermatol Surg. 2003;29(4):325–32. discussion 332.
12. Fritz M, Counters JT, Zelickson BD. Radiofrequency treatment for middle and lower face laxity. Arch Facial Plast Surg. 2004;6(6):370–3.
13. Dover JS, Zelickson B. Results of a survey of 5,700 patient monopolar radiofrequency facial skin tightening treatments: assessment of a low-energy multiple-pass technique leading to a clinical end point algorithm. Dermatol Surg. 2007;33(8):900–7.
14. Friedman DJ, Gilead LT. The use of hybrid radiofrequency device for the treatment of rhytides and lax skin. Dermatol Surg. 2007;33(5):543–51.
15. Dierickx C. The role of deep heating for noninvasive skin rejuvenation. Lasers Surg Med. 2006;38:799–807.
16. Dierickx CC, Altshuler GA, Erofeev A, et al. Deep dermal optical/island damage as a novel approach to skin tightening. Lasers Surg Med. 2006;S18:80.
17. Kennedy JE, Ter Haar GR, Cranston D. High intensity focused ultrasound: surgery of the future? Br J Radiol. 2003;76(909):590–9.
18. Alam M, White LE, Martin N, Witherspoon J, Yoo S, West DP. Ultrasound tightening of facial and neck skin: a rater-blinded prospective cohort study. J Am Acad Dermatol. 2010;62(2):262–9.
19. Gliklich R, White M, Slayton M, Barthe P, Makin I. Clinical pilot study of intense ultrasound therapy to deep facial skin and subcutaneous tissues. Arch Facial Plast Surg. 2007;9:88–95.
20. Laubach H, Makin I, Barthe P, Slayton M, Manstein D. Intense focused ultrasound: evaluation of a new treatment modality for precise microcoagulation within the skin. Dermatol Surg. 2008;34(5):729–34.
21. White M, Makin I, Barthe P, Slayton M, Gliklich R. Selective creation of thermal injury zones in the superficial musculoaponeurotic system using intense ultrasound therapy. Arch Facial Plast Surg. 2007;9:22–9.
22. Doshi SN, Alster TS. Combination radiofrequency and diode laser for treatment of facial rhytides and skin laxity. J Cosmet Laser Ther. 2005;7(1):11–5.
23. Yu CS, Yeung CK, Shek SY, et al. Combined infrared light and bipolar radiofrequency for skin tightening in Asians. Lasers Surg Med. 2007;39:471–5.
24. Fitzpatrick R, Geronemus R, Goldberg D, et al. Multicenter study of noninvasive radiofrequency for periorbital tissue tightening. Lasers Surg Med. 2003;33:232–42.
25. Alster TS, Tanzi E. Improvement of neck and cheek laxity with a nonablative radiofrequency device: a lifting experience. Dermatol Surg. 2004;30(4):503–7.
26. Kushikata N, Negishi K, Tezuka Y, Takeuchi K, Wakamatsu S. Non-ablative skin tightening with radiofrequency in Asian skin. Lasers Surg Med. 2005;36(2):92–7.
27. Bogle MA, Ubelhoer N, Wiess RA, et al. Evaluation of the multiple pass, low fluence algorithm for radiofrequency tightening of the lower face. Lasers Surg Med. 2007;39:210–7.
28. Hsu TS, Kaminer MS. The use of nonablative radiofrequency technology to tighten the lower face and neck. Semin Cutan Med Surg. 2003;22(2):115–23.
29. Biesman BS, Sterling SB, Carruthers J, et al. Monopolar radiofrequency treatment of human eyelids: a prospective, multicenter, efficacy trial. Lasers Surg Med. 2006;38:890–8.
30. Alexiades-Armenakas M, Dover JS, Arndt KA. Unipolar versus bipolar radiofrequency treatment of rhytides and laxity using a mobile painless delivery method. Lasers Surg Med. 2008;40:446–53.
31. Goldberg DJ, Hussain M, Fazeli A, Berlin AL. Treatment of skin laxity of the lower face and neck in older individuals with a broad-spectrum infrared light device. J Cosmet Laser Ther. 2007;9(1):35–40.
32. Chua SH, Ang P, Khoo LS, Goh CL. Nonablative infrared skin tightening in type IV to V Asian skin: a prospective clinical study. Dermatol Surg. 2007;33(2):146–51.
33. Chan HH, Yu CS, Shek S, et al. A prospective, split face, single blinded study looking at the use of an infrared device with contact cooling in the treatment of skin laxity in Asians. Lasers Surg Med. 2008;40:146–52.
34. Taylor MB, Prolopenko I. Split-face comparison of radiofrequency versus long-pulse Nd-YAG treatment of facial laxity. J Cosmet Laser Ther. 2006;8:17–22.
35. Key DJ. Single-treatment skin tightening by radiofrequency and long-pulsed, 1064-nm Nd: YAG laser compared. Lasers Surg Med. 2007;39(2):169–75.

## Self-Assessment

1. Radiofrequency devices can be used safely in patients with metal braces and pacemaker devices.

2. Photographs are the FDA-approved method of measurement for skin tightening.

3. RF and IR devices are safe to use in all skin phototypes.

4. A high energy, low pass algorithm will ensure safe and effective treatment for skin laxity.

5. Cooling mechanisms are essential in preventing epidermal damage during the use of IR devices.

6. IUS cannot be used for skin types IV–VI.

## Answers

1. False
2. False
3. True
4. False
5. True
6. False

# Nonlaser Superficial Resurfacing Techniques: Superficial Chemical Peels and Microdermabrasion

**17**

John Starling III and Darius J. Karimipour

## Introduction

Superficial skin resurfacing is the application of various modalities to the skin with the goal of achieving a partial thickness skin injury that penetrates no deeper than the superficial papillary dermis. The approaches to superficial skin resurfacing may be classified into laser based and nonlaser techniques. Some of the most commonly used nonlaser, superficial resurfacing techniques include superficial chemical peels and microdermabrasion (MDA). Indications for superficial resurfacing include photoaging, fine rhytides, ichthyosis, acne vulgaris, melasma, solar lentigenes, and postinflammatory hyperpigmentation. Objective gains from superficial resurfacing are often modest, but these techniques continue to remain extremely popular with patients because of rapid healing ("minimal downtime"), low cost, and minimal risk. Typically, no anesthesia is required. Superficial resurfacing may also be

combined with laser modalities. Superficial resurfacing techniques may be used on all Fitzpatrick skin types. These techniques yield the best results when used as a series of treatments combined with diligent use of a home topical regimen and daily photoprotection. As with any esthetic surgical procedure, careful patient selection, thorough patient education, and a mutual understanding of realistic outcomes will lead to the most satisfactory results.

## Alpha Hydroxy Acid Peels

Alpha hydroxy acids (AHAs) have achieved widespread use in the last 2 decades. Their benefits have been well known since the time of Cleopatra who applied sour milk (lactic acid) to her face for antiaging properties. Yogurt was also used historically as a source of lactic acid, and women from varying nationalities historically used lemon juice (citric acid), dregs of red wine (tartaric acid), and sugar cane juice (glycolic acid) to esthetically improve the skin [1].

AHAs are nontoxic acids formed naturally in foods, and those occurring naturally are inherently impure and lack the quality control seen in the uniformly consistent chemically produced preparations [2]. AHAs include glycolic, lactic, malic, citric, and tartaric acids which differ in molecular structure, carbon chain length, and molecular weight. Glycolic acid represents the smallest AHA and is a commonly used agent for chemical peeling. In recent years, AHAs have

J. Starling III (✉)
Department of Dermatology, University of Michigan
Hospitals, 1910 Taubman Center, 1500 E. Medical
Center Drive, Ann Arbor, MI 48109-0314, USA

Dermatology Associates of Wisconsin, S.C.,
Oshkosh, WI 54904, USA
e-mail: johnthree@gmail.com

D.J. Karimipour
Department of Dermatology, University of Michigan
Hospitals, 1910 Taubman Center, 1500 E. Medical
Center Drive, Ann Arbor, MI 48109-0314, USA

M. Alam (ed.), *Evidence-Based Procedural Dermatology*,
DOI 10.1007/978-0-387-09424-3_17, © Springer Science+Business Media, LLC 2012

been widely recommended by dermatologists and others for facial rejuvenation and treatment of photodamaged skin, acne vulgaris, postinflammatory hyperpigmentation, and melasma.

When performing AHA peels, it is important to properly select patients who will most likely benefit from superficial peels. The ideal patients include those who are willing to go through a series of chemical peels and do not have expectations out of proportion to what these agents can accomplish. As best results come with a series of chemical peels, it is best to choose a patient who can undergo at least six treatments at a frequency of at least every 2–4 weeks. While improvement may be experienced at the end of a series of peels, the process is unlike the one-time treatments seen in more aggressive medium and deep chemical peels. It is often helpful to counsel patients that AHA peels do not require a great deal of prepeel preparation or postpeel care and that significant "downtime" is not required.

It is often helpful if patients are "primed" with home use of either a topical glycolic acid product or topical tretinoin for at least 2–3 weeks prior to a glycolic acid peel experience. This home prepeel regimen not only may enhance the results of the peel, but may also be helpful in identifying patients who will have a hypersensitivity to the peeling procedure or ingredients. Glycolic acid peels are available in concentrations ranging from 20 to 70% either as free acid or partially neutralized/buffered peels, and often are available in premoistened pads or towelettes. These peels should be performed in a gradual "step up" of the applied concentration to ensure that the patient does not have any untoward side effects from the treatment. The peel is performed by applying the glycolic acid solution to the skin via pad, towelette, or brush method and is applied starting at the forehead and moving down over the cheeks, chin, and nose. A glycolic acid peel is usually timed on the skin for 5 min at any given concentration and then neutralized with a postpeel neutralizer. However, if epidermolysis or significant discomfort happens prior to 5 min, the peel is immediately neutralized with the postpeel neutralizer. Application of the postpeel neutralizer yields a foaming reaction, and the postpeel

neutralizer should be applied until foaming ceases. After the peel has been neutralized, the patient may be offered application of cool water and a postpeel mild moisturizer.

Recent interest in AHAs was stimulated by early studies that demonstrated diminished corneocyte cohesion above the granular layer leading to abrupt loss of abnormal stratum corneum and decreased epidermal thickness. These observed histologic changes led to the first clinical studies of AHAs which were performed on patients with disorders of keratinization including patients with ichthyosiform disorders. AHAs subjectively improved the skin appearance of patients with ichthyosiform disorders of several types [3, 4] (III/B).

Clinical and histopathologic studies on AHA peel effects on photoaged skin soon followed (Table 17.1). Many investigators have suggested that AHA chemical peels can improve rhytides based on the results of the following studies demonstrating new collagen deposition. AHAs (25% glycolic, lactic, or citric acid) were shown in an early study to subjectively improve the appearance of photoaged forearm skin, and among the changes seen in the epidermis and dermis of AHA treated skin was a qualitative increase in dermal collagen [5] (II/A). A disproportionate increase in dermal collagen deposition with minimal nonspecific reaction has also been demonstrated in serial biopsies of mini-pig skin treated with 50 and 70% glycolic acid relative to other peeling agents [6] (III/B). However, skin biopsies of Skh:HR-hairless mice photoaged with ultraviolet B irradiation prior to 50% glycolic acid peeling showed an elevation in dermal collagen that was not statistically significant [7] (III/B). A recent double-blind, vehicle-controlled study showed that AHA peels produced significant improvement in rough texture, fine rhytides, solar keratoses, and lightening of solar lentigines. Histopathology showed thinning of the stratum corneum, enhancement of the granular layer, and epidermal thickening [8] (II/A).

AHA peels are believed to have maximum efficacy when a series of treatments are performed at the highest concentrations that a given patient can tolerate. Although "lunchtime" low

**Table 17.1** Peer-reviewed literature of AHA chemical peel treatment of ichthyosis and photoaging

| References | No. of patients | Study design | Indication and macroscopic assessment | Microscopic assessment | Evidence level |
|---|---|---|---|---|---|
| Van Scott and Yu [4] | 14 | Prospective controlled study | Ichthyosiform disorders Subjective: 3+ (disappearance of scale from lesions) to 4+ (restoration to normal looking skin) | Abrupt loss of abnormal stratum corneum, ↓ epidermal thickness | III/B |
| Ditre et al. [5] | 17 | Randomized controlled study | Photoaged skin Subjective: "plumper" appearance of skin, less apparent macular dyspigmentation | ↑ Epidermal thickness, ↓ basal cell atypia, ↓ melanin clumping, ↑ dermal mucopolysac-charides, ↑collagen density | II/A |
| Moy et al. [6] | 2 (mini-pig) | Prospective controlled study | Not performed | Minimal nonspecific reaction, ↑ collagen deposition | III/B |
| Butler et al. [7] | 20 (mice) | Prospective controlled study | Photoaged skin Not performed | ↑ Normal horizontal arrangement of elastic fibers | III/B |
| Newman et al. [8] | 41 | Double-blind vehicle-controlled study | Photoaged skin Subjective: ↓ rough texture/fine wrinkling, ↓ solar keratoses, ↑ lightening of lentigenes | Thinning of stratum corneum, ↑ granular layer, ↑ epidermal thickness | II/A |
| Alam et al. [9] | 10 | Unblinded randomized controlled trial | General appearance Subjective: no significant improvement from baseline | Not performed | II/A |

**Table 17.2** Peer-reviewed literature of AHA chemical peel treatment of melasma

| References | No. of patients | Study design | Indication and macroscopic assessment | Evidence level |
|---|---|---|---|---|
| Lim and Tham [10] | 10 | Split-faced prospective controlled study (20% GA) | Melasma Subjective: trend in greater lightening vs. controls, not statistically significant | III/B |
| Lawrence et al. [11] | 11 | Split-faced controlled clinical trial (70% GA vs. JS) | Melasma Objective: statistically significant improvement in colorimeter analysis and MASI score in both groups, no significant difference between groups Subjective: patients rated GA as more painful than JS, 75% of patients rated >50% improvement in melasma with both agents | III/B |
| Sarkar et al. [12] | 40 | Randomized controlled study (30–40% GA) | Melasma Objective: statistically significant improvement in MASI score in peel group vs. controls | II/A |
| Hurley et al. [13] | 18 | Split-faced randomized investigator masked clinical trial (20–30% GA) | Melasma Subjective: no significant difference in linear analog scale, or physician global evaluation vs. controls Objective: no significant difference in mexameter readings or MASI score in peel group vs. controls | II/A |
| Coleman and Brody [14] | N/A | Expert clinical experience | Subjective: improvement in melasma with GA 50–70% peels alone without hydroquinone | VI/C |
| Erbil et al. [15] | 28 | Randomized controlled study (20–70% GA) | Objective: statistically significant improvement in MASI score in peel group vs. controls | II/A |
| Sharquie et al. [16] | 12 | Prospective controlled study (92% LA) | Melasma Objective: statistically significant improvement in MASI score and visual analog scale | III/B |
| Sharquie et al. [17] | 24 | Split-faced controlled comparison study (92% LA vs. JS) | Melasma Objective: statistically significant improvement in MASI score and visual analog scale in both groups, no significant difference between groups | III/B |

*GA* glycolic acid; *LA* lactic acid; *JS* Jessner's solution; *MASI* melasma area severity index

concentration 20% glycolic acid peels are quite popular with patients because of "minimal downtime," these peels have been shown along with low-intensity MDA in a randomized, controlled trial to have no significant improvement in overall skin rejuvenation from baseline [9] (II/A). Regardless of overall results, a trend in patient preference towards glycolic acid peels over MDA approached significance in this study.

AHA peels have also been studied in the treatment of melasma (Table 17.2). Glycolic acid peels (20–70%) initially were shown to hasten improvement in melasma and fine facial rhytides when compared to application of 10% glycolic acid and 2% hydroquinone gel alone [10] (III/B). A split-faced study of glycolic acid and Jessner's solution peels showed that glycolic acid was equally as effective as Jessner's solution in hastening the effects of topical therapy in melasma, but patients perceived glycolic acid peels as more painful [11] (III/B). An open pilot study showed that the addition of serial 30–40% glycolic acid peels to a regimen of topical modified Kligman's formula (hydroquinone 5%, tretinoin 0.05%, and hydrocortisone acetate 1% in cream base) showed a trend towards more rapid and greater improvement in treatment of melasma in dark-skinned patients than Kligman's formula alone [12] (II/A). One randomized study has shown that the addition of four 20–30% glycolic acid peels did not enhance the effects of hydroquinone treatment alone in melasma treatment [13] (II/A). However, lower strength glycolic acid was chosen to avoid visible frosting and epidermolysis which in the authors' experience lead to significant postinflammatory hyperpigmentation. It was hypothesized that the lack of significant results was because the low 20–30% concentration of glycolic acid used only produced erythema and not epidermolysis. The reviewers who generated this hypothesis stated clinical observations of improvement in melasma when 50–70% glycolic acid solutions were used monthly in the absence of hydroquinone [14] (VI/C). Serial applications of 20–70% glycolic acid peels in increasing concentrations were studied with a topical regimen of azelaic acid 20% cream b.i.d. and adapalene 0.1% gel q.h.s. in the treatment of melasma. The peel group showed a statistically better result in melasma area severity index (MASI) scores vs. control patients who used topical treatment alone. The timing of statistically better results in MASI scores at 12, 16, and 20 weeks corresponded to treatment with 50% glycolic acid which suggests that a final concentration of 50% glycolic acid may be ideal for melasma treatment [15] (II/A). Superficial glycolic peels appear to be effective in the treatment of this often frustrating condition.

Although glycolic acid has been the most extensively studied AHA in melasma, lactic acid has also been examined as a novel therapeutic peeling agent in melasma and has been found in one study to yield responses in MASI scores and visual analog scale that were highly statistically significant [16] (III/B). A follow-up study [17] (III/B) demonstrated that lactic acid was as effective as Jessner's solution in treating patients with melasma.

AHAs have also been studied as a treatment of acne and postinflammatory hyperpigmentation (Table 17.3), and of all the AHA compounds used in clinical practice, glycolic acid has been most extensively studied for these skin disorders. One of the earliest well-designed studies of serial glycolic acid peels effects on acne was performed on Asian patients. The peels were performed in conjunction with the use of glycolic acid home care products, and the authors found significant resolution of comedones, papules, and pustules in the peel-treated group compared to controls who used only 15% glycolic acid home care products during the study. Follicular pores were reported to become smaller with treatment. An overall improvement in skin texture with "brighter and lighter" looking skin was reported (III/B) [18]. A similar study found that glycolic acid peels produced the most rapid improvement in comedonal acne; however, patients in this study applied a topical antibiotic twice daily which may have contributed to some of the observed efficacy, particularly in papulopustular lesions [19] (III/B). Glycolic acid was found in a split-faced study to be as effective as Jessner's solution for improving mild-to-moderate acne vulgaris, and patients were seen to have lesser exfoliation with glycolic acid peels than treatment with Jessner's solution, perhaps making it a more suitable treatment when "downtime" is an issue [20] (II/A). Glycolic acid has also been evaluated head to head in a split-faced study with salicylic acid in the treatment of mild-to-moderate acne vulgaris. Both were significantly effective in treating active acne, while salicylic acid showed more sustained effects in decreasing the total number of acne lesions [21] (II/A). However, this study is limited in that patients were allowed to continue stable regimens of physician-prescribed and over-the-counter therapy with no changes allowed during the study period (25% used a topical retinoid, 25% were taking oral antibiotics, and 55% were on other topical therapy at enrollment). It has been hypothesized that AHA peel efficacy in the treatment of acne is due to AHA peels' ability to decrease sebum secretion. However, Lee et al. demonstrated that sebum levels are not significantly changed after two peels with either glycolic acid or Jessner's solution [22] (III/B).

**Table 17.3** Peer-reviewed literature of AHA chemical peel treatment of acne

| References | No. of patients | Study design | Indication and macroscopic assessment | Evidence level |
|---|---|---|---|---|
| Wang et al. [18] | 40 | Prospective controlled study (35–50% GA) | Moderate-to-severe acne vulgaris Subjective: significant resolution of comedones, papules, pustules. Significant shrinking of follicular pores | III/B |
| Atzori et al. [19] | 80 | Prospective controlled study (70% GA) | Acne vulgaris Subjective: most rapid significant improvement in comedonal acne. Significant improvement in papulopustular acne | III/B |
| Kim et al. [20] | 26 | Split-faced randomized clinical trial (79% GA vs. JS) | Mild-to-moderate acne vulgaris Objective: significantly improved acne scores with both treatments. No significant differences between treatment effects. ↑ exfoliation with JS vs. GA | II/A |
| Kessler et al. [21] | 17 | Split-faced double-blind randomized controlled study (30% GA vs. 30% SA) | Mild-to-moderate acne vulgaris Objective: significant ↓ in number of acne lesions with both treatments. SA showed ↑ sustained effect in reduction of acne lesion number | II/A |
| Lee et al. [22] | 38 | Prospective controlled study (30% GA vs. JS) | Sebum secretion Objective: no significant change in sebum levels after two peels with either agent | III/B |
| Burns et al. [23] | 16 | Randomized controlled study (68% GA in maximum concentration) | Postinflammatory hyperpigmentation Subjective: trend toward more rapid and greater improvement vs. controls. ↑ lightening of normal skin Objective: trend toward more rapid and greater improvement in colorimetric analysis | II/A |
| Garg et al. [24] | 44 | Prospective controlled study (35% GA vs. 20%/10% SMA) | Objective: significant reduction in active acne lesions in both groups. SMA was more effective in reducing total acne score. Significant reduction in icepick and boxcar scars in both groups Subjective: higher visual analog score for SMA vs. GA | III/B |

*GA* glycolic acid; *JS* Jessner's solution; *SA* salicylic acid; *SMA* salicylic-mandelic acid

Papulopustular acne is often associated with postinflammatory hyperpigmentation particularly in those with Fitzpatrick Type IV, V, and VI skin. This is a common complaint of patients with darker Fitzpatrick skin types and is often considered acne scarring by the layperson. The use of glycolic acid peels in the treatment of postinflammatory hyperpigmentation in black patients (Fitzpatrick Type IV, V, and VI skin) was studied by Burns et al. This group compared glycolic acid peels to the application of a home regimen of containing 2% hydroquinone/10% glycolic acid gel b.i.d. and 0.05% tretinoin q.h.s. Subjects receiving glycolic acid peels demonstrated a trend toward more rapid and greater improvement in postinflammatory hyperpigmentation and increased lightening of normal skin [23] (II/A).

Though glycolic acid has been studied most in AHA peel treatment of acne, mandelic acid has also shown efficacy in treating active acne vulgaris and postinflammatory hyperpigmentation. Mandelic acid has been studied clinically in the form of salicylic-mandelic acid peels (SMPs). Both SMP and glycolic acid peels have been shown to be effective in the treatment of acne vulgaris and related postinflammatory hyperpigmentation; however, SMPs were significantly better than glycolic acid in reducing the total acne score [24] (III/B). On the basis of this study, it is difficult to determine how much of the observed efficacy is due to either the salicylic acid or mandelic acid portion of the combination. Further studies will need to be performed to better evaluate the utility of mandelic acid in the treatment of acne.

## Salicylic Acid Peels

Salicylic acid is a commonly used agent in office peels. Although salicylic acid is commonly described as a beta hydroxy acid, the correct chemical structure is that of *ortho*-hydroxybenzoic acid as the hydroxyl group is at the carbon adjacent to the carboxyl containing carbon. Salicylic acid is well known in its acetylated form, aspirin, which is ingested orally for various maladies. Although no investigators have studied topical salicylic acid treatment in pregnant patients, it is considered FDA Pregnancy Class C as aspirin has been shown to cause birth defects in animal models when absorbed systemically [25]. Physician-administered salicylic acid peels are commonly performed at a concentration of 20–30%, and home concentrations range from 0.5 to 10% [26]. Salicylic acid has been studied in myriad clinical applications including acne vulgaris, postinflammatory hyperpigmentation, melasma, and photodamaged skin. However, the bulk of peer-reviewed literature has examined salicylic acid peeling effects on acne vulgaris (Table 17.4).

Salicylic acid is an organic solvent that removes intercellular lipids covalently linked to the cornified envelope that surrounds keratinized cells [27]. Organic acids are known to extract desmosomal proteins including desmogelins and thus destroy cohesion of epidermal cells [28]. The histologic effects of salicylic acid peeling have been investigated by applying increasing concentrations of salicylic acid (up to 30%) to the backs of hairless mice for 20 min followed by histologic evaluation at various times postpeel [29] (III/B). The peel produced significant desquamation of the upper lipophilic layers of the stratum corneum, and the epidermal thinning was accompanied by residual epidermal cell rearrangement into a more regular configuration. Salicylic acid also macerated cornified follicular plugs and gradually dilated follicular pores to yield extrusion of plugs at 48 h postpeel. Postpeel levels of PCNA (proliferating cell nuclear antigen) positive epidermal basal cells were increased after salicylic treatment consistent with epidermal basal cell activation and regeneration of the epidermal cornified layer. No significant inflammation or degenerative changes were seen on histologic sections.

The safety and clinical effect of salicylic acid peels was first studied in patients with skin types V and VI who had varying indications for peeling including acne vulgaris, postinflammatory hyperpigmentation, melasma, and textural changes. Moderate (51–75% clearance) to significant (>75% clearance) improvement was observed in 88% of the patients studied [30] (III/B). Salicylic acid has also been studied specifically in the treatment of mild-to-moderate facial acne in Asian patients and noted to significantly decrease inflammatory and noninflammatory acne lesions. Gradual skin lightening in the peel group was also observed during the course of the study [31] (III/B). The side effects were generally well tolerated, and there was no significant postpeel difference in stratum corneum hydration, skin surface lipid, skin pH, and transepidermal water loss (TEWL) from baseline. A follow-up study from the same institution further investigated the whitening effect of salicylic acid peels in Asian patients with acne [32] (III/B). There was a clear trend during treatment towards continual and gradual skin lightening that did not reach significance, but improvement in erythema was statistically significant. The split-face comparison study by Kessler et al. [21] (II/A) of glycolic acid and salicylic acid peels in treatment of mild-to-moderate acne vulgaris (see Table 17.3) showed both to be significantly effective in treating active acne, and salicylic acid-treated sides showed more sustained effects in decreasing total number of acne lesions. It was hypothesized that this sustained effect was secondary to the lipophilicity of salicylic acid. Salicylic acid peels have been studied in comedonal acne specifically and achieved a

**Table 17.4** Peer-reviewed literature of salicylic acid peel treatment of acne vulgaris

| References | No. of patients | Study design | Indication and macroscopic assessment | Microscopic assessment | Evidence level |
|---|---|---|---|---|---|
| Imayama et al. [29] | 12 (mice) (7.5–30% SA) | Prospective controlled study | Not performed | No inflammation or degeneration, desquamation of upper lipophilic layers of stratum corneum, ↑ regular configuration of basal cell layer, ↑ basal cell activation, maceration/extrusion of follicular plugs | III/B |
| Grimes [30] | 25 (20–30% SA) | Prospective controlled study | Acne vulgaris, postinflammatory hyperpigmentation, melasma, rough/oily skin, enlarged pores; Subjective: moderate (51–75% clearing) to significant (>75% clearing) in 88% of patients | Not performed | III/B |
| Lee and Kim [31] | 35 (30% SA) | Single-blinded prospective controlled study | Mild-to-moderate acne vulgaris; Objective: ↓ number of active acne lesions, ↓ mean acne grade, no difference in hydration, skin surface lipid, skin pH, or TEWL; Subjective: 77.1% pts. reported good to moderate improvement | Not performed | III/B |
| Ahn and Kim [32] | 24 (30% SA) | Prospective controlled study | Skin lightening; Objective: trend of ↑ lightening in treated skin ($p = 0.0286$), Significant ↓ erythema | Not performed | III/B |
| Hashimoto et al. [33] | 16 (30% SA) | Prospective controlled study | Acne vulgaris; Objective: average ↓ mean total comedone count of 75% | Not performed | III/B |
| Dainichi et al. [34] | 6 (mice), 44 (aging), 436 (acne) (20–30% SA) | Prospective controlled study | Aging; Subjective: ↑ skin smoothness, ↑ elasticity, ↑ color improvement; Acne; Subjective: ↓ development of comedones and papules | Histology (mice): ↓ epidermal thickness, ↑ maceration and detachment of follicular cornified plugs, ↑ new, fine, regularly arranged cells; EM: restoration of regular grooves in skin surface with removal of cornified cells from hair follicles | III/B |

*SA* salicylic acid; *TEWL* trans epidermal water loss; *EM* electron microscopy mean comedone count reduction of 75% in patients who completed the study. The peels were also deemed equivalent to the sustained remission achieved by topical retinoids in comedonal acne [33] (III/B). One of the most recent studies of salicylic acid peeling examined clinical effects in photoaged skin. Histologic studies were also performed on mouse skin, and confirmed findings found in previous studies. These histologic observations are included in Table 17.4. Ninety-eight percent of patients treated for photoaged skin achieved a desired rejuvenated appearance characterized by smoother skin texture, increased elasticity, and improvement in color. There was also a considerable reduction in development of comedones and papules in patients with active acne vulgaris [34] (III/B).

## Jessner's Solution

Jessner's solution is composed of lactic acid 14%, salicylic acid 14%, and resorcinol 14% in ethyl alcohol. It has been used for well over 100 years and has a long history of safety and efficacy [35]. Jessner's solution traditionally has been used as an epidermal exfoliating agent to enhance peeling depth of another agent such as 35% trichloroacetic acid (TCA), 70% glycolic acid, or solid carbon dioxide slush. However, Jessner's solution alone has been used to treat common conditions including melasma and acne vulgaris. Despite the long history of Jessner's solution peeling, there are relatively few controlled studies on the overall efficacy of this peel, and there are few studies comparing Jessner's solution with other superficial peeling agents.

Jessner's solution has been discussed above as being equally effective as AHAs in the treatment of patients with melasma and moderate-to-severe acne vulgaris [12, 14, 22] (Tables 17.2 and 17.3). Jessner's solution peels have been compared most recently with 30% glycolic acid in treatment of melasma. Patients were blinded to the treatment received and were treated every 2 weeks for 12 weeks with nightly application of tretinoin 0.05% cream, daily sunscreen, and regular use of a moisturizer. Both peels achieved

highly significant improvement in patients' MASI scores, but the difference between treatments was not statistically significant [36] (II/A).

## Microdermabrasion

Developed in Italy by Marini and Lo Brutto in 1985 and introduced by Monteleone [37], MDA has become an extremely popular method of superficial skin resurfacing. Approximately 830,000 cases of MDA were performed in the United States in 2007 [38]. MDA has been classified by the US Food and Drug Administration as a Type I device (nonlife sustaining). MDA manufacturers are therefore not required to establish expertise for marketing the unit and do not require clearance from the FDA for MDA sales. There are many different types of MDA systems. Most MDA units are closed-loop negative pressure systems that pass aluminum oxide crystals over the skin. Some systems use sodium chloride crystals and positive pressure, and some systems are crystal-free using a handpiece with an abrasive diamond-studded tip. MDA has been popularized not only as a method for facial rejuvenation, but also as a treatment for a variety of skin conditions including photodamage, acne scarring, superficial rhytides, dull skin tone, enlarged pores, and mottled hyperpigmentation.

MDA appears to be safe to perform in patients of all Fitzpatrick skin types. Appropriate candidates for MDA include those patients who not only seek a procedure with minimal to no "downtime," but also understand that this procedure produces more modest results than those gained with more invasive resurfacing procedures. Patients seeking improvement in overall blending of skin color and/or texture are more likely to experience improvement than patients who desire removal of specific skin lesions. Patients seeking improvement in more advanced disorders of collagen including deep rhytides and deep atrophic scarring are unlikely to benefit from this procedure.

MDA is typically performed as a series of weekly to biweekly treatments, and depending on the condition being treated, approximately 4 to 8 treatments are recommended. The treatment area of choice is divided up into smaller zones that may be easily treated in a sequential manner. A minimum of 2–3 passes of the handpiece across the skin surface are applied in different directions before treating the next area which achieves an even and complete treatment to each zone. The dominant hand should be used to stretch the patient's skin between the thumb and index finger to allow for even contact of the handpiece with the skin. While higher pressures and increased number of passes may be used for deeper pathology, passes and pressures should be decreased when treating sensitive areas such as the periorbital skin, temples, and upper cutaneous lip. The desired clinical endpoint is that of mild-to-moderate erythema of the patient's skin without discrete abrasions or petechiae. After treatment is completed, a mild cleanser is applied by the treating clinician followed by application of a damp washcloth. A light moisturizer may be gently applied to the patient's skin as long as the patient is not prone to development of acne.

Despite the increasing popularity of MDA, there continues to be a paucity of peer-reviewed literature on the clinical efficacy of MDA in treating various skin conditions (Table 17.5). MDA has been studied most extensively in treating disorders of collagen such as photodamage, scarring, and fine rhytides. The first reported scientific study of MDA showed that a series of treatments achieved good to excellent improvement in patients with different types of facial scarring from acne, trauma, varicella, and burns [39] (III/B). However, the treatments were quite aggressive (up to 79 mmHg) and varying amounts of treatments were required to achieve desired results. Early investigation of MDA treatment of photoaging showed that a series of treatments seemed to achieve clinical improvement in roughness/textural irregularities of skin, mottled pigmentation, and overall complexion satisfaction, while fine wrinkling, comedones, and milia were not significantly improved [40] (III/B). MDA has also been reported to improve oiliness, skin thickness, dilated pores, and fine rhytides [41] (III/B). Coimbra et al. demonstrated using expert and lay evaluation of MDA-treated photodamaged skin that the procedure may improve

hyperchromic discoloration and fine rhytides [42] (III/B). The effectiveness of MDA in treating disorders of collagen seems to be proportional to both the aggressiveness of treatments, i.e., level of skin penetration achieved, and the number of treatments performed. For example, a series of low-intensity MDA treatments in a randomized, controlled trial was shown to have no significant improvement in overall skin rejuvenation from baseline [9] (II/A). This is also the opinion of the authors of this chapter and the subject of a soon-to-be-published manuscript at the time of this chapter's inception.

The microscopic effects of MDA have been studied in the hope of elucidating how MDA achieves clinical improvement of disorders of collagen, and these studies are detailed in Table 17.5. Although histopathologic evaluation suggests that MDA acutely thins the stratum corneum, some of this thinning may be secondary to transient compaction and homogenization. Chronic epidermal changes in MDA-treated photoaged skin include increased epidermal thickness, decreased melanization, and increased elastin [40]. This increase in epidermal thickness in MDA-treated photoaged skin has been strikingly significant and has ranged from 0.01 to 0.1 mm [41]. MDA appears to restore the epidermal polarity of photoaged skin while decreasing basal cell liquefaction and dermal elastosis of photoaged skin [41]. Dermal changes observed histologically in MDA-treated photoaged skin include increased perivascular infiltrate, edema, and vascular ectasia [43]. MDA has also been reported in one study to increase total and organized dermal collagen [42]. A recent immunohistological and ultrastructural study confirmed that MDA-treated skin showed mild increases in epidermal thickness, fibroblast count, dermal vascular ectasia, patchy and perivascular inflammation, and densely arranged thick collagen fibers [44] (III/B).

Photodamaged skin treated with MDA has been shown to have transient temperature increase and decrease in sebum along with decreased skin stiffness and increased skin compliance. These changes are felt to be consistent with mild abrasion and increased local perfusion [45]. MDA appears to induce molecular events conducive to

**Table 17.5** Peer-reviewed literature on microdermabrasion

| References | No. of patients | Study design | Indication and macroscopic assessment | Microscopic assessment | Evidence level |
|---|---|---|---|---|---|
| Tsai et al. [39] | 41 | Prospective controlled study | Facial scarring Subjective: good to excellent improvement | Not performed | III/B |
| Shim et al. [40] | 14 | Prospective controlled study | Photoaging Subjective: ↓ roughness textural irregularities, pigmentation, ↑ complexion satisfaction | Acute: ↓ stratum corneum thickness, ↑ compaction and homogenization Chronic: ↑ epidermal thickness, ↓ melanization, ↑ elastin | III/B |
| Hernandez–Perez and Ibiett [41] | 7 | Prospective controlled study | Oiliness, thickness, general appearance Subjective: oiliness, thickness, and dilated pores – good to excellent improvement. Fine wrinkles – moderate-to-good improvement | Epidermal: ↓ atrophy, ↓ horny plugs, ↑ epidermal polarity, ↓ basal cell liquefaction, ↑ epidermal thickness Dermal: ↓ elastosis, ↓ edema, ↓ telangiectasia, ↓ inflammation | III/B |
| Coimbra et al. [42] | 25 | Prospective controlled study | Photoaging and fine rhytides Objective: improvement in discoloration Subjective: satisfactory improvement | Epidermal: ↑ thickness Dermal: ↑ total and organized collagen | IV/B |
| Freedman et al. [43] | 10 | Prospective controlled study | Not performed | Epidermal: ↑ thickness, flattening of rete Dermal: ↑ vascular ectasia, ↑ inflammation, collagen, elastin | III/B |
| Hussein et al. [44] | 45 | Prospective controlled study | Not performed | Epidermal: ↑ thickness Dermal: ↑ fibroblast count, patchy and perivascular inflammation, vascular ectasia, collagen fibers | III/B |
| Tan et al. [45] | 10 | Prospective controlled study | Photoaging Objective: mild improvement Subjective: mild improvement | Epidermal: slight ↑ orthokeratosis, flattening of rete Dermal: perivascular infiltrate, slight ↑ edema, ↑ vascular ectasia | III/B |
| Karimipour et al. [46] | 49 | Prospective controlled study | Not performed | Stratum corneum thickness–no change, ↑ transcription factors, cytokines. MMPs. ↑ type I procollagen mRNA in two subjects | III/B |
| Karimipour et al. [47] | 10 | Prospective controlled study | Not performed | Negative pressure + abrasion: ↑ c-Jun of AP-1, IL-1β, TNFα, MMPs (1, 3, 9) Negative pressure only: ↑ MMP1, MMP3 | III/B |
| Lloyd [48] | 25 | Prospective study | Acne vulgaris Objective: good to excellent improvement Subjective: ↑ patient reports of skin improvement | Not performed | IV/B |
| Bhalla and Thami [49] | 30 | Open randomized clinical trial (MDA±topical retinoid) | Subjective Postacne scarring: 5–20% improvement Melasma: 5–15% improvement Facial rejuvenation: 20–40% improvement | Not performed | II/A |

Adapted from Bhalla and Thami [49]

*MDA* microdermabrasion; *MMPs* matrix metalloproteinases; *AP-1* activator protein-1; *IL* interleukin; *TNF* tumor necrosis factor dermal modeling and repair, and some of these molecular events include elevation of transcription factors, primary cytokines, type I procollagen mRNA and protein levels, and matrix metalloproteinases in skin [46] (III/B). A follow-up study found that the abrasive component of MDA was necessary for stimulating genes involved in dermal matrix remodeling [47] (III/B). However, it is unclear that these observed changes directly result in significant clinical improvement in patient appearance.

The use of MDA in treating acne is quite sparse, and one study has evaluated the effects of MDA in treating acne vulgaris. While 72% of the patients who completed the study had "excellent" or "good" results, the patients entered the study under dermatologic care for their acne and remained on acne medications during the study. Most patients were treated with not only oral antibiotics, but also topical retinoids, and medi-

cations were changed during the course of the study. It is therefore difficult from this study alone to determine if MDA has true efficacy in treating active acne [48] (IV/B). It is the opinion of the authors of this chapter that MDA is not a viable treatment for acne vulgaris and a randomized, controlled, split-faced trial needs to be performed to address this question.

The clinical efficacy of MDA treatment in pigmentary disorders other than the hyperpigmentation and mottled pigmentation seen with photodamage is quite sparse. One recent study examined the clinical effect of MDA in treating patients with many skin conditions including melasma. Patients were treated either with MDA alone or in conjunction with topical adapalene 0.1%. Treatment with MDA and topical adapalene 0.1% showed greater overall improvement (30–40%) in melasma vs. treatment with MDA alone (5–15%) [49] (II/A).

### Evidence-Based Summary

| Findings | Evidence level |
|---|---|
| Commonly used nonlaser superficial resurfacing procedures include chemical peels (α-hydroxy acids, salicylic acid, Jessner's solution) and microdermabrasion | |
| α-hydroxy acids are effective in treating photodamage and ichthyosiform disorders of the skin | (II/A to III/B) |
| α-hydroxy acids are effective in hastening resolution of melasma | (II/A to III/B) |
| α-hydroxy acids and salicylic acid are effective in treating active acne | (II/A to III/B and III/B, respectively) |
| α-hydroxy acids have been shown to induce the following histopathologic findings: abrupt loss of normal stratum corneum, increased epidermal thickness, decreased basal cell atypia, and decreased melanin clumping | (II/A to III/B) |
| Salicylic acid is effective in treating active acne vulgaris | (III/B) |
| Salicylic acid has been shown to induce the following histopathologic findings without inflammation or degeneration: desquamation of the upper lipophilic layers of the stratum corneum, maceration/extrusion of follicular keratin plugs, increased regular configuration of the basal cell layer, and increased epidermal thickness | (III/B) |
| Microdermabrasion has been shown to show subtle improvement in photoaging and overall skin appearance, and patients often are somewhat pleased with results obtained from serial microdermabrasion treatments | (II/A to III/B) |
| Microdermabrasion has been shown to induce the following epidermal histopathologic changes in photodamaged skin: increased epidermal thickness, decreased melanization of the basal layer, decreased basal cell liquefaction, normalization of epidermal polarity | (III/B to IV/B) |
| Microdermabrasion has been shown to induce the following dermal histopathologic changes in photodamaged skin: decreased dermal elastosis, increased perivascular infiltrate, increased edema and vascular ectasia, and increased dermal collagen | (III/B to IV/B) |
| Microdermabrasion appears to induce molecular events conducive to dermal modeling and repair, and some of these molecular events include elevation of transcription factors, primary cytokines, type I procollagen mRNA and protein levels, and matrix metalloproteinases in skin. However, it is unclear that these observed changes directly result in significant clinical improvement in patient appearance | (III/B) |

# References

1. Slavin JW. Considerations in alpha hydroxyl acid peels. Clin Plast Surg. 1998;25(1):45–52; review.
2. Murad H, Shamban AT, Premo PS. The use of glycolic acid as a peeling agent. Dermatol Clin. 1995;13(2):285–307; review.
3. Van Scott EJ, Yu RJ. Hyperkeratinization, corneocyte cohesion, and alpha hydroxy acids. J Am Acad Dermatol. 1984;11(5 Pt 1):867–79.
4. Van Scott EJ, Yu RJ. Control of keratinization with alpha-hydroxy acids and related compounds. I. Topical treatment of ichthyotic disorders. Arch Dermatol. 1974;110(4):586–90.
5. Ditre CM, Griffin TD, Murphy GF, Sueki H, Telegan B, Johnson WB, et al. Effects of alpha-hydroxy acids on photoaged skin: a pilot clinical, histologic, and ultrastructural study. J Am Acad Dermatol. 1996;34 (2 Pt 1):187–95.
6. Moy LS, Peace S, Moy RL. Comparison of the effect of various chemical peeling agents in a mini-pig model. Dermatol Surg. 1996;22(5):429–32.
7. Butler PE, Gonzalez S, Randolph MA, Kim J, Kollias N, Yaremchuk MJ. Quantitative and qualitative effects of chemical peeling on photo-aged skin: an experimental study. Plast Reconstr Surg. 2001;107(1): 222–8.
8. Newman N, Newman A, Moy LS, Babapour R, Harris AG, Moy RL. Clinical improvement of photoaged skin with 50% glycolic acid. A double-blind vehicle-controlled study. Dermatol Surg. 1996;22(5):455–60.
9. Alam M, Omura NE, Dover JS, Arndt KA. Glycolic acid peels compared to microdermabrasion: a right-left controlled trial of efficacy and patient satisfaction. Dermatol Surg. 2002;28(6):475–9.
10. Lim JT, Tham SN. Glycolic acid peels in the treatment of melasma among Asian women. Dermatol Surg. 1997;23(3):177–9.
11. Lawrence N, Cox SE, Brody HJ. Treatment of melasma with Jessner's solution versus glycolic acid: a comparison of clinical efficacy and evaluation of the predictive ability of Wood's light examination. J Am Acad Dermatol. 1997;36(4):589–93.
12. Sarkar R, Kaur C, Bhalla M, Kanwar AJ. The combination of glycolic acid peels with a topical regimen in the treatment of melasma in dark-skinned patients: a comparative study. Dermatol Surg. 2002;28(9):828–32; discussion 832.
13. Hurley ME, Guevara IL, Gonzales RM, Pandya AG. Efficacy of glycolic acid peels in the treatment of melasma. Arch Dermatol. 2002;138(12):1578–82.
14. Coleman WP III, Brody HJ. Efficacy of low-strength glycolic acid application in the treatment of melasma. Arch Dermatol. 2003;139(6):811; author reply 811–2.
15. Erbil H, Sezer E, Tastan B, Arca E, Kurumlu Z. Efficacy and safety of serial glycolic acid peels and a topical regimen in the treatment of recalcitrant melasma. J Dermatol. 2007;34(1):25–30.
16. Sharquie KE, Al-Tikreety MM, Al-Mashhadani SA. Lactic acid as a new therapeutic peeling agent in melasma. Dermatol Surg. 2005;31(2):149–54; discussion 154.
17. Sharquie KE, Al-Tikreety MM, Al-Mashhadani SA. Lactic acid chemical peels as a new therapeutic modality in melasma in comparison to Jessner's solution chemical peels. Dermatol Surg. 2006;32(12): 1429–36.
18. Wang CM, Huang CL, Hu CT, Chan HL. The effect of glycolic acid on the treatment of acne in Asian skin. Dermatol Surg. 1997;23(1):23–9.
19. Atzori L, Brundu MA, Orru A, Biggio P. Glycolic acid peeling in the treatment of acne. J Eur Acad Dermatol Venereol. 1999;12(2):119–22.
20. Kim SW, Moon SE, Kim JA, Eun HC. Glycolic acid versus Jessner's solution: which is better for facial acne patients? A randomized prospective clinical trial of split-face model therapy. Dermatol Surg. 1999; 25(4):270–3.
21. Kessler E, Flanagan K, Chia C, Rogers C, Glaser DA. Comparison of alpha- and beta-hydroxy acid chemical peels in the treatment of mild to moderately severe facial acne vulgaris. Dermatol Surg. 2008;34(1): 45–50; discussion 51.
22. Lee SH, Huh CH, Park KC, Youn SW. Effects of repetitive superficial chemical peels on facial sebum secretion in acne patients. J Eur Acad Dermatol Venereol. 2006;20(8):964–8.
23. Burns RL, Prevost-Blank PL, Lawry MA, Lawry TB, Faria DT, Fivenson DP. Glycolic acid peels for postinflammatory hyperpigmentation in black patients. A comparative study. Dermatol Surg. 1997;23(3): 171–4; discussion 175.
24. Garg VK, Sinha S, Sarkar R. Glycolic acid peels versus salicylic-mandelic acid peels in active acne vulgaris and post-acne scarring and hyperpigmentation: a comparative study. Dermatol Surg. 2009;35(1):59–65.
25. Kempiak SJ, Uebelhoer N. Superficial chemical peels and microdermabrasion for acne vulgaris. Semin Cutan Med Surg. 2008;26(3):212–20.
26. Akhavan A, Bershad S. Topical acne drugs: review of clinical properties, systemic exposure, and safety. Am J Clin Dermatol. 2003;4(7):473–92.
27. Lazo ND, Meine JG, Downing DT. Lipids are covalently attached to rigid corneocyte protein envelop existing predominantly as beta-sheets: a solid-state nuclear magnetic resonance study. J Invest Dermatol. 1995;105(2):296–300.
28. Rawlings A, Harding C, Watkinson A, Banks J, Ackerman C, Sabin R. The effect of glycerol and humidity on desmosome degradation in stratum corneum. Arch Dermatol Res. 1995;5:457–64.
29. Imayama S, Ueda S, Isoda M. Histologic changes in the skin of hairless mice following peeling with salicylic acid. Arch Dermatol. 2000;136(11):1390–5.

30. Grimes PE. The safety and efficacy of salicylic acid chemical peels in darker racial-ethnic groups. Dermatol Surg. 1999;25(1):18–22.

31. Lee HS, Kim IH. Salicylic acid peels for the treatment of acne vulgaris in Asian patients. Dermatol Surg. 2003;29(12):1196–9; discussion 1199.

32. Ahn HH, Kim IH. Whitening effect of salicylic acid peels in Asian patients. Dermatol Surg. 2006;32(3): 372–5; discussion 375.

33. Hashimoto Y, Suga Y, Mizuno Y, Hasegawa T, Matsuba S, Ikeda S, et al. Salicylic acid peels in polyethylene glycol vehicle for the treatment of comedogenic acne in Japanese patients. Dermatol Surg. 2008;34(2):276–9; discussion 279.

34. Dainichi T, Ueda S, Imayama S, Furue M. Excellent clinical results with a new preparation for chemical peeling in acne: 30% salicylic acid in polyethylene glycol vehicle. Dermatol Surg. 2008;34(7):891–9; discussion 899.

35. Monheit GD. Chemical peels. Skin Therapy Lett. 2004;9:6–11.

36. Ejaz A, Raza N, Iftikhar N, Muzzafar F. Comparison of 30% salicylic acid with Jessner's solution for superficial chemical peeling in epidermal melasma. J Coll Physicians Surg Pak. 2008;18(4):205–8.

37. Monteleone G. Microdermabrasion with aluminum hydroxide powder in scar camouflaging. In: Proceedings of the 3rd meeting of Southern Italy Plastic Surgery Association, Benevento, 9–10 Dec 1988.

38. ASAPS. 2007 ASAPS statistics: 11.7 million cosmetic procedures in 2007: American Society for Aesthetic Plastic Surgery reports 8% increase in surgical procedures. http://www.surgery.org/press/statistics-2007.php. Accessed 3 Feb 2009.

39. Tsai RY, Wang CN, Chan HL. Aluminum oxide crystal microdermabrasion. A new technique for treating facial scarring. Dermatol Surg. 1995;21(6):539–42.

40. Shim EK, Barnette D, Hughes K, Greenway HT. Microdermabrasion: a clinical and histopathologic study. Dermatol Surg. 2001;27(6):524–30.

41. Hernandez-Perez E, Ibiett EV. Gross and microscopic findings in patients undergoing microdermabrasion for facial rejuvenation. Dermatol Surg. 2001;27(7): 637–40.

42. Coimbra M, Rohrich RJ, Chao J, Brown SA. A prospective controlled assessment of microdermabrasion for damaged skin and fine rhytides. Plast Reconstr Surg. 2004;113(5):1438–43; discussion 1444.

43. Freedman BM, Rueda-Pedraza E, Waddell SP. The epidermal and dermal changes associated with microdermabrasion. Dermatol Surg. 2001;27(12):1031–3; discussion 1033–4.

44. Hussain MR, Ab-Deif EE, Abdel-Motaleb AA, Zedan H, Abdel-Mequid AM. Chemical peeling and microdermabrasion of the skin: comparative immunohistological and ultrastructural studies. J Dermatol Sci. 2008;52(3):205–9.

45. Tan MH, Spencer JM, Pires LM, Ajmeri J, Skover G. The evaluation of aluminum oxide crystal microdermabrasion for photodamage. Dermatol Surg. 2001;27(11):943–9.

46. Karimipour DJ, Kang S, Johnson TM, Orringer JS, Hamilton T, Hammerberg C, et al. Microdermabrasion: a molecular analysis following a single treatment. J Am Acad Dermatol. 2005;52(2):215–23.

47. Karimipour DJ, Kang S, Johnson TM, Orringer JS, Hamilton T, Hammerberg C, et al. Microdermabrasion with and without aluminum oxide crystal abrasion: a comparative molecular analysis of dermal remodeling. J Am Acad Dermatol. 2006;54(3):405–10.

48. Lloyd JR. The use of microdermabrasion for acne: a pilot study. Dermatol Surg. 2001;27(4):329–31.

49. Bhalla M, Thami GP. Microdermabrasion: reappraisal and brief review of the literature. Dermatol Surg. 2006;32(6):809–14.

## Self-Assessment

1. $\alpha$-hydroxy acids have been shown to be effective in treatment of which of the following conditions?
   (a) Acne vulgaris
   (b) Ichthyosis
   (c) Melasma
   (d) Photoaging
   (e) All of the above

2. Which of the following are histolopathologic changes that are *specifically* seen in salicylic acid peels?
   (a) Lack of inflammation or degeneration
   (b) Partial epidermal desquamation
   (c) Maceration and extrusion of follicular horny plugs
   (d) Decreased basal layer atypia
   (e) All of the above
   (f) Both A and C

3. Which of the following is NOT a component of Jessner's Solution?
   (a) Lactic acid
   (b) Salicylic acid
   (c) Ethanol
   (d) Resorcinol
   (e) Glycolic acid

4. Which of the following is NOT a superficial resurfacing technique?
   (a) Salicylic acid peel
   (b) Glycolic acid peel
   (c) Microdermabrasion
   (d) Jessner's solution peel
   (e) Jessner's-trichloroacetic acid peel

5. Which of the following is true regarding microdermabrasion?
   (a) Rated as a nonlife sustaining (Type I) device by the FDA
   (b) Crystals passed over the skin include aluminum oxide and sodium chloride
   (c) Abrasive component has been found to be necessary in stimulating genes involved in dermal matrix remodeling
   (d) Low-intensity microdermabrasion has no significant posttreatment differences in skin appearance from controls when used for facial rejuvenation.
   (e) All of the above

## Answers

1. e: All of the above
2. f: Both a and c
3. e: Glycolic acid
4. e: Jessner's-trichloroacetic acid peel
5. e: All of the above

# Cosmeceuticals

Zoe Diana Draelos

## Introduction

The terms cosmeceutical and evidence-based may not belong in the same phrase. Cosmeceuticals are considered by many scientists to represent fluff without stuff and indeed the reader may come to a similar conclusion at the end of this chapter. Nevertheless, it is worthwhile to examine the state of the science for cosmeceuticals as they represent an ever-expanding field in dermatology with perhaps much yet unrealized promise. Cosmeceuticals extend beyond cosmetics to enhance skin functioning, usually aiming to return the skin to a more youthful state. For example, wrinkle-reducing moisturizers, antioxidant serums, and skin-lightening salves all fall into this category. Cosmeceuticals are somewhat confusing, however, as both prescription and OTC products have been labeled by this term. Drug cosmeceuticals include topical retinoids for improving dermal collagen production, topical minoxidil for enhanced scalp hair growth, and eflornithine for facial hair growth reduction. These products will not be discussed, as they are not available to the consumer except by prescription. The second category of cosmeceuticals includes OTC drugs, such as sunscreens and antiperspirants. These also are outside the realm of this chapter. The discussion will focus on cosmeceuticals that are topically applied for the purpose of improving skin appearance.

## Cosmeceutical Development

The marketing of new ingredients and formulations with captivating advertising claims drives the cosmeceutical realm. The unending introduction of new products on a monthly basis makes generalization difficult, yet there are some basic concepts that apply to cosmeceutical development. These will be reviewed to help the reader better interpret the evidence to support cosmeceutical efficacy. First, cosmeceuticals are basically cosmetics and as such must be safe. This means that the best source of new materials for formulation would be substances derived from either plants or food components. Second, cosmeceutical additives must be available as a powder or liquid, since the majority of cosmeceuticals must be elegantly applied to the external body. Third, cosmeceuticals must have some easily identifiable benefit upon which to base a functional claim. For all of these reasons, the majority of cosmeceutical ingredients have their origin in the botanical realm or in foods.

New cosmeceuticals ingredients in the botanical realm are identified based on the algorithm presented in Table 18.1. Once the botanical active is identified and synthesized, it is typically applied

Z.D. Draelos (✉)
Department of Dermatology, Duke University School of Medicine, 2444 North Main Street, High Point, NC 27262, USA
e-mail: zdraelos@northstate.net

**Table 18.1** Steps in cosmeceutical ingredient development

1. New botanical material received in the laboratory
2. Various fractions of the botanical extracted
3. Fractions analyzed for relationship to known chemical compounds
4. Purified fraction exposed to gene array chip
5. Analysis completed for upregulation or downregulation of key events in cellular oxidation, inflammation, or irritation
6. New isolate studied in an in vitro model of cell culture for confirmation of gene array results
7. Positive in vitro findings lead to isolate analysis in mouse model focusing on markers of possible cutaneous benefit
8. Positive mouse findings lead to formulation in a vehicle suitable for human use
9. Human model testing conducted to determine if active has any cutaneous value
10. Formulation fine-tuned and patented
11. New ingredient licensed to cosmetic manufacturer
12. New technology enters the marketplace

**Table 18.2** Sources of cosmeceutical actives

| |
|---|
| Plant source |
|   Leaves, roots, fruits, berries, stems, twigs, barks, flowers |
| Growing conditions |
|   Soil composition, amount of available water, climate variations, plant stress |
| Harvesting conditions |
|   Time from harvest to transport, care of plant materials during shipping, storage conditions prior to manufacture |
| Preparation method |
|   Crushing, grinding, boiling, distilling, pressing, drying |
| Final extract status |
|   Liquid, powder, paste, syrup, crystal |
| Concentration |
|   Sufficient amount of active to produce biologic effect |

to a fibroblast gene chip to determine if it affects any key cellular event. After demonstration of a presumed physiologic effect, the active is tested in vitro to determine an effect on cultured fibroblasts. If positive data are obtained, the active is studied in a mouse model for confirmation. The active is then placed in a vehicle suitable for human application and clinical studies are undertaken. Successful human clinical studies pave the way for successful introduction into the marketplace via ingredient licensing arrangements.

The search for botanicals suitable for formulation into cosmeceuticals has led to the gathering of flowers, seeds, roots, leaves, twigs, and berries from plants all over the world. It is important to remember, however, that the constituents of a plant component are influenced by the season in which the plant material was picked, the growing conditions, and the processing of the agent. These variables are summarized in Table 18.2.

## Cosmeceutical Efficacy

Cosmeceuticals have been introduced for many different purposes including improving skin texture, radiance, smoothness, tone, and pigmentation.

The main benefit of most cosmeceutical formulations is a reduction in transepidermal water loss from the application of occlusive and humectant ingredients to the skin surface. Occlusive substances include petrolatum, mineral oil, vegetable oils, lanolin, and silicone oils. Humectant substances include glycerin, sodium PCA, hyaluronic acid, propylene glycol, and proteins. There is no doubt that skin hydration is an important cosmeceutical benefit known as moisturization. Most cosmeceutical ingredients are placed in a moisturizing vehicle making placebo-controlled studies inadequate. Cosmeceutical efficacy must be determined based on a double-blind comparison between the vehicle plus the cosmeceutical active as compared to the vehicle alone. This study design would provide the most compelling evidence that the cosmeceutical ingredient produced a documented benefit. As the reader will discover, few cosmeceutical ingredients are studied with this methodology.

The claims pertaining to skin texture, radiance, and smoothness are moisturizer claims. These are primarily derived from vehicle effects. The more novel antiaging claims that this chapter will investigate are improvements in skin tone and pigmentation. Skin tone is a somewhat ambiguous term by design to allude to improvement in the characteristics of the skin associated with aging. Most of the ingredients that deliver on this benefit are antioxidants. The claim of pigmentation improvement is related to the ability of the cosmeceutical to lighten melasma and lentigenes while overall improving skin color. The rest of this chapter will be devoted to the evidence surrounding the efficacy of antioxidants and pigment-lightening ingredients in cosmeceutical formulations.

## Antioxidants

Antioxidants form one of the most popular categories of cosmeceutical ingredients. This is due to the fact that the major cause of cutaneous aging is oxidation of skin structures from highly reactive oxygen molecules present in our oxygen rich environment. It is amazing to think that the life-giving oxygen required to survive is also the same oxygen responsible for aging the human body. The primary source of cosmeceutical antioxidant ingredients is botanical extracts, since all plants must protect themselves from oxidation following UV exposure.

Antioxidant botanicals function by quenching singlet oxygen and reactive oxygen species, such as superoxide anions, hydroxyl radicals, fatty peroxy radicals, and hydroperoxides. There are many botanical antioxidants available from raw material suppliers to the cosmeceutical industry, which can be classified into one of three categories as carotenoids, flavonoids, and polyphenols. Carotenoids are chemically related to retinoids, while flavonoids possess a polyphenolic structure that accounts for their antioxidant, UV protectant, and metal chelation abilities. Lastly, polyphenols represent a chemical subset of flavonoids. These classes of antioxidants are discussed utilizing popular ingredients to take an evidence-based approach.

## Carotenoids

Carotenoids are derivatives of vitamin A and have found widespread use in cosmeceuticals due to the established topical antiaging benefits associated with the prescription retinoid tretinoin. The carotenoids are a large family of orange-, red-, and yellow-appearing substances that perform vital antioxidant roles when ingested and are less well established as topical antioxidants.

## Astaxanthin

Astaxanthin is a pink carotenoid found in high concentration in salmon, accounting for the characteristic pink color of the fish. This is the rationale for antiaging diets recommending the ingestion of a serving of salmon 5 times weekly [1] (IV,B). For topical application purposes, astaxanthin is obtained from the marine microalgae *Haematococcus pluvialis.* The efficacy of astaxanthin is attributed to its cell membrane, composed of two external lipid layers, which has been touted to possess stronger antioxidant abilities than vitamin E [2] (IV,B). It is both water and oil soluble only being produced by algae when exposed to intense UV radiation.

Few topical studies exist to confirm the topical effect of astaxanthin [3] (VI,C), but it has been studied extensively as an oral supplement [4] (IV,B). It is used as a homeopathic treatment for macular degeneration because; unlike canthaxanthin, another carotenoid, it does not crystallize in the eye. It crosses the blood–brain barrier and has been studied in brain dysfunction to include spinal cord injuries and Parkinson's disease [5] (VI,C). Even though other carotenoids, such as beta-carotene, have been proven ineffective in reducing the oxidative stress associated with cardiovascular disease, astaxanthin is currently undergoing further investigation [6] (IV,B).

Astaxanthin in concentrations of 0.03–0.07% produces a pink-colored cream. This limits the concentration that can be used, but no topical adverse reactions have been associated with this carotenoid. The topical antioxidant benefits of astaxanthin have not been established.

## Lutein

Another carotenoid found in topical cosmeceuticals is lutein. It is naturally found in green leafy vegetables, such as spinach and kale. Lutein is an antioxidant in the plant kingdom, also being used for blue light absorption. In the animal kingdom, lutein is found in egg yolks, animal fats, and the corpus luteum. It is a lipophilic molecule, not soluble in water, characterized by a long polyene side chain composed of conjugated double bonds. These double bonds are degraded by light and heat, a universal characteristic of carotenoids to a greater or lesser degree [7] (IV,B).

Lutein is used as a natural colorant due to its orange-red color resulting from the absorption of blue light. Its largest use is as a food supplement for chickens, which results in more vivid yellow yolks. In humans, lutein is concentrated in the macula and has been linked to the prevention of macular degeneration [8] (IV,B). It has been available as a nutritional supplement since 1996 and can be administered as a sublingual spray for elderly patients with macular degeneration. Most well-conducted studies evaluating the benefit of lutein for macular degeneration have been inconclusive [9] (IV,B). No recommended daily allowance has been established for lutein, but 6 mg/day has been published [10] (VI,C). Most of the lutein used for food additives is derived from marigolds.

The question remains as to whether lutein topically is of value. Again data are lacking, but excess lutein intake can result in carotenodermia and excess topical application results in bronzing of the skin. It may be of interest that lutein fed to chickens results in the characteristic yellow appearance of chicken skin, which is felt to be more attractive than the natural white skin. I am not sure that this would be the case in humans.

## Lycopene

Another potent carotenoid is lycopene, found in most fruits and vegetables with a red color including tomatoes, watermelon, pink grapefruit, papaya, gac, red bell pepper, and pink guava. The highest lycopene containing food is ketchup, but lycopene is not an essential human nutrient. The Mayo Clinic website rates the evidence for the use of lycopene as an antioxidant as a C, since it is not clear if lycopene has these effects on the human body [11] (IV,B). Lycopene oral supplements have been purported to reduce the risk of prostate cancer, but the FDA concludes there is little scientific evidence to support this claim [12] (VI,C).

Lycopene is a highly unsaturated hydrocarbon containing 11 conjugated and 2 unconjugated double bonds, which makes it a longer molecule than any other carotenoid. This makes its absorption into the skin doubtful. It undergoes *cis*-isomerization possible when exposed to sunlight. Even though lycopene was the new oral supplement

**Table 18.3** Cutaneous effects of topical retinoids

| Gross dermatologic effects |
| --- |
| Improvement in fine and coarse facial wrinkling |
| Decreased tactile roughness |
| Reduction of actinic keratoses |
| Lightening of solar lentigenes |

| Histologic dermatologic effects |
| --- |
| Reduction in stratum corneum cohesion |
| Decreased epidermal hyperplasia |
| Increased production of collagen, elastin, and fibronectin |
| Reduction in tonofilaments, desmosomes, melanosomes |
| More numerous Langerhans cells |
| Angiogenesis |
| Decreased glycosaminoglycans |
| Reduced activity of collagenase and gelatinase |
| Normalization of keratinization of the pilosebaceous unit |

added to many commercial multivitamins this year, its topical value has never been documented. It is safe for skin application, but may stain the skin in high concentration.

## Retinol

Of all the topical carotenoids, retinol is the best understood, since it is necessary for vision and possesses a well-characterized skin receptor [13] (II,A). Prescription retinoids, such as tazarotene and tretinoin, are well studied for their ability to induce the skin changes noted in Table 18.3; however, OTC retinoids may demonstrate some of the same effects, to a lesser degree [14, 15] (II,A).

It is theoretically possible to interconvert the retinoids from one form to another. For example, retinyl palmitate and retinyl propionate, chemically known as retinyl esters, can become biologically active following cutaneous enzymatic cleavage of the ester bond and subsequent conversion to retinol. Retinol is the naturally occurring vitamin A form found in red, yellow, and orange fruits and vegetables. It is the pigment responsible for vision, but is highly unstable. Retinol can be oxidized to retinaldehyde and then oxidized to retinoic acid, also known as prescription tretinoin. It is this cutaneous conversion of retinol to retinoic acid that is responsible for the biologic activity of some of the new stabilized over-the-counter vitamin A preparations designed to improve the appearance of benign

**Table 18.4** Biologic activity of flavonoids

| |
| --- |
| Photoprotection against UVB |
| Quenching of reactive oxygen species |
| Metal chelation |
| Inhibition of targeted enzymes |
| Hormonal modulation |
| Anti-inflammatory activity |
| Microorganism growth inhibition |
| Antioxidant effect of multiple organ systems |

photodamaged skin [16] (II,A). Unfortunately, only small amounts of retinyl palmitate and retinol can be converted by the skin, accounting for the increased efficacy seen with prescription preparations containing retinoic acid.

The main problem with prescription retinoids is their irritancy. Unfortunately, as the biological efficacy of the retinoid increases, so does the irritancy. This is also the case with the OTC retinoids. Retinol is more irritating than the retinyl esters and also more unstable. It is for this reason that cosmeceutical formulations not manufactured under strict oxygen-free conditions prefer to add retinyl palmitate to moisturizing creams. However, the retinyl palmitate may present to act as an antioxidant for the lipids present in the moisturizer.

The topical benefit of retinol has been documented by well-controlled studies [17] (II,A). It is commonly felt among dermatologists that retinol is of benefit [18] (IV,B), but it is difficult in moisturizer studies that do not include vehicle control to separate the retinol benefit from the moisturizer benefit. Nevertheless, of all the carotenoids available for formulation, retinol has the most evidence to support topical application efficacy.

## Flavonoids

Flavonoids are aromatic compounds, frequently with a yellow color, that occur in higher plants. Five-thousand flavonoids have been identified with a similar chemical structure possessing 15 carbon atoms and possessing a variety of biologic activities (Table 18.4) [19] (VI,C). Flavonoids can be divided into flavones, flavonols, isoflavones, and flavanones, each with a slightly different chemical structure. Currently, the most common isoflavones incorporated into cosmeceuticals are daidzein and genistein derived from soybeans. Other sources of flavonoids include curcumin, silymarin, pycnogenol, and gingko. These will be discussed next.

### Soy

The soybean-derived isoflavones genistein and daidzein function as phytoestrogens when orally consumed and have been credited with the decrease in cardiovascular disease and breast cancer seen in Asian women [20] (III,B). These isoflavones are present when the soy is fermented [21] (II,B). Other purported systemic benefits include improvement in immunity [22] (IV,C), reduction of prostate cancer [23] (IV,C), and improvement in cognition [24] (IV,C). Some of the cutaneous effects of soy have linked to its estrogenic effect in postmenopausal women. Topical estrogens have been shown to increase skin thickness and promote collagen synthesis [25] (II,A). It is interesting to note that genistein increases collagen gene expression in cell culture; however, there are no published reports of this collagen-stimulating effect in topical human trials. Genestein has also been reported to function and a potent antioxidant scavenging peroxyl radicals and protecting against lipid peroxidation in vivo [26] (III,B). The only studies that document the ability of soy to protect against UVB-induced skin damage are in mice where a topical application of nondenatured soy extracts reduced UVB-induced cyclooxygenase-2 expression, prostaglandin-E2 secretion, and inhibited p38 MAP kinase activation [27] (II,B).

### Curcumin

Curcumin is a popular natural yellow food coloring used in everything from prepackaged snack foods to meats. It is sometimes used in skin care products as a natural yellow coloring in products that claim to be free of artificial ingredients. Curcumin comes from the rhizome of the tumeric plant and is consumed orally as an Asian spice, frequently found in rice dishes to color the otherwise white rice yellow. However, this yellow color is undesirable in cosmetic preparations, since yellowing of products is typically associated with oxidative spoilage. Tetrahydrocurcumin, a hydrogenated form of curcumin, is off-white in color and can be added to skin care product not only to function as a skin antioxidant, but also to prevent the lipids in the moisturizer from becoming rancid. The antioxidant effect of tetrahydrocurcumin is said to be greater than vitamin E by cosmetic chemists. It is said to provide antioxidant skin benefits by quenching oxygen radicals and inhibiting nuclear factor-KB [28, 29] (V,C).

The effects of curcumin as a topical antioxidant in the skin have not been as well studied as its oral ingestion in rodents for the correction of cystic fibrosis defects and inhibition of tumor proliferation [30, 31] (V,C).

## Silymarin

Silymarin is an extract of the milk thistle plant (Silbum marianum), which belongs to the aster family of plants including diasies, thistles, and artichokes. The plant is named milk thistle because the oldest recorded use of the extract was to enhance human lactation and the plant produces a white milky sap. The extract consists of three flavinoids derived from the fruit, seeds, and leaves of the plant. These flavonoids are silybin, silydianin, and silychristine. Homeopathically, silymarin is used to treat liver disease, but it is a strong antioxidant preventing lipid peroxidation by scavenging free radical species. Its antioxidant effects have been demonstrated topically in hairline mice by the 92% reduction of skin tumors following UVB exposure [32, 33] (VI,C). The mechanism for this decrease in tumor production is unknown, but topical silymarin has been shown to decrease the formation of pyrimidine dimers in a mouse model [34] (VI,C). It has also been found to improve the healing of burns in albino rats [35] (VI,C).

Silymarin is found in a number of high-end moisturizer for benign photoaging to prevent cutaneous oxidative damage and to reduce facial redness. A double-blind placebo-controlled study in 46 subjects with stage I–III rosacea found improvement in skin redness, papules, itching, hydration, and skin color [36] (III,B). This was felt to be due to its direct activity on modulating cytokines and angiokines. Other well-controlled human trials are lacking.

## Pycnogenol

Pycnogenol is an extract of French marine pine bark (*Pinus pinaster*), which grows only on the southwest coast of France in Les Landes de Gascongne. The extract is a water-soluble liquid containing several phenolic constituents, including taxifolin, catechin, and procyanidins. It also contains several phenolic acids, including p-hydroxybenzoic, protocatechuic, gallic, vanillic, p-couric, caffeic, and ferulic [37] (VI,C). It is a trade-marked ingredient that is sold for oral consumption as a preventative for cardiovascular disease [38], a treatment for diabetic microangiopathy [39], and a pain reliever for muscle cramps [40] (IV,B). It is a potent free radical scavenger that can reduce the vitamin C radical, returning the vitamin C to its active form [41] (VI,C). The active vitamin C in turn regenerates vitamin E to its active form maintaining the natural oxygen scavenging mechanisms of the skin intact.

Pycnogenol is the ideal antiaging additive since it demonstrates no chronic toxicity, no mutagenicity, no teratogenicity, and no allergenicity [42] (VI,C). It is consumed orally to enhance the production of nitric oxide, which inhibits platelet aggregation in coronary artery disease, thus it is also deemed safe for topical use. Its use for skin indications is less well documented, however. In B16 melanoma cells, it was shown to inhibit tyrosinase activity and melanin biosynthesis [43] (IV,B). Many discussions of antioxidant flavonoids include a mention of pycnogenol, but little quality data are presented [44] (VI,C).

## Ginkgo

Ginkgo biloba, also named the maidenhair tree, is the last member of the Ginkgoaceae family, which grew on earth some 200–250 million years ago. For this reason, ginkgo contains flavonoids not found in other botanicals. It possesses bilobalide (a sequiterpene), ginkgolides (diterpenes with 20 carbon atoms), and other aromatic substances such as ginkgol, bilobdol, and ginkgolic acid. It is a plant with numerous purported benefits which is a common part of homeopathic medicine in the Orient for 4,000 years. The plant leaves are said to contain unique polyphenols such as terpenoids (ginkgolides, bilobalides), flavinoids, and flavonol glycosides that have anti-inflammatory effects. These anti-inflammatory effects have been linked to antiradical and antilipoperoxidant effects in experimental fibroblast models [45] (IV,C). Ginkgo flavonoid fractions containing quercetin, kaempferol, sciadopitysin, ginkgetin, and isoginkgetin have been demonstrated to induce human skin fibroblast proliferation in vitro. Increased collagen and extracellular fibronectin were also demonstrated by radioisotope assay [46] (IV,C). Thus, ginkgo extracts are added to many cosmeceuticals to function as antioxidants and promoters of collagen synthesis based on nonhuman models of oxidative damage.

## Polyphenols

Polyphenols are a subset of flavonoids used in many cosmeceuticals. Two main sources of polyphenols are teas and fruits. This section presents green tea and pomegranate as examples of the evidence available to support polyphenol biologic activity.

### Green Tea

Tea, also known as Camellia sinensis, is botanically popular in the Orient for 5,000 years used both topically and orally. Teas are a rich part of the Oriental culture used to stay alert during extended meditation. An Indian legend tells of a Prince Siddhartha Guatama, the founder of Buddhism, who tore off his eyelids in frustration over his inability to stay awake during meditation. A tea plant is said to have sprouted from where his eyelids fell providing the ability to stay awake, meditate, and reach enlightenment. Tea reached western cultures during the sixth century from Turkish traders.

There are several different types of teas: green, black, oolong, and white. The different teas come from the same plant, but different processing imparts different properties. Green tea is made from unfermented tea leaves and contains the highest concentration of polyphenol antioxidants [47] (VI,B). Black tea leaves are fermented days before heating. Oolong tea originates in the Fukien province of China and the leaves are treated much like black tea, except the withering and fermentation times are minimized. White tea comes from young tea leaves that are harvested for a few days each spring when the plant emerges from the ground. These leaves are said to be very high in antioxidants. The highest quality white tea is obtained from buds that are just ready to open known as needles or tips.

The evidence to support the anticancer benefits of topical and oral green tea use was felt to be inadequate by the FDA. On June 30, 2005, the FDA concluded, "that there is no credible evidence to support qualified health claims for green tea consumption and a reduced risk of gastric, lung, colon/rectal, esophageal, pancreatic, ovarian, and combined cancers. Thus, the FDA is denying these claims. However, FDA concludes that there is very limited credible evidence for qualified health claims specifically for green tea and breast cancer and for green tea and prostate cancer, provided the claims are appropriately worded so as not to mislead consumers" [48] (VI,C). In addition, the evidence to support cardiovascular benefits was inadequate. On May 9, 2006, in response to "Green Tea and Reduced Risk of Cardiovascular Disease," the FDA concluded "there is no evidence to support qualified health claims for green tea or green tea extract and a reduction in a number of risk factors associated with cardiovascular disease" [49] (VI,C). Some FDA advisers have voiced concern that teas may contain high levels of pesticides and heavy metals.

Green tea is manufactured from both the leaf and bud of the plant. Orally, green tea is said to contain beneficial polyphenols, such as epicatechin, epicatechin-3-gallate, epigllocatechin, and eigallocatechin-3-gallate (EGCG), which function as potent antioxidants [50] (IV,B). EGCG is the most potent of the polyphenols sold as a white caffeine-free powder [51] (VI,C). Oral studies with EGCG have demonstrated the increased fat oxidation and improvements in heart rate and serum glucose levels with 300 mg [52, 53] (V,B).

Other alkaloids present in green tea include caffeine, theobromine, and theophylline.

Green tea can be easily added to topical creams and lotions designed to combat the signs of photoaging, but it must be stabilized itself with an antioxidant, such as butylated hydroxytoluene. The Mayo Clinic Drugs and Supplements rates the evidence to support green tea as a photoprotectant as a C [54] (VI,C).

A study by Katiyar et al. demonstrated the anti-inflammatory effects of topical green tea application on C3H mice. A topically applied green tea extract containing GTP ((−)-epigallocatechin-3-gallate) was found to reduce UVB-induced inflammation as measured by double skin-fold swelling [55] (IV,B). They also found protection against UV-induced edema, erythema, and antioxidant depletion in the epidermis. This work was further investigated by applying GTP to the back of humans 30 min prior to UV irradiation, which resulted in decreased myeloperoxidase activity and decreased infiltration of leukocytes as compared to untreated skin [56] (III,B).

The application of topical green tea polyphenols prior to UV exposure has also been shown to decrease the formation of cyclobutane pyrimidine dimers [57] (IV,B). These dimers are critical in initiating UV-induced mutagenesis and carcinogenesis, which represent the end stage of the aging process. Thus, green tea polyphenols can function topically as antioxidants, anti-inflammatories, and anti-carcinogens making them a popular cosmeceutical additive [58, 59] (III,B).

## Pomegranate

Similar to lycopene, another oral supplement appearing in health drinks and vitamin is pomegranate extract. Pomegranate, botanically known as *Punica granatum*, is a deciduous tree bearing a red fruit native to Afghanistan, Pakistan, Iran, and northern India [60]. It was brought to California by the Spanish settlers in 1769 and is commercially cultivated for its juice. The pomegranate became famous in Greek mythology when Persephone was kidnapped by Hades and taken to the Underworld to be his wife. Persephone had consumed four pomegranate seeds while in the Underworld and thus had to spend 4 months every year in Hades, during which time nothing would grow. This gave rise to the season of winter.

Pomegranate juice, commonly consumed in the Middle East, provides about 16% of the adult requirement of Vitamin C per 100 mg serving. It also contains pantothenic acid, also known as Vitamin B5, potassium, and antioxidant polyphenols. These substances have been demonstrated to protect against UVA- and UVB-induced cell damage in SKU-1064 human skin fibroblasts [61] (IV,B). Pomegranate juice has also been purported to reduce oxidative stress, affect LDL, and platelet aggregation in humans and apolipoprotein e-deficient mice [62, 63] (IV,B). It has also been studied for improving hyperlipidemia in diabetic patients [64] (IV,B).

## Other Antioxidants

### Aloe Vera

Probably the most widely used cutaneous botanical anti-inflammatory is aloe vera. The mucilage is released from the plant leaves as a colorless gel and contains 99.5% water and a complex mixture of mucopolysaccharides, amino acids, hydroxy quinone glycosides, and minerals. Compounds isolated from aloe vera juice include aloin, aloe emodin, aletinic acid, choline, and choline salicylate [65] (VI,C). Reported cutaneous effects of aloe vera include increased blood flow, reduced inflammation, decreased skin bacterial colonization, and enhanced wound healing [66] (VI,C). The anti-inflammatory effects of aloe vera may result from its ability to inhibit cyclooxygenase as part of the arachidonic acid pathway.

The MedlinePLus Herbs and Supplements rates the evidence to support the use of aloe vera in the treatment of dry skin and burns as a C. Other studies have evaluated the effect of aloe vera on burn wounds and acne [67, 68] (V,C). Aloe vera cream was found to show no tanning or sunburn protection and no efficacy in sunburn treatment as compared to placebo [69] (III,B). Reuter et al. studied a 97.5% concentration of aloe vera for its anti-inflammatory effects and demonstrated positive results in a sunburn cell assay as compared to 1% hydrocortisone [70] (III,B). These data provide evidence for the anti-inflammatory effect of pure aloe vera gel; however, most products sold over-the-counter for under $10 do not contain a high enough percentage of aloe vera to induce clinically relevant inflammation reduction.

## CoEnzyme Q10

An endogenous antioxidant that has been incorporated into antiaging moisturizers is CoEnzyme Q10, also known as ubiquinone or CoQ10. For a topical antioxidant to be clinically effective, it must penetrate into the skin. Hoppe and colleagues from Beiersdorf demonstrated the topical penetration of CoEnzyme Q10 into the viable epidermis and a reduction in oxidation as measured by weak photon emission. They were also able to show a significant decrease in the expression of collagenase in human dermal fibroblasts following UVA radiation and improvement in orbital wrinkling [71, 72] (III,B). However, oral supplementation had no effect on the main antioxidant defenses or prooxidant generation in tissues in mice. It also did not affect the life span in mice according to Sohal et al. [73] (III,B). A human study by Passi et al. administered 50 mg Vitamin E and 50 mg CoEnzyme Q10 and 50 mg selenium. An increase in stratum corneum CoEnzyme Q10 was noted after 15 and 30 days of ingestion, but the significance of this finding was not evaluated [74] (II,B).

Other evidence suggests that topical CoEnzyme Q10 may provide additive antioxidant benefits when combined with colorless carotenoids phytoene and phytofluene. This effect was demonstrated in fibroblast cultures [75] (IV,C).

## Pigment-Lightening Agents

Facial hyperpigmentation is one of the most common signs of photoaging. Many different patterns can be seen. Focal hyperpigmentation in the form of small lentigenes across the lateral cheeks usually begins about age 25–30, depending on cumulative sun exposure, with continued accumulation of lesions throughout life. Pigmentation can also present in the form of melasma with reticulated pigment over the sides of the forehead lateral

jawline and upper lip. Lastly, hyperpigmentation can present as overall darkening of the skin from a combination of melanin pigment, fragmented elastin fibers, and residual hemosiderin. Cosmeceutical treatments for hyperpigmentation are problematic. A successful treatment must remove existing pigment from the skin, shut down the manufacture of melanin, and prevent the transfer of existing melanin to the melanosomes.

Many cosmetic products are available to lighten skin and improve even skin tone. These products typically do not contain hydroquinone, but rather other botanically derived products that interrupt melanin synthesis. These botanicals include ascorbic acid, licorice extract, alpha lipoic acid, kojic acid, aleosin, and arbutin. Hydroquinone has been eliminated from most cosmetics, since the European Union and Asia have removed hydroquinone from the over-the-counter market. Most cosmetic companies are international in their distribution and formulate for the global market and not the United States market specifically, where over-the-counter hydroquinone is still allowed. This section evaluates the data to support the efficacy of the most popular botanicals in skin lightening.

## Ascorbic Acid

Ascorbic acid, also known as Vitamin C, is used in cosmeceuticals for hyperpigmentation because it interrupts melanogenesis by interacting with copper ions to reduce dopaquinone and blocks dihydrochinindol-2-carboxyl acid oxidation [76] (II,A). Ascorbic acid, an antioxidant, is rapidly oxidized when exposed to air with limited stability. For this reason, many cosmeceuticals are using the more stable magnesium ascorbyl phosphate, which is metabolized to ascorbic acid in the skin. High concentrations of ascorbic acid must be used with caution, however, as the low pH can be irritating to the skin. Pigment-lightening cosmeceuticals may contain ascorbic acid as a pH adjustor or to function as an antioxidant preservative. It is important to recognize that ascorbic acid is a multifunctional ingredient with very minimal pigment-lightening capabilities.

## Licorice Extract

Licorice extracts are found in cosmeceuticals to decrease facial redness and reduce pigmentation. The extract contains liquiritin and isoliquertin, which are glycosides containing flavenoids [77] (III,B), which induce skin lightening by dispersing melanin. To see clinical results, the liquiritin must be applied in the dose of 1 g/day for 4 weeks. Irritation is not a side effect as is so frequently observed with hydroquinone and ascorbic acid, but efficacy is minimal.

## Alpha Lipoic Acid

Alpha lipoic acid is found in a variety of antiaging cosmeceuticals to function as an antioxidant [78] (II,B), but it may also have very limited pigment-lightening properties. It is a disulfide derivative of octanoic acid that is able to inhibit tyrosinase. However, it is a large molecule and cutaneous penetration to the level of the melanocyte is challenging significantly reducing its efficacy.

## Kojic Acid

Kojic acid, chemically known as 5-hydroxymethyl-4H-pyrane-4-one, is one of the most popular cosmeceutical skin lightening agents found in cosmetic counter skin lightening cream distributed worldwide. It is a hydrophilic fungal derivative obtained from Aspergillus and Penicillium species. It is the most popular agent employed in the Orient for the treatment of melasma; however, it is highly unstable [79] (IV,B). Newer formulations have incorporated kojic dipalmitate, but the efficacy of this derivative has not been well studied. Some research indicates that kojic acid is equivalent to hydroquinone in pigment-lightening ability [80] (IV,B). The activity of kojic acid is attributed to its ability to prevent tyrosinase activity by binding to copper.

## Aleosin

Aleosin is a low-molecular-weight glycoprotein obtained from the aloe vera plant. It is a natural hydroxymethylchromone functioning to inhibit tyrosinase by competitive inhibition at the DOPA oxidation site [81, 82] (IV,B). In contrast to hydroquinone, it shows no cell cytotoxicity; however, it has a limited ability to penetrate the skin due to its hydrophilic nature. The effects of aleosin have been largely demonstrated in pigmented skin equivalents, not human use studies [83] (IV,B). It is sometimes mixed with arbutin, our next topic of discussion, to enhance its skin-lightening abilities.

## Arbutin

Arbutin, chemically known as 4-hydroxyphenyl-beta-glucopyranoside, is obtained from the leaves of the Vaccinicum vitis-idaca and other related plants. It is a naturally occurring gluconopyranoside that causes decreased tyrosinase activity without affecting messenger RNA expression [84] (IV,C). It also inhibits melanosome maturation. Arbutin is not toxic to melanocytes and is used in a variety of pigment-lightening preparations in Japan at concentrations of 3%. Higher concentrations are more efficacious than lower concentrations, but a paradoxical pigment darkening may occur. Arbutin-beta-glycosides have been produced that are less cytotoxic than arbutin [85] (VI,C).

## Summary

Cosmeceuticals form an important part of the over-the-counter skin treatment market, but evidence for efficacy is clearly lacking. This chapter has scanned the reputable literature looking for research to substantiate the use of topical antioxidants and pigment-lightening agents to improve skin functioning and appearance. It may be surprising that so little good research has been conducted on products that are ubiquitous in the current marketplace. While there is never a good rationale for product sales without documentation, many cosmetic manufacturers are slow to engage in this type of research. Data that demonstrate convincing efficacy in large double-blind, vehicle-controlled trials would possibly raise the specter that a previously classified over-the-counter formulation could be reclassified as a drug.

An excellent example of reclassification is a lash growing cosmetic that was removed from the market by the FDA. A liquid for stimulating lash growth was recently marketed by a physician and spa dispensed cosmeceutical company. The product performed amazingly well, resulting in documentable lash lengthening after 3 months of use. The product enjoyed high sales until it was discovered that the product contained a chemical similar to a prescription glaucoma drug. The product was removed from the market because the FDA felt that the drug had been misbranded as a cosmetic. Products that perform too well are subject to inspection.

Development of a cosmeceutical category, similar to the quasi-drug category in Japan, would pave the way for better evidence in the cosmeceutical realm. This would provide an open opportunity for manufacturers to fully understand the efficacy or lack thereof for specific ingredients and final formulations. Until this legislation in enacted, cosmeceuticals will lack the evidence-based knowledge required for legitimacy.

### Evidence-Based Summary

1. Cosmeceuticals are unregulated cosmetics that do not always adhere to evidence-based scientific methods of study.
2. The most active ingredients in cosmeceuticals are the moisturizing ingredients that compose the vehicle, which is challenging when conducting vehicle-controlled studies as part of an evidence-based approach.
3. Antioxidants are a major category of cosmeceuticals, which include carotenoids, flavonoids, and polyphenols.
4. Developing evidence-based therapeutic antioxidants is challenging because antioxidants provide protection against future oxidative skin insults and cannot repair past damage requiring large sample size multiyear longitudinal studies.

# References

1. Hussein G, Sankawa U, Goto H, Matsumoto K, Watanabe H. Astaxanthin, a carotenoid with potential in human health and nutrition. J Nat Prod. 2006;69(3): 443–9.
2. Karppi J, Rissanen TH, Nyyssonen K, Kaikkonen J, Olsson AG, Voutilaninen S, et al. Effects of astaxanthin supplementation of lipid peroxidation. Int J Vitam Nutr Res. 2007;77(1):3–11.
3. Seki T. Effects of astaxanthin on human skin. Frag J. 2001;12:98–103.
4. Higuera-Ciapara I, Felix-Valenzuela L, Goycoolea FM. Astaxanthin: a review of its chemistry and applications. Crit Rev Food Sci Nutr. 2006;46(2): 185–96.
5. Tso MO, Lam TT. Method of retarding and ameliorating central nervous system and eye damage. US Patent #5527533. Board of trustees of the University of Illinois, USA; 1996.
6. Pashkow FJ, Watumull DG, Campbell CL. Astaxanthin: a novel potential treatment for oxidative stress and inflammation in cardiovascular disease. Am J Cardiol. 2008;101(10A):58D–68.
7. Alves-Rodrigues A, Shao A. The science behind lutein. Toxicol Lett. 2004;150(1):57–83.
8. Barclay L. Lutein improves visual function in age-related macular degeneration. Medscape Medical News. http://www.medscape.com Accessed 13th June 2011.
9. Hahn A, Mang B. Lutein and eye health-current state of discussion. Med Monatsschr Pharm. 2008;31(8): 299–308.
10. Semba RD, Dagnelie G. Are Lutein and zeaxanthin conditionally essential nutrients for eye health? Med Hypotheses. 2003;61(4):465–72.
11. www.MayoClinic.com.
12. American Association for Cancer Research Newsletter May 17; 2007, "No Magic Tomato?"
13. Kligman LH, Do CH, Kligman AM. Topical retinoic acid enhances the repair of ultraviolet damaged dermal connective tissue. Connect Tissue Res. 1984;12:139–50.

14. Goodman DS. Vitamin A and retinoids in health and disease. N Engl J Med. 1984;310(16):1023–31.
15. Noy N. Interactions of retinoids with lipid bilayers and with membranes. In: Livrea MA, Packer L, editors. Retinoids. Marcel Dekker: New York; 1993. p. 17–27.
16. Duell EA, Derguini F, Kang S, Elder JT, Voorhees JJ. Extraction of human epidermis treated with retinol yields retro-retinoids in addition to free retinol and retinyl esters. J Invest Dermatol. 1996;107:178–82.
17. Kafi R, Swak HS, Schumacher WE, Cho S, Hanft VN, Hamilton TA, et al. Improvement of naturally aged skin with vitamin A (retinol). Arch Dermatol. 2007; 143(5):606–12.
18. Hruza GJ. Retinol benefits naturally aged skin. J Watch Dermatol. 2007;6(6).
19. Arct J, Pytokowska K. Flavonoids as components of biologically active cosmeceuticals. Clin Dermatol. 2008;26:347–57.
20. Glazier MG, Bowman MA. A review of the evidence for the use of phytoestrogens as a replacement for traditional estrogen replacement therapy. Arch Intern Med. 2001;161:1161–72.
21. Friedman M, Brandon DL. Nutritional and health benefits of soy proteins. J Agric Food Chem. 2001;49(3):1069–86.
22. Sakai T, Kogiso M. Soy isoflavones and immunity. J Med Invest. 2008;55(3–4):167–73.
23. Sarkar FH, Li Y. Soy isoflavones and cancer prevention. Cancer Invest. 2003;21(5):817–8.
24. Omoni AO, Aluko RE. Soybean foods and their benefits: potential mechanisms of action. Nutr Rev. 2005;63(8):272–83.
25. Maheux R, Naud F, Rioux M, Grenier R, Lemay A, Guy J, et al. A randomized, double-blind, placebo-controlled study on the effect of conjugated estrogens on skin thickness. Am J Obstet Gynecol. 1994;170: 642–9.
26. Wiseman H, O'Reilly JD, Adlercreutz H, Mallet AL, Bowey EA, Rowland IR, et al. Isoflavone phytoestrogens consumed in soy decrease F-2-isoprostane concentrations and increase resistance of low-density lipoprotein to oxidation in humans. Am J Clin Nutr. 2000;72:395–400.
27. Chen N, Scarpa R, Zhang L, Seiberg M, Lin CB. Nondenatured soy extracts reduce UVB-induced skin damage via multiple mechanisms. Photochem Photobiol. 2008;84(6):1551–9.
28. Hatcher H, Planalp R, Cho J, Torti FM, Torti SV. Curcumin: from ancient medicine to current clinical trials. Cell Mol Life Sci. 2008;65(11):1631–52.
29. Jagetia GC, Aggarwal BB. "Spicing up" of the immune system by curcumin. J Clin Immunol. 2007;27(1):19–35.
30. Egan ME, Pearson M, Weiner SA, Rajendran V, Rubin D, glockner-Pagel J, et al. Curcumin, a major constituent of turmeric, corrects cystic fibrosis defects. Science. 2004;304(5670):600–2.
31. Kunnumakkara AB, Anand P, Aggarwal BB. Curcumin inhibits proliferation, invasion, angiogenesis and metastasis of different cancers through interaction with multiple cell signaling proteins. Cancer Lett. 2008;269(2):199–225.
32. Katiyar SK, Korman NJ, Mukhtar H, Agarwal R. Protective effects of silymarin against photocarcinogenesis in a mouse skin model. J Natl Cancer Inst. 1997;89:556–66.
33. Katiyar SK. Silymarin and skin cancer prevention: anti-inflammatory, antioxidant and immunomodulatory effects (review). Int J Oncol. 2005;26(1):169–76.
34. Chatterjee L, Agarwal R, Mukhtar H. Ultraviolet B radiation-induced DNA lesions in mouse epidermis: an assessment sing a novel 32P-postlabeling technique. Biochem Biophys Res Commun. 1996;229: 590–5.
35. Toklu HZ, Tunali-Akbay T, Erkanli G, Yuksel M, Ercan F, Sener G. Silymarin, the antioxidant component of Silybum marianum, protects against burn-induced oxidative skin injury. Burn. 2007;33(7):908–16.
36. Berardesca E, Cameli N, Cavallotti C, Levy JL, Pierard GE, de Paoli Ambrosi G. Combined effects of silymarin and methylsulfonylmethane in the management of rosacea: clinical and instrumental evaluation. J Cosmet Dermatol. 2008;7(1):8–14.
37. Pycnogenol. Drug information online: http://www.drugs.com/npp/pycnogenol.html. Accessed 7 Dec 2008.
38. Devaraj S, Vega-Lopez S, Kaul N, Schonlau F, Rohdewald P, Jialal I. Supplementation with a pine bark extract rich in polyphenols increases plasma antioxidant capacity and alters the plasma lipoprotein profile. Lipids. 2002;37:931–4.
39. Cesarone MR, Belcaro G, Rohdewald P, Pellegrini L, Ledda A, Vinciguerra G, et al. Improvement of diabetic microangiopathy with pycnogenol: a prospective, controlled study. Angiology. 2006;57(4):431–6.
40. Vinciguerra G, Belcaro G, Cesarone MR, Rohdewald P, Stuard S, Ricci A, et al. Cramps and muscular pain: prevention with pycnogenol in normal subjects, venous patients, athletes, claudicants and in diabetic microangiopathy. Angiology. 2006;57(3):331–9.
41. Cossins E, Lee R, Packer L. ESR studies of vitamin C regeneration, order of reactivity of natural source phytochemical preparations. Biochem Mol Biol Int. 1998;45:583–98.
42. Schonlau F. The cosmetic pycnogenol. J Appl Cosmetol. 2002;20:241–6.
43. Kim YJ, Kang KS, Yokozawa T. The anti-melanogenic effect of pycnogenol by its anti-oxidative actions. Food Chem Toxicol. 2008;46(7):2466–71.
44. Rona C, Vailati F, Berardesca D. The cosmetic treatment of wrinkles. J Cosmet Dermatol. 2004;3(1):26–34.
45. Joyeux M, Lobstein A, Anton R, Mortier F. Comparative antilipoperoxidant, antinecrotic and scavenging properties of terpenes and biflavones from Ginkgo and some flavonoids. Planta Med. 1995;61:126–9.
46. Kim SJ, Lim MH, Chun IK, Won YH. Effects of flavonoids of Ginkgo biloba on proliferation of human skin fibroblast. Skin Pharmacol. 1997;10:200–5.
47. Hsu S. Green tea and the skin. J Am Acad Dermatol. 2005;52:1049–59.

48. US FDA/CFSAN Letter Responding to Health Claim Petition dated January 27, 2004: Green tea and Reduced Risk of Cancer Health Claim (Docket number 2004Q-0083).

49. US FDA/CFSAN Qualified Health Claims: Letter of Denial Green Tea and Reduced Risk of Cardiovascular Disease (Docket number 2005Q-0297).

50. Katiyar SK, Elmets CA. Green tea and skin. Arch Dermatol. 2000;136:989–94.

51. Geria NM. Green, black or white, it fits beauty to a "t". HAPPI. 2006:46–50.

52. Abstract 6 Journal of the American College of Nutrition 2006;25(5).

53. Abstract 7 Journal of the American College of Nutrition 2006;25(5).

54. Chui AD, Chan JL, Kern DG, et al. Double-blinded, placebo-controlled trial of green tea extracts in the clinical and histologic appearance of photoaging skin. Dermatol Surg. 2005;31(7 Pt 2):855–60.

55. Katiyar SK, Elmets CA, Agarwal R, et al. Protection against ultraviolet-B radiation-induced local and systemic suppression of contact hypersensitivity and edema responses in C3H/HeN mice by green tea polyphenols. Photochem Photobiol. 1995;62: 855–61.

56. Elmets CA, Singh D, Tubesing K, Matsui MS, Katiyar SK, Mukhtar H. Green tea polyphenols as chemopreventive agents against cutaneous photodamage. J Am Acad Dermatol. 2001;44:425–32.

57. Katiyar SK, Afaq F, Perez A, Mukhtar H. Green tea polyphenol treatment to human skin prevents formation of ultraviolet light B-induced pyrimidine dimers in DNA. Clin Cancer Res. 2000;6:3864–9.

58. Ahmad N, Mukhtar H. Cutaneous photochemoprotection by green tea. A brief review. Skin Pharmacol Appl Skin Physiol. 2001;14:69–76.

59. Mukhtar H, Katiyar SK, Agarwal R. Green tea and skin – anticarcinogenic effects. J Invest Dermatol. 1994;102:3–7.

60. Jurenka JS. Therapeutic applications of pomegranate (*Punica granatum* L.): a review. Altern Med Rev. 2008;13(2):128–44.

61. Pacheco-Palencia LA, Noratto G, Hingorani L, Talcott ST, Mertens-Talcott SU. Protective effects of standardized pomegranate (*Punica granatum* L.) polyphenolic extract in ultraviolet-irradiated human skin fibroblasts. J Agric Food Chem. 2008;56(18): 8434–41.

62. Aviram M, Rosenblat M, Gaitini D, Nitecki S, Hoffman A, Dornfeld L, et al. Pomegranate juice consumption for 3 years by patients with carotid artery stenosis reduces common carotid intima-media thickness, blood pressure and LDL oxidation. Clin Nutr. 2004;23(3):423–33.

63. Aviram M, Dornfeld L, Rosenblat M, et al. Pomegranate juice consumption reduces oxidative stress, atherogenic modifications to LDL, and platelet aggregation: studies in humans and in atherosclerotic apolipoprotein e-deficient mice. Am J Clin Nutr. 2000;71:1062–76.

64. Esmaillzadeh A, Tahbaz F, Gaieni I, Alavi-Majd H, Azadbakht L. Concentrated pomegranate juice improves profiles in diabetic patients with hyperlipidemia. J Med Food. 2004;7(3):305–8.

65. McKeown E. Aloe vera. Cosmet Toilet. 1987;102: 64–5.

66. Waller T. Aloe vera. Cosmet Toilet. 1992;107:53–4.

67. Maenthaisong R, Chaiyakunapruk N, Niruntraporn S, Kongkaew C. The efficacy of aloe vera for burn wound healing: a systematic review. Burns. 2007;33(6):713–8.

68. Orafidiya LO, Agbani EO, Oyedele AO, Babalola OO, Onayemi O, Aiyedun FF. The effect of aloe vera gel on the anti-acne properties of the essential oil of Ocimum gratissimum Linn leaf-a preliminary clinical investigation. Int J Aromather. 2004;14(1):15–21.

69. Puvabanditsin P, Vongtongsri R. Efficacy of aloe vera cream in prevention and treatment of sunburn and suntan. J Med Assoc Thai. 2005;88 Suppl 4:S173–6.

70. Reuter J, Jocher A, Stump J, Grossjohann B, Franke G, Sshempp CM. Investigation of the anti-inflammatory potential of aloe vera gel (97.5%) in the ultraviolet erythema test. Skin Pharmacol Physiol. 2008;21(2): 106–10.

71. Hoppe U, Bergemann J, Diembeck W, Ennen J, Gohla S, Harris I, et al. Coenzyme Q10, a cutaneous antioxidant and energizer. Biofactors. 1999;9(2–4):371–8.

72. Blatt T, Mundt C, Mummert C, Maksiuk T, Wolber R, Keyhani R, et al. Modulation of oxidative stresses in human aging skin. Z Gerontol Geriatr. 1999;32(2): 83–8.

73. Sohal RS, Kamzalov S, Sumien N, Ferguson M, Rebrin I, Heinrich KR, et al. Effect of coenzyme Q10 intake on endogenous coenzyme Q content, mitochondrial electron transport chain, antioxidant defenses, and life span of mice. Free Radic Biol Med. 2006;40(3):480–7.

74. Passi S, DePita O, Grandinetti M, Simotti C, Littarru GP. The combined use of oral and topical lipophilic antioxidants increases their levels both in sebum and stratum corneum. Biofactors. 2003;18(1–4):289–97.

75. Fuller B, Smith D, Howerton A, Kern D. Anti-inflammatory effects of coQ10 and colorless carotenoids. J Cosmet Dermatol. 2006;5(1):30–8.

76. Espinal-Perez LE, Moncada B, Castanedo-Cazares JP. A double blind randomized trial of 5% ascorbic acid vs. 4% hydroquinone in melasma. Int J Dermatol. 2004;43(8):604–7.

77. Amer M, Metwalli M. Topical liquiritin improves melasma. Int J Dermatol. 2000;39(4):299–301.

78. Beitner H. Randomized, placebo-controlled, double blind study on the clinical efficacy of a cream containing 5% alpha-lipoic acid related to photoageing of facial skin. Br J Dermatol. 2003;149(4):841–9.

79. Lim JT. Treatment of melasma using kojic acid in a gel containing hydroquinone and glycolic acid. Dermatol Surg. 1999;25:282–4.

80. Garcia A, Fulton Jr JE. The combination of glycolic acid and hydroquinone or kojic acid for the treatment of melasma and related conditions. Dermatol Surg. 1996;22(5):443–7.

81. Choi S, Lee SK, Kim JE, et al. Aloesin inhibits hyper-pigmentation induced by UV radiation. Clin Exp Dermatol. 2002;27:513–5.

82. Jones K, Hughes J, Hong M, et al. Modulation of mel-anogenesis by aloesin: a competitive inhibitor of tyro-sinase. Pigment Cell Res. 2002;15:335–40.

83. Wang Z, Li X, Yang Z, He X, Tu J, Zhang T. Effects of aloesin on melanogenesis in pigmented skin equiv-alents. Int J Cosmet Sci. 2008;30(2):121–30.

84. Hori I, Nihei K, Kubo I. Structural criteria for depig-menting mechanism of arbutin. Phytother Res. 2004;18:475–9.

85. Jun SY, Park KM, Choi KW, Jang MK, Kang HY, Lee SH, et al. Inhibitory effects of arbutin-beta-glycosides synthesized from enzymatic trans-glycosylation for melanogenesis. Biotechnol Lett. 2008;30(4):743–8.

## Self-Assessment

1. How do antioxidants function to prevent oxidative damage?
   - (a) Antioxidants quench singlet oxygen through electron translocation.
   - (b) Antioxidants donate an electron to reactive oxygen species.
   - (c) Antioxidants consume oxygen to stabilize reaction oxygen species.
   - (d) a and b
   - (e) b and c
   - (f) a and b and c

2. The carotenoids include
   - (a) Astaxanthin
   - (b) Soy
   - (c) Lutein
   - (d) Lycopene
   - (e) a and b and c
   - (f) a and c and d

3. Cosmeceutical pigment-lightening agents function by
   - (a) Inhibiting tyrosinase
   - (b) Stabilizing melanin
   - (c) Providing photoprotection
   - (d) a and b
   - (e) a and c
   - (f) a and b and c

4. Cosmeceuticals are classified in the United States as
   - (a) Over-the-counter drugs
   - (b) Quasi drugs
   - (c) Prescription drugs
   - (d) No classification currently exists
   - (e) a and b
   - (f) a and d

5. Cosmeceutical ingredients are derived from
   - (a) Leaves
   - (b) Twigs
   - (c) Animals
   - (d) Algae
   - (e) a and b
   - (f) All of the above

## Answers

1. b: Antioxidants donate an electron to reactive oxygen species
2. f: a and c and d
3. e: a and c
4. d: No classification currently exists
5. f: All of the above

# Botulinum Toxin

# 19

## Berthold Rzany and Alexander Nast

## Introduction

Three BoNT-A preparations dominate the international markets: Botox (aka Vistabel, Vistabex), Dysport (aka Azzalure), and Xeomin (aka Bocouture).

There are a multitude of questions that could be answered in that field. For the purpose of clarity of the chapter, the review will focus on three questions:

1. What is the evidence for using saline *with* preservatives for dilution?
2. What is the evidence for the optimal dosage for the glabella?
3. What is the evidence for the safety of switching from one to another BoNT-A preparation?

## What Is the Evidence for Using Saline with Preservatives for Dilution?

Why is this question interesting at all? Because there is the hypothesis that the addition of a preservative reduces injection pain.

### Consensus Documents

Several consensus statements for two of the three products are available. All guidelines are consensus guidelines; however, none of the guidelines followed a structured consensus approach (nominal group technique) (Table 19.1).

Based on the consensus statements, we do have a comment on the usage of preserved saline. The US-American group called it the "preferred" method [1]. However, no strong recommendation is given. In the German guidelines, no recommendation for preserved saline is given [2–4]. However, in one of the papers, the US consensus is mentioned (VI/C) [2].

### Case Series and Cohort Studies

Case series and cohorts may reflect "real life" scenarios. Therefore, they may be helpful in seeing how a drug is used outside clinical trials.

B. Rzany (✉) • A. Nast
Division of Evidence Based Medicine (dEBM),
Klinik für Dermatologie, Charité – Universitätsmedizin
Berlin, Campus Charité mitte, Charitéplatz 1,
D-10117 Berlin, Germany
e-mail: berthold.rzany@charite.de

M. Alam (ed.), *Evidence-Based Procedural Dermatology*,
DOI 10.1007/978-0-387-09424-3_19, © Springer Science+Business Media, LLC 2012

**Table 19.1** Overview on consensus statements for using saline with or without a preservative

| Guidelines | Carruthers et al. [1] (VI/C) | Sommer et al. [2] (VI/C) | Rzany [3] (VI/C) | Rzany et al. [4] (VI/C) |
|---|---|---|---|---|
| Level | Level 1 (consensus-based, no formalized consensus) | Level 1 (consensus-based, no formalized consensus) | Level 1 (consensus-based, no formalized consensus) | Level 1 (consensus-based, no formalized consensus) |
| Botulinum toxin A discussed | Botox | Botox/Vistabel | Dysport | Dysport |
| Recommendation | Preserved saline *can be used* to dilute botulinum toxin type A. Mentioned as "preferred" in the consensus statement | Mentioning of the US consensus. No clear statement from the German experts. General recommendation for nonpreserved saline | No mentioning of preserved saline | No mentioning of preserved saline |

**Table 19.2** Case series focusing on the use of saline with a preservative

| References, country | Study type, no. of patients | Outcome criteria | Results | Comment |
|---|---|---|---|---|
| Alam et al. [5], USA (III/B) | Retrospective study 5 mL dilution, $n = 18$ | % of change of discomfort | 18 (90%) of 20 patients reported that treatment with exotoxin reconstituted with preserved saline was less painful than prior treatment with exotoxin reconstituted with preservative free saline | The 5 mL dilution used is for procedures in esthetic dermatology unusual The outcome criteria is not validated |

We were able to find only one paper [5] describing a small case series. In the case series, a quite high volume for injection was used. Most patients reported the treatment to be more painful when the exotoxin was reconstituted with preservative free saline (III/B) (Table 19.2).

## Randomized Controlled Trials and Meta-Analyses

There is no meta-analyses available so far. A total of two clinical trials can be found.

Two studies focus on the effect of adding a preservative to the saline used for the dilution of BoNT-A. One is a small randomized double-blinded RCT using a 5 mL dilution, and the other is a larger nonrandomized single blinded trial using a 2 mL dilution [5, 6]. Both trials point to a decreased pain sensation when adding a preservative (9 mg benzyl alcohol per mL). However,

one has to be aware that the addition of benzyl alcohol as a preservative may carry a small risk of contact sensitization [7] (Table 19.3).

## What Is the Evidence for the Optimal Dosage for the Glabella?

## Consensus Documents

All guideline papers focus on the treatment of the glabella. In contrast to the available clinical trials with defined injection points and dosages, a range of injection points and dosages is offered (Table 19.4).

The number of the injection points for the glabella vary from 3 to 7. For Botox, gender-specific dosages are given ranging from 20 to 50 U [1, 2]. In contrast for Dysport, no gender-based dosages are given. The range lies between 30 and 60 (70) U [2–4] (EL VI).

**Table 19.3**  Controlled trials focusing on the use of saline with a preservative

| References, country | Study type, no. of patients | Outcome criteria | Results | Comment |
|---|---|---|---|---|
| Alam et al. [5] (III/B), USA | RCT Double blind, $n=15$ Multiple locations BoNT-A diluted with 5 mL (9 mg of benzyl alcohol per mL) | % of change of discomfort | 15 (100%) of patients reported (54%) less pain in the side of their face treated with the exotoxin reconstituted with preservative containing saline ($p=0.001$) | Small trial The outcome criteria is not validated |
| Sarifakioglu and Sarifakioglu [6] (III/B), Turkey | CT Single blinded Multiple locations (upper face, crow's feet, $n=60$, neck) 2 mL dilution (9 mg of benzyl alcohol per mL)[a] | VAS (0–10) | 1.2 (with preservative) vs. 4.5 for the upper face 0.6 (with preservative) vs. 3.9 for the neck ($p=0.000$) | The preservative containing solution was always applied on the right side. The trial was not randomized |

[a] Probably (the source of the benzyl alcohol was United States Pharmacopeia, Abbot Laboratories, North Chicago, IL, USA)

**Table 19.4**  Consensus statements focusing on the optimal dosage for the glabella

| Guidelines | Carruthers et al. [1] (VI/C) | Sommer et al. [2] (VI/C) | Rzany [3] (VI/C) | Rzany et al. [4] (VI/C) |
|---|---|---|---|---|
| Level | Level 1 (consensus-based, no formalized consensus) | Level 1 (consensus-based, no formalized consensus) | Level 1 (consensus-based, no formalized consensus) | Level 1 (consensus-based, no formalized consensus) |
| Botulinum toxin A discussed | Botox | Botox/Vistabel | Dysport | Dysport |
| Recommendation for the usage of BoNT-A in the glabella area | 5–7 injection points Men might require more points Women: 20–30 U Men: 30–40 U | 4–6 injection points, two different injection pattern given Women: 22 U (10–50 U) Men: 29 U (12–50 U) | 3–5 injection points 30–60 U | 3–5 injection points 30–50 U in patients with weak- or medium-strength muscles 40–60 U, in rare cases, 70 U in patients with strong muscles |

## Case Series and Cohort Studies

There is a multitude of case reports and case series on the treatment with BoNT-A in the area of the glabella. However, in the view of the excellent evidence from randomized clinical trials, there is no benefit from looking at the smaller case series. Therefore, the focus should go to the larger case series.

We were able to find two large case series, one retrospective cohort and one trial without a comparator.

### Dysport aka Azzalure

The trial as well as the case series confirm the safety of BoNT-A in the treatment of glabellar lines in a real life scenario. Fifty Dysport U were the chosen dose for the glabella in the study of Moy et al. [8] (II/A). However, in the real life study, it became clear that there was a range of dosing with a median dose of 50–70 Dysport U (III/B) [9] (Table 19.5).

### Botox aka Vistabel aka Vistabex and Xeomin aka Bocouture

We could not find similar large case series for either Botox or Xeomin.

## Randomized Controlled Trials and Meta-Analyses

There are no meta-analyses available so far. However, several good controlled trials can be

**Table 19.5** Cases series focusing on the BoNT-A (Dysport) dosage for the glabella

| References, country | Study type, dosage used, no. of patients | Efficacy | Safety | Comment |
|---|---|---|---|---|
| Moy et al. [8] (III/B), USA | CT Open label 50 Dysport U 1,200 patients receiving at least 5 injections of 50 U Dysport in the glabella region | By investigator assessment, the response rate (patients reporting none or mild glabellar line severity scale scores on day 30) ranged from 80 to 91% during cycles 1–5 | The most frequently occurring related AEs were injection site disorders (18%), nervous system disorders (14 and 12% headache), and eye disorders (9%). A total of 45 patients had a total of 55 instances of ptosis across all cycles. The rates of ptosis decreased during successive cycles from 2.4% in cycle 1 to 0.6% in cycle 5 | In this study, for the first time the onset of the effect of Dysport treatment examined. An effect was seen within 1 day in some cases, and the median time to onset was 3 days for all cycles Safety: Reported ptosis does not differentiate between brow ptosis and eyelid ptosis! |
| Rzany et al. [9], Germany and Austria (II/A) | Retrospective cohort Variable regions were treated with variable doses $n=945$ | The glabella was treated most frequently (93.9%), with the majority (81.5%) of patients receiving treatment in more than one areas of the face. The median BoNT-A dose in the glabella was 50–60 units (25th to 75th percentile, 40–70 units); for those who received injections in the glabella only, the median BoNT-A dose was 50–70 units (25th to 75th percentile, 50–100 units) | Of the 945 patients, 90.6% ($n=856$) did not experience any AEs over any treatment cycle. The total AE rate per treatment cycle was 4.1% ($n=39/945$) in Cycle 1, decreasing to 2.0% ($n=11/553$) in Cycle 5, giving an overall mean incidence of 2.5% per treatment cycle. Lid or brow ptosis was uncommon (0.46% of treatment cycles; range, 0.85–0.1%) and generally mild | Safety: Reported ptosis does not differentiate between brow ptosis and eyelid ptosis! |

found. The trials will be discussed for each brand separately.

## Botox aka Vistabel aka Vistabex

There are several trials focusing on the optimal dosage for Botox in the glabella area. In the first large placebo-controlled trial, patients with moderate-to-severe glabellar lines at maximum frown received intramuscular injections of 20 U Botox or placebo into five glabellar sites. A total of 264 patients were enrolled (203 treated with Botox, 61 with placebo). There was a significantly greater reduction in glabellar line severity with Botox than with placebo (all measures, every follow-up visit; $p<0.02$) [10]. The same authors investigated

in another double-blind, randomized clinical trial the efficacy, safety, and duration of the effect of four different dosages of Botox in the treatment of glabellar rhytids in females. Eighty female subjects with moderate-to-severe wrinkles at maximum frown entered the study. Patients were randomly administered 10, 20, 30, or 40 Botox U in seven injection points. Objectively, 10 U of Botox was significantly less effective than 20, 30, or 40 U. The relapse rate at 4 months was significantly higher in the 10 U group (83%) vs. the 40, 30, or 20 U groups (28, 30, and 33% respectively). The authors concluded that 20–40 Botox U were significantly more effective at reducing glabellar lines than 10 U and suggested 20 Botox U

**Table 19.6**  Randomized controlled trials focusing on the BoNT-A dosage (here Botox) for the glabella

| References, country | Study type, no. of patients, % female, injection points | Outcome criteria | Results | Comment |
|---|---|---|---|---|
| Carruthers et al. [10], USA (II/A) | RCT Double blind Randomized 203 BoNT-A and 61 placebo patients 85.2% respect. 77% female 5 injection points | Physician assessment Responder: grade 0 or 1 at maximum frown | Responder rate at day 30 Placebo: 1.6% 20 Botox U: 83.7% | |
| Carruthers et al. [13], USA (II/A) | RCT Double blind Randomized 202 BoNT-A and 71 placebo patients 79.7% respect. 83.1% female patients 5 injection points | Physician assessment Responder: grade 0 or 1 at maximum frown | Responder rate at day 30 Placebo: 7% 20 Botox U: 76.7% | Placebo rate from graph estimated may be a bit lower |
| Carruthers et al. [11], USA (II/A) | RCT Double blind Randomized 80 BoNT-A 100% female 7 injection points | Physician assessment Responder: grade 0 or 1 at maximum frown | Responder rate at 4 weeks 10 Botox U: 68% 20 Botox U: 78% 30 Botox U: 98% 40 Botox U: 100% | All female study 10, 20, and 30 estimated from the graphs |
| Carruthers and Carruthers [12], USA (II/A) | RCT Double blind Randomized 80 BoNT-A 0% female 7 injection points | Physician assessment Responder: grade 0 or 1 at maximum frown | Responder rate at 1 month 20 Botox U: 65% 40 Botox U: 90% 60 Botox U: 95% 80 Botox U: 100% | All male study |

as the most appropriate Botox dosage for female patients [11].

A similar study in male patients was published the same year. In this study, eighty men were randomized to receive a total dose of either 20, 40, 60, or 80 U of Botox distributed in 7 points in the glabellar and lower forehead area. The 40, 60, and 80 U dosages of BoNT-A were consistently more effective in reducing glabellar lines than the 20 U dose (duration, peak response rate, improvement from baseline). There was a dose-dependent increase in both the response rate at maximum frown and the duration of effect assessed by the trained observer. The authors conclude that male participants with glabellar rhytids benefit from starting dosages of at least 40 U of Botox [12] (Table 19.6).

### Dysport aka Azzalure

So far, there are four trials published focusing on the optimal dosage for the glabella [14–17]. The base is a dose ranging study from Ascher et al. [15] comparing 25, 50, and 75 Dysport U compared to placebo. A total of 119 patients with moderate-to-severe glabellar lines at rest were treated. The dosage was distributed over five intramuscular glabellar sites forming a bird-shaped pattern. Outcome measures included evaluations of glabellar lines by independent experts from blinded standardized photographs at rest 1 month after treatment, physician evaluations, and patient assessments during a 6-month period. A significant efficacy was reported for the three BoNT-A groups for at least 3 months after injection (at least $p < 0.015$). Investigator and patient evaluations suggested that 50 U was the optimal dosage [15]. These results are supported by the large US study which was published in January 2007 [16] (Table 19.7).

### Xeomin aka Bocouture

So far there is no published data from RCTs on the use of Xeomin in the glabella area available. Therefore, the product cannot be discussed in this overview.

Summing up, based on these studies (where a majority of female patients were included),

**Table 19.7** Randomized controlled trials focusing on the BoNT-A dosage (here Dysport) for the glabella

| References, country | Study type, no. of patients, % female, injection points | Outcome criteria | Results | Comment |
|---|---|---|---|---|
| Ascher et al. [15], France (II/A) | RCT Randomized Double blind 119 95.8% females 5 injection points | Physician assessment Responder: grade 0 or 1 at rest | Responder rate at 1 month Placebo: 6.7% 25 Dysport U: 44.8% 50 Dysport U: 44.8% 75 Dysport U: 55.2% | Assessment was done at rest. This makes the study difficult to compare |
| Ascher et al. [14], France (II/A) | RCT Randomized Double blind 100 patients 94% females 5 injection points | The time between the first and second injections | At months 3 and 4 after the first injection (50 Dysport U), the cumulative percentage of patients having a second injection (50 Dysport U) was lower in the BoNT-A group compared to the placebo group, with a significant difference at month 4 | |
| Rzany et al. [17], Germany (II/A) | RCT Double blind 3 or 5 injection points 110 and 111 patients 89.9 and 90.1% female patients | Assessment by experts based on photographs Responder: a reduction of at least 1 point between weeks 0 and 4 at maximum frown | Responder rate at 4 weeks Placebo: 18.9% 30 Dysport U: 86.1% Placebo: 7.9% 50 Dysport U: 86.3% | This was not a dose-finding study. Two different injection point distributions and dosages were compared to placebo |
| Monheit et al. [16], USA (II/A) | Clinical trial Randomized Double blind 373 patients 83.9% females 5 injection points | Physician assessment Responder: grade 0 or 1 at maximum frown | Responder rate at day 30 Placebo: 9% 20 Dysport U: 68% 50 Dysport U: 79% 75 Dysport U: 84% | Data not given in paper, the proportions are estimated from a PP from Gary Monheit. 50 Dysport U were determined to be the optimal dosage |

20 Botox U respectively 50 Dysport U seems to be the optimal dose for the glabella. This corresponds to a 1:2.5 ratio between both products. When treating the glabella and additionally the forehead (two further points), the optimal dosage seems to be somewhat higher. Here, in men [12], 40 Botox U is suggested to be the optimal dosage.

## What Is the Evidence for the Safety of Switching from One to Another BoNT: A Preparation?

We are not living in a one toxin world anymore. With multiple toxins on the market, the question arises if we switch between several BoNT-A preparations, how should we do this and how safe is this?

## Consensus Documents

Astonishingly, the consensus documents are not really helpful. In Germany where two BoNT-A preparations were available on the market at the time of the publication of the consensus statements, no recommendations for switching between one and the other toxin were given [2–4]. In the US, naturally with only one toxin on the market, no switching recommendations were given [1] (EL VI). So we do have consensus statements; however, they do not focus on the rules from switching from one brand to the other.

## Case Series and Cohort Studies

There is only one case series [18] (EL VI) with severe methodological problems [19]. The results of this study are not helpful.

## Randomized Controlled Trials and Meta-Analyses

There are no meta-analyses and randomized controlled trials on that subject.

So far, there is no good study on how patients should be switched from one BoNT-A preparation to another. Would we need such a study? Probably not. We do have or will have (in case of Xeomin) good evidence on efficacy and safety for all the available toxins. However, especially new users have to be aware that the units of the toxins are not comparable. There is a considerable confusion on the units and potential ratios when switching from one toxin to the other [20]. Therefore, we would recommend that new and – even more important – advanced users refer to the consensus statements or text books before treating their patients with a brand that they are not familiar with [21].

## Not Discussed Questions

For this chapter, we could not discuss all questions that would have been interesting to discuss. Therefore, we would like to give some rule of thumbs which hopefully are helpful when approaching new questions.

1. Make sure you have clinically meaningful questions!
2. Consensus statements may be helpful – especially if the consensus statements are from evidence-based guidelines.
3. Be aware that nonevidence-based guidelines may contain some advice that is based on erroneous assumptions.
4. The best evidence comes from randomized controlled trials.
5. Placebo-controlled trials designed for the regulatory agencies are usually best.
6. Be very critical when looking at SMALL comparative trials. There results might be based on statistical chance and might not reflect real differences or comparability [22].
7. Mistrust all kind of clinical data that are not based on a clinical trial in a situation where a clinical trial could have been done [18, 19].

## Conclusions

There is some evidence that the addition of preservative may decrease the injection pain. Based on this evidence, the usage of saline with preservatives (benzyl alcohol) may be suggested. However, larger clinical trials are necessary to turn this into a sound recommendation.

Concerning the optimal dosage for the glabella, we do have a vast amount of evidence arising from large cohort studies as well as clinical trials for the two main products. Based on these trials, 50 Dysport U or 20 Botox U can be recommended as the basic dosage for the glabella. Nevertheless, one has to be aware that all except one study were performed in overwhelmingly female populations. Therefore, this dosage may be considered a starting dose in men and may be adjusted to muscle mass and muscle activity.

Last but not the least: what is the evidence for efficacy and safety for switching from one BoNT-A brand to the other. The evidence is nil. Therefore, when switching patients from one to the other BoNT-A brand, the user should be advised to rely on the various consensus papers or on hands-on books for dosing instructions.

## References

1. Carruthers J, Fagien S, Matarasso SL. Consensus recommendations on the use of botulinum toxin type a in facial aesthetics. Plast Reconstr Surg. 2004;114 (6 Suppl):1S–22S.
2. Sommer B, Bergfeld D, Sattler G. Consensus recommendations on the use of botulinum toxin type A in

aesthetic medicine. J Dtsch Dermatol Ges. 2007;5 Suppl 1:S1–S29.

3. Rzany B. Bericht zum 1. Expertentreffen zur Anwendung von Botulinumtoxin A in der Ästhetischen Dermatologie. Kosmetische Medizin. 2003;24:2–8.

4. Rzany B, Fratila A, Heckmann M. 2. Expertentreffen zur Anwendung von Botulinumtoxin A (Dysport®) in der Ästhetischen Dermatologie. Kosmetische Medizin. 2005;26:134–41.

5. Alam M, Dover JS, Arndt KA. Pain associated with injection of botulinum A exotoxin reconstituted using isotonic sodium chloride with and without preservative: a double-blind, randomized controlled trial. Arch Dermatol. 2002;138(4):510–4.

6. Sarifakioglu N, Sarifakioglu E. Evaluating effects of preservative-containing saline solution on pain perception during botulinum toxin type-a injections at different locations: a prospective, single-blinded, randomized controlled trial. Aesthetic Plast Surg. 2005;29(2):113–5.

7. Amado A, Jacob SE. Letter: benzyl alcohol preserved saline used to dilute injectables poses a risk of contact dermatitis in fragrance-sensitive patients. Dermatol Surg. 2007;33(11):1396–7.

8. Moy R, Maas C, Monheit G, Huber MB. Long-term safety and efficacy of a new botulinum toxin type A in treating glabellar lines. Arch Facial Plast Surg. 2009;11(2):77–83.

9. Rzany B, Dill-Muller D, Grablowitz D, Heckmann M, Caird D. Repeated botulinum toxin A injections for the treatment of lines in the upper face: a retrospective study of 4,103 treatments in 945 patients. Dermatol Surg. 2007;33(1 Spec No.):S18–25.

10. Carruthers JA, Lowe NJ, Menter MA, Gibson J, Nordquist M, Mordaunt J, et al. A multicenter, double-blind, randomized, placebo-controlled study of the efficacy and safety of botulinum toxin type A in the treatment of glabellar lines. J Am Acad Dermatol. 2002;46(6):840–9.

11. Carruthers A, Carruthers J, Said S. Dose-ranging study of botulinum toxin type A in the treatment of glabellar rhytids in females. Dermatol Surg. 2005;31(4):414–22. discussion 22.

12. Carruthers A, Carruthers J. Prospective, double-blind, randomized, parallel-group, dose-ranging study of botulinum toxin type A in men with glabellar rhytids. Dermatol Surg. 2005;31(10):1297–303.

13. Carruthers JD, Lowe NJ, Menter MA, Gibson J, Eadie N. Double-blind, placebo-controlled study of the safety and efficacy of botulinum toxin type A for patients with glabellar lines. Plast Reconstr Surg. 2003;112(4):1089–98.

14. Ascher B, Zakine B, Kestemont P, Baspeyras M, Bougara A, Niforos F, et al. Botulinum toxin A in the treatment of glabellar lines: scheduling the next injection. Aesthet Surg J. 2005;25(4):365–75.

15. Ascher B, Zakine B, Kestemont P, Baspeyras M, Bougara A, Santini J. A multicenter, randomized, double-blind, placebo-controlled study of efficacy and safety of 3 doses of botulinum toxin A in the treatment of glabellar lines. J Am Acad Dermatol. 2004; 51(2):223–33.

16. Monheit G, Carruthers A, Brandt F, Rand R. A randomized, double-blind, placebo-controlled study of botulinum toxin type A for the treatment of glabellar lines: determination of optimal dose. Dermatol Surg. 2007;33(1 Spec No.):S51–9.

17. Rzany B, Ascher B, Fratila A, Monheit GD, Talarico S, Sterry W. Efficacy and safety of 3- and 5-injection patterns (30 and 50 U) of botulinum toxin A (Dysport) for the treatment of wrinkles in the glabella and the central forehead region. Arch Dermatol. 2006;142(3): 320–6.

18. de Boulle K. Patient satisfaction with different botulinum toxin type A formulations in the treatment of moderate to severe upper facial rhytids. J Cosmet Laser Ther. 2008;10(2):87–92.

19. Pickett A, Rzany B. Botulinum toxin in aesthetic applications: "How often misused words generate misleading thoughts". J Cosmet Laser Ther. 2009; 11(3):178–9.

20. Pickett A, Dodd S, Rzany B. Confusion about diffusion and the art of misinterpreting data when comparing different botulinum toxins used in aesthetic applications. J Cosmet Laser Ther. 2008;10(3):181–3.

21. De Maio M, Rzany B. Botulinum toxin in aesthetic medicine. Heidelberg: Springer; 2007, ISBN-10: 3540340947; ISBN-13: 978–3540340942.

22. Rzany B, Nast A. Head-to-head studies of botulinum toxin A in aesthetic medicine: which evidence is good enough? J Am Acad Dermatol. 2007;56(6): 1066–7.

## Self-Assessment

1. With what should BoNT-A be diluted?
   (a) With distilled water
   (b) With saline mixed with lidocain
   (c) With saline with or without preservative
   (d) With saline mixed with lidocain and epinephrine
   (e) It should be injected undiluted

2. What is the recommended dose for BoNT-A when treating the glabella?
   (a) 50 Botox and 50 Dysport U
   (b) 20 Botox and 50 Dysport U
   (c) 20 Botox and 20 Dysport U
   (d) There is no recommended dose
   (e) 50 Botox and 20 Dysport U
      Please note: Botox aka Vistabel aka Vistabex and Dysport aka Azzalure

3. When should you get suspicious about the validity of the results of a study?
   (a) When the study was not conducted in the US
   (b) When the study was placebo-controlled
   (c) When the study was randomized
   (d) When it is a small trial comparing two different BoNT-A preparations
   (e) When it a study for the regulatory agencies

4. The recommendations when switching from one BoNT-A product to another are so far based on:
   (a) Meta-analyses
   (b) Randomized controlled clinical trials with a cross-over design
   (c) Randomized controlled clinical trials with another BoNT-A product as a comparator
   (d) Expert opinion
   (e) Consensus statements

## Answers

1. c: With saline with or without preservative
2. b: 20 Botox and 50 Dysport U
3. d: When it is a small trial comparing two different BoNT-A preparations
4. d: expert opinion

# Soft Tissue Augmentation

Kenneth Beer and Shivani Nanda

## Introduction

Soft tissue augmentation is one of the most common nonsurgical procedures performed in dermatology. Its popularity among practitioners and patients continues to grow, as is evidenced by the 400% increase in the number of procedures completed between 2001 and 2007 [1] (V/B). Areas frequently treated by soft tissue augmentation include the nasolabial crease, marionette lines, tear troughs, mental crease, glabellar lines, and lips (Fig. 20.1). Soft tissue augmentation is administered via injection of dermal fillers, which restore tissue or subcutaneous fat lost to disease or aging processes.

Dermal fillers can be classified as permanent or temporary fillers according to the duration of their indicated effect. Permanent fillers include silicone- or polymethylmethacrylate (PMMA)-containing products. Temporary fillers can be categorized into three types, based on the source of their active product: (1) synthetic materials, which include calcium hydroxylapatite (CaHA) and poly-L-lactic acid (PLA), (2) autografts (derived from the same person), made up of autologous fat, and (3) xenografts (derived from another species), consisting of porcine collagen, bovine collagen, and animal-based hyaluronic acid (HA). However, unlike permanent fillers, temporary fillers undergo biological degradation of their active products. Thus, they must periodically be readministered to maintain soft tissue augmentation. Although the overall complication rates for fillers are low [2] (V/B), permanent fillers are responsible for many of the long-term complications associated with adverse filler events.

To enhance patient satisfaction and minimize complications during the administration of any dermal filler, a common set of guidelines has been compiled from evidence-based consensus recommendations for soft tissue augmentation (Table 20.1). Preoperative considerations include discussion of realistic patient expectations when planning treatment, procurement of informed consent, examination of the treatment site for the presence of active dermatological conditions, and a thorough review of the patient's medical history, especially regarding allergic reactions, history of cold sores, and previous dermal filler treatments. Further, patients should be advised to avoid nonprescription anticoagulants, such as aspirin and NSAIDS, for 7–10 days before treatment. Subsequently, dermal fillers can be injected through a number of techniques, which include linear threading, serial puncture, fanning, cross-hatching, or combinations of these techniques (Fig. 20.2). The choice of injection technique

K. Beer (✉)
Esthetic Surgical and General Dermatology,
1500 North Dixie Highway Suite 303,
West Palm Beach, FL 33401
e-mail: kenbeer@aol.com

S. Nanda
Feinberg School of Medicine, Northwestern University,
Arthur J. Rubloff Building, 420 East Superior Street,
Chicago, IL 60611, USA
e-mail: s-nanda@northwestern.edu

M. Alam (ed.), *Evidence-Based Procedural Dermatology*,
DOI 10.1007/978-0-387-09424-3_20, © Springer Science+Business Media, LLC 2012

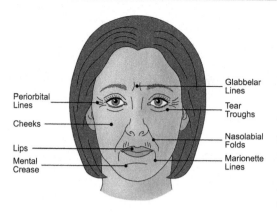

Periorbital Lines

Cheeks

Lips

Mental Crease

Glabbelar Lines

Tear Troughs

Nasolabial Folds

Marionette Lines

**Fig. 20.1** Areas frequently treated by soft tissue augmentation

**Table 20.1** Consensus guidelines for soft tissue augmentation

Preoperative considerations
  Discuss patient goals and expectations
  Obtain informed consent
  Record patient medical history, with particular emphasis on
    History of allergies, herpes simplex, cold sores
    Current/recent medications
    Prior use of dermal fillers
  Conduct physical examination, including
    Inspection of site of planned injection for active dermatological conditions
    Evaluation of skin thickness and texture at site of planned injection
  Administer skin test for
    Bovine/porcine collagen fillers
    Animal-based hyaluronic acids
  Photograph "before" pictures
Operative considerations
  Thoroughly cleanse site of injection with antiseptic
  Mark the area to be treated
  If desired, administer anesthetic
Postoperative considerations
  Photograph "after" pictures
  If swelling is observed, apply an ice pack

depends on the filler being used, treatment site, and depth of injection placement. It is advised that anesthetics be utilized during treatment to reduce patient discomfort. The physician and patient should also discuss any expected erythema, bruising, and swelling following treatment with any dermal filler.

To achieve optimal cosmetic results, physicians must understand the unique properties regarding the longevity and mechanism of action of each dermal filler. FDA-approved dermal fillers and their associated properties are listed in Table 20.2. In this chapter, we evaluate the most commonly used fillers in the United States, including collagens, HAs, CaHA, and PLA, to better understand the evidence-based literature regarding the practice, efficacy, and safety of soft tissue augmentation.

## Collagen

### Prior Evidence-Based Consensus Reports

Consensus documents published by the American Academy of Dermatology in 1996 outline evidence-based guidelines for soft tissue augmentation using bovine-derived collagen fillers. Specifically, the recommendations are compiled for three FDA-approved bovine collagen fillers, Zyderm I® (35 mg/mL of collagen), Zyderm II® (65 mg/mL of collagen), and Zyplast® (35 mg/mL of collagen that is cross-linked to improve longevity of action). According to the consensus panel, all three fillers are indicated for the treatment of age-related wrinkles/lines, dermal atrophy, angular cheilitis, and depressed scars. The fillers are ineffective in the treatment of viral pockmarks, ice pick scars, abdominal stretch marks, and conditions resulting in a loss of subcutaneous tissue. Prior to administration, the authors specify that skin testing with the Collagen Test Implant is required and must be assessed for the presence of erythema, induration, or pruritus at 48 or 72 h, and at 4 weeks. Collagen injections can be delivered only following negative test results at the 4-week mark. Even after a negative skin test result, it is reported that 1–3% of individuals experience an allergic reaction following treatment. The likelihood of such a hypersensitivity reaction can be reduced with the use of cross-linked bovine collagen. Evidence-based recommendations for proper administration of bovine collagen fillers emphasize the use of a 30-gauge needle which "should pierce the skin, usually at a 45° angle, and then be advanced once within the dermis to the proper level of implantation (upper dermis for

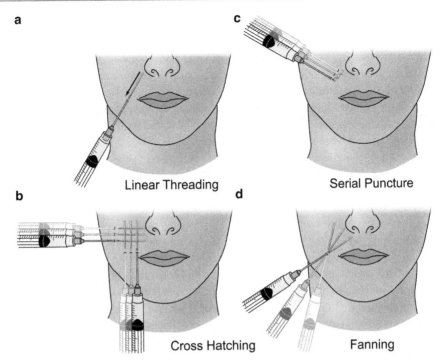

**a** Linear Threading

**c** Serial Puncture

**b** Cross Hatching

**d** Fanning

**Fig. 20.2** Dermal filler injection techniques. (**a**) Linear threading: filler is injected evenly throughout needle withdrawal or insertion. (**b**) Serial puncture: filler is injected in closely spaced aliquots. (**c**) Cross-hatching: needle is advanced and filler is injected with each withdrawal. The process is repeated as needle direction is altered continuously, without ever completely withdrawing the needle from the skin. (**d**) Fanning: filler is injected as two series of linear threads, orientated 90° apart

**Table 20.2** Summary of dermal filler properties

| Filler | Composition | Site of placement | FDA-approved uses |
|---|---|---|---|
| Bovine collagen | | | |
| Zyderm I® | 35 mg/mL bovine collagen | Upper dermis | Facial wrinkles/lines, angular cheilitis, |
| Zyderm II® | 65 mg/mL bovine collagen | Upper dermis | dermal atrophy, depressed scars |
| Zyplast® | 35 mg/mL cross-linked bovine collagen | Dermis | |
| Porcine collagen | | | |
| Evolence® | 35 mg/mL cross-linked porcine collagen | Mid-dermis | Moderate-to-severe facial wrinkles/folds, depressed scars |
| Hyaluronic acid | | | |
| Captique®, Hylaform®, Hylafrom Plus® Restylane® Perlane® Juvederm® Plus and Ultra Plus | 4.5–6 mg/mL hyaluronic acid 20 mg/mL hyaluronic acid 20 mg/mL hyaluronic acid 24 mg/mL hyaluronic acid | Mid-dermis Mid-dermis Deep dermis Mid-dermis | Moderate-to-severe facial wrinkles/folds |
| Calcium hydroxylapatite | | | |
| Radiesse® | Synthetic calcium hydroxylapatite | Subdermal | Moderate-to-severe facial wrinkles/folds HIV-related facial lipoatrophy |
| Poly-L-lactic acid | | | |
| New Fill®, Sculptra® | Synthetic poly-L-lactic acid | Subdermal | HIV-related facial lipoatrophy |

Note: At this time, these products are no longer available in the US noncross-linked bovine collagen, deep dermis for cross-linked bovine collagen)" [3] (VI/C).

In 1996, the American Academy of Dermatology also published guidelines for the use of porcine-based collagen fillers, finding their use safe and effective for moderate-to-severe facial wrinkles/folds and depressed scars. Like bovine collagen, porcine-based collagen is deemed ineffective for the treatment of viral pockmarks, ice pick scars, abdominal stretch marks, and conditions resulting in a loss of subcutaneous tissue. To evaluate preexisting allergies to the gelatin matrix component of the filler, the consensus panel states that skin testing with an intradermal injection, consisting of a solution of 0.05 mL of gelatin and ε-aminocaproic acid in saline, is required. Subsequently, the site of injection needs to be assessed for "induration and erythema lasting more than 5 h after administration, or commencing more than 24 h after implantation." Following a negative test result at week 4, it is appropriate for treatment to begin. Panel members also conclude that administration of porcine collagen is most effective with a 27–20-gauge needle injected intradermally [4] (VI/C).

## Case Series and Cohort Studies

The newest collagen product in the United States is Evolence®, a cross-linked porcine-based collagen with a collagen concentration of 35 mg/mL. Commonly used for the treatment of deep facial wrinkles and folds, Evolence® is formulated to mimic human collagen to enhance its biological compatibility. To address concerns about its immunogenicity, skin testing was performed to document any clinical or laboratory evidence of allergenicity. Shoshani et al. evaluated 530 subjects who received two injections of 0.1 mL of Evolence® in their forearms 30 days apart. Patients were assessed at various time intervals for erythema and induration. In addition, antibody testing was performed to evaluate the production of IgG, IgM, IgA, and IgE. No moderate or severe reactions were noted in this study. Three subjects (0.6%) developed mild erythema and one subject

(0.2%) had a 2+ serum antibody reaction. Due to the low percentage of hypersensitivity observed in this study, the authors concluded that skin testing was not necessary prior to treatment with Evolence® [5] (IV/B).

Evidence supporting the efficacy of Evolence® was presented in the form of a histological evaluation of the product following its injection. In this study, Pitaru et al. assessed the three-dimensional and histologic appearance of Evolence®, Zyderm®, and Zyplast® after injection into rabbits. Using biopsies of the various products at 1, 6, 12, and 24 months postinjection, they demonstrated that Zyderm® and Zyplast® were present at minute concentrations at 6 months, while Evolence® persisted for up to 24 months. After analysis of the immune response to the various products, the authors posit that the low degree of immunogenicity of the porcine collagen is responsible for the persistence noted [6] (IV/B).

## Randomized Controlled Trials

A multicenter, randomized controlled trial was conducted to evaluate the safety and efficacy of Evolence® in comparison with a HA filler (Restylane®) of proven safety and efficacy, for the treatment of nasolabial creases. The study randomized 149 subjects, with approximately symmetrical nasolabial creases, to receive the porcine-based collagen filler or the HA filler on contralateral sides of the face. Subjects were evaluated by a blinded investigator at the time of screening and after treatment. Statistically significant improvement in scores on the Modified Fitzpatrick Wrinkle Scale after treatment, in comparison to the screening visit, was observed for both fillers. At 6-month follow-up, mean scores for both fillers continued to display statistically significant improvement. However, statistical significance in the differences between scores for the two fillers was not observed. Subjects in this trial had mild complications that included swelling, bruising, discomfort, and induration. Of note, the swelling and bruising were more significant on the side of the face treated with HA, but induration was seen more commonly on the collagen-injected side. Thus, the data for Evolence® demonstrate that it is a safe and effective soft tissue augmentation product, of equal safety and efficacy to HA fillers for treatment of the nasolabial folds [7] (II/A).

## Hyaluronic Acid

HA fillers are quickly replacing collagen fillers for use in soft tissue augmentation as cosmetic results for HA fillers persist up to 3 months longer than results for bovine collagen fillers, for which the cosmetic effect persists for an average of 3–4 months [8] (II/A). These cross-linked polymers are naturally found in all adult animal tissues and exhibit no tissue or species specificity, decreasing immunological reactions upon injection. Due to their hydrophilic nature, HA fillers enhance the structure and volume of soft tissues by readily attracting water molecules to the site of injection. Various HA fillers differ in concentrations of HA; Hylaform®, Hylaform Plus®, and Captique® contain 4.5–6 mg/mL of HA, Restylane® and Perlane® contain 20 mg/mL, and Juvederm® Ultra and Ultra Plus contain 24 mg/mL.

## Prior Evidence-Based Consensus Reports

In 2006, the American Society of Plastic Surgeons published a consensus report outlining guidelines for the use of Restylane®. The report concludes that HA fillers are most effective for the treatment of the nasolabial folds, lips, and marionette lines. The majority of the panel found that a 2 mL dose of Restylane®, administered every 4–6 months, results in optimal correction of facial wrinkles/folds in their average patients. Based on evaluation of data through 2006, the panel members observed that 0.02% of individuals experienced posttreatment complications that included inflammation, needle marks, edema, erythema, palpable lumps, bruising, and over- or undercorrection. Cessation of aspirin and other anticoagulants

is recommended to decrease the incidence of complications. In addition, the use of antiviral prophylaxis is advocated prior to the treatment of patients with a history of herpes simplex. Further, this report reveals that minorities account for approximately 20% of those injected with Restylane®. There does not appear to be any significant increase in keloids or hyperpigmentation following the use of HA fillers in this population [9] (VI/C).

## Randomized Controlled Trials

Because evidence-based literature on HA fillers is separately generated for each of the leading fillers, it is not possible to make broad conclusions, but rather it is more appropriate to separately discuss some of the trends for each of the leading HA fillers, Restylane®, Perlane®, and Juvederm®.

## Restylane® and Perlane®

A comparison of Restylane® vs. Zyplast® was performed in 188 patients with moderate or severe nasolabial creases. This multicenter, randomized controlled trial was pivotal for evaluating HAs with the gold standard (bovine collagen) for soft tissue augmentation. Using a split-face comparison in a double-blinded manner, the authors concluded that Restylane® was superior to Zyplast® in both the degree of correction offered and the duration of correction provided. At 6-month follow-up, 67% of Zyplast®-treated sites had returned to baseline. In comparison, only 29% of Restylane®-treated sites had reverted to baseline at follow-up. Initial reports of swelling were greater with Restylane® than with Zyplast® (87 vs. 73.9%). However, the authors concluded that the long-term safety profile of the HA filler was superior, as only 26.8% of Restylane® patients experienced an adverse event at follow-up compared with 39.1% of those treated with Zyplast®. All reported adverse events were minor, consisting of erythema and/or induration [8] (II/A).

Persistence of Restylane® following correction has also been evaluated in another multi-center trial. In this trial, 75 patients were randomized to either receive retreatment of one nasolabial crease at 4.5 or 9 months following initial correction. Assessment by a blinded evaluator revealed significant improvement, lasting up to 18 months, after initial treatment for both regimens. However, there was no difference in efficacy between the two retreatment schedules [10] (II/A). As with other studies that use repeated injections to measure duration of filler effects, the results of this study are of limited clinical value since most patients lack the time and financial resources to return for several treatments in short succession. A cost/benefit analysis that includes the cost of adverse events, in addition to costs associated with the treatment regimens proposed by this study, is needed to determine the utility of the data gathered.

Many patients undergoing soft tissue augmentation also choose other facial rejuvenation modalities, such as lasers and light sources. Thus, data to evaluate the safety of utilizing these procedures in combination with soft tissue augmentation are clinically relevant. In one study, 33 subjects were treated with HA fillers on one side of the face and HA fillers followed by either nonablative laser, radiofrequency (RF), or intense pulsed light (IPL) therapies on the contralateral side of the face. The results showed no appreciable difference in the correction attained by dermal fillers alone in comparison with those preceding laser, RF, or IPL treatment. Moreover, no statistically significant increase was observed in the number of adverse events reported with HA fillers used in conjunction with laser/RF/IPL treatment. However, the sample size of this study limited extensive conclusions from being drawn in regard to the effects of specific lasers, such as the 1,450 nm diode laser, on the safety and utility of HA fillers. These data suggest that the most commonly performed laser and light source treatments do not impact the safety or efficacy of HA fillers [11] (II/A).

Perlane® is chemically identical to Restylane®, differing only in the size of the particles of HA it contains. Whereas Restylane® has approximately

**Table 20.3** Wrinkle severity rating scale (WSRS)

| Score | Description |
|---|---|
| 5 | Extreme: Extremely deep and long folds detrimental to facial appearance; 2–4 mm visible V-shaped fold when stretched |
| 4 | Severe: Very long and deep folds; prominent facial feature; less than 2 mm visible fold when stretched |
| 3 | Moderate: Moderately deep folds; clear facial feature visible at normal appearance but not when stretched |
| 2 | Mild: Shallow but visible fold with a slight indentation; minor facial feature |
| 1 | Absent: No visible fold; continuous skin line |

Adapted from Carruthers et al. [12]

100,000 particles/mL, Perlane® has 20,000 particles/mL. This difference affords Perlane® the characteristics to treat deeper creases than can be treated by Restylane®. One randomized, double-blind study compared Perlane® with Hylaform®, a HA filler containing a weaker concentration of HA. The study evaluated 150 patients injected with Perlane® on one nasolabial crease and Hylaform® on the contralateral side. Perlane® provided a durable correction lasting at least 6 months after the final treatment. In 75% of patients treated with Perlane®, at least a one-grade improvement in the Wrinkle Severity Rating Scale (Table 20.3) was observed by a blinded evaluator, compared with 38% of those treated with Hylaform®. Side effects for both Perlane®- and Hylaform®-treated sides were mostly mild, consisting of swelling, pain, and erythema. However, there was an increased incidence of complications with Perlane® (41.3%) compared with the incidence of such events with Hylaform® (21.3%). The authors hypothesize that this result may be due to the higher viscosity of Perlane®, which warranted the use of a higher gauge needle [12] (II/A). Thus, Perlane® may offer time and cost advantages to patients owing to the greater longevity of its esthetic correction in comparison with HA fillers of lower concentrations, with the caveat of compromising patient comfort.

Hamilton et al. conducted two multicenter, randomized trials to assess the immunogenicity in 433 subjects injected at the nasolabial fold with either Restylane® or Perlane®, two nonani-mal-stabilized hyaluronic acid (NASHA) fillers. Evaluation of immune responses to the dermal fillers was performed by immunoassay tech-niques and histopathological analysis at various time points up to 24 weeks following treatment. 91.8% of subjects had negative IgG anti-NASHA titers. Interestingly, approximately 7.8% of patients had IgG anti-NASHA antibodies at enrollment. However, these antibody titers remained stable over the time course of the study. The authors concluded that no cellular or humoral responses were present in 98% of enrolled sub-jects, providing evidence that both Restylane® and Perlane® have low rates of immunogenic and allergenic responses [13] (II/A).

## Juvederm®

Juvederm® is a HA filler of greater concentration and cross-linking than Restylane®. The pivotal study for Juvederm® was a multicenter, double-blind, randomized controlled trial, in which the safety and efficacy of Juvederm® 30, Ultra, and Ultra Plus were compared with Zyplast®, a cross-linked bovine collagen, for the treatment of moderate-to-severe nasolabial creases. Four hundred and thirty-nine subjects with approxi-mately symmetrical, bilateral nasolabial folds were randomized to receive either Juvederm® 30, Ultra, or Ultra Plus and Zyplast® on contralateral sides of their faces. This study demonstrated that treatment with Juvederm® resulted in sustained improvement in a greater proportion of subjects than treatment with Zyplast® at 24-week follow-up. Further, Juvederm® was preferred by between 78 and 88% of patients 6 months postinjection [14] (II/A). A limitation to this study is that, unlike clinical practice, this trial provided touch-up injections of either filler following initial treatment, obscuring the efficacy measurements obtained in this study.

Another multicenter, double-blinded trial assessing the long-term safety and efficacy of Juvederm® Plus and Ultra Plus concluded that Juvederm® Ultra and Ultra Plus provided effec-tive soft tissue augmentation for up to 1 year [15]

(II/A). However, this conclusion was based upon a treatment regimen, involving up to three treat-ments, that is not typical of most clinical situa-tions, in which only a single treatment session is offered. Thus, further investigation in a clinically relevant context is needed to verify the longevity of correction offered by Juvederm®.

To assess the benefit of Juvederm® Ultra incor-porated with an anesthetic on patient comfort, one multicenter, double-blind, European trial treated 60 patients, on contralateral sides of the face, with Juvederm® Ultra preincorporated with lidocaine and Juvederm® Ultra without lidocaine. Patients rated the degree of pain, associated with injections of the lidocaine-product, as mild in 72.4% of the cases. Those injected without lido-caine evaluated the discomfort as strong or very strong in 63.8% of the cases. Thus, lidocaine-incorporating fillers appear to enhance patient comfort during soft tissue augmentation [16] (II/A).

## Calcium Hydroxyapatite

### Prior Evidence-Based Consensus Reports

A consensus report published in 2007 by the American Society of Plastic Surgeons states that synthetic CaHA fillers are effective and safe treatments for age-related facial wrinkles/folds and lipoatrophy related to human immunodefi-ciency virus (HIV). CaHA fillers are identical in composition to the CaHA found in bones. As such, consensus guidelines have concluded that "injectable CaHA is biocompatible, nontoxic, nonirritating, and nonantigenic." Upon subder-mal injection using a 27-gauge needle, the cal-cium hydroxylapatite causes steady migration of collagen molecules to the target site, producing long-term soft tissue correction. Prior to treat-ment, the consensus panel recommends the use of anesthetics to enhance patient comfort. However, care should be taken to mark the treat-ment area prior to administration of anesthetic, as the anesthetic may alter properties of the skin surface [17] (VI/C).

## Case Series and Cohort Studies

In a pilot study to examining the safety and longevity of CaHA, three patients were injected with 0.1 mL of CaHA gel in the postauricular area and bilateral nasolabial folds. Three mm punch biopsies were obtained 1 and 6 months postinjection and examined by histopathology and electron microscopy for inflammatory cell reaction, fibrosis, ossification, and/or granuloma formation. No such adverse events were observed following implantation. Further, formation of a matrix of collagen occurred early around the implant and persisted for at least 6 months postinjection. Thus, CaHA appears to remain in the body for long periods of time without significant adverse events [18] (V/B).

In a larger study of 1,000 patients treated with CaHA, the persistence of CaHA was analyzed over the span of 4 years. The procedure was largely performed in the nasolabial creases, but marionette lines and other facial areas were also treated. More than 80% of patients reported persistence of results at 12 months. Thus, CaHA appears to be effective for soft tissue augmentation up to 1 year postinjection at various anatomical locations. Complications of CaHA injection reported in this study were low, with the most frequent adverse events including redness, swelling, itching, and bruising. Less frequently observed was a 1.7% rate of nodule formation following injection with CaHA. However, nodule formation was noted in 5.9% of patients injected with CaHA for lip augmentation during the author's earlier experiences. The incidence of nodule formation declined to 2% for the last 100 lip augmentations performed. This suggests that the learning curve for CaHA treatment of the lips is sharp, and lip augmentation with CaHA should be reserved for those who have had ample experience with the procedure [19] (IV/B).

Due to their potential for long-term persistence in the body, CaHA fillers have also been indicated in the treatment of lipoatrophy observed in patients with HIV. Carruthers and Carruthers treated 30 patients with HIV-related lipoatrophy using CaHA and conducted follow-up at 3, 6, and 12 months to assess changes in cheek thickness. Results indicated a statistically significant increase in cheek thickness at all three time points. The most commonly reported complications included edema (93%), echhymosis (83%), and erythema (77%). However, data from this study require several caveats when considering its application to clinical use. First, the average volume injected per subject over 6 months was 13.3 mL; substantially greater than the 8.4 mL utilized in other studies [20] (IV/B). In addition, touch-up treatments were offered at 6- and 12-month follow-up, potentially confounding the interpretation of data in this study. However, even with these caveats, it is clear that CaHA has a role to play for some patients with HIV-related lipoatrophy and that it can offer long-term correction with minimal posttreatment complications [21] (IV/B).

## Randomized Controlled Trials

A randomized, split-face study evaluated the safety and efficacy of CaHA against nonanimal-stabilized HA on the treatment of nasolabial folds at two medical clinics in Europe. Blinded evaluators used the Wrinkle Severity Rating Scale (Table 20.3) and the Global Esthetic Improvement Scale (Table 20.4) to evaluate 60 patients at 6-, 9-, and 12-month follow-up visits. 79% of CaHA-treated folds continued to display acceptable cosmetic results at 12 months, compared with 43% of folds treated with HA fillers. This result was statistically significant. However, while adverse events were similar and minimal for both products, lip nodules were observed following treatment with CaHA [22] (II/A).

Another multicenter, randomized, split-face trial studied 117 subjects with moderate-to-deep nasolabial folds. CaHA was administered to one nasolabial fold, while human collagen was injected to the other nasolabial fold in each patient. Following initial and follow-up visits, blinded raters utilized photographs to evaluate the esthetic appearance of each subject, finding superior cosmetic results in CaHA-treated folds at

**Table 20.4** Global esthetic improvement scale (GAIS)

| Rating | Description |
|---|---|
| Very much improved | Optimal cosmetic result from the implant |
| Much improved | Marked improvement in appearance from the initial condition, but not completely optimal. A touch-up would slightly improve the result |
| Improved | Obvious improvement in appearance from the initial condition, but a touch-up or retreatment is indicated |
| No change | The appearance is essentially the same as the original condition |
| Worse | The appearance is worse than the original condition |

Adapted from Carruthers et al. [12]

6 months postinjection. Moreover, fewer injections with CaHA, as compared with human collagen, were required to achieve optimal cosmetic results. The authors concluded that CaHA achieved longer-lasting esthetic results than human collagen and decreased the time and cost required for treatment [23] (II/A).

## Poly-L-Lactic Acid (PLA)

PLA (Sculptra®) is a synthetic polymer suspended in a carboxymethylcellulose gel that is manufactured as a lyophilized powder. Since its FDA-approval in 2004 for treatment of HIV-related facial lipoatrophy, PLA has been used to replace volume lost with aging or disease. Its mechanism of action involves an increase in volume via induction of collagen synthesis and delayed fibroplasia.

### Prior Evidence-Based Consensus Report

A 2006 consensus panel, summarizing treatment guidelines for PLA, recommends pretreatment counseling of patients to highlight the delay in esthetic transformation that occurs following PLA injection, with results becoming apparent weeks to months after the initial treatment.

Moreover, patients should be made aware that multiple treatment sessions will be required to achieve optimal correction. The consensus panel also finds use of PLA to be associated with the formation of subcutaneous papules at a rate of 3.2% for nonvisible nodules and 1.2% for visible nodules. To minimize these complications, the authors recommend higher volume dilution (8–12 mL) of the product with water 12 h before injection, fewer vials (1–2) used at each session, adequate time between injection sessions (at least 6 weeks), and posttreatment patient massage. The consensus panel also advises strict adherence to the subcutaneous placement of the dermal filler, as intradermal injections have been associated with granulomatous inflammatory responses [24] (VI/C).

## Case Series and Cohort Studies

The use of PLA in the treatment of HIV-related lipoatrophy was investigated in a prospective, open-label study by VEGA. Fifty patients received 3–5 treatments with PLA, with each treatment session spaced 2 weeks apart. Patients were evaluated intermittently for 96 weeks by photographs, facial ultrasonography, and clinical examination. Upon 48-week follow-up, there was a statistically significant, threefold increase in skin thickness that was sustained throughout the 96-week study. Although patients were treated with higher mean doses of PLA per treatment session than are commonly used for the treatment of wrinkles/folds, adverse events were minimal. The primary complications reported were edema and ecchymosis. Nonvisible subcutaneous nodules were present in 44% (22/50) of subjects, but resolved in 24% of cases by the 96-week follow-up visit. The authors concluded that PLA was a safe and efficacious treatment option for HIV-related lipoatrophy, with potentially longer-lasting results than other treatment options, including autologous fat transplants or HA fillers [25] (IV/B).

Subjective assessment of skin thickening and satisfaction was performed as part of a prospective clinical trial that used PLA to treat 61

HIV-infected patients with facial lipoatrophy over a 5-month period. Upon follow-up, 100% of subjects and physicians in this trial reported "Excellent" results corresponding to achievement of the desired appearance [26] (IV/B). Thus, PLA appears to be an effective treatment modality that can enhance quality of life for patients with HIV-related lipoatrophy.

## Randomized Controlled Trials

In a single-site, open-label trial, 30 patients with HIV-related facial lipoatrophy were randomized to either an immediate or delayed treatment regimen, consisting of three bilateral injections of PLA administered 2 weeks apart. The immediate arm received injections at 0, 2, and 4 weeks, while the delayed arm received treatment at 12, 14, and 16 weeks. At 12 weeks, there was a statistically significant increase in mean skin thickness in the immediate treatment group compared with the delayed treatment group, who had not received any treatment at this time. Further, the study assessed the efficacy of PLA treatment via subjective assessments of patient satisfaction by visual analog scales (VASs) and by the Hospital Anxiety and Depression Scale (HADS). In both groups, there was an increasing trend in patient satisfaction from baseline to final follow-up visit, 18 months after final treatment with PLA. However, these data did not achieve statistical significance. The most frequent adverse event reported at follow-up was the presence of nonvisible nodules in 31% of cases, which the authors attribute to the overstimulation of fibroblasts as a result of uneven dispersal of PLA in the dermis. Apart from the presence of these subcutaneous nodules, only minor adverse events were reported after treatment. Consequently, PLA was characterized as a safe and efficacious treatment for HIV-related lipoatrophy [27] (II/A).

Overall, the data for volumetric correction with PLA support its utility. As with all other soft tissue augmentation procedures, its use may be associated with adverse events, such as the formation of subcutaneous papules, bruising, erythema, and tenderness. Although PLA is currently only FDA-approved to treat HIV-related lipoatrophy, its off-label use for cosmetic soft tissue augmentation is growing. This trend will likely potentiate the evidence-based data available in this field.

## Conclusion

The growing popularity of soft tissue augmentation in recent years [28] (V/B) has led to a rapid increase in the development of novel dermal fillers, designed to enhance longevity of action and biocompatibility. Well-designed clinical trials assessing the safety and efficacy of all marketable dermal fillers are a requirement for FDA approval. Evidence for the most widely used products currently available supports their use for the treatment of dermal atrophy, depressed scars, HIV-associated lipoatrophy, and/or age-related wrinkles/folds, with high degrees of confidence. Moreover, trials assessing the safety of collagen, HA, CaHA, and PLA fillers have found these products to be associated with only minor complications, primarily including erythema, bruising, and inflammation. However, information regarding the exact duration of esthetic outcomes with these dermal fillers is somewhat obscured by the design of studies that include treatment regimens that do not parallel real-world, patient care situations.

Thus, when evaluating the evidence-based data for soft tissue augmentation, it is necessary to scrutinize the methodology employed and the statistical significance obtained. The continuous development of injectable dermal fillers in the coming years will warrant that the conscientious medical practitioner thoroughly review and analyze the evidence-based literature evaluating the safety and efficacy of these products for soft tissue augmentation.

## Evidence-Based Summary

| Findings | Evidence level |
| --- | --- |
| Bovine collagen fillers are indicated for facial wrinkles/lines, angular cheilitis, dermal atrophy, and depressed scars | VI/C |
| Porcine collagen fillers are FDA-approved to treat moderate-to-severe facial wrinkles/folds and depressed scars and produce results that persist for longer periods than after injection with bovine fillers | II/A |
| Porcine-based collagen fillers (Evolence®) have similar safety and efficacy profiles as nonanimal-stabilized hyaluronic acid fillers for the treatment of nasolabial creases | II/A |
| Patients should be administered skin testing prior to treatment with bovine or porcine-based collagen fillers. Evolence® does not require skin testing | IV/B |
| Hyaluronic acid fillers can be used to treat moderate-to-severe facial wrinkles/folds, with results lasting upwards to 1 year | II/A |
| Hyaluronic acid fillers (Juvederm®, Restylane®) have longer-lasting results in the treatment of nasolabial folds than do bovine collagen fillers (Zyplast®), without an increase in incidence of adverse events | II/A |
| Hyaluronic acid fillers (Juvederm®) preincorporated with lidocaine are more easily tolerated by patients than are hyaluronic acid fillers alone | II/A |
| Hyaluronic acid fillers can be used in combination with laser/RF/IPL therapies without a significant increase in adverse events | II/A |
| Calcium hydroxylapatite fillers are FDA-approved for the treatment of moderate-to-severe facial wrinkles/folds and HIV-related facial lipoatrophy | VI/C |
| Calcium hydroxylapatite fillers (Radiesse®) offer longer-lasting esthetic improvement for the nasolabial folds than nonanimal-stabilized hyaluronic acid fillers and human collagen fillers | II/A |
| Calcium hydroxylapatite fillers result in soft tissue augmentation for HIV-related lipoatrophy, with results lasting upwards to 1 year | IV/B |
| Poly-L-lactic acid fillers are FDA-approved for the treatment of HIV-related facial lipoatrophy only | VI/C |
| Poly-L-lactic acid produces statistically significant increases in skin thickness in patients with HIV-related lipoatrophy with minimal complications | II/A |
| The most frequent long-term adverse event observed after treatment of HIV-related facial lipoatrophy with PLA was the presence of subcutaneous nodules | II/A |

# References

1. Tierney EP, Hanke CW. Recent trends in cosmetic and surgical procedure volumes in dermatologic surgery. Dermatol Surg. 2009;35(9):1324–33.
2. Cohen JL. Understanding, avoiding, and managing dermal filler complications. Dermatol Surg. 2008;34:S92–9.
3. Drake LA et al. Guidelines of care for soft tissue augmentation collagen implants. J Am Acad Dermatol. 1996;34:698–702.
4. Drake LA. Guidelines of care for soft tissue augmentation: gelatin matrix implant. J Am Acad Dermatol. 1996;34:695–7.
5. Shoshani D, Markovitz E, Cohen Y, Heremans A, Goldlust A. Skin test hypersensitivity study of a cross-linked, porcine collagen implant for aesthetic surgery. Dermatol Surg. 2007;33:S152–8.
6. Pitaru S, Noff M, Blok L, Nir E, Pitaru S, Goldlust A, et al. Long-term efficacy of a novel ribose cross-linked collagen dermal filler: a histologic and histo-morphometric study in an animal model. Dermatol Surg. 2007;33:1045–54.
7. Narins RS, Brandt FS, Lorenc ZP, Maas CS, Monheit GD, Smith SR, et al. A randomized, multicenter study of the safety and efficacy of Dermicol-P35 and non-animal-stabilized hyaluronic acid gel for the correction of nasolabial folds. Dermatol Surg. 2007;33:S213–21.

8. Narins RS, Brandt F, Leyden J, Lorenc ZP, Rubin M, Smith S. A randomized, double-blind multicenter comparison of the efficacy and tolerability of Restylane versus Zyplast for the correction of nasolabial folds. Dermatol Surg. 2003;29:588–99.

9. Matarasso S, Carruthers J, Jewell M. Restylane Consensus Group. Consensus recommendations for soft tissue augmentation with nonanimal stabilized hyaluronic acid (Restylane). Plast Reconstr Surg. 2006;117:S3–31.

10. Narins RS, Dayan SH, Brandt FS, Baldwain EK. Persistence and improvement of nasolabial fold correction with non animal hyaluronic acid 100,000 gel particles/mL filler on two retreatment schedules: results up to 18 months on two retreatment schedules. Dermatol Surg. 2008;34:S2–8.

11. Goldman MP, Alster TS, Weiss R. A randomized trial to determine the influence of laser therapy, monopolar radiofrequency treatment and intense pulsed light therapy administered immediately after hyaluronic acid gel implantation. Dermatol Surg. 2007;33:535–42.

12. Carruthers A, Carey W, De Lorenzi C, Remington K, Schachter D, Sapra S. Randomized, double-blind comparison of the efficacy of two hyaluronic acid derivatives, Restylane Perlane and Hylaform in the treatment of nasolabial folds. Dermatol Surg. 2005;31:1591–8.

13. Hamilton R, Strobos J, Adkinson N. Immunogenicity of cosmetically administered nonanimal-stabilized hyaluronic acid particles. Dermatol Surg. 2007;33:S176–85.

14. Baumann LS, Shamban AT, Lupo MP, Monheit GD, Thomas JA, Murphy DK, et al. Comparison of smooth- gel hyaluronic acid dermal fillers with cross-linked bovine collagen: a multicenter, double-masked, randomized within-subject study. Dermatol Surg. 2007;33:S128–35.

15. Pinsky MA, Thomas JA, Murphy DK, Walker PS. Juvederm vs. Zyplast nasolabial Fold Study Group. Juvederm injectable gel: a multicenter double blind randomized study of safety and effectiveness. Aesthet Surg J. 2008;28:17–23.

16. Levy P, DeBoulle K, Raspaldo H. Comparison of injection comfort of a new category of cohesive hyaluronic acid filler with pre-incorporated lidocaine and a hyaluronic acid filler alone. Dermatol Surg. 2009;35:332–7.

17. Graivier MH, Bass LS, Busso M, Jasin ME, Narins RS, Tzikas TL. Calcium hydroxylapatite (Radiesse) for correction of the mid- and lower face: consensus recommendations. Plast Reconstr Surg. 2007;120:S55–66.

18. Marmur ES, Phelps R, Goldberg D. Clinical, histologic, and electron microscopic findings after injection of a calcium hydroxylapatite filler. J Cosmet Laser Ther. 2004;6:223–6.

19. Tzikas T. A 52 month summary of results using calcium hydroxylapatite for facial soft tissue augmentation. Dermatol Surg. 2008;34:S9–15.

20. Silvers SL, Eviatar JA, Echavez MI, Pappas AL. Prospective, open-label, 18-month trial of calcium hydroxylapatite (Radiesse) for facial soft-tissue augmentation in patients with human immunodeficiency virus-associated lipoatrophy: one-year durability. Plast Reconstr Surg. 2006;118:S34–45.

21. Carruthers A, Carruthers J. Evaluation of injectable calcium hydroxylapatite for the treatment of facial lipoatrophy associated with human immunodeficiency virus. Dermatol Surg. 2008;34:1486–99.

22. Moers-Carpi MM, Tufet JO. Calcium hydroxylapatite versus nonanimal stabilized hyaluronic acid for the correction of nasolabial folds: a 12-month, multicenter, prospective, randomized, controlled, split-face trial. Dermatol Surg. 2008;34:210–5.

23. Smith S, Busso M, McClaren M, Bass LS. A randomized, bilateral, prospective comparison of calcium hydroxylapatite microspheres versus human-based collagen for the correction of nasolabial folds. Dermatol Surg. 2007;33:S112–21.

24. Lam SM, Azizzadeh B, Graivier M. Injectable poly-L-lactic acid (Sculptra): technical considerations in soft-tissue contouring. Plast Reconstr Surg. 2006;118:S55–63.

25. Valantin MA, Aubron-Olivier C, Ghosn J, Laglenne E, Pauchard M, Schoen H, et al. Polylactic acid implants (new fill) to correct facial lipoatrophy in HIV infected patients: results of the open label study VEGA. AIDS. 2003;17:2471–7.

26. Burgess C, Quiroga RM. Assessment of the safety and efficacy of poly-L-lactic acid for the treatment of HIV associated facial lipoatrophy. J Am Acad Dermatol. 2005;52:223–9.

27. Moyle GJ, Brown S, Lysakova L, Barton SE. Long-term safety and efficacy of poly-L-lactic acid in the treatment of HIV-related facial lipoatrophy. HIV Med. 2006;7:181–5.

28. Wise JB, Greco T. Injectable treatments for the aging face. Facial Plast Surg. 2006;22:140–6.

## Self-Assessment

1. Which of the following dermal fillers require skin testing prior to their use in soft tissue augmentation?
   (a) Calcium hydroxylapatite
   (b) Poly-L-lactic acid
   (c) Bovine collagen
   (d) Nonanimal-stabilized hyaluronic acid

2. Calcium hydroxylapatite fillers are FDA-approved for which of the following indications?
   (a) Moderate-to-severe facial wrinkles/folds
   (b) Depressed, acne scars
   (c) HIV-associated facial lipoatrophy
   (d) a and c

3. The mechanism of action by which poly-L-lactic acid fillers produce volume expansion is:
   (a) By attracting water to the target site due to their hydrophilic nature
   (b) By delayed fibroplasia
   (c) Through the induction of new collagen synthesis
   (d) b and c
   (e) a and b

4. Data reported in clinical trials suggest that which of the following dermal fillers produce results that last for the shortest duration of time?
   (a) Calcium hydroxylapatite
   (b) Poly-L-lactic acid
   (c) Bovine collagen
   (d) Porcine collagen
   (e) Nonanimal-stabilized hyaluronic acid

5. (True or False) IPL treatment following use of hyaluronic acid fillers for soft tissue augmentation increases the incidence of adverse events.

6. (True or False) Cross-linked dermal fillers have been shown to display greater longevity of treatment outcomes in comparison to noncross-linked dermal fillers.

## Answers

1. c: Bovine collagen
2. d: a and c
3. d: b and c
4. c: Bovine collagen
5. False
6. True

# Liposuction

# 21

## Shari A. Nemeth and Naomi Lawrence

## Introduction

Liposuction is the surgical removal of subcutaneous adipose tissue using aspiration cannulas introduced through small skin incisions. Tumescent liposuction refers to the technique of infiltrating the subcutaneous compartment with dilute concentrations of lidocaine and epinephrine as described by Klein [1]. By definition tumescent liposuction excludes the use of additional anesthetics that have a risk of suppressing the respiratory system. It is done completely under local anesthesia. Prior to development of the tumescent technique, excess adipose had been removed by a combination of en bloc resection with skin excision or curettage through small incisions. Today, liposuction may be performed in the outpatient setting under local tumescent anesthesia, which allows for the removal of large volumes of fat with minimal blood loss, low postoperative morbidity, and excellent cosmesis. It has been used to successfully treat undesired adipose tissue from nearly all body sites (Table 21.1), and it is also an effective treatment for noncosmetic adipose collections including lipomas, gynecomastia, and hyperhidrosis.

## Consensus Documents

### American Academy of Dermatology [2] (VI/C)

The American Academy of Dermatology (AAD) convened a task force in 2000 to provide guidelines for the safe performance of tumescent liposuction. Their recommendations were published in 2001 and are summarized in Table 21.2.

### American Society for Dermatologic Surgery [3] (VI/C)

The ASDS Guidelines of Care for Tumescent Liposuction were published in 2006. These guidelines are similar to the early ones established by the AAD with a few exceptions. The ASDS guidelines are listed in Table 21.3.

### Indian Association of Dermatologists, Venereologists, and Leprologists Dermatosurgery Task Force [4] (VI/C)

The Recommendations of the IADVL Dermatosurgery task force on tumescent liposuction mirror

S.A. Nemeth (✉)
Division of Dermatologic Surgery, Cooper University Hospital, 10000 Sagemore Drive, Suite 10103, Marlton, NJ 08053, USA

Department of Dermatology, Mayo Clinic Arizona, Scottsdale, AZ 85259, USA
e-mail: nemeth.shari@mayo.edu

N. Lawrence
Division of Dermatologic Surgery, Cooper University Hospital, 10000 Sagemore Drive, Suite 10103, Marlton, NJ 08053, USA

**Table 21.1** Regional consideration for liposuction

| Neck |
|---|
| Forward placed hyoid bone may limit ability to fully contour the anterior neck |
| Enlarged thyroid or submandibular glands may contribute to neck fullness |
| Micrognathia contributes to chin deformity and skin redundancy |
| Have patient contract platysma in a grimace to define the preplatysmal fat pad |

| Abdomen |
|---|
| Lateral hip-flexed (diver's) position helps delineate superficial fat from muscle and omental fat |

| Outer thigh |
|---|
| Determine the extent to which the buttocks weight contributes to the outer thigh deformity |
| Flexion of gluteal musculature defines the contribution of adipose in the buttocks to the protuberance of the outer thigh – if the outer thigh decreased on gluteal contraction the weight of the buttocks is significant |

those of the AAD and ASDS. They differ only in the maximum cannula size which they recommended be 3.5 mm and the maximum amount of fat to be removed in a single operative session which they recommend not exceed 5 L. They offer the additional recommendation of preoperative antibiotics starting 5 days before surgery. Differences in the recommendations of these three organizations are summarized in Table 21.4.

## Guidelines for Liposuction in Hyperhidrosis

In 2004, the Multi-Specialty Working Group on the Recognition, Diagnosis, and Treatment of Primary Focal Hyperhidrosis outlined recommendations for

**Table 21.2** Recommendations of AAD task force on tumescent liposuction 2001

| Physician qualification |
|---|
| Completed residency and board certification in a specialty recognized by the ABMS that provides education in liposuction and training in cutaneous surgery |
| Documented liposuction training in residency or experience at the surgical table under the supervision of a trained liposuction surgeon |
| In addition to surgical technique, training should include instruction on fluid and electrolyte balance, liposuction complications, tumescent anesthesia, and other forms of anesthesia employed |

| Facility |
|---|
| Liposuction can be safely performed in a physician's office surgical facility, ambulatory surgical facility, or hospital operating room |
| Liposuction surgeons and designated staff should have training in the management of acute cardiac emergencies |
| Hospital privileges should not be required; however, a written plan for management of medical emergencies, including possible transfer, should be in place |

| Preoperative evaluation |
|---|
| Liposuction is contraindicated in patients with severe cardiovascular disease, severe coagulation disorders, including thrombophilia, and during pregnancy |
| A thorough medical history including history of bleeding diatheses, emboli, thrombophlebitis, infectious diseases, poor wound healing, and diabetes mellitus. Patients with a history of these conditions should receive medical clearance. History should also include prior abdominal surgery and problems with past surgical procedures |
| All medications, vitamins, and herbs should be documented, noting medications that affect coagulation, or interact with lidocaine, epinephrine, or other sedatives or anesthetics used |
| Physical evaluation of patient's general physical health, and examination of specific sites under consideration for liposuction |
| Psychosocial evaluation of diet and exercise habits, history of weight change, familial body shape, patient's emotional ability to endure the procedure and their understanding of the limitations of liposuction, and whether they have reasonable expectations |
| Preoperative labs depend on type and extent of planned liposuction and conditions revealed in the history and physical |
| If indicated, complete blood count, platelet count, prothrombin time, partial thromboplastin time, chemistry profile, including liver function tests, and pregnancy tests in women of childbearing age |

(continued)

**Table 21.2**  (continued)

Type of anesthesia employed

Lidocaine is the preferred type of local anesthesia

Medications that inhibit lidocaine metabolism should be discontinued prior to liposuction or the total dosage of lidocaine should be reduced

The maximum dose of lidocaine should be 55 mg/kg, dependent on appropriate epinephrine concentration in the tumescent solution

The concentration of epinephrine in the tumescent solution is 0.25–1.5 mg/L. The total dosage should not exceed 50 µg/kg

If the maximum dose of lidocaine is exceeded, the surgeon should consider dividing the liposuction into separate procedures

Oral anxiolytics, sedatives, or narcotics at dosages that do not induce respiratory depression may be used

Intramuscular anxiolytics, sedatives, or narcotics may be used with caution, due to the risk of respiratory depression

Intravascular anxiolytics, sedatives, or narcotics should only be used in an accredited surgical facility or hospital operating room with appropriate monitoring by credentialed personnel

Inhalation (general) anesthesia is not recommended

Surgical technique/procedure

Performing liposuction in conjunction with other procedures should be done with caution unless all are done with the patient under local anesthesia and the recommended dose of tumescent lidocaine is not exceeded

Cannulae should be no larger than 4.5 mm in diameter

Volume of fat removed should generally not exceed 4,500 mL in a single operative session

The dry technique is contraindicated

Liposuction as treatment for obesity is considered experimental and not recommended

Intraoperative and postoperative monitoring

Baseline vital signs, blood pressure, and pulse should be recorded pre- and postoperatively

If removing >100 mL of aspirate, continues blood pressure, cardiac and pulse oximetry monitoring should be available along with supplemental oxygen

Sedated patients should have postoperative monitoring until fully recovered

A plan for medical emergencies should be in place

Postoperative compression

Use of compression garments, binders, and tape is recommended to reduce bruising, hematomas, seromas, and pain. Antiphlebitis hose may be useful for cases involving the lower leg

Duration of compression should be based on physician judgment, location of surgery, and rate of recovery

**Table 21.3**  ASDS guidelines for care of tumescent liposuction 2006

Safety

The maximum safe dose of tumescent lidocaine is 55 mg/kg

Education/training

Physicians performing liposuction should have completed residency training and be board-certified in a specialty that provides extensive training in cutaneous surgery

Physicians should have documentation of training in liposuction either as a resident or through certification through a liposuction training course, and documentation of experience at the surgical table under an experienced physician

The physician should also have an in-depth understanding of fluid and electrolyte balance, knowledge of tumescent anesthesia and its complications, and an understanding of the skin and subcutaneous tissues

Indications

Patients at or near ideal body weight who desire selective contouring of excess subcutaneous fat that are resistant to diet and exercise

Patients not at their ideal body weight may benefit from selective liposuction to improve overall body silhouette and ability to fit more comfortably into clothing

Tumescent liposuction is also safe and effective for treating lipomas, gynecomastia or pseudogynecomastia, lipodystrophy, and axillary hyperhidrosis and bromhidrosis

Mobilization of flaps and subcutaneous fat debulking during reconstruction and scar revision may also be facilitated by tumescent liposuction

(continued)

**Table 21.3**  (continued)

Preoperative evaluation

History and physical should focus on diet and exercise patterns, familial body shape, and specific regions the patient wants treated

Wound healing problems, bleeding diatheses, poor scarring, and past surgeries; infectious diseases including hepatitis and HIV should be documented

Family history that may signal coagulation disorders including thrombophlebitis, pulmonary embolism, and multiple miscarriages

Medications should be documented and drugs that affect the hemostasis or lidocaine metabolism should be noted

The procedure should be explained, including risks, benefits, reasonable expectations of results, and potential for additional procedures

The physical exam should evaluate the patient's general physical health as well as the sites amenable to liposuction, noting the distribution of muscle and fat as android or gynecoid

Close examination of the skin focusing on scars from previous surgeries or trauma, hernias, and varicosities. Skin quality, tone, and elasticity should be assessed in the areas of proposed treatment. Any asymmetry of body sites should be documented and pointed out to the patient. Specific areas have unique features to be examined (Table 21.3)

Laboratory studies

Surgeons performing a significant liposuction surgery may want to obtain complete blood count, platelet count, prothrombin time, partial thromboplastin time, chemistry profile including liver function tests, and urinalysis

Consider preoperative beta-HCG as well as urine pregnancy test on the day of the procedure for women of childbearing age

Order screening studies for HIV, hepatitis B and C based on local standards of care and physician preference

Tumescent anesthesia

Should be prepared on day of the procedure by trained personnel

Recommended maximum dose of lidocaine is 35–55 mg/kg. Concentration of lidocaine is recommended between 0.05 and 0.1% depending on the area to be infused

Epinephrine between 0.5 and 1.5 mg should be added per 1 L bag

Approximately 12.55 cc of sodium bicarbonate should be added to a 1 L bag

Triamcinolone 10 mg/1 L bag may also be added

Medications that inhibit the metabolism of lidocaine through the cytochrome P450 system should be discontinued 2 weeks before surgery. If the patient is unable to eliminate these medications, the total dose of lidocaine should be decreased

Tumescent liposuction: surgical technique and volume removal

Liposuction may be performed safely in the office setting or ambulatory surgical center

Oral anxiolytics may be used to alleviate patient concerns over having the procedure. IM or IV sedation is usually unnecessary when the area to be suctioned has been adequately tumesced

Maximum volume of supernatant fat removed per liposuction session should not exceed 4 L

Maximum cannula diameter should typically not exceed 4 mm

Monitoring

Baseline vital signs should always be recorded pre- and postoperatively

Intraoperative monitoring typically varies with local standards of care, but if patients are consciously sedated intraoperative monitoring should include pulse oximetry, continuous cardiac monitoring and intermittent blood pressure, and pulse and respiratory rate readings. Resuscitation equipment should be immediately available when using conscious sedation and the operative team should be certified in ACLS and supplemental oxygen should be available

Replacement fluids are not necessary with the tumescent technique as there is sufficient absorption through hypodermoclysis

Postoperative care

In the postoperative period patients should typically wear compression garments for 1–4 weeks to improve aesthetic results

Patients should remain ambulatory following tumescent liposuction and they should return to their usual exercise activities as comfort allows

**Table 21.4** Major variations in guidelines for tumescent liposuction

|  | AAD | ASDS | IADVL |
| --- | --- | --- | --- |
| Maximum volume per session (mL) | 4,500 | 4,000 | 5,000 |
| Maximum cannula size (mm) | 4.5 | 4 | 3.5 |
| Preoperative antibiotics | Not addressed | Not addressed | Should be given based on physician preference |

treatment of axillary hyperhidrosis [5] (V/B). "Failure to respond or intolerance to other treatments may be an indication for referral for a surgical procedure." This includes subcutaneous curettage (SEC) and tumescent liposuction.

In 2007 the Canadian Hyperhidrosis Advisory Committee developed recommendations for treatment of axillary hyperhidrosis based on the severity of the hyperhidrosis using the Hyperhidrosis Disease Severity Scale [6] (V/B). For patients with more mild hyperhidrosis, surgical intervention in the form of suction curettage (SC) or tumescent liposuction is recommended only if the patient does not respond to botulinum toxin A. Otherwise, the committee concluded that local surgery should only be considered in severe cases of hyperhidrosis in which the patient fails to respond to all other treatment options.

## Case Series and Cohort Studies

### Tumescent Anesthesia

Since Klein first introduced the concept of tumescent liposuction in 1987, several groups have looked at the metabolism and maximum concentration of lidocaine used in tumescent liposuction. In 1990, Klein [7] (V/B) established that a conservative guideline for the maximum lidocaine dose in tumescent anesthesia is 35–45 mg/kg. He also demonstrated that peak serum lidocaine levels are reached around 12 h postinfusion.

Ostad et al. [8] (IV/B) demonstrated that doses as high as 55 mg/kg are safe in their study of 60 patients who underwent liposuction. The mean dose of lidocaine used in these patients was 57 mg/kg. The patients were evaluated for signs of lidocaine toxicity over a 24-h period. Another ten patients had serial plasma lidocaine level measurements over a 24-h period following liposuction. The lidocaine level of the lipoaspirate was also measured. No evidence of lidocaine toxicity was found based on subjective evaluation of the 60 patients or as determined by the plasma sampling. The peak plasma lidocaine concentration occurred at approximately 4–8 h after infusion of tumescent anesthesia. A negligible amount of lidocaine was removed by liposuction as determined by the lidocaine level in the aspirate.

A Swedish group led by Nordstrom and Stange [9] (V/B) evaluated lidocaine plasma levels and objective and subjective symptoms of lidocaine toxicity during the 20 h following tumescent anesthesia with 35-mg/kg lidocaine for abdominal liposuction. They infiltrated 3 L of buffered 0.08% lidocaine with epinephrine over the abdomens of eight females. The patients did not receive any IV fluids. Plasma lidocaine levels were recorded. Subjective symptoms such as digital/circumoral paresthesias, facial fasciculations, numbness in nontreated areas, lightheadedness, tinnitus, and objective symptoms such as nystagmus, hypotension, arrhythmia, and unnatural drowsiness were recorded every 3 h for 20 h after the procedure by a nurse anesthetist. Peak plasma levels were 2.3 mg/mL and were reached between 5 and 17 h postinfusion. There was no correlation between peak levels of lidocaine and dose per kg body weight or total amount of lidocaine. Patients experienced no objective symptoms of fluid overload or lidocaine toxicity.

In 2005, Rubin et al. [10] (IV/B) compared serum lidocaine levels in eight healthy women who underwent tumescent anesthesia in the neck in one session and the thighs during a separate session at least 1 week apart. They demonstrated that peak serum lidocaine levels are reached sooner above the clavicles (5.8 h) than with infusion of equivalent tumescent anesthesia in the thighs (12.0 h).

## Conclusions

Tumescent anesthesia should not exceed a lidocaine dose of 55 mg/kg. The surgeon should anticipate that peak serum lidocaine levels will occur around 12 h postprocedure. In liposuction procedures above the clavicles, there may be a higher risk of toxic reactions when combined with other tumescent procedures, due to the more rapid absorption of lidocaine in this location.

## Female Breast Liposuction

Patients seek treatment for large breasts for several reasons including neck, shoulder, and back pain, intertrigo, postural issues, and difficulty purchasing clothing. In 1991, Matarasso and Courtiss introduced the use of liposuction alone for breast reduction [11] (V/B). They reported on nine patients and 14 breasts in which suction-assisted lipectomy was the only technique used to reduce breast volume. The amount of fat removed ranged from 75 to 475 g. Follow up ranged from 1 to 5 years and no evidence of fat reaccumulation, as indicated by breast enlargement, had occurred.

In 2001, Gray retrospectively evaluated 204 breast reductions by liposuction performed between 1996 and 1998 by a single surgeon [12] (V/B). The average aspirate per breast was 850 mL. He reported improvement in nipple ptosis and contraction of enlarged areolae. He did not report any cases of skin infection, but one patient developed a seroma and another a hematoma.

In 2004 Moskovitz et al. [13] (V/B) published an outcome study on breast liposuction. Seventy-eight patients who had undergone liposuction breast reduction over a 4-year period were surveyed. Eighty percent were very or completely satisfied with their outcomes, 87% said they would choose the procedure again, and 92% would recommend it to a friend. Patients reported alleviation or elimination of shoulder pain (93%), intertrigo (96%), shoulder ruts (88%), and reported better fitting clothes (91%), and improved posture (72%). The women reported returning to work an average of 5 days postoperatively and

resumed full activities at around 2 weeks. These results compare favorable to the outcomes seen with traditional mammoplasty.

Moskovitz et al. [14] (V/B) recruited 20 African American women to examine the effectiveness of liposuction breast reduction in this population. Patients completed a questionnaire both pre- and postoperatively, and objective measures of nipple/sternal and inframammary crease/nipple distances were recorded. Seventeen patients completed the study, and average follow up was 12 months. The average volume of lipoaspirate was 1,075 cc per breast. There were no major or minor complication and no patient suffered hypertrophic or keloidal scarring. Complaints of pain and other breast-related symptom all decreased significantly postoperatively. No statistically significant change in nipple sensation was reported. All patients obtained measurable elevation of the nipple/areola complex postoperatively with an average elevation of 4 cm.

In 2006, Mellul et al. [15] (V/B) published a series of 14 patients with breast hyperplasia treated with tumescent liposuction. The mean volume lost per breast after liposuction as measured by the dip test was 713 mL from the right breast and 696 mL from the left breast. At 6 months postprocedure nipple ptosis had improved, with an average elevation of the nipple/areola complex of 2.89 cm on the right and 2.25 cm on the left. There was no significant change in mammography images postprocedure. Thirteen patients (93%) were satisfied with the procedure and only one pursued further reduction.

## Conclusions

Breast reduction by liposuction is a safe and effective procedure for treatment of gigantomastia and related symptoms. Most patients note improvement in symptoms associated with large breasts, and the risk of developing worsened nipple ptosis as a result of the procedure has been soundly refuted. Furthermore, patients do not appear to develop any significant changes in their mammograms that would obscure detection of malignancy in the future.

## Axillary Hyperhidrosis and Bromhidrosis/Osmidrosis

Axillary hyperhidrosis results from excess secretion by eccrine glands. Axillary bromhidrosis or osmidrosis is the unpleasant odor that results when skin bacteria decompose apocrine sweat.

In 2005, Lee and Ryman [16] (V/B) published a case series of ten patients who underwent axillary tumescent liposuction for treatment of hyperhidrosis. Of the ten patients, four relapsed and required additional liposuction in the same area. Patients who relapsed did so between 4 and 15 months postprocedure. Six patients did not require further treatment with the longest reported remission being 7 years. Two patients reported bruising in the axillae, but no other major complications were reported.

Tsai and Lin [17] (IV/B) studies 20 female patients with osmidrosis, 10 were treated with simple tumescent liposuction and 10 were treated with tumescent liposuction combined with curettage. An average of 100–150 mL was aspirated per side. Among the ten patients treated with simple liposuction, 10% (1 patient) was satisfied, 70% (7 patients) were partially satisfied, and 20% (2 patients) were dissatisfied. Among the ten patients treated in combination, 80% (8 patients) were satisfied and 20% (2 patients) were partially satisfied. There were no major complications reported following either procedure except for mild bruising and swelling.

Darabaneanu et al. [18] (III/B) treated 56 axillae of 28 consecutive patients with axillary hyperhidrosis with subcutaneous sweat gland SC during a 20-month period. All patients had failed to respond to topical treatments. Follow-up examinations were performed on day 1, and 1, 3, 6, and 12 months postoperatively. Sweat rates were determined by gravimetry. A group of 17 healthy volunteers without a history of abnormal sweating served as controls. Controls had an average sweat rate of 7 mg/min under resting conditions and 7.9 mg/min under exercise conditions. The patients with axillary hyperhidrosis had a preoperative sweat rate of 48.3 mg/min at rest and 152.7 mg/min under exercise conditions. Patients were subdivided into groups based on their preoperative sweating rates. Group A were those with resting sweat rates less than 25 mg/min, Group B were those with a rate between 25 and 50 mg/min, and Group C were those with rates greater than 50 mg/min. After surgical intervention, sweat rates during rest decreased an average of 58% after 1 year, and decreased an average of 87% during exercise after 1 year. However, the degree of postoperative sweat reduction was dependent upon the preoperative baseline rates. The results in patients in Group A, with relatively low sweat rates preoperatively, were not significantly different between baseline and 12 months. By contrast, patients in Groups B and C had statistically significant decreases at 12 months. Patient satisfaction was highest in patients with the best clinical results. The complications included bruising, which resolved in all cases. Four patients developed wound infections which all resolved with treatment. One patient developed hypertrophic scarring that required excision and skin grafting.

Perng et al. [19] (V/B) retrospectively reviewed 134 patients who underwent superficial liposuction and curettage for axillary osmidrosis. The overall complication rate was 3.73%, which included hematoma, local infection, and partial skin necrosis. This rate is lower than the 11% complication rate of open surgical treatment with excision of skin and soft tissue. Eighty percent of the patients were satisfied with their results after liposuction-curettage; however, the number of patients with a poor outcome was higher with liposuction-curettage (19%) than with en bloc excision (9%).

In the study by Lee et al. [20] (V/B), 25 patients with axillary osmidrosis or hyperhidrosis were treated with tumescent liposuction and curettage. Results were assessed by the patients and their family or close friends. Of the 50 axillae treated, 49 (98%) reported good to excellent results. Axillary sweating decreased in 42 axillae. No patients reported excessive scarring from the procedure and no serious complications were reported, but two patients developed wound infections. Overall, 62% reported being very satisfied and 36% were satisfied with the results. Histologic examination of the curette specimens showed large and numerous apocrine glands. Biopsies done postoperatively at 2 weeks showed decreased number and degeneration of apocrine glands.

In a study by Seo et al. [21] (V/B), 43 patients underwent tumescent liposuction with curettage for treatment of axillary bromhidrosis. The follow-up period averaged 15.8 months. Thirty-one (72.1%) patients showed excellent to good results based on patient and medical staff evaluation. Transient ecchymosis was the most common postoperative complication, followed by focal skin necrosis, induration, and hematoma/seroma which were noted in 4, 3, and 1 patient, respectively. No local infections, permanent contractures, or nerve damage occurred. Postoperative, histologic evaluation of axillary skin showed decreased apocrine and eccrine glands as compared to preoperative specimens.

Bechara et al. [22] (IV/B) compared efficacy of different surgical cannulas used in liposuction-curettage for treatment of axillary hyperhidrosis. Sweat rates were measured by gravimetry before and 6 months after surgery in 42 patients who had failed conservative therapy. Fourteen patients were operated on with a 1-hole liposuction cannula with flattened tip, 14 patients with a larger 3-hole liposuction cannula with rounded tip, and 14 with a sharp SC cannula with flattened, rostriform tip with three sharpened openings with sharp rasps in between. At 6 months, sweat rates decreased 44% in the 1-hole group, 49% in the 3-hole cannula group, and 63% in the sharp cannula group. The sharp cannula group had a statistically significant decrease in sweating when compared to the other groups. All three groups experienced complications including hematoma, superficial skin erosion, bridle formation, paresthesia, and partial alopecia. These were all more common in the sharp cannula group. There was no significant difference in pain or patient satisfaction across the three groups.

In 2007, Bechara et al. [23] (V/B) investigated the efficacy and side-effects of a second liposuction-curettage procedure with an aggressive rasping cannula in 19 patients with an insufficient response to prior surgery. Gravimetry was performed before and 8 months after surgery. Sweat

rates reduced an average of 69% in 17 (89%) of patients, and two patients did not respond. Eighty-four percent of patients were completely satisfied or satisfied with the results. The most common side effect was bruising, followed by superficial skin erosion (6 subjects), paraesthesia (4 subjects), and seroma (2 subjects). Bridle formation was present up to 14 weeks in 6 subjects, but had resolved in all affected patients by 8 months. The surgeons did report slightly increased difficulty during dissection of the dermis from the subcutaneous fat in three patients.

Bechara et al. [24] (V/B) intended to enroll 20 patients in a study comparing efficacy of liposuction-curettage to liposuction-curettage with subsequent manual shaving for hyperhidrosis. They aborted the study after four patients due to complications. All four developed moderate to severe hematoma and one showed flap necrosis on the combined treatment side, but only slight bruising was noted on the liposuction-curettage side with one patient developing a superficial erosion. Although the complication rate was higher on the combined side, at 15 weeks no significant differences were found in sweat reduction as measured by gravimetry in the eight axilla of these four patients.

## Conclusions

Tumescent liposuction with curettage is an effective treatment for patients with hyperhidrosis or osmidrosis refractory to standard medical therapy. In order to assess the treatment efficacy, pre- and postoperative gravimetry studies should be considered. Patients with higher sweat rates respond better to liposuction-curettage than those with normal to slightly elevated sweat rates.

Patients undergoing liposuction-curettage with a rasping cannula have a higher rate of side effects, such as hematoma and erosion, due to the more aggressive nature of the procedure vs. conventional liposuction with blunt-tipped cannula. Most patients will experience some postoperative bruising in the area suctioned. Patients should be counseled on the additional risks of infection, skin necrosis, seroma/hematoma, and hypertrophic scarring. In patients who do not attain their desired level of improvement, it is safe to perform the procedure a second time, which often provides the desired results.

## Other Uses for Liposuction

Tumescent liposuction has been described as an alternative to surgical excision of large, diffuse lipomas. Choi et al. [25] (V/B) reported a series of 21 patients presenting with 31 lipomas ranging in size from 1.2 to 11 cm that were treated with tumescent liposuction followed by extraction of the fibrous capsule with blunt dissection and a hemostat. Twenty-three lipomas were removed successfully, but in three cases fatty tissue remained. Hematoma and skin dimpling were noted in three cases but these resolved. In 12 patients no recurrence was found after 2 years, but the remaining patients were lost to follow up.

Babovic et al. [26] (V/B) reported two cases of patients with neurofibromatosis type 1 with plexiform neurofibromas successfully debulked with liposuction. Postoperative follow up at 6 months showed no evidence of tumor regrowth in either case.

## Diet and Exercise

It is well documented that obesity is a risk factor for cardiovascular disease and type II diabetes mellitus. It has been hypothesized that removal of subcutaneous fat with liposuction may decrease a patient's risk of these conditions by decreasing their overall adiposity. Robles-Cervantes et al. [27] (V/B) measured the preoperative glucose, insulin, and cholesterol levels of 15 healthy, non-obese women who underwent liposuction. They repeated these labs 3 weeks postoperatively. Serum glucose and cholesterol decreased significantly. Estimated insulin secretion increased without significant change in insulin sensitivity. Patients did not have a statistically significant weight change.

Giugliano et al. [28] (IV/B) studied 30 healthy premenopausal obese women who underwent liposuction and compared them to 30 healthy age-matched normal-weight controls. The control group had lower fasting glucose and insulin concentrations and lower levels of inflammatory markers and higher levels of adiponectin. The average lipoaspirate volume was 3,540 mL. Six months after liposuction, the obese women were less insulin resistant, had reduced concentrations of inflammatory markers, and increased serum levels of adiponectin and HDL. They did not compare postprocedure values to the control group.

Klein et al. [29] (V/B) evaluated 15 obese women before and 10–12 weeks after abdominal liposuction. They did not note any significant change in insulin sensitivity, inflammatory markers, adiponectin or improvement in other risk factors of coronary heart disease including blood pressure, plasma glucose, insulin, or lipid concentrations.

## Conclusions

Although, follow up in all of these studies did not exceed 6 months, in the early postoperative period liposuction does not appear to be detrimental to the patient's metabolic health, and they may even experience some health benefits. Liposuction is still not recommended as a treatment for obesity or obesity-related metabolic conditions.

## Side Effects

Yun et al. [30] (V/B) retrospectively reviewed 73 liposuction cases and 34% of these patients reported subjective breast enlargement. Frew et al. [31] (V/B) interviewed 70 women 6–28 months after having tumescent liposuction to determine incidence of breast enlargement postliposuction. Thirty-seven percent (26 of 70) reported an increase in breast size after liposuction.

In a retrospective review of 44 patients who had undergone traditional tumescent liposuction, Finzi [32] (V/B) reported breast enlargement in 43% of patients (19 of 44) vs. only one patient reporting breast enlargement out of 27 women who had other cosmetic procedures. Seventy-four percent (14 of 19) of these patients had liposuction of the abdomen or abdomen and flanks. There was also a positive correlation between the increase in breast size and the total amount of supranatant fat removed. Those with breast enlargement weighed more preprocedure, and had more total fat removed; however, these patients did not gain weight after the procedure.

## Conclusions

Patients undergoing tumescent liposuction should be counseled on the potential for breast enlargement after the procedure, and that this may occur in the absence of significant weight gain postprocedure. Whether liposuction of specific body sites is associated with an increased likelihood of postoperative breast enlargement requires further study.

## Patient Expectations/Complications/Safety

Broughton et al. surveyed 209 patients who had undergone liposuction during a 5-year period [33] (V/B). The majority of patients (80%) were satisfied with their results. Fifty-three percent thought that their appearance was either excellent or very good. Weight gain was reported in 43% of the respondents. Among those patients who gained weight, 73% were either very satisfied or satisfied, compared with 82% of responders who did not gain weight.

Butterwick studied the number of touch-up procedures done in a large liposuction practice [34] (V/B). She found that over a 2-year period 12.3% of 954 liposuction procedures had a touch-up procedure. Men and women had an equal number of touch-up procedures. The most common areas for touch-up were the neck and abdomen. These were also the most commonly treated sites. The weight pattern after liposuction may play a role as 47% of these patients had increased weight.

In 1988, Bernstein and Hanke [35] (V/B) surveyed 55 dermatologists who had performed 9,478 liposuction cases. The risk of systemic complications was 0.07%. Five patients had excessive intraoperative or postoperative bleeding, and two patients developed infections. There were no reports of death. The rate of local complications was also low with contour irregularities (2.1%), hematoma (0.47%), and persistent edema (0.46%) being the most common. In 1996, Hanke surveyed ASDS fellows and evaluated data on 15,336 patients who had liposuction [36] (V/B). There were no serious complications reported. In 1999, Coleman et al. reviewed malpractice data between 1995 and 1997 from the National Database of the Physicians Insurance Association of America [37] (V/B). They found that the rate of hospital-based malpractice settlements was three times that of office-based liposuction. Less than 1% of defendants were dermatologists even though 33% of liposuction cases in the United States are performed by dermatologic surgeons.

In 2002, Houseman et al. [38] (V/B) reported the results of a survey of ASDS members on the liposuction cases they performed between 1994 and 2000. The overall response rate was 89% (450/505). Of the respondents 78% perform liposuction. The data encompassed 267 surgeons, and 261 provided data on 66,570 liposuction procedures. No deaths were reported. The overall serious adverse event (SAE) rate was 0.68/1,000 and this rate was higher for hospitals and ambulatory surgery centers than for nonaccredited office settings. SAE rates were also higher for tumescent liposuction combined with intravenous or intramuscular sedation than when combined with oral or no sedation.

Power liposuction complications were compared to those of traditional and tumescent liposuction by Katz et al. [39] (V/B). They showed an overall complication rate of power liposuction of 1.4% and fewer complications than traditional liposuction with general anesthesia and no significant difference between power liposuction and tumescent liposuction.

In 2004, Hanke et al. [40] (V/B) used self-reported data collected by the AAAHC Institute for Quality Improvement from 39 study centers and 688 patients who had tumescent liposuction. The overall clinical complication rate was 0.7% (5 of 702). There was a minor complication rate of 0.57%. The major complication rate was 0.14% with one patient requiring hospitalization. Seventy-five percent of the patients reported no discomfort during their procedures. Fifty-nine percent of patients responded to a survey 6 months after their procedure and 91% were positive about their decision to have the procedure and 85% had a high level of satisfaction with the procedure.

Perhaps, some of the most convincing evidence on the safety of tumescent liposuction has come from Coldiron's review of the Florida adverse event data [41]. (V/B) In 2000, the Florida Agency for Health Care Administration (AHCA) made reporting of adverse events occurring after office procedures mandatory. Although underreporting is a potential problem with this system, AHCA crosschecks these reports with malpractice claims and spontaneous complaints. In 7 years, there were 174 reported events occurring in association with office surgical procedures, 31 resulted in death, and 143 in reportable complications and hospital transfers. Eighteen deaths were associated with a cosmetic procedure. Eight of the deaths occurred after liposuction performed by a plastic surgeon, which was the single most common cause of death. Of these 7 were performed under general anesthesia and deaths were attributed to pulmonary emboli in 4 and unknown causes in 3 cases. One death occurred after liposuction with IV sedation. All deaths occurred several hours to 9 days after liposuction. Of the surgical deaths, 22.6% were associated with liposuction under general anesthesia and 13.6% of the adverse incidents requiring hospital transfer were associated with liposuction under general anesthesia. There were no liposuction deaths or injuries associated with tumescent anesthesia. Of the 143 surgical procedures that resulted in a reportable incident, 60.8% were in association with a cosmetic procedure. Eighty-six percent of these cosmetic procedures occurred with the use of general anesthesia. Twenty incidents associated with liposuction were reported by plastic surgeons, 1 by a facial plastic surgeon, 1 by a dermatologist, and 2 by a physician who was not board certified.

Klein and Kaassarjdian [42] (V/B) reported a case of lidocaine toxicity in a patient that was attributed to coadministration of medications. A 39-year-old woman underwent liposuction of the inner thighs, inner knees, and buttocks. She received 58 mg/kg of tumescent lidocaine. She was concurrently taking sertraline and was given fluazepam preoperatively. She presented 10 h after the procedure with symptoms of lidocaine toxicity and a blood lidocaine level of 6.1 mg/mL (6 mg/mL is associated with increased risk of toxicity). Medications that inhibit lidocaine metabolism by the cytochrome P450 3A4 pathway are listed in Table 21.5.

Martinex et al. [43] reported the death of a 38-year-old woman who had tumescent liposuction of her abdomen, hips, and thighs. Thirty minutes after administration of anesthesia, which included lidocaine and mepivacaine, the patient seized and then went into cardiopulmonary arrest. Attempts to revive here were unsuccessful. Postmortem studies demonstrated that she had a serum concentration of 4.9 mg/mL of lidocaine, and toxic 16.2 mg/mL of mepivacaine. The cause of death was ruled an overdose of local anesthetic agents.

In 1998, the department of surgery at Madigan Army medical center reported a case of necrotizing fasciitis after tumescent liposuction [44] (V/B). A previously healthly, 31-year-old female presented 4 days after tumescent liposuction of her thoracic roll, flanks, hips, abdomen, medial thighs, and knees with weakness, fevers, and a red, painful nodule on her left flank. Total fat removed during the procedure was 2,551 mL. She was a cigarette smoker. She had been treated with cephalexin postoperatively. The patient ultimately recovered after multiple surgical debridements and staged full thickness skin grafts.

In 1997 Gilliland and Coates [45] (V/B) reported a case of pulmonary edema in a healthy 55-year-old male who received 7,900 mL of subcutaneous and 2,200 mL of intravenous fluid. He was placed under general anesthesia, and 3,900 mL was aspirated from the abdomen and flanks.

**Table 21.5** Drug interactions with lidocaine

| Alprazolam | Clarithromycin | Erythromycin | Lovastatin | Paroxetine | Tacrine |
|---|---|---|---|---|---|
| Amiodarone | Clomipramine | Felodipine | Mexiletine | Phenytoin | Tamoxifen |
| Amiodarone | Cyclosporine | Fluconazole | Miconazole | Propofol | Triazolam |
| Amitriptyline | Danazol | Fluoxetine | Midazolam | Propranolol | Valproic acid |
| Atazanavir | Diazepam | Flurazepam | Nefazodone | Quinidine | Verapamil |
| Atorvastatin | Diethyldithiocarbamate | Fluvoxamine | Nelfinavir | Quinupristin | Zileuton |
| Carbamazepine | Diltiazem | Grapefruit | Nevirapine | Ritonavir | |
| Cervivastatin | disopyramide | Indinavir | Nicardipine | Saquinavir | |
| Cimetidine | Divalproex | Itraconazole | Nifedipine | Sertraline | |
| Ciprofloxacin | Enoxacin | Ketoconazole | Norfloxacin | Simvastatin | |

Adapted from Heuther and Brodland [51] and http://www.Liposuction.com

Twenty minutes postoperatively, the patient developed shortness of breath and decreased oxygen saturation, and physical exam was consistent with pulmonary edema. The patient was transferred to the intensive care unit and treated with IV diuretics. He recovered without sequelae.

In 2002, Jacob and Weisenborn [46] (V/B) reported the results of a prospective study that examined the relationship between volumes of adipose extracted, volume of tumescent anesthesia, or lidocaine dosages used in liposuction and the early onset of menses postoperatively. Twenty-three surgeries were performed on 17 premenopausal patients by one dermatologic surgeon. Patient ages ranged from 27 to 47. Four patients were on oral contraceptives and two were menstruating at the time of surgery. Four patients, ages 38–46, experienced early onset of menses. The areas treated in these patients were the upper abdomen and waist, upper abdomen and flanks, and two patients had the upper and lower abdomen treated. There was no correlation between volumes of anesthesia, amounts of lidocaine or volumes of adipose removed, and early onset of menses. Two of the four patients had a second liposuction procedure on the flanks/waist and flanks/hips but not the anterior abdomen and did not have menstrual disturbances. The authors did not comment on when in their menstrual cycle the patients who did and did not experience early onset of menses were. It would also be valuable to know how the ovulatory cycle of these patients were affected, as this could have implications in the patients' postliposuction contraceptive choices.

Andrews et al. [47] (V/B) reported a case of herpes zoster following liposuction in a 58-year-old woman who had bilateral back- and mid-flank liposuction with a combination of ultrasonic and traditional tumescent liposuction. A total of 1,400 mL was aspirated. Eight days postoperatively, she presented with burning pain of the left flank and on exam had a vesicular eruption in that area. She was treated with oral acyclovir and analgesics and the remainder of her postoperative course was uncomplicated.

## Conclusions

Tumescent liposuction when performed by trained dermatologic surgeons has a very low complication rate. Major complications are typically associated with aggressive liposuction, large volume procedures, general anesthesia, or IV sedation. Liposuction under general anesthesia has a higher than acceptable complication rate and should be abandoned in practice.

## Randomized Controlled Trials and Meta-Analyses

Chilean surgeons, Prado et al. [48] (II/A), published a prospective, randomized, double-blind controlled clinical trial comparing laser-assisted lipoplasty with suction-assisted lipoplasty. Between July 2004 and February 2005, 25 patients with localized lipodystrophy and body mass index (BMI) in the normal range (20–20 kg/m$^2$) were randomly assigned to have suction-assisted lipoplasty and laser-assisted lipoplasty on the left and right body halves in one or more comparable body areas. All procedures were performed by the same surgeon with local anesthesia in an outpatient facility. Laser-assisted lipoplasty was done with the SmartLipo laser. The patients were tumesced and then a 2-mm optical fiber was introduced through the skin puncture sites. After each zone was treated with 500 J, the adipose was aspirated through a multifenestrated 3-mm cannula until the volume was equal to the infiltration volume. The same tumescent infiltration and suction ratio was used on the suction-assisted lipoplasty side. The sides were compared with preoperative photos on postoperative days 3–5, 12–15, and 6–11 months. All 25 female patients completed the postoperative visits and their results were sent to two blinded plastic surgeons for evaluation.

The cosmetic results were graded on the Strasser scale measuring malposition, distortion, asymmetry, contour deformity, and scar. Postoperative pain was evaluated at 24 h and 3–5 days postoperatively, and was assessed by the senior surgeon. Recovery time was measured in days and recovery was defined as the day after which the patient was able to work with no pain. They assessed BMI preoperatively and at the last follow up visit. Surgical operative time was measured for each side separately. The infranatant specimens were evaluated histologically by a blinded pathologist to determine the level of disruption of the fatty aspirate reflecting the level of damage to the tissue.

There were no differences on the Strasser scale for the evaluation of cosmetic results and the scores did not change significantly at subsequent follow-up visits. Ecchymosis, edema, and retraction did not differ between the groups or between the first and second postoperative visits. Overall, there was less postoperative pain in the laser-assisted lipoplasty side when compared to the suction-assisted side. Recovery after the surgery was $16.6 \pm 4$ days; there was no comparison between modalities as patients had both interventions. There was no difference in the pre- and postoperative BMI of patients. Surgical time was longer on the laser-assisted vs. the suction-assisted side (60 vs. 45 min median). Lipocrits were lower on the laser-assisted side.

Issues with this study include the small patient number. They did not do standardized measurements of the treated body sites before and after liposuction. Since patients had both interventions, no comment could be made on the difference in recovery time between the two modalities. There were no significant complications in this study, although the sample size was small. The authors did not comment or provide data on whether different sites responded better to one method or the other. It is possible that one modality may be more efficacious in a given anatomic location because of differences in adipose density, fibrous tissue, vascularity, etc.

For a new technology to compete with or supplant an existing safe and effective modality, it must be at least equal to or superior to current techniques. In this study, laser-assisted lipoplasty required the use of an expensive laser, longer operating times, disposable fiber optics, and after the laser was applied suction was still required. This study failed to demonstrate clinical advantages of laser-assisted lipoplasty. The only statistically significant difference was less pain on the laser-assisted side, but there was not a clear explanation for this. As technology evolves, this may become a cost-effective alternative to suction-assisted liposuction but it has not done so thus far.

A Taiwanese group led by Yang et al. [49] (II/A) randomized 36 patients with axillary osmidrosis into three groups to evaluate if the temperature and pH of tumescent anesthesia affected the perceived pain during infiltration. Group A received warm neutral (40°C) and room temperature neutral (22°C) tumescent anesthesia to either axilla. Group B received warm neutral (pH 7.35, 40°C) and warm non-neutral (nonbuffered) (pH 4.78) tumescent anesthesia. Group C received warm non-neutral and room temperature non-neutral tumescent injections. Pain associated with the infiltration of anesthesia was rated on a visual analog scale. An average of 150 mL of anesthesia was used per axilla. The non-neutral solution consisted of 0.1% lidocaine, 1:1,000,000 epinephrine in normal saline at pH 4.78. Neutral tumescent anesthesia was 0.1% lidocaine, with 1:1,000,000 epinephrine and 10 mEq of sodium bicarbonate in 1 L of normal saline at pH 7.35. Immediately after injection of the axillary region, each patient quantified the degree of pain induced by the infiltration. In Group A, there was significantly less pain on the side injected with warm neutral solution vs. the room temperature neutral solution. In Group B, the patients reported less pain on the side injected with warm neutral solution than warm non-neutral solution. In group C, there was significantly more pain on the side injected with room temperature non-neutral solution vs. the warm non-neutral solution.

The authors of this study confirmed what several others have reported that warm tumescent anesthesia is less painful. Buffering tumescent anesthesia is already a standard practice by many liposuction surgeons as a way to decrease discomfort of the infusion. The authors did not evaluate how warming the tumescent fluid may accelerate break down of epinephrine. This is a known effect of buffering with sodium bicarbonate as epinephrine concentrations decrease by about 25% in 1 week. Therefore, it is recommended that tumescent anesthesia be prepared on the day of the procedure. This was a small study and the authors did not comment on the demographic characteristics of the three groups and if there was any significant differences between them. It would have been useful if the authors had attempted to quantify the difference in pain between the groups. From this study, it seems reasonable to buffer and warm tumescent anesthesia prior to infusion.

Wollina et al. [50] (II/A) looked at 163 patients with focal axillary hyperhidrosis as assessed by Minors starch iodide test and compared minor skin resection with SEC to SC. Patients ranged in age from 16 to 61, and there were 33 men and 129 women. One hundred and twenty-five patients were treated with SEC and 37 patients were treated with LC. Outcome was measured by patients' global assessment and Minors starch iodide test.

In SEC, the rate of residual sweating was 12% and relapse rate was 1% of patients. In LC the relapse rate was 16.2% of patients within 12 months. Patients who had LC had significantly less pain, no scarring, wound infections, bleeding, or delayed healing. The SEC group had an average hospital stay of 5.8 days and the mean time to return to work as 8.8 days. For LC the procedure was done on an outpatient basis, and return to work was 1.3 days. Total satisfaction rate was 97% in the SEC group and 89.2% in the LC group. Although SEC is somewhat more effective in permanent reduction of hyperhidrosis, LC is less invasive, has less scarring, and less downtime. In the SEC group, one axilla was operated on first then the other side was done a minimum of 4 weeks later, which required a second hospital stay and recovery period. In the LC group, three patients had an en bloc resection previously. The first patient's procedure had failed and the other two patients' primary surgery was effective but they were unhappy with their scars and pain after resection. Twenty-seven patients had both axilla treated on the same day with LC and 5 had them done on different days and in 5 only one side was done. Follow up was at 1–58 months for SEC and 51 months for LC.

In this study, SEC was more effective but had a higher complication rate than LC. It is possible that the higher patient satisfaction with SEC was due in part to the fact that SEC was covered by insurance and patients who had LC had to pay for it. An objective measure of sweat rate, such as gravimetry, could have been used to more accurately assess clinical improvement in both patient groups. Although SEC was more effective, there was significantly less downtime and scarring in the LC group favoring it as the surgical treatment of choice for focal axillary hyperhidrosis.

## Conclusions

Tumescent liposuction is a safe and effective treatment for removing undesired adipose tissue from nearly all body sites with minimal blood loss, low postoperative morbidity, and excellent cosmesis. It is also an effective treatment for non-cosmetic adipose collections including lipomas, gynecomastia, and hyperhidrosis.

The recommendations for tumescent liposuction presented in this chapter are summarized in the Evidence-Based Summary at the end of this chapter. There are few randomized controlled clinical trials on liposuction parameters. Given this paucity of strong evidence-based data, recommendations on the practice of liposuction will continue to be based on consensus opinions of expert practitioners and cohort data.

## Evidence-Based Summary

| Findings | Evidence level |
|---|---|
| Physicians performing liposuction should have appropriate training and board certification as outlined by the AAD and ASDS | (IV/C) |
| Liposuction should be used for contouring and improvement in body silhouette. It is not a treatment for obesity or obesity-related conditions | (VI/C) |
| Extensive preoperative history and physical examinations should be performed with special attention to chronic medical conditions and previous surgeries, particularly in the area to be suctioned | (VI/C) |
| Psychosocial status of the patient should be assessed. Patient expectations for what liposuction can accomplish for them should be established in the initial preoperative assessment. Physicians should discuss the potential side effects and complications with the patient and obtain informed consent | (VI/C) |
| Liposuction can be performed safely in an outpatient office surgical suite, ambulatory surgical center, or hospital operating room | (V/B) |
| All personnel involved in liposuction should be trained in management of acute cardiac emergencies (e.g., ACLS), and a plan for hospital transfer should be in place | (IV/C) |
| Tumescent anesthesia with no sedation or oral sedation is the recommended anesthesia in liposuction. Use of IM or IV anesthesia is discouraged because of the increased risk of complication and should only be used in monitored settings by trained personnel. Liposuction should not be performed under general anesthesia | (V/B) |
| Maximum dosage of lidocaine in tumescent anesthesia should not exceed 55 mg/kg | (IV/B) |
| Medications that affect the metabolism of lidocaine should be discontinued 2 weeks prior to liposuction, and if the medication cannot be stopped the total dose of lidocaine should be decreased | (V/B) |
| Preoperative labs should be ordered according to local surgical culture, but at a minimum should include complete blood count, platelet count, prothrombin time, partial thromboplastin time, and chemistry profile including liver tests. Premenopausal women should have a urine pregnancy test on the day of the procedure | (VI/C) |
| Pre- and postoperative vital signs should be recorded, and in larger volume procedures the ability for continuous cardiac and pulse oximetry monitoring should be available | (VI/C) |
| Maximum cannula size should range between 3.5 and 4.5 mm | (VI/C) |
| Maximum volume aspirated per session should not exceed 4,000–5,000 mL | (VI/C) |
| Postoperative compression garments should be worn for a period of time determined by the physician based on location and extent of liposuction | (VI/C) |
| Use of perioperative antibiotics should be based on physician judgment on a case by case basis | (VI/C) |
| Patients should remain ambulatory following the procedure and return to their normal physical activities as comfort allows | (VI/C) |
| Liposuction-curettage is safe and effective for hyperhidrosis and osmidrosis in patients who failed conservative medical therapy | (II/A) |
| Liposuction is an effective treatment for gigantomastia, and does not result in worsened nipple ptosis | (V/B) |

# References

1. Klein JA. The tumescent technique for liposuction surgery. Am J Cosmet Surg. 1987;4:263–7.
2. Coleman WP, Glogau RG, Klein JA, Moy RL, Narins RS, Chuang T, et al. Guidelines for care of liposuction. J Am Acad Dermatol. 2001;45:438–47.
3. Coldiron B, Coleman WP, Cox SE, Jacob C, Lawrence N, Kaminer M, et al. ASDS guidelines of care for tumescent liposuction. Dermatol Surg. 2006;32: 709–16.
4. Mysore V et al. Tumescent liposuction: standard guidelines of care. Indian J Dermatol Venereol Leprol. 2008;74:S54–60.
5. Hornberger J, Grimes K, Naumann M, et al. Recognition, diagnosis, and treatment of primary focal hyperhidrosis. J Am Acad Dermatol. 2004;51: 274–86.
6. Solish N, Bertucci V, Dansereau A, et al. A comprehensive approach to the recognition, diagnosis, and severity-based treatment of focal hyperhidrosis: recommendations of the Canadian hyperhidrosis advisory committee. Dermatol Surg. 2007;33: 908–23.
7. Klein JA. Tumescent technique for regional anesthesia permits lidocaine doses of 35–45mg/kg for liposuction. Peak plasma are diminished and delayed 12 hours. J Dermatol Surg Oncol. 1990;16:248–63.
8. Ostad A, Kageyama N, Moy RL. Tumescent anesthesia with a lidocaine dose of 55mg/kg is safe for liposuction. Dermatol Surg. 1996;22:921–7.
9. Nordstrom H, Stange K. Plasma lidocaine levels and risks after liposuction with tumescent anaesthesia. Acta Anaesthesiol Scand. 2005;49:1487–90.
10. Rubin JP, Xie Z, Davidson C, Rosow CD, Chang Y, May JW. Rapid absorption of tumescent lidocaine above the clavicles: a prospective clinical study. Plast Reconstr Surg. 2005;115:1744–51.
11. Matarasso A, Courtiss EH. Suction mammoplasty: the use of suction lipectomy to reduce large breasts. Plast Reconstr Surg. 1991;87:709–17.
12. Gray LN. Update on experience with liposuction breast reduction. Plast Reconstr Surg. 2001;108(4): 1006–10.
13. Moskovitz MJ, Muskin E, Baxt SA. Outcome study in liposuction breast reduction. Plast Reconstr Surg. 2004;114(1):55–60.
14. Moskovitz MJ, Baxt SA, Jain AK, Hausman RE. Liposuction breast reduction: a prospective trial in African American women. Plast Reconstr Surg. 2007;119:718–26.
15. Mellul SD, Dryden RM, Remigio DJ, Wulc AE. Breast reduction performed by liposuction. Dermatol Surg. 2006;32:1124–33.
16. Lee MR, Ryman WJ. Liposuction for axillary hyperhidrosis. Australas J Dermatol. 2005;46(2):76–9.
17. Tsai RY, Lin JY. Experience of tumescent liposuction in the treatment of osmidrosis. Dermatol Surg. 2001;27:446–8.
18. Darabaneanu S, Darabaneanu HA, Niederberger U, Russo PA, Lischner S, Hauschild A. Longterm effectiveness of subcutaneous sweat gland suction curettage for axillary hyperhidrosis: a prospective gravimetrically controlled study. Dermatol Surg. 2008;34:1170–7.
19. Perng CK, Yeh FL, Ma H, et al. Is the treatment of axillary osmidrosis with liposuction better than with open surgery? Plast Reconstr Surg. 2004;114:93.
20. Lee D, Cho SH, Kim YC, Park JH, Lee SS, Park SW. Tumescent liposuction with dermal curettage for treatment of axillary osmidrosis and hyperhidrosis. Dermatol Surg. 2006;32:505–11.
21. Seo SH, Jang BS, Oh CK, Kwon KS, Kim MB. Tumescent superficial liposuction with curettage for treatment of axillary bromhidrosis. J Eur Acad Dermatol Venereol. 2008;22(1):30–5.
22. Bechara FG, Sand M, Sand D, Altmeyer P, Hoffmann K. Surgical treatment of axillary hyperhidrosis. A study comparing liposuction cannulas with a suction-curettage cannula. Ann Plast Surg. 2006;56: 654–7.
23. Bechara FG, Sand M, Tomi NS, Altmeyer P, Hoffmann K. Repeat liposuction curettage treatment of axillary hyperhidrosis is safe and effective. Br J Dermatol. 2007;157:739–43.
24. Bechara FG, Sand M, Hoffmann K, Altmeyer P. Aggressive shaving after combined liposuction curettage for axillary hyperhidrosis leads to more complications without further benefit. Dermatol Surg. 2008;34:952–3.
25. Choi CW, Kim J, Moon SE, Youn SW, Park KC, Huh CH. Treatment of lipomas assisted with tumescent liposuction. J Eur Acad Dermatol Venereol. 2007;21: 243–6.
26. Babovic S, Bite U, Karnes PS, Babovic-Vuksanovic D. Liposuction: a less invasive surgical method of debulking plexiform neurofibromas. Dermatol Surg. 2003;29:785–7.
27. Robles-Cervantes JA, Yanez-Diaz S, Cardenas-Camarena L. Modification of insulin, glucose and cholesterol levels in nonobese women undergoing liposuction – is liposuction metabolically safe? Ann Plast Surg. 2004;52(1):64–7.
28. Giugliano G, Nicoletti G, Grella E, Giugliano F, Esposito K, Scuderi N, et al. Effect of liposuction on insulin resistance and vascular inflammatory markers in obese women. Br J Plast Surg. 2004;57:190–4.
29. Klein S, Fontana L, Young VL, Coggan AR, Kilo C, Patterson BW, et al. Absence of an effect of liposuction on insulin action and risk factors for coronary heart disease. N Engl J Med. 2004;350:2549–57.
30. Yun PL, Bruck M, Felsenfeld L, Katz BE. Breast enlargement after liposuction: comparison of incidence between power liposuction versus traditional liposuction. Dermatol Surg. 2003;29:165–7.
31. Frew KE, Rossi A, Bruck MC, Katz BE, Narins RS. Breast enlargement after liposuction: comparison of incidence between power liposuction versus traditional liposuction. Dermatol Surg. 2005;31:292–6.

32. Finzi E. Breast enlargement induced by liposuction. Dermatol Surg. 2003;29:928–30.

33. Broughton G, Horton B, Lipschitz A, Kenkel JM, Brown SA, Rohrich RJ. Lifestyle outcomes, satisfaction, and attitudes of patients after liposuction: a Dallas experience. Plast Reconstr Surg. 2006;117:1738–49.

34. Lawrence L, Butterwick KJ. Immediate and long-term postoperative care and touch ups. In: Narins RS, editor. Safe liposuction and fat transfer. New York: Marcel Dekker; 2003. p. 329–41.

35. Bernstein G, Hanke CW. Safety of liposuction: a review of 9478 cases performed by dermatologists. J Dermatol Surg Oncol. 1988;14:1112–4.

36. Hanke CW, Bernstein G, Bullock S. Safety of tumescent liposuction in 15,336 patients. Dermatol Surg. 1995;21:459–62.

37. Coleman III WP, Hanke CW, Lillis P, et al. Does the location of the surgery or the specialty of the physician affect malpractice claims in liposuction. Dermatol Surg. 1999;25:343–7.

38. Houseman TS, Lawrence N, Mellen BG, et al. The safety of liposuction: results of a national survey. Dermatol Surg. 2002;28:971–8.

39. Katz BE, Bruck MC, Felsenfeld L, Frew KE. Power liposuction: a report on complications. Dermatol Surg. 2003;29:925–7.

40. Hanke W, Cox SE, Kuznets N, Colemann WP. Tumescent liposuction report performance measurement initiative: national survey results. Dermatol Surg. 2004;30:967–78.

41. Coldiron BM, Healy C, Bene NI. Office surgery incidents. What seven years of Florida data show us. Dermatol Surg. 2008;34(3):258–91.

42. Klein JA, Kassarjdian N. Lidocaine toxicity with tumescent liposuction. A case report of probably drug interactions. Dermatol Surg. 1997;23(12):1169–74.

43. Martinex MA, Ballesteros S, Segura LJ, Garcia M. Reporting a fatality during tumescent liposuction. Forensic Sci Int. 2008;178(1):e11–6.

44. Gibbons MD, Lim RB, Carter PL. Necrotizing fasciitis after tumescent liposuction. Am Surg. 1998;64(5): 458–60.

45. Gilliland MD, Coates N. Tumescent liposuction complicated by pulmonary edema. Plast Reconstr Surg. 1997;99(1):215–9.

46. Jacob CI, Weisenborn EJ. Liposuction and menstrual Irregularities. Dermatol Surg. 2004;30:1035–7.

47. Andrews TR, Perdikis G, Shack RB. Herpes zoster as a rare complication of liposuction. Plast Reconstr Surg. 2004;113(6):1838–40.

48. Prado A, Andrades P, Danilla S, Leniz P, Castillo P, Gaete F. A prospective, randomized, double-blind, controlled clinical trial comparing laser-assisted lipoplasty with suction assisted lipoplasty. Plast Reconstr Surg. 2006;118:1032–45.

49. Yang CH, Hsu HC, Shen SC, Juan WH, Hong HS, Chen CH. Warm and neutral tumescent anesthetic solutions are essential factors for a less painful injection. Dermatol Surg. 2006;32:1119–23.

50. Wollina U, Kostler E, Schonlebe J, Haroske G. Tumescent suction curettage versus minimal skin resection with subcutaneous curettage of sweat glands in axillary hyperhidrosis. Dermatol Surg. 2008;34: 709–16.

51. Heuther MJ, Brodland DG. Local anesthetics. In: Wolverton SE, editor. Comprehensive dermatologic drug therapy. China: Saunders Elsevier; 2007. p. 825–49.

## Self-Assessment

1. What key aspects of the medical and surgical history should be documented during the preoperative evaluation?
   (a) Previous surgeries with special attention to surgeries performed in the area to be suctioned
   (b) Psychosocial history including history of Body Dysmorphic Disorder
   (c) Recent fluctuations in weight
   (d) Chronic medical conditions (i.e., cardiovascular disease, diabetes)
   (e) All of the above

2. In whom is liposuction absolutely contraindicated?
   (a) Diabetics
   (b) Personal history of lidocaine allergy
   (c) Family history of breast cancer
   (d) Women of childbearing age
   (e) History of surgery in the area to be suctioned

3. How long after tumescent anesthesia is infused do plasma lidocaine levels peak?
   (a) 1 h
   (b) 4 h
   (c) 8 h
   (d) 12 h
   (e) 24 h

4. What is the recommended maximum volume that should be aspirated during a single liposuction session?
   (a) 1,000 mL
   (b) 3,000 mL
   (c) 5,000 mL
   (d) 7,500 mL
   (e) 10,000 mL

5. What are the recommended qualifications of a physician performing liposuction?
   (a) Advance Cardiac Life Support certification
   (b) Board certification in a specialty that emphasize training in cutaneous surgery
   (c) Evidence of liposuction surgery training in residency or documented liposuction-specific training postresidency
   (d) All of the above

# Answers

1. e: All of the above
2. b: Personal history of lidocaine allergy
3. d: 12 h
4. c: 5,000 m
5. d: All of the above

# Hair Transplantation

Jane Unaeze and David H. Ciocon

## Introduction

Hair transplantation surgery has evolved radically since its introduction in the German literature by Dieffenbach in the early nineteenth century. Since that time, from the first report of successful punch graft transplantation for alopecia by Okuda in the 1930s, to Norman Orentreich's use of larger 6–8 mm punch grafts and his description of the concept of donor site dominance in the 1950s, to the definition of the follicular unit by Headington and the development of follicular unit transplantation by Limmer and its subsequent championing by Bernstein and Rassman in the 1990s, the field has trended towards developing techniques that achieve more natural-appearing and esthetic end-results [1–5]. Alternate techniques such as scalp reduction and scalp flaps have been described but they have become largely obsolete because outcomes that were too frequently esthetically unpleasing. Developing an evidence-based approach to hair restoration surgery is difficult, however, because most hair restoration techniques have been described in case series, anecdotal reports, position papers, and colloquium guidelines, and have not been compared in large, prospective, randomized controlled trials [6].

J. Unaeze • D.H. Ciocon (✉)
Division of Dermatology, Albert Einstein College of Medicine, Yeshiva University, 3411 Wayne Avenue, 2nd Floor, Bronx, NY 10467, USA
e-mail: dhciocon@gmail.com

In this chapter we attempt to summarize current guidelines and recommendations regarding more common methods of hair restoration such as the combined mini-and micrografting technique and the follicular unit transplantation technique as well as less common procedures such as scalp reduction, scalp advancement with tissue expansion, and scalp flaps. With each summary, we include data from the most current literature, rating the strength of evidence for each recommendation or guideline. Similar taxonomies have been used by editors of the US family medicine and primary care journals, and the critical model is supported by the Clinical Guidelines Task Force [7].

## Patient Selection

Although many patients benefit from hair restoration surgery, selecting the proper patient is vital to optimizing therapeutic outcome, since hair loss can typically continue throughout an individual's life. Most experts agree that the ideal candidates for hair restoration surgery are individuals with patterned androgenetic alopecia [4, 8–10] [V/C]. The most common pattern of male androgenetic alopecia is the "regular" Norwood pattern, in which two areas of hair loss – a bitemporal recession and thinning crown – gradually enlarge and coalesce until the entire front, top, and crown of the scalp are bald [10]. The different stages of the regular Norwood pattern are shown in Fig. 22.1. A second, less common pattern, Norwood class A, is characterized by

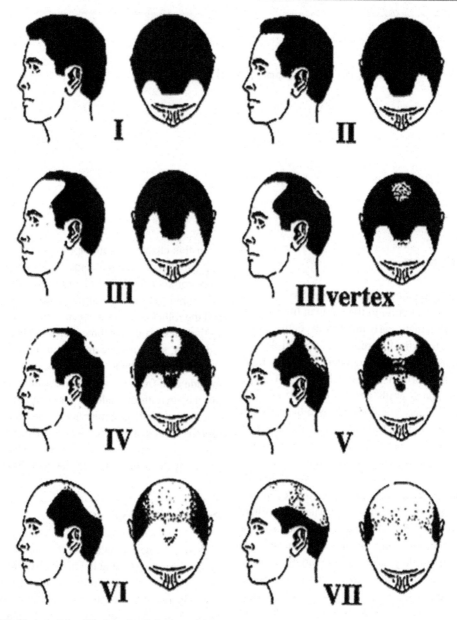

**Fig. 22.1** Norwood classification of male pattern alopecia

a distinctly anterior to posterior progression, usually resulting in baldness on the front and top of the scalp but with more limited involvement of the crown. A third type of male pattern alopecia known as diffuse pattern alopecia (DPA) is characterized by diffuse thinning in the front, top, and vertex. In all three patterns, the sides and back are preserved, though the sides may become thinned with age. Most experts agree that occipital and parietal scalp hairs form a stable permanent zone in all three patterns of androgenetic alopecia and provide the optimal donor site for hair restoration surgery [2, 11, 12] [V/C].

Individuals with unpatterned forms of alopecia do not make good transplant candidates because they lack predictable and stable hair growth zones. Unfortunately, differentiating unpatterned and patterned forms of male androgenetic alopecia can be difficult. Two key clinical differences, however, are the slower rate of hair loss progression in patterned alopecia and an almost "transparent" appearance to the side and occipital hairs in unpatterned alopecia. Other features of unpatterned hair loss include the maintenance of an adolescent hair pattern, a persistent frontal hairline, greater than 35% miniaturization of hairs in the usual donor area, and a donor area hair density less than 1.5 hairs/mm² [4] [V/C].

Women tend to suffer from an unpattterned type of alopecia. Such individuals are poor candidates for hair restoration surgery. However, many women with patterned hair loss can be considered for hair restoration, as long as other secondary causes of female pattern hair loss, including iron deficiency, thyroid disorders, and excessive androgen production, are ruled out [13, 14] [V/C]. All patients regardless of gender must be screened preoperatively for potential surgical contraindications, including a history of bleeding diathesis, medications, or supplements that promote bleeding such as acetylsalicylic acid, nonsteroidal anti-inflammatory medications, vitamin E, and a history of implantable metal devices. With regard to lifestyle modification, all patients are encouraged to avoid alcohol 2–3 days before surgery to minimize bleeding and to avoid tobacco for at least 24 h before and 1–2 weeks after the procedure for optimal wound healing. Finally, most patients are routinely encouraged to discontinue topical minoxidil 4–5 days before surgery because of its vasodilatory properties. Physicians also routinely place patients on finasteride before surgery to minimize the chance of a postsurgical effluvium, although there are no controlled studies confirming this benefit [15] [VI/C].

## Preoperative Planning

Various opinions have been expressed with regard to the optimal timing of hair transplantation with respect to the stage of alopecia. Bernstein has argued that hair restoration should not be contemplated for any male patient until they reach at least a Norwood class III stage, with the understanding that early class III patients often benefit from

medications such as finasteride and minoxidil, alone. Conversely, extensive balding should not preclude one from being a hair restoration candidate, so long as the donor zone is stable with miniaturization of less than 20% and the patient's expectations are realistic. With regard to age, most experts agree that transplantation should be postponed until the mid-twenties (age 23–25) so that medications, particularly finasteride, are given adequate time to work [9] [VI/C]. As most patients show regrowth for up to 2 years after medical treatment is initiated, finasteride should be given at least this long before surgery is considered. Finasteride exerts its effects by inhibiting the conversion of testosterone to dihydrotestosterone, which blocks the androgen-mediated pathway of follicle miniaturization, the hallmark of androgenetic alopecia [12]. Controlled studies have shown that it not only increases the number of functioning hair follicles but also increases hair caliber and length [16]. It also functions synergistically with minoxidil, which increases hair growth by increasing blood flow to the treated follicles [15, 17] [I/A]. Rawnsley has argued that hair transplantation should not be attempted before the age of 27. Waiting to this age, he argues, allows clinicians to better identify patients with unpatterned forms of alopecia who would respond poorly to hair transplantation surgery as well as patients who will develop more severe grades of alopecia that require more comprehensive counseling regarding long-term outcomes [4] [VI/C].

## Informed Consent

Preoperative planning for surgical hair restoration not only includes careful patient selection but also obtaining informed consent and assessing the patient's expectations, both realistic and unrealistic. Discussion of the process must include a description of the process of pattern hair loss, nonsurgical pharmaco-therapeutic management options, postoperative complications, and reassurance that most results are not appreciable until 8–9 months after the procedure. In particular, young patients must be instructed that their existing hair can still be lost in the future and that drug therapy is usually advantageous in preserving existing hair. Patients must also be counseled not to expect the same hair density and thickness they had before balding [9] [VI/C].

## Surgical Technique

Hair transplantation involves relocation of hairs from the occiput and parietal areas to bare areas, typically the crown or vertex, the top, and front of the scalp. Mini-and micrografting is a method of hair transplantation widely practiced in the 1980s that involves the harvesting and transplantation of randomly assorted groups of hair without consideration for the natural configuration of follicular units [1, 4, 18]. The transplanted grafts are sectioned from a donor strip from the back of the scalp according to the number of hairs they contain. Minigrafts consist of 4–6 hairs while micrografts consist of 1–3 hairs. As one expert argues, a more accurate term for the procedure is "mini-micrografts cut to size," since the grafts are cut to a predetermined size rather than dissected according to how the hairs naturally grow [4]. The minigrafts are placed into small circular recipient sites made with punch blades, 1.5–2.5 mm in size, and sometimes into slit recipient sites made with a small linear blade. The micrografts are typically placed into smaller incisions in front of the minigrafts to create the frontal hairline. The donor strip that provides the mini- and micrografts is harvested using a multibladed knife that cuts 3–5 strips, each 1.5–2 mm in width [19]. From these strips the grafts are dissected under loupe-assisted magnification or direct visualization with good lighting.

The minigrafting technique was described in 1981 by Nordstrom et al. who reported using 3–6 haired grafts anterior to punch grafts to improve the appearance of the frontal hairline. Bradshaw extended the use of these smaller 3–6-hair grafts throughout the restored scalp to achieve a more refined and natural appearance [1, 4]. As mentioned previously, the relative disadvantage of this technique is that the grafts do not necessarily correspond to the naturally occurring follicular units (see below), so that individual follicular units may not be fully intact in a single graft. Second, the use of the multibladed knife for harvesting can result in the destruction of up to 20% of the naturally occurring follicular units in the donor area, injuring potential sites for future harvesting. Finally, with this technique, all the tissue from the donor site is transplanted since trimming of the tissue would result in loss of the hair fragments within the grafts. As a result, an excess of intervening bald skin in the donor area is often transplanted along with the hairs. This can result in grafts that are larger than necessary in the recipient area. This not only could produce decreased optical density in the recipient area (which gives the area an undesirable "see-through quality") but also potentially compromise the blood supply of the grafts and limit their survival.

The idea of follicular unit transplantation that emerged in the late 1980s was dependent on the recognition by Headington that scalp hair grows in natural clusters or "follicular units," rather than as single hairs [20, 21]. These units are best appreciated by clipping scalp hair to 1 mm in length and viewing them with a magnifying densitometer. Each unit is a discrete, anatomic and physiologic grouping of 1–4 terminal hair follicles with 1 or 2 associated vellus follicles, nine sebaceous lobules, and arrector pili muscles surrounded by its own neurovascular bundle and circumferential adventitial collagen sheath. Limmer was the first to describe the clinical use of follicular unit grafts in the mid-1990s using stereoscopic dissection, while Bernstein and Rasmann elaborated on its rationale and optimal techniques in a series of respected publications [8, 9, 22–27]. In contrast to mini- and micrografting (Table 22.1), each follicular unit graft is dissected out individually under stereomicroscopic visualization to permit careful removal of surrounding, nonhair-bearing skin. These grafts are then placed into very tiny recipient sites, many of which are less than 1 mm [26, 28, 29]. In a typical procedure 1,800–2,200 of these follicular unit grafts are transplanted, but as many as 5,000 grafts can sometimes be transferred in a single session. The number of follicular units transferred is limited, however, by the hair density, scalp laxity, and local blood supply. As recipient

**Table 22.1** Comparison of follicular unit transplantation and mini- and micrografting transplantation

| Grafts | Follicular unit transplantation | Mini- and micrografting transplantation |
|---|---|---|
| Follicular units used exclusively | Yes | No |
| Graft size | Uniformly small | Larger |
| Number of hairs/graft | 1–4 | 1–6 (or more) |
| Hair/skin ratio in graft | High | Variable |
| Extra skin transplanted | No | Yes |
| Recipient wound size | Uniformly small | Variable |
| Techniques | | |
| Harvesting types | Single strip or follicular unit extraction | Multibladed knife |
| Microscopic dissection required | Yes/variable | No |
| Preservation of follicular units | Yes | No |
| Follicular transection | No | Yes |
| Maximizes donor supply | Yes | No |
| Results | | |
| Healing time | Fast | Slower |
| Maximum optical density | Yes | No |
| Cost and convenience | | |
| Staff requirements | Moderate | Small |
| Duration of individual procedure | Long | Short |
| Time for complete restoration | Short if few sessions | Long |
| Cost per procedure | More | Less |
| Total cost for restoration | Similar | Similar |

Adapted from New Hair Institute [72]

sites are made closer together, the likelihood of compromising their local microvascular integrity increases, threatening the viability of the grafts [30–32]. The current recommended standard for graft density is approximately 25–30 follicular units per centimeter squared per session, although there have been successful reports of up to 100 follicular units per centimeter in a single session [27, 33–36] [V/C]. Dense packing is more suited to the completely bald recipient site. Among the factors that have been shown to improve overall optical density in the transplanted area are large hair shaft diameter, reduced contrast between hair color and scalp, the presence of curl, and lighter colored hair [4].

The follicular unit grafts can be harvested from the donor site on the occiput either through standard single strip excision or through follicular unit extraction (FUE) [37]. In standard strip excision, an elliptical incision is made over the external occipital protuberance after infiltration with tumescent anesthesia [38, 39]. To make the incision, experts have reported using either a single blade to excise with a free hand ellipse or a scalpel handle loaded with two parallel ten blades, with tapering of the ends into corners of an ellipse [4, 40]. To minimize scar formation in the donor area, most experts agree that the width of the ellipse should usually not exceed 1 cm and that its length be proportional to the number of grafts needed [41, 42] [V/C]. In most reports, closure of the donor site is achieved without undermining to minimize bleeding and with a running nonabsorbable suture or staples. However, some experts argue that reducing tension by undermining is essential for minimizing scar formation [9, 36] [IV/C]. Various opinions have been expressed with regard to the appropriate size of the nonabsorbable suture to be used to close the donor sites, but most prefer a suture caliber in the range of 3–0 to 5–0 [43] [V/C]. Once the strip is extracted, it is dissected under stereo-magnification into slivers that are each 1.5–2 mm wide. Each sliver can then be dissected into 1–2 hair follicular unit grafts or 3–4 hair follicular unit grafts, which are held on normal saline-soaked nonadherent gauze or on Petri dishes filled with normal saline. While most hair restoration surgeons dissect these slivers under stereomicroscopic magnification [44, 45] [III/B], several reports from the literature have described successful follicular unit graft dissection using standard loupe magnification or naked eye visualization [46] [IV/B]. Furthermore, whether the follicular unit graft should be "chubby" or "skinny" has been a matter of intellectual debate, and not tested in randomized controlled trials [32, 47]. Skinny grafts require smaller recipient sites and can be packed densely, but overly fine dissection can injure the arrector pili muscles, sebaceous glands, telogen hairs, and the follicles themselves which may be crucial to optimal hair growth. Once harvested, grafts must be protected from desiccation [48, 49] [V/C]. The timing from harvest to transplantation to the recipient site is important since graft survival rates have been demonstrated to drop from 95% at 2 h from harvest to transplantation to 86% after 6 h from harvest [4] [V/C]. Therefore, experts universally agree that preparation of these grafts requires a well-trained, efficient, and well-coordinated ancillary staff and a surgeon meticulously trained in the expedient performance of proper follicular transplantation technique.

An alternative approach to follicular unit graft harvesting has been described and is known as "follicular unit extraction" or FUE [50] [V/C]. With this technique, each individual follicular unit is harvested under stereoscopic magnification using a small circular incision created by a trephine [51] [V/C]. Each circular incision is left open to heal by secondary intention. Although more time consuming, the advantage to this technique over standard ellipse incision is avoidance of a linear scar. Furthermore, for patients with loose or tight donor skin, or limited donor tissue because of previous transplantation surgeries, FUE permits the removal of less tissue with an optical cosmetic outcome. The technique is particularly suited for hair transplant patients who wish to maintain a very short or "buzzed" hairstyle after surgery without a visible scar. The disadvantages include fewer grafts being transplanted per procedure, an increase in overall operative time and cost because of longer harvesting times, as well as an increased risk of transecting harvested hair follicles [50].

Various methods for recipient bed preparation have been described. In the "stick and place" method, each recipient site is created by the physician, followed by immediate insertion of a graft into each site by an assistant with a Jeweler's forceps. Alternatively, all recipient sites can be created first, followed by placement of grafts into each site. While the relative merits of each technique have been described, including shorter operative times and lower rates of graft-recipient site mismatch for the "stick and place" method, they have not been compared in randomized controlled trials. The most commonly reported instruments to create these sites include a 19 or 20-gauge needle for one-hair and two-hair follicular unit grafts and an 18-gauge needle for thick two-hair or 3–4 unit hair grafts [1, 4, 52] [VI/C]. Slits are made by puncturing the scalp to a 4 mm depth and can have either a coronal or sagittal orientation depending on the growth pattern of the surrounding native hair. Recipient sites can be created with the aid of loupe magnification or naked eye visualization, although Avram et al. have reported improved results when creating the sites with polarized light emitting diode magnification [53] [IV/C]. If the recipient scalp is bare, site orientation should follow the normal angulation of 20–40° from the plane of the scalp, with a tendency to more acute angulation along the frontal hairline and the temporal area. Sites anterior to the vertex transition line are typically oriented anteriorly and more inferiorly towards the lateral aspect. Hairs posterior to this line are more randomly configured and are oriented to match the natural whorl of the crown. It is generally agreed that placement of the recipient sites in the frontal hairline must include consideration for hairline design, feathering, and achievement of optical density [25, 54, 55] [V/C]. To achieve a more natural-appearing frontal hairline, Epstein has argued for the use of "one and two-hair grafts arranged in an irregular pattern with micro-zones of alternating greater and lower density" [1]. Finally, most experts agree that the goal of any first transplantation session should be to maximize optical density in the frontal regions of the scalp by forward weighting, which includes placing recipient sites closely together at a typical density of 30 follicular units per centimeter

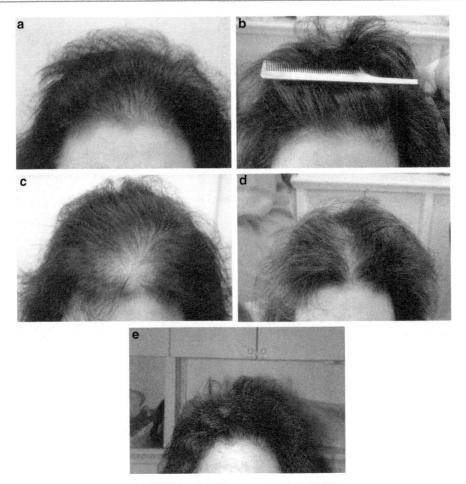

**Fig. 22.2** (**a**) Before treatment with the hair combed back for critical evaluation. (**b**) Twelve months after frontal hair transplant with 934 follicular units with the hair combed for critical evaluation. (**c**) Before treatment, caudal view with the hair parted for critical evaluation. (**d**) Three and a half years after second follicular unit transplantation session (posterior to frontal area treated 1 year earlier) with the hair parted for critical evaluation. (**e**) Photo taken at the same time as the one shown in (**d**)

squared, and placing larger follicular units in the front, particularly in the forelock region [35].

Although the mini- and microgroft technique and the follicular unit transplantation technique are different in both theory and practice (Table 22.1), they should not be considered mutually exclusive. In fact many recognized authorities have reported using both types of grafts in their practices, depending on the desired density for the areas they are transplanting [36, 56, 57] [V/C]. To avoid confusion, however, members of the International Society of Hair Restoration Surgery have published consensus guidelines emphasizing that, whatever method be employed, hair restoration surgeons be vigilant about documenting a precise description of both the type and number of grafts they are using, and whether they are dissecting the grafts on the basis of size, number of hairs, or number of follicular units [24] [VI/C]. The legendary Unger has published extensively on hair restoration, and in an excellent review from 2005, demonstrated that grafts harvested using both techniques can be elegantly combined depending on the desired cosmetic outcome (Figs. 22.2–22.5) [58] [V/C].

Artificial hair transplantation has been reported in cases where the donor site has been depleted, but historically, has been marred by poor quality fiber, untrained operators, and inadequate technique. A recent pilot study of ten patients by

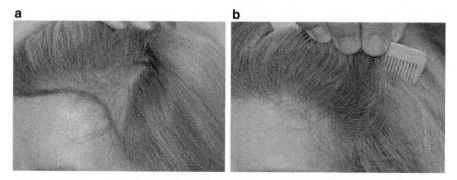

**Fig. 22.3** (a) Before first transplant. (b) Eight months after first follicular unit transplant (consisting of 1,573 follicular units)

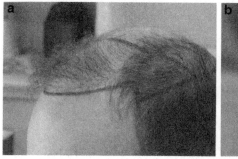

**Fig. 22.4** (a) A patient before his first transplant at our office. Grafts that had too many hairs and too coarse hairs for a hairline had been used by the prior surgeon. There had also been no attempt to treat adjacent areas with thinning hair. The *black* crayon outlines the proposed recipient area for our session. (b) Eleven months after a session of 1,973 follicular units showing a more typical result of current hair transplanting techniques and appropriate planning

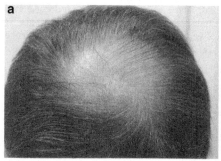
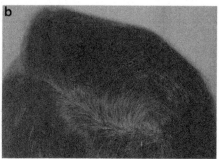

**Fig. 22.5** (a) Crown area before first hair transplant. Patient was 45 years old with no evidence or family history of vertex male pattern baldness. (b) One year post- hair transplant (consisting of 2,132 follicular units). This patient had particularly good results because of his excellent hair characteristics for hair transplanting

Agrawal has reported promising results when patients received synthetic copolyamide grafts; however, the data on this technique is still limited and largely experimental [59] [V/C].

Finally, follicular transplantation has also been described for other parts of the body, including the eyebrow, beard, mustache, eyelash area, and areas of scarring alopecia. Most reports have described a few cases only that do not conform to the standard clinical profiles of most hair restoration patients. As result, techniques such as this are still considered anecdotal [60–62] [VI/C].

## Excisional Surgery

In addition to hair transplantation, less common surgical options for androgenetic alopecia include scalp reduction, scalp extension and scalp flap surgery [1, 63]. Scalp reduction is defined as the excision of an area of alopecia or prospective alopecia. The size of the area that can be excised varies with the degree of natural scalp laxity and the extent of surgical undermining and/or the amount of prior stretching of the hair bearing rim or "biological creep" created by scalp expansion or extension prior to alopecia reduction. The larger the area that can be removed, the smaller the remaining area of alopecia will be, with the result that fewer grafts will be required to transplant it. Unger has recommended that scalp reduction be employed at anytime the objective is "complete" coverage of frontal, mid-third, and vertex alopecia [VI/C] [64]. The more scalp reduction that is done the more likely one can conserve available donor tissue before the entire area of alopecia is treated.

A variety of scalp reduction patterns have been described but the most common patterns employed are the ellipse, inverted Y, and more recently a flattened S shape [64]. The inverted Y pattern is typically used when one anticipates insufficient donor tissue to transplant the entire bald area even after scalp reduction. This design prevents the production of scar in areas that cannot later be covered with transplanted hair. Usually, scalp reduction is carried out after the first two transplants have been completed, but occasionally, scalp reduction will be done before any transplanting is started. This occurs most often in the following situations: (1) in the setting of great scalp laxity, making it likely that the shape of the hairline will be altered by the scalp reduction (2) the area of alopecia is particularly large and therefore requires several scalp reductions to raise the superior border of the temporo-parietal hair to an appropriate level (3) the crown is the recipient area and the patients is relatively young and might need the grafts saved by scalp reduction for other areas of future alopecia (4) one is correcting poorly planned transplantation in which new areas of alopecia have developed without sufficient donor grafts having been left

to treat them (5) one is treating large areas of cicatricial alopecia [64].

Scalp extension refers to a procedure described by Frechet in 1993 in which a conventional scalp reduction is combined with the use of a scalp extender [65, 66]. A scalp extender consists of a Silastic sheet with metal hooks at either end that is stretched to double its original width and hooks into the underside of the galea beneath the left and right side "permanent" rim hair. Over a period of approximately 30 days, the Silastic sheet attempts to revert to its original size bringing both sides of fringe hair closer together in the process. During a second scalp reduction, after 30 days, twice the amount of alopecic skin can be removed in a conventional scalp reduction. Using scalp extension, as much as 12 cm of alopecic skin can be removed. The object of scalp extension is the removal of "all" alopecic skin. The subsequent slot of alopecic hair that remains after multiple scalp reductions and extension can be corrected by another type of surgery Frechet described and called a "three flap corrective procedure." Results of the procedure are impressive (VI/C). Unger has recently suggested that Frechet shorten his excision to stop just posterior to the middle of the vertex and limit his objectives to eliminating all but an approximately 5 cm wide area of alopecia [63]. This would allow for a rapid major reduction in the area of alopecia while avoiding the formation of a slot defect that would require the technically demanding three flap procedure that has deterred many from employing scalp extension.

Scalp flap surgery, most notably the Juri flap and the Fleming Mayer flap have been described but are no longer as popular as they were in the 1980s [67]. They are temporo-parietal flaps, pedicled on the posterior branch of the temporal artery, can be as long as 24 cm, and are sufficient for creating an entire frontal hairline 3–4 cm wide. Because of the level of surgical manipulation involved, the procedures are typically performed by a small number of plastic and facial surgeons and not dermatologists. Although the direction of hair growth in the hairline is primarily posterior, the density achieved by such flaps, according to Epstein "is unsurpassed." It is estimated that a single flap can provide 10,000 hairs. For further coverage behind the flap, a second flap from the contralateral side or hair grafting can be performed. These flap procedures are rarely performed today because of their limitations, the incidence of scarring, and because they have been largely supplanted by grafting techniques that yield more natural appearing results. Flap hairlines are typically abrupt, and donor and recipient site scarring often require that hair be worn long [VI/C]. However, the most significant disadvantage to flap surgery is that it cannot be used for individuals with Norwood class 4 or greater hair loss patterns, since the advancement of hair loss may increase the visibility of donor site scars.

## Complications

Complications from hair restoration surgery are extremely low and are much more frequently associated with scalp advancement and scalp flap surgeries than with grafting [68, 69] [V/C]. Most of these complications have already been discussed in the preoperative planning section of this chapter. Typical ones are complications inherent to any outpatient surgery procedure, including bleeding, infection, reactions to lidocaine or epinephrine, and scarring. With regard to grafting techniques, swelling over the forehead may occur 3 days postoperatively due to intravascular-to-interstitial electrolyte effects and large amounts of injected tumescent anesthesia fluid pooling. Use of short courses of oral corticosteroids or local injections of a dilute solution of intralesional corticosteroids have been advocated for this complication. Prolonged recipient scalp erythema and transient numbness due to donor or recipient site neuropraxia have been infrequently reported. Postoperative recipient telogen effluvium has also been reported but can be prevented, according to anecdotal reports, by early use of finasteride. A folliculitis can happen as hair growth occurs in follicles that have been buried by epidermal overgrowth during the second month after grafting but usually resolves spontaneously or can be treated by unroofing the skin with a hypodermic needle. Finally, long-term complications include poor graft survival and unpleasant cosmetic outcomes. Many of these complications can be avoided however, through careful attention to design,

minimizing time between graft harvesting and transplantation, and delicate handling of graft tissue [29] [V/C]. Most of all, poor patient selection and inadequate preoperative counseling can account for the majority of patient dissatisfaction after the procedure.

## Photobiomodulation

In recent years, the use of laser/light sources to improve hair growth in areas of alopecia has been investigated. Photobiomodulation is the commonly used term to describe the effect of lower light energy on the cellular level. The mechanism by which photobiomodulation stops or reverses male or female pattern hair loss is unknown. One theory suggests that such laser/light devices increase blood flow to the dermal papilla [70]. Clinical examples of photobiomodulation include the paradoxical growth of hair that occurs in a small percentage of patients undergoing laser hair removal and PUVA to treat alopecia totalis. Treatment protocols include 15–30 min treatments on alternating days for 2–4 weeks, tapering to 1–2 treatments per week for 6–12 months, followed by biweekly and once monthly maintenance treatments. A review of these new devices and the evidence that supports their use has been written by Avram et al., however much of the cited data is primarily anecdotal and nonscientific [71].

## Conclusion

Hair restoration surgery is a safe and effective means of redistributing hair to areas of alopecia in individuals with patterned hair loss whose medical options have been exhausted. Although scalp advancement and scalp flap surgeries can accomplish similar ends, their results are far inferior to grafting techniques with respect to postoperative scarring, perioperative bleeding, and achieving a "natural" cosmetic outcome [73]. While efforts to standardize hair transplantation techniques have arisen in recent years, particularly with regard to the classification of the mini- and micrografting and follicular unit transplantation procedures, many hair restoration surgeons continue to impose their own personal "stamps" on the techniques, making them inconsistent consistent across centers. Proper training of the surgeon and the assisting team as well as judicious preoperative planning and patient selection are essential to an optimal functional and cosmetic outcome. Large, prospective randomized controlled trials are needed to compare the relative advantages and disadvantages of each technique as most of the data comes from anecdotal reports, cases series, small retrospective trials, and position papers.

### Evidence-Based Summary

| Recommendation | Level of evidence |
| --- | --- |
| For men, hair restoration surgery should be reserved for individuals with regular Norwood class, Norwood class A, or diffuse pattern alopecia | V/C |
| Women with patterned alopecia may be candidates for hair restoration surgery if secondary causes of alopecia including iron deficiency, thyroid disease, and hyper-androgenism are excluded | V/C |
| Features of unpatterned hair loss include the maintenance of an adolescent hair pattern, a persistent frontal hairline, miniaturization of hairs in the occipital donor area >35%, and a donor area hair density less than 1.5 hairs/mm$^2$ | V/C |
| Hair transplantation should be postponed in men until the mid-twenties (age 23–25) after a minimum of a 2-year trial of finasteride and/or minoxidil | VI/C |
| Minoxidil should be discontinued 4–5 days preoperatively to minimize bleeding risk | VI/B |
| Finasteride should be started on all patients prior to surgery as it minimizes the likelihood of a postoperative telogen effluvium | VI/B |
| Detailed informed consent, preoperative counseling, and careful patient selection are key predictors of patient satisfaction after surgery | VI/C |
| Mini- and micrografting and follicular unit transplantation are the most widely practiced methods of hair transplantation and are associated with superior cosmetic outcomes compared to scalp reduction, flap, or advancement surgery | V/B |
| For follicular unit transplantation, the current recommended standard for grafted density is 25–30 follicular units per centimeter per session | V/C |
| Transplanting 5,000 or more follicular units in a single session (mega session) is associated with decreased graft survival | V/C |
| Graft survival decreases as the time between harvesting and transplantation increases | V/C |
| For follicular unit transplantation, the grafts can be harvested through either elliptical strip excision or follicular unit extraction | V/C |
| Follicular unit extraction is best reserved for individuals with limited donor tissue or who desire to wear their hair short postoperatively | V/C |
| For elliptical donor excision, the width of the donor strip should not exceed 1 cm to minimize scarring and facilitate closure | V/C |
| Dissection of follicular unit grafts is best accomplished under stereomicroscopic magnification | III/B |
| Preparation of the recipient bed must include a consideration of native hair growth patterns and hairline design | V/C |
| The recipient area can be prepared using 16–21 gauge needles under direct visualization, with loupe magnification, or the assistance of polarized light emitting diode magnification | IV/C |
| A well-trained ancillary staff and a well-trained surgeon are associated with optimal outcomes in follicular grafting | VI/C |
| Optimal results may not seen until up to a year after surgery | V/C |
| Complications from follicular grafting are minimal and are similar to those associated with standard outpatient excisional surgery | V/C |
| Artificial hair transplantation with synthetic fibers may be used successfully in cases where donor tissue is limited or nonexistent | V/C |
| Laser/light technology may have clinical benefit in stimulating hair growth in patients with alopecia | V/C |

**Acknowledgments** We would like to extend our deepest gratitude to Dr. Walter Unger who not only provided representative clinical photographs for the chapter but also generously assisted in the preparation of the manuscript.

# References

1. Epstein JS. Evolution of techniques in hair transplantation: a 12-year perspective. Facial Plast Surg. 2007; 23:51–9.
2. Orentreich N. Autografts in alopecias and other selected dermatological conditions. Ann N Y Acad Sci. 1959;83:463–79.
3. Rassman WR, Bernstein RM, McClellan R, Jones R, Worton E, Uyttendaele H. Follicular unit extraction: minimally invasive surgery for hair transplantation. Dermatol Surg. 2002;28:720–8.
4. Rawnsley JD. Hair restoration. Facial Plast Surg Clin North Am. 2008;16:289–97.
5. Unger WP. The history of hair transplantation. Dermatol Surg. 2000;26:181–9.
6. Patwardhan N, Mysore V. IADVL Dermatosurgery Task Force. Hair transplantation: standard guidelines of care. Indian J Dermatol Venereol Leprol. 2008;74(Suppl):S46–53.
7. Ebell MH, Siwek J, Weiss BD, Woolf SH, Susman JL, Ewigman B, et al. Simplifying the language of evidence to improve patient care: strength of recommendation taxonomy (SORT): a patient-centered approach to grading evidence in medical literature. J Fam Pract. 2004;53:111–20.
8. Bernstein RM, Rassman WR. Follicular unit transplantation. Dermatol Clin. 2005;23:393–414.
9. Bernstein RM, Rassman WR. Follicular transplantation. Patient evaluation and surgical planning. Dermatol Surg. 1997;23:771–84.
10. Olsen EA, Messenger AG, Shapiro J, Bergfeld WF, Hordinsky MK, Roberts JL, et al. Evaluation and treatment of male and female pattern hair loss. J Am Acad Dermatol. 2005;52:301–11.
11. Rebora A. Pathogenesis of androgenetic alopecia. J Am Acad Dermatol. 2004;50:777–9.
12. Whiting DA. Possible mechanisms of miniaturization during androgenetic alopecia or pattern hair loss. J Am Acad Dermatol. 2001;45:S81–6.
13. Chartier MB, Hoss DM, Grant-Kels JM. Approach to the adult female patient with diffuse nonscarring alopecia. J Am Acad Dermatol. 2002;47:809–18.
14. Unger WP, Unger RH. The art of hair transplantation in women. Dermatology. 2004;4:26–8.
15. Avram MR, Cole JP, Gandelman M, Haber R, Knudsen R, Leavitt MT, et al. Roundtable consensus meeting of the 9th annual meeting of The International Society of Hair Restoration Surgery. The potential role of minoxidil in the hair transplantation setting. Dermatol Surg. 2002;28:894–900.
16. Thompson IM, Goodman PJ, Tangen CM, Lucia MS, Miller GJ, Ford LG, et al. The influence of finasteride on the development of prostate cancer. N Engl J Med. 2003;349:215–24.
17. Bouhanna P. Androgenetic alopecia: combining medical and surgical treatments. Dermatol Surg. 2003;29:1130–4.
18. Lam SM, Karamanovski E. Surgical hair restoration. Oper Tech Otolaryngol. 2007;18:195–202.
19. Arnold J. Mini-blades and a mini-blade handle for hair transplantation. Am J Cosm Surg. 1997;14:195–200.
20. Headington JT. Transverse microscopic anatomy of the human scalp. A basis for a morphometric approach to disorders of the hair follicle. Arch Dermatol. 1984;120:449–56.
21. Choi YC, Kim JC. Single hair transplantation using the Choi hair transplanter. J Dermatol Surg Oncol. 1992;18:945–8.
22. Bernstein RM, Rassman WR, Rashid N. A new suture for hair transplantation: poliglecaprone 25. Dermatol Surg. 2001;27:5–11.
23. Bernstein RM. Measurements in hair restoration. Hair Transplant Forum Int. 1998;8:27.
24. Bernstein RM, Rassman WR, Seager D, Shapiro R, Cooley JE, Norwood OT, et al. Standardizing the classification and description of follicular unit transplantation and mini-micrografting techniques. Dermatol Surg. 1998;24:957–63.
25. Bernstein RM, Rassman WR. The aesthetics of follicular transplantation. Dermatol Surg. 1997;23:785–99.
26. Bernstein RM, Rassman WR. The logic of follicular unit transplantation. Dermatol Clin. 1999;17:277–95.
27. Bernstein RM, Rassman WR. What is delayed growth? Hair Transplant Forum Int. 1997;7:22.
28. Stough D, Whitworth JM. Methodology of follicular unit hair transplantation. Dermatol Clin. 1999;17:297–306.
29. Tan Baser N, Cigsar B, Balci Akbuga U, Terzioglu A, Aslan G. Follicular unit transplantation for male-pattern hair loss: evaluation of 120 patients. J Plast Reconstr Aesthet Surg. 2006;59:1162–9.
30. Leavitt M, Perez-Meza D, Barusco M. Research symposium 1999–2000: clinical update on research studies reported at the world hair restoration society/international society of hair restoration surgery live surgery workshop. Int J Cosm Surg Aesthet Derm. 2001;3:135–8.
31. Mayer and Keene. Study comparing follicular unit growth with different planting densities. In: Presented at the 2003 annual meeting of the International Society of Hair Restoration Surgery.
32. Mayer and Keene. Hair transplant study. In: Presented at the 2005 annual meeting of the International Society of Hair Restoration Surgery.
33. Alhaddab M, Kohn T, Mark S. Effect of graft size, angle, and intergraft distance on dense packing in hair transplants. Dermatol Surg. 2004;31:650–4.
34. Marritt E. The death of the density debate. Dermatol Surg. 1999;25:654–60.
35. Unger WP. Density issue in hair transplantation. Dermatol Surg. 1998;24:297.
36. Unger RH, Unger WP. What's new in hair transplants? Skin Therapy Lett. 2003;8:5–7.

37. Seery GE. Hair transplantation: management of donor area. Dermatol Surg. 2002;28:136–42.
38. Brandy DA. Intricacies of the single-scar technique for donor harvesting in hair transplantation surgery. Dermatol Surg. 2004;30:837–44.
39. Seager DJ, Simmons C. Local anesthesia in hair transplantation. Dermatol Surg. 2002;28:320–8.
40. Brandy DA. New instrumentation for hair transplantation surgery. Dermatol Surg. 1998;24:629–31.
41. Chang SC. Estimation of number of grafts and donor area. Hair Transplant Forum Int. 2001;11:101–3.
42. Jimenez F, Ruifernández JM. Distribution of human hair in follicular units. A mathematical model for estimating the donor size in follicular unit transplantation. Dermatol Surg. 1999;25(4):294–8.
43. Unger WP. Suturing of donor sites. In: Unger WP, editor. Hair transplantation. New York: Marcel Dekker; 1979. p. 64.
44. Bernstein RM, Rassman WR. Dissecting microscope versus magnifying loupes with transillumination in the preparation of follicular unit grafts. A bilateral controlled study. Dermatol Surg. 1998;24:875–80.
45. Seager D. Binocular stereoscopic dissecting microscopes: should we use them? Hair Transplant Forum Int. 1996;6:2–5.
46. Brandy DA. A technique for hair-grafting in between existing follicles in patients with early pattern baldness. Dermatol Surg. 2000;26:801–5.
47. Beehner ML. A comparison of hair growth between follicular-unit grafts trimmed "skinny" vs. "chubby". Dermatol Surg. 1999;25:339–40.
48. Kurata S, Ezaki T, Itami S, Terashi H, Takayusu S. Viability of isolated single hair follicles preserved at 4 degrees C. Dermatol Surg. 1999;25:26–9.
49. Raposio E, Cella A, Panarese P, Mantero S, Nordstrom REA, et al. Effects of cooling micrografts in hair transplantation surgery. Dermatol Surg. 2001;25:705–9.
50. Harris JA. Follicular unit extraction. Facial Plast Surg. 2008;24:404–13.
51. Onda M, Igawa HH, Inoue K, Tanino R. Novel technique of follicular unit extraction hair transplantation with a powered punching device. Dermatol Surg. 2008;34:683–8.
52. Brandy DA, Meshkin M. Utilization of No-Kor needles for slit-micrografting. J Dermatol Surg Oncol. 1994;20:336–9.
53. Avram MR. Polarized light-emitting diode magnification for optimal recipient site creation during hair transplant. Dermatol Surg. 2005;31:1124–7.
54. Beehner M. Hairline design in hair replacement surgery. Facial Plast Surg. 2008;24:389–403.
55. Lam SM, Hempstead BR, Williams EF. A philosophy and strategy for surgical hair restoration: a 10-year experience. Dermatol Surg. 2002;28:1035–42.
56. Brandy DA. The art of mixing follicular units and follicular groupings in hair restoration surgery. Dermatol Surg. 2004;30:846–56.
57. Unger W. Different grafts for different purposes. Am J Cosm Surg. 1997;14:177–83.
58. Unger WP. Hair transplantation: current concepts and techniques. J Investig Dermatol Symp Proc. 2005;10:225–9.
59. Agrawal M. Modern artificial hair implantation: a pilot study of 10 patients. J Cosmet Dermatol. 2008;7:315–23.
60. Marritt E. Transplantation of single hairs from the scalp as eyelashes. Review of the literature and a case report. J Dermatol Surg Oncol. 1980;6:271–3.
61. Al-Bdour MD. Eyebrow to eyelid cilia transplant: a case report. Case Rep Clin Pract Rev. 2005;6:351–3.
62. Straub PM. Replacing facial hair. Facial Plast Surg. 2008;24:446–52.
63. Unger WP. Hair transplantation. In: Arndt KA, Dover JS, Kaminer MS, editors. Atlas of cosmetic surgery. Philadelphia: WB Saunders; 2002. p. 231–63.
64. Unger M. Scalp reduction. In: Unger W, editor. Hair transplantation. 3rd ed. New York: Marcel Dekker; 1995. p. 549–69.
65. Epstein JS, Kabaker SS, Puig C, Maas C. Scalp extension in the treatment of male pattern baldness. Am J Cosm Surg. 1996;13:135–9.
66. Frechet P. Scalp extension. In: Unger W, editor. Hair transplantation. 3rd ed. New York: Marcel Dekker; 1995. p. 642–62.
67. Mangubat EA. Scalp reconstruction and repair. Facial Plast Surg. 2008;24:428–45.
68. Perez-Meza D, Niedbalski R. Complications in hair restoration surgery. Oral Maxillofac Surg Clin North Am. 2009;21:119–48.
69. Vogel JE. Hair restoration complications: an approach to the unnatural-appearing hair transplant. Facial Plast Surg. 2008;24:453–61.
70. Cooley J, Vogel J. Loss of the dermal papilla during graft dissection and placement: another cause of x-factor? Hair Transplant Forum Int. 1997;7:20–1.
71. Avram MR, Leonard Jr RT, Epstein ES, Williams JL, Bauman AJ. The current role of laser/light sources in the treatment of male and female pattern hair loss. J Cosmet Laser Ther. 2007;9:27–8.
72. New Hair Institute. Follicular unit transplants. www.newhair.com/treatment/follicular-unittransplants.asp. Accessed 14 March 2009.
73. Limmer BL. The density issue in hair transplantation. Dermatol Surg. 1997;23:747–50.

## Self-Assessment

1. True/False. Follicular unit grafting including mini- and micrografting and follicular unit transplantation results in superior cosmetic results compared to scalp advancement, scalp flaps, and scalp reduction surgery.

2. All of the following patients make excellent candidates for hair transplantation EXCEPT
   (a) A 29-year-old male with regular Norwood class IV male pattern alopecia who has tried finasteride for 2 years, with ideal donor density
   (b) A 25-year-old male with regular Norwood class II alopecia who has never tried finasteride, with ideal donor density
   (c) A 35-year-old man with Norwood class A alopecia who has been on finasteride since the age of 27, with ideal donor density
   (d) A 34-year-old woman with patterned alopecia who has normal androgen levels, iron levels, and thyroid hormone levels, with ideal donor density
   (e) A 35-year-old man with regular Norwood class IV alopecia, who has taken finasteride for 3 years, and who has 18% miniaturized hair follicles in the donor region

3. The recommended density of transplanted follicular units during a first session of follicular unit transplantation is as follows:
   (a) 15 follicular units/cm$^2$
   (b) 25 follicular units/cm$^2$
   (c) 35 follicular units/cm$^2$
   (d) 45 follicular units/cm$^2$

4. The maximum recommended number of follicular units transferred in a single session is as follows:
   (a) 2,000 follicular units
   (b) 3,000 follicular units
   (c) 4,000 follicular units
   (d) 5,000 follicular units

5. True/False. Controlled studies have shown that optimal graft viability can be achieved if follicular unit grafts are dissected with the aid of stereomicroscopic magnification.

6. To minimize scar formation, the maximum recommended width of the donor ellipse harvested during follicular unit transplantation is as follows:
   (a) 5 mm
   (b) 10 mm
   (c) 20 mm
   (d) 30 mm

## Answers

1. True
2. b: A 25-year-old make with regualr Norwood class II alopecia who has never tried finasteride with ideal donor density.
3. b: 25 follicular units/cm$^2$
4. d: 5,000 follicular units
5. True
6. b: 10 mm

# Face Lifting

**23**

## Elizabeth Grossman, Roberta D. Sengelmann, and Murad Alam

## Introduction

The face lift, as performed by dermatologic surgeons, encompasses a number of ambulatory, office-based, surgical facial rejuvenation procedures that can be performed under local anesthesia with optional sedation.

## Consensus Documents

The aging face is characterized by loss of skin elasticity, fat resorption, loss of muscle tone and volume, and loss of bone volume. As facial soft tissue ptosis develops with aging, the vector of

E. Grossman (✉)
Department of Dermatology,
Northwestern University, 676 N. St. Clair Street,
Suite 1600, Chicago, IL 60611, USA
e-mail: dfife@surgical-dermatology.com

R.D. Sengelmann
504 W. Pueblo Street, Suite 202, Santa Barbara,
CA 93105, USA

Department of Dermatology, University of California,
15374 Alton Parkway, Irvine, CA 92618, USA

M. Alam
Department of Dermatology,
Northwestern University, 676 N. St. Clair Street,
Suite 1600, Chicago, IL 60611, USA

Section of Cutaneous and Aesthetic Surgery,
Feinberg School of Medicine, Northwestern University,
Chicago, IL, USA

descent is primarily downward. Surgical management seeks to reverse this descent through elevation of the superficial musculoaponeurotic system (SMAS), which underlies the skin and subcutis, and overlies the muscle and deep neurovascular structures. A number of techniques are employed to specifically address the individual patient's specific needs; these are summarized in Table 23.1. The simplest approach is achieved via SMAS plication [1]. Using this technique, the SMAS is folded upon itself and secured, without additional undermining. A primary advantage to this approach is that there are minimal complications as the sub-SMAS structures, including the facial nerve, are left undisturbed and intact. The lateral SMASectomy approach, popularized by Baker [2], is similar to plication in that there is no undermining of the SMAS. With the lateral SMASectomy, a strip of the SMAS overlying the parotid gland is resected. Using large absorbable sutures, the resected edges of the SMAS are joined, thereby elevating the lower portions of the SMAS. Using Baker's technique, the facial nerve is protected by the parotid gland in the area of SMAS resection. More extensive rhytidectomies are performed by creating a limited SMAS flap (conventional SMAS face lift) or an extended SMAS flap. The SMAS flap is created in addition to the skin flap, and is separately repositioned. This process is sometimes referred to as a "deep-plane" rhytidectomy and does require careful localization and avoidance of deep neurovascular structures, such as the facial nerve and its branches.

M. Alam (ed.), *Evidence-Based Procedural Dermatology*,
DOI 10.1007/978-0-387-09424-3_23, © Springer Science+Business Media, LLC 2012

**Table 23.1** Facelift techniques

| Facelift technique | Essential features | Comments |
| --- | --- | --- |
| SMAS plication | Skin flap created. SMAS is folded on itself with no undermining | Straight forward, limited anesthetic requirements |
| Lateral SMASectomy | Skin flap created. SMAS overlying parotid is resected and tightened. No SMAS undermining | Little risk of nerve injury. Limited recovery time |
| SMAS lift (extended/conventional) | Skin flap created. Separate SMAS flap created. Flaps advanced independently | Benefit over plication alone is uncertain Extended SMAS lift enables greater degree of SMAS flap mobility |
| S-lift and variants | Skin flap created. No SMAS undermining. SMAS is plicated with purse string-type sutures | Similar to SMAS plication with sutures elevating the SMAS and platysma. Limited anesthetic requirements |

At the opposite extreme, the continued desire for a less invasive face lift prompted the development of even less minimally invasive approaches than the standard SMAS plication face lift. These so-called "short-scar" or "mini-lifts" include procedures such as Saylan's "S-lift" [3] and Tonnard's "Minimal Access Cranial Suspension" [4]. The common features of these approaches are reliance upon a limited facelift incision, conservative skin flap creation, and the use of sutures in a loop configuration to plicate the deeper tissues.

Two obvious advantages to the short-scar rhytidectomy procedure, compared to the traditional rhytidectomy procedure, are the quicker time to recovery and the potentially decreased expense to the patient. Despite these benefits, an important question is whether the less invasive procedure achieves comparable results. At the time of this writing, there does not exist a consensus statement from a major dermatologic organization offering guidance or direction with regard to the facelift procedure.

## Case Series and Cohort Studies

That being said, a few large retrospective cohort studies and case series assessing safety and efficacy have been published. Tanna and Lindsey [5] have published one of the largest series of short-scar rhytidectomies, in which they assessed their experience of 1,000 short-scar rhytidectomies (V, C). In this study, all patients safely underwent the procedure with local anesthesia. Although one third of patients also required oral sedation, none required general or intravenous anesthesia.

Postoperatively, suture extrusion was the most frequently observed complication, occurring in 148 patients, while hematomas occurred in ten patients. Hyperpigmentation and hypertrophic scarring occurred with an incidence of less than 1%, and there were no episodes of nerve injury, skin flap necrosis, alopecia, or parotid injury. Although the cosmetic results from this series were not systematically analyzed, the authors assert that their patients were pleased with their results. They conclude that the short-scar rhytidectomy is an excellent option for patients with mild to moderate aging of the face.

In addition to large retrospective series assessing face lifts for overall safety and efficacy, in recent years, there have been multiple case series and cohort studies that have examined more specific features of face lifts. These include studies that describe and test novel techniques, improvements upon existing methods, and methods to avoid potential complications.

## Suspension Suture Techniques

One variant of the limited face lift uses suspension sutures to achieve tissue lifting via a minimally invasive approach. Placement of these sutures without necessarily making an incision purports to be not only less time intensive, but also potentially safer than more conventional face lifting. However, there are sparse data confirming the safety, efficacy, and longevity of suspension suture lifts. Table 23.2 summarizes four publications that evaluated suspension sutures.

A retrospective study by Kaminer et al. [6] (V, B) assessed the long-term patient satisfaction

**Table 23.2**  Recent studies on suspension suturing techniques

| Type of suture | References | Level of evidence | Conclusion |
| --- | --- | --- | --- |
| *Contour lift* – Barbed, anchored, unidirectional, nonabsorbable | Kaminer et al. [6] | V, B | The barbed suture lift provides moderate long-term improvement for facial laxity up to 16 months postprocedure |
| *Silhouette suture* – a 3-0 polypropylene suture with ten absorbable hollow cones equally interspersed with knots | Bisaccia et al. [7] | V, B | In appropriately selected patients, excellent correction of ptotic facial and neck tissues was achieved |
| *Monograms suture* – 2-0 absorbable monofilament with 5–9 equally spaced knots through which are secured 7–9 mm bits of 0 thickness similar suture material | Eremia and Willoughby [8] | III, B | In conjunction with open face lifts excellent results are achieved at 1 year. Results from pure suspension lift were lost in 80–100% of patients after 1 year |
| *2-0 Polypropylene* – using a Khawaja–Hernandez or Keith needle | Khawaja and Hernandez-Perez [9] | V, B | Nearly 80% of patients were satisfied with their results at 1 year |

and longevity of improvement following a lifting procedure utilizing barbed, anchored, unidirectional, nonabsorbable sutures. In this series, both patients and independent dermatologists assessed the results after 6 months. Interestingly, patients rated their average satisfaction as 6.9 on a scale of 1–10, while independent scorers rated the average improvement as 4.6 out of 10. This discrepancy prompted the authors to question what defines a successful operation; however, based upon patient satisfaction scores, they advocated the continued use of barbed, anchored, unidirectional, nonabsorbable sutures.

In a case series by Bisaccia et al. [7] (V, B), the Silhouette suture (a 3-0 polypropylene suture with ten absorbable hollow cones equally interspersed with knots) is described for the elevation of sagging tissues of the face and neck. Patients who underwent rhytidectomy with this procedure experienced improvements, leading the authors to conclude that the Silhouette suture will become a useful addition to facial rejuvenation. However, this data was obtained using nonrandom selection techniques and further validation is warranted.

Recently, Eremia and Willoughby [8] (III, B) published a controlled study evaluating the use of the Monogram suture technique. The Monogram suture is a 2-0 absorbable monofilament; in the procedure, 5–9 equally spaced knots are placed to secure 7–9 mm portions of 0 thickness similar

suture material. In this comparative study, one group of patients had suspension suture elevation with no skin excision and the other group had suspension suture elevation in combination with conservative open surgical face lifts. Patients for whom the Monogram suture was used in conjunction with open face lifts experienced excellent results that persisted for up to 1 year. Conversely, the benefits from the pure suspension lift were lost in 80–100% of patients after the 1-year mark.

Khawaja and Hernandez-Perez [9] (V, B) published a series of 19 patients who underwent a transcutaneous face lift. In their procedure, a 2-0 polypropylene suture was anchored to the periosteum of the temporal bone and is then utilized to pull up the SMAS. Follow up was from 6 months to 1 year. Based upon a satisfaction survey, nearly 80% of patients were pleased with their results.

## Minimally Invasive Techniques for Particular Facial Subunits

Traditional facelift procedures address aging associated with the entire face. However, such invasive procedures may not be appropriate for younger patients with specific concerns. Furthermore, avoiding the possible morbidity of an invasive operation is extremely desirable. Limited facelift procedures aimed at addressing

**Table 23.3** Recent studies on facial subunit lifting procedures

| Facial subunit/technique | References | Level of evidence | Conclusion |
| --- | --- | --- | --- |
| *Middle face* – preauricular incision with SMAS plication and removal of skin laxity | Bisaccia et al. [10] | VI, C | Patients are pleased with results, and maintenance of correction achieved with this technique persists up to 2 years |
| *Middle face* – S-lift face lift utilizing purse string sutures placed in SMAS from the zygoma to the jawline | Fulton et al. [3] | VI, C | After a follow-up period of 6 months, there were no episodes of recurrence or skin necrosis |
| *Upper face/brow* – extreme beveled incision 4–5 mm into the anterior hairline, with excision of 1.5–2 cm of excess skin | Niamtu [11] | VI, C | At 30 months, there was no reported relapse; and the use of a beveled incision encourages hair regrowth |

specific facial subunits have been developed to provide patients with tailored results while decreasing overall complications. Table 23.3 summarizes published data pertaining to such procedures.

In 2004, Columbia University published their 2-year experience [10] (VI, C) with 30 patients who underwent a minimally invasive facelift procedure to correct mid-facial aging. Although the results were not systematically analyzed, the authors asserted that most patients were pleased with the results, and maintenance of correction achieved with this technique persisted for up to 2 years. Similarly, Fulton et al. [3] published a series of 23 patients who underwent an S-lift face lift utilizing purse string sutures placed in SMAS from the zygoma to the jaw line (VI, C). They concluded that after a follow-up period of 6 months, there were no episodes of skin necrosis or patients requiring repeat correction.

For patients with specific desires pertaining to upper facial rejuvenation, a subcutaneous brow and forehead lift may be preferable. Niamtu [11] recently published a series of 50 female patients who underwent such a procedure (VI, C). After 30 months, there were no reported cases of relapse, and only two patients experienced flap necrosis. However, it is worth noting that the results were not well categorized or systematized.

## Potential Complications and Avoidance Strategies

A variety of complications are seen in association with rhytidectomy. These include hematoma formation, infection, skin necrosis, disfiguring scar, and alopecia. There is little dermatologic research on estimating the quality and quantity of these risks.

Temporal alopecia resulting from traumatized hair follicles is an unpleasant complication that detracts from the final appearance following rhytidectomy. In an attempt to prevent temporal hair loss, Eremia et al. [12] studied the use of minoxidil (III, B). In their series, 60 women underwent either standard SMAS/flap technique or plication, and were treated with either 2 or 5% topical minoxidil for 2 weeks prior to surgery and 4 weeks postoperatively. Subjects were followed for 3–6 months. The use of minoxidil resulted in a 0% incidence of permanent alopecia, and a 1.7% incidence of temporary alopecia (one patient developed alopecia that resolved upon resuming 5% minoxidil). In comparison, historical controls [13] reported the incidence of temporary alopecia at 8.4%. Therefore, minoxidil appeared to provide a protective benefit when used before and after face lift. However, since the historical controls were from 1977, it is uncertain to what extent the two groups of patients were comparable.

Although alopecia is an upsetting complication of rhytidectomy, hematoma formation may be associated with greater morbidity. Postoperative hematomas can cause facial edema, tissue ischemia, and hyperpigmentation, and may necessitate the placement of drains. Drain placement is not without risk, as drains can serve as a conduit for introduction of bacteria into the wound leading to wound infection and possible scarring. It is therefore desirable to prevent hematomas intraoperatively. Fibrin glue has been widely studied in the plastic surgery community for this purpose. Zoumalan and Rizk [14] studied whether spraying fibrin glue underneath the flap prior to closure reduced hematoma formation (III, B). A significant difference ($p=0.01$) in risk was detected across the two groups (600 patients total) compared in this nonrandomized study, with a notable decrease in hematoma formation with the use of fibrin glue. Patients who did not receive fibrin glue developed hematomas at a rate of 3.4%, compared to 0.4% in those who did receive the fibrin glue. In this study, all the hematomas, from both groups, were minor, managed with needle aspiration, and did not require repeat operation.

## Randomized Controlled Trials and Meta-Analyses

Due to the elective nature of the facelift procedure, patients are reluctant to be randomized to a given treatment modality. Furthermore, the private practice settings in which many of these procedures are performed, and differences in operative technique across surgeons, have impeded the completion of multiple large studies or meta-analyses. Nonetheless, a few such trials have been published, primarily those focusing on the treatment of complications associated with face lifts. This section will discuss their design, conclusions, and limitations.

The first such study, published nearly 15 years ago, randomized 21 patients to undergo limited/conventional SMAS face lift on one side of their face, and extended SMAS/composite rhytidectomy on the other [15] (II, A). In this trial, 20 women and 1 man were enrolled and followed for 1 year postoperatively. The results were photographed and assessed by three independent facelift surgeons, the operating surgeons, and the patients. The specific surgical combinations used in this publication are outlined in Fig. 23.1.

At 24 h postoperatively, there were no noticeable differences between the two facial halves. Additionally, at both 6 months and 1 year follow up, neither the independent surgeon evaluator, nor the operating surgeon, nor the patient, could detect a difference in facelift result between the two sides. The results of this study support the use of less invasive techniques. However, differences may become evident with longer follow up. In a similar, although nonrandomized, study, Prado

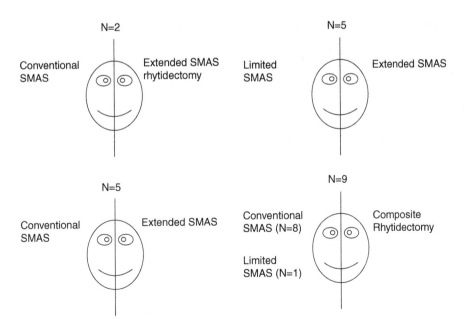

**Fig. 23.1** Treatment arms for a split-face study on face-lifting techniques. Patients were randomized to receive either limited or conventional SMAS face lift on one side of their face, and extended SMAS or composite rhytidectomy on the other [15]

et al. [16] compared the outcomes of minimal access cranial suspension to lateral SMASectomy (III, B). There was no difference in cosmetic results between the two techniques at 1 month and 2 year follow up, but the very long-term persistence of efficacy was not compared.

An additional, prospective, randomized study was undertaken by Owsley et al. [17] to ascertain whether the use of steroid medication could reduce facial edema following facelift surgery (II, A). Fifteen patients were treated with methylprednisolone 500 mg preoperatively followed by a 6-day tapering course. When compared to 15 patients who did not receive steroids, there was no difference in facial edema. The potential risk for decreased wound healing encountered in patients on steroids was not assessed in this chapter. Based upon the equivocal results, steroids may not be routinely recommended as prophylaxis for facial edema reduction.

Finally, in one of the few meta-analyses published pertaining to face lifts, Por et al. [18] (I, A) systematically evaluate the use of tissue sealants in face lifts. The majority of the data is derived from the Plastic Surgery literature; however, the results are revealing. Utilizing Medline, EMBASE, and Cochrane, three randomized controlled studies [19–21] were identified and included for analysis. Although not statistically significant, the use of tissue sealants demonstrated a strong trend toward reduction of postoperative drainage at 24 h and ecchymosis at 1 week. Conversely, tissue sealants did not decrease postoperative edema. These data, combined with the series published by Zoumalan and Rizk [14], strengthen the argument for routinely using tissue sealants intraoperatively during facelift procedures.

The modern face lift is a complex procedure that is continually evolving. Although there is more data regarding face lifting under general anesthesia, there remains little data on the procedure as performed by the dermatologic surgeon. In particular, more research would facilitate the selection of appropriate facelifting procedures for particular indications, and to minimize complications, speed recovery, and provide a long-lasting benefit.

**Evidence-Based Summary**

| Findings | Level of evidence |
|---|---|
| Short-scar rhytidectomy is a safe procedure with a 1% risk of hematoma, and a less than 1% risk of hyperpigmentation, hypertrophic scarring, nerve injury, and skin necrosis | V/B |
| The cosmetic results between limited and conventional face lifts are equivalent | II/A |
| Suspension sutures provide excellent short-term results; however, their long-term efficacy is yet to be proven | III/B |
| Postrhytidectomy temporal alopecia can be avoided with the use of minoxidil | III/B |
| Perioperative steroid administration does not reduce facial edema following rhytidectomy | II/A |
| Fibrin glue may decrease hematoma formation; however, its clinical relevance is not proven | I/A |

# References

1. Webster RC, Smith RC, Smith KF. Face lift, part 3: plication of the superficial musculoaponeurotic system. Head Neck Surg. 1983;6:696–701.
2. Baker DC. Lateral SMASectomy. Plast Reconstr Surg. 1997;100:509–13.
3. Fulton JE, Saylan Z, Helton P, Rahimi AD, Golshani M. The S-lift facelift featuring the U-suture and O-suture combined with skin resurfacing. Dermatol Surg. 2001;27:18–22.
4. Tonnard P et al. Minimal access cranial suspension lift: a modified S-lift. Plast Reconstr Surg. 2002;109: 2074–86.
5. Tanna N, Lindsey WH. Review of 1,000 consecutive short-scar rhytidectomies. Dermatol Surg. 2008;34:196–202. discussion 202–3.
6. Kaminer MS, Bogart M, Choi C, Wee SA. Long-term efficacy of anchored barbed sutures in the face and neck. Dermatol Surg. 2008;34:1041–7.
7. Bisaccia E, Kadry R, Saap L, Rogachefsky A, Scarborough D. A novel specialized suture and inserting device for the resuspension of ptotic facial tissues: early results. Dermatol Surg. 2009;35:645–50.
8. Eremia S, Willoughby MA. Novel face-lift suspension suture and inserting instrument: use of large anchors knotted into a suture with attached needle and inserting device allowing for single entry point placement of suspension suture. Preliminary report of 20 cases with 6-to 12-month follow-up. Dermatol Surg. 2006;32:335–45.
9. Khawaja HA, Hernandez-Perez E. Transcutaneous face-lift. Dermatol Surg. 2005;31:453–7.
10. Bisaccia E, Khan AJ, Scarborough DA. Anterior face-lift for correction of middle face aging utilizing a minimally invasive technique. Dermatol Surg. 2004; 30:769–76.
11. Niamtu III J. The subcutaneous brow- and forehead-lift: a face-lift for the forehead and brow. Dermatol Surg. 2008;34:1350–61. discussion 1362.
12. Eremia S, Umar SH, Li CY. Prevention of temporal alopecia following rhytidectomy: the prophylactic use of minoxidil. A study of 60 patients. Dermatol Surg. 2002;28:66–74.
13. Leist FD, Masson JK, Erich JB. A review of 324 rhytidectomies, emphasizing complications and patient dissatisfaction. Plast Reconstr Surg. 1977;59:525–9.
14. Zoumalan R, Rizk SS. Hematoma rates in drainless deep-plane face-lift surgery with and without the use of fibrin glue. Arch Facial Plast Surg. 2008;10: 103–7.
15. Ivy EJ, Lorenc ZP, Aston SJ. Is there a difference? A prospective study comparing lateral and standard SMAS face lifts with extended SMAS and composite rhytidectomies. Plast Reconstr Surg. 1996;98:1135–43. discussion 1144–7.
16. Prado A, Andrades P, Danilla S, Castillo P, Leniz P. A clinical retrospective study comparing two short-scar face lifts: minimal access cranial suspension versus lateral SMASectomy. Plast Reconstr Surg. 2006;117:1413–25. discussion 1426–7.
17. Owsley JQ, Weibel TJ, Adams WA. Does steroid medication reduce facial edema following face lift surgery? A prospective, randomized study of 30 consecutive patients. Plast Reconstr Surg. 1996;98:1–6.
18. Por YC, Shi L, Samuel M, Song C, Yeow VK. Use of tissue sealants in face-lifts: a metaanalysis. Aesthetic Plast Surg. 2009;33:336–9.
19. Marchac D, Greensmith AL. Early postoperative efficacy of fibrin glue in face lifts: a prospective randomized trial. Plast Reconstr Surg. 2005;115:911–6. discussion 917–8.
20. Oliver DW, Hamilton SA, Figle AA, Wood SH, Lamberty BG. A prospective, randomized, double-blind trial of the use of fibrin sealant for face lifts. Plast Reconstr Surg. 2001;108:2101–5. discussion 2106–7.
21. Powell DM, Chang E, Farrior EH. Recovery from deep-plane rhytidectomy following unilateral wound treatment with autologous platelet gel: a pilot study. Arch Facial Plast Surg. 2001;3:245–50.

## Self-Assessment

1. Which of the following are true of the SMAS plication?
   (a) It must be performed under general anesthesia
   (b) It involves extensive dissection and mobilization of the sub-superficial musculoaponeurotic system structures, such as the facial nerve
   (c) It is a complicated, and difficult to learn procedure
   (d) The procedure relies upon folding the SMAS in upon itself and securing it without additional undermining

2. What distinguishes the SMAS plication from the lateral SMASectomy?
   (a) In the lateral SMASectomy, there is undermining of the SMAS
   (b) In the lateral SMASectomy, a strip of the SMAS overlying the parotid gland is resected
   (c) In the lateral SMASectomy, the facial nerve is divided
   (d) In the lateral SMASectomy, no effort is made to elevate the lower portions of the SMAS

3. The most frequently reported complication following short-scar rhytidectomies is?
   (a) Suture extrusion
   (b) Hematomas
   (c) Hyperpigmentation and hypertrophic scarring
   (d) Nerve injury

4. Which of the following is true regarding the Silhouette suture?
   (a) It is a barbed, anchored, unidirectional, nonabsorbable suture
   (b) It is 2-0 absorbable monofilament with 5–9 equally spaced knots through which are secured 7–9 mm bits of 0 thickness similar suture material
   (c) It is a 3-0 polypropylene suture with ten absorbable hollow cones equally interspersed with knots
   (d) It is a multidirectional suture

5. What methods have been described to prevent temporal alopecia resulting from traumatized hair follicles following rhytidectomy?
   (a) Either 2 or 5% topical minoxidil for 2 weeks prior to surgery and 4 weeks postoperatively
   (b) Phototherapy
   (c) Ethanol injection
   (d) Topical steroids

## Answers

1. d: The procedure relies upon folding the SMAS in upon itself and securing it without additional undermining.

   When performing the SMAS plication, the SMAS is folded upon itself and secured, without additional undermining. A primary advantage to this approach is that there are minimal complications as the sub-SMAS structures, including the facial nerve, are left undisturbed and intact. This is a straight forward procedure with limited anesthetic requirements.

2. b: In the lateral SMASectomy, a strip of the SMAS overlying the parotid gland is resected.

   The lateral SMASectomy approach is similar to plication in that there is no undermining of the SMAS. With the lateral SMASectomy, a strip of the SMAS overlying the parotid gland is resected. Effort is made to elevate the lower portions of the SMAS. The facial nerve is protected by the parotid gland in the area of SMAS resection.

3. a: Suture extrusion

   Postoperatively after short-scar rhytidectomies, suture extrusion was the most frequently observed complication, while hematomas occurred in 1% of patients. Hyperpigmentation and hypertrophic scarring occurred with an incidence of less than 1%, and there were no episodes of nerve injury, skin flap necrosis, alopecia, or parotid injury reported in the series from Tanna and Lindsey.

4. c: It is a 3-0 polypropylene suture with ten absorbable hollow cones equally interspersed with knots.

   The Silhouette suture is a 3-0 polypropylene suture with ten absorbable hollow cones equally interspersed with knots described for the elevation of sagging tissues of the face and neck.

   The contour lift suture is a barbed, anchored, unidirectional, nonabsorbable suture.

   The monograms suture is 2-0 absorbable monofilament with 5–9 equally spaced knots through which are secured 7–9 mm bits of 0 thickness similar suture material.

5. a: Either 2 or 5% topical minoxidil for 2 weeks prior to surgery and 4 weeks postoperatively.

   Eremia and colleagues studied the use of minoxidil. Subjects were followed for 3–6 months. The use of minoxidil resulted in a 0% incidence of permanent alopecia, and a 1.7% incidence of temporary alopecia. In comparison, historical controls reported the incidence of temporary alopecia at 8.4%. Therefore, minoxidil appeared to provide a protective benefit when used before and after face lift.

# Blepharoplasty

Anjali Butani

## Introduction and Definition

The recent popularity of cosmetic surgery has cultivated a renewed interest in understanding the components of the aging face. While much attention has focused on the glabellar complex and the lower third of the face, the periorbital region continues to play an important role in facial rejuvenation.

The upper third of the face, consisting of the forehead, eyebrows, upper and lower eyelids, and eyes, typically displays characteristics of aging before the middle and lower thirds of the face. These changes include lowering of the brow and the development of dermatochalasis of the upper eyelid. Flattening of the lateral brow results in lateral hooding. Canthal laxity may arise along with lateral canthal descent, leading to a decreased canthal tilt angle and shortening of the horizontal palpebral fissure. Fat pseudoherniation or atrophy can occur. Malar fat pad descent results in the secondary appearance of a nasojugal groove. Rhytids appear over the forehead, glabella, and lateral periorbital region. The skin may become dyspigmented. Overall, there is a relative ptosis of the anatomical structures, a loss of the convexity of the eyelids and a perceived smaller appearance of the globe. These changes can vary from being extremely subtle to being incredibly prominent.

Of these indicative signs of aging, changes in the eyelids have received the most attention from patients. Patients with eyelid dermatochalasis, lateral hooding and fat pseudoherniation often seek medical advice for appearing fatigued, sad, or older than their actual age. Blepharoplasty can correct for these changes and restore a more alert and youthful appearance.

Blepharoplasty continues to be one of the most popular cosmetic surgery procedures. The minimally invasive nature of the procedure, relatively short recovery time and rare incidence of complications make blepharoplasty an appealing choice for both patients and surgeons. According to a 2006 survey by the American Academy of Facial Plastic and Reconstructive Surgery, blepharoplasty represented the most common cosmetic surgical procedure performed on women, while it was the third most common cosmetic surgical procedure in men (VI/C) [1].

Blepharoplasty is generally performed as an outpatient procedure. Both upper and lower blepharoplasty begins with a thorough periorbital evaluation. A detailed ophthalmologic history should be obtained. Many surgeons require a full ophthalmologic examination by an ophthalmologist prior to operating. Medical conditions, especially those that may be contributing to the changing periorbital anatomy or may affect surgical outcome, should be reviewed.

A. Butani (✉)
Butani Dermatology, 170 South Main Street, Suite 200, Orange, CA 92868, USA
e-mail: ButaniDerm@gmail.com

M. Alam (ed.), *Evidence-Based Procedural Dermatology*,
DOI 10.1007/978-0-387-09424-3_24, © Springer Science+Business Media, LLC 2012

Prior to the procedure, standard photographs are taken. A gentle antiseptic agent is used to clean the surgical site. Areas of excessive skin and fat prolapse are marked with sterile marking ink. The area is then anesthetized with a local injection of 1 or 2% lidocaine with or without epinephrine. Some surgeons may give an oral sedative, such as clonidine or diazepam, or use intravenous conscious sedation for additional comfort.

In its simplest form, upper eyelid blepharoplasty is performed by excising redundant skin. Along with the skin, a variable amount of orbicularis oculi muscle is sometimes also removed. Various modalities can be used to perform this excision, including cold steel scalpel, radiofrequency devices, electrocautery, and $CO_2$ laser. If there is protrusion of the upper lid fat pads, these fat pads can be destroyed after exposing them by making a small incision through the orbital septum. Some literature suggests gentle pressure applied to the globe may induce herniation through a surgically weakened orbital septum. After hemostasis is achieved, the site is closed with sutures, glue, or steristrips, depending on the surgeon's preference.

Lower eyelid blepharoplasty can be performed using two distinct techniques. The transcutaneous method involves excising redundant skin with a subciliary incision under the lower eyelash line. After removal of the skin-orbicularis oculi muscle flap, pseudoherniated fat pads can be removed by incising through the orbital septum and destroying them. The transconjunctival technique involves a retroseptal approach. The lower eyelid is retracted in a superolateral fashion with a Desmarres retractor while using a nonconductive eyelid plate (Pyrex plate or Jaeger plate) to protect the globe. An incision is made in the tarsoconjunctival aspect of the lower tarsal plate. The lower eyelid fat pads herniate through this incision. Impeccable hemostasis should be attained when employing either lower eyelid blepharoplasty technique.

Currently, there are no meta-analyses available on this procedure. There are also no consensus statements available through the American Academy of Dermatology, American Society for Dermatologic Surgery, American Academy of Cosmetic Surgery, American Society of Plastic Surgeons, American Society of Ophthalmic Plastic and Reconstructive Surgery (ASOPRS), or the American Academy of Facial Plastic and Reconstructive Surgery. This is expected as there are few controversies regarding the procedure. A report by the American Academy of Ophthalmology and a practice parameter by the American Society of Plastic Surgeons are discussed below.

The remainder of the chapter is divided into different aspects of blepharoplasty, as many published works address similar issues.

## Indications

Blepharoplasty is typically performed as an elective procedure for those who desire a more youthful or less fatigued appearance [2, 3].

In 1995, the American Academy of Ophthalmology defined the functional indications for upper and lower blepharoplasty. The Committee on Ophthalmic Procedures Assessment reported the most common functional indication for upper blepharoplasty is a superior visual field defect secondary to dermatochalasis of the eyelid, with redundant tissue extending inferiorly past the eyelid margin. Functional blepharoplasty may also be required for treatment of trauma. In addition, blepharoplasty may be necessary to treat the resulting changes of inflammatory disorders of the orbit and eyelids. The lower eyelid may need functional blepharoplasty in cases of significant eyelid edema resulting from medications or metabolic and inflammatory disorders. Entropion (inversion of the eyelid margin) and epiblepharon (a congenital lid anomaly in which a fold of pretarsal skin and underlying orbicularis oculi muscle force the lashes against the cornea) may also require functional correction of the eyelid (VI/C) [4]. The American Society of Plastic Surgeons Practice Parameter for Blepharoplasty also includes ptosis, floppy eyelid syndrome, and herniated orbital fat as reasons for functional blepharoplasty. In addition, blepharochalasis (chronic recurrent edema of the eyelids with subsequent degeneration of the internal eyelid structures and laxity of the eyelid) is also an indication for surgical correction of the eyelid (VI/C) [3].

Rizk and Matarasso [5] conducted a retrospective study of 100 patients to analyze the indications and treatment of lower eyelid blepharoplasty. They concluded that orbicularis oculi muscle hypertrophy is also an absolute indication for lower lid transcutaneous blepharoplasty as this requires resection of the preseptal orbicularis muscle (V/B).

## Preoperative Evaluation

The preoperative evaluation should include a thorough medical history. A review by Trussler and Rohrich [6] recommends the history also include a lifestyle history. History of chronic illnesses, hypertension, diabetes mellitus, cardiac disease, bleeding or hematologic disorders, and thyroid disturbances should be documented. Previous surgeries and medications, especially those that affect bleeding, should be reviewed. A proper ophthalmologic history should include information on vision, prior trauma, glaucoma, allergic reactions, and problems with dry eyes or excessive tearing. Patients must be asked about prior laser-assisted in situ keratomileusis (LASIK) and other similar refractive surgeries. The authors recommend no cosmetic surgery of the periorbital region be performed in the 6 months following refractory surgery, given the increased incidence of postblepharoplasty dry-eye syndrome and related visual changes. They also recommend patients with dry eyes should be referred to an ophthalmologist for a Schirmer's test (VI/C).

Alterations in tear secretion and tear film stability after LASIK and subsequent blepharoplasty were studied by Griffin et al. [7]. They performed blepharoplasty on nine patients that had undergone bilateral LASIK in the previous 18 months. This group was compared to a control group of nine patients with no history of LASIK, dry eyes, or contact lens use. The authors found no statistically significant difference in tear characteristics after blepharoplasty between both groups. They concluded that blepharoplasty may be performed after LASIK after an interval of time (III/B).

The role of the Schirmer's test in predicting the development of dry-eye syndrome following blepharoplasty was evaluated by Rees and LaTrenta [8] in a prospective analysis of 100 patients. Because blepharoplasty can mechanically alter eyelid closure and impair the lubricating mechanism, subclinical dry-eye syndrome is an important consideration in any patient contemplating blepharoplasty, especially those with morphologically prone eyes. The authors found the Schirmer's test could not reliably predict the development of postoperative dry-eye syndrome. They state the morphology of the orbit is a more reliable indicator to signal the predilection to develop this complication (V/B).

Many surgeons require a full preoperative ophthalmologic exam to assess visual fields, visual acuity, adequacy of the tear film, functionality of the periocular muscles, and underlying glaucoma or macular disease.

Trussler and Rohrich [6] recommend a detailed periorbital physical examination. This should include evaluation of the surrounding skeletal support and any degree of brow ptosis. The amount of upper and lower eyelid dermatochalasis and lateral hooding should be noted. The eyelid should be evaluated, including ptosis of the lid, the angle of the lateral canthal tilt, and lower lid laxity. Hypertrophy or relaxation of the orbicularis oculi, fat herniation, and any asymmetry of the eyes should be noted (VI/C).

## Preoperative Markings

Fincher and Moy [9] summarized the steps of preoperative markings in their comprehensive review on cosmetic blepharoplasty. Preoperative markings should be performed with the patient sitting up with the eyebrows in a neutral position. The inferior incision markings for an upper blepharoplasty excision are placed in the position of the future pretarsal crease. The superior incision markings are determined by using the pinch test. Progressively more tissue is grasped using the pinch test method until the upper eyelashes begin to evert (VI/C).

**Table 24.1** Cutting devices used for blepharoplasty: evidence-based advantages and disadvantages

| $CO_2$ laser | Colorado needle | Radiofrequency (RF) | Cold steel scalpel |
|---|---|---|---|
| Advantages | | | |
| Simultaneous incision and hemostasis | Simultaneous incision and hemostasis | Simultaneous incision and hemostasis | Decreased inflammation |
| Improved intraoperative visibility | Decreased operative time | Decreased collateral damage | Allows tactile feedback |
| Decreased operative time | Decreased thermal damage | Allows tactile feedback | |
| Decreased collateral damage | Allows tactile feedback | | |
| Increased patient comfort | | | |
| Decreased ecchymosis/edema | | | |
| Decreased recuperation time | | | |
| Disadvantages | | | |
| Possible increased inflammation | | | Requires separate device to achieve hemostasis |
| No tactile feedback | | | |

## Postoperative Care

Postoperative management varies greatly according to the surgeon's preference. A review by Rohrich et al. [2] recommends the use of a chilled light gel compress, saline eye drops, and lubricating eye ointment. Antibiotic eye drops may be used prophylactically. The patient's head should be elevated. The authors note that lagophthalmos resolves in 1–2 weeks and is generally due to postoperative periorbital edema. Consistent use of eye drops and lubricating eye ointment is necessary to prevent corneal abrasions during this time (VI/C).

## Techniques

Blepharoplasty can be performed using a number of cutting devices. Each instrument offers its own advantages and disadvantages, as listed in Table 24.1. Blepharoplasty with a cold steel scalpel was discussed by Coleman [10]. The author points out that while there may be less bleeding during the incision with laser blepharoplasty, whether this results in less postoperative bruising has not been determined. A cutting laser creates a controlled burn with increased inflammation compared to the minimal inflammatory response of a scalpel (VI/C). A review by Gladstone [11] notes that lasers are associated with greater hemostasis and less collateral damage (VI/C).

The $CO_2$ laser was compared to cold steel by David and Sanders [12]. Thirteen patients were studied. Eyes were randomly assigned to each device. The laser resulted in reduced operative time, less bleeding, and decreased ecchymosis and edema. Scars were indistinguishable at 30 days in both groups (II/A). Morrow and Morrow [13] conducted a similar randomized study between $CO_2$ laser blepharoplasty and cold steel blepharoplasty. No difference in healing was appreciated with either method. In addition to the previously mentioned advantages of the laser technique, the authors noted superior intraoperative visibility, increased patient comfort, and shorter recuperation time with the laser (II/A).

Biesman [14] has published a similar review comparing the $CO_2$ laser with cold steel for blepharoplasty. The author believes the laser offers the advantage of improved efficiency as the handpiece acts as a cutting tool, a blunt dissection device, and a cautery unit (VI/C). In this work, Biesman also summarized his prospective multicenter study which compared laser surgery directly to cold steel surgery. Although no significant difference in swelling or wound appearance was found, surgeons preferred using the laser for its improved hemostasis.

Laser blepharoplasty with the $CO_2$ laser was compared with a diamond laser scalpel in a randomized control trial of ten patients by Baker et al. [15]. Each eyelid was assigned to each technique. Masked observers found no statistically significant difference in outcome between the two sides. The author did note that compared to the free beam $CO_2$ laser, the diamond laser scalpel provides subtle tactile feedback to surgeons and allows the ability to incise with varying levels of hemostasis (II/A).

The short pulse $CO_2$ laser was compared to the Colorado needle tip with electrocautery in a randomized trial by Rokhsar et al. [16]. Twelve patients were studied. Mean intraoperative time with the Colorado needle was shorter. Histologic examination revealed less thermal damage of the tissue harvested with the Colorado needle. However, no difference in healing parameters was noted by patient or physician 1 month postoperatively. The Colorado needle offers the advantages of the short pulse $CO_2$ laser along with greater tactile feedback (II/A).

A review of laser blepharoplasty by Lessner and Fagien [17] found the same advantages to the laser technique as mentioned above. The authors caution surgeons to remove less skin during blepharoplasty if resurfacing is planned for the same site as thermal collagen contracture will occur after laser resurfacing (VI/C).

A randomized control trial of 30 patients was conducted by Niamtu [18] to compare a radiowave device with an ultrapulse $CO_2$ laser for upper blepharoplasty. Each eye was randomly treated with one modality. Five blinded board-certified surgeons could not appreciate any statistically significant difference in scar quality at 12 months. The author concluded that both devices incise and provide coagulation simultaneously, minimize collateral damage, and produce indistinguishable scars (II/A).

Radiosurgery was compared with conventional scalpel surgery in opposite eyelids by Ritland et al. [19]. This prospective study of 13 patients found better wound healing and a higher Hollander score at 1 week ($p = 0.014$) with radiosurgery, but no statistically significant difference at 3 months (V/B).

Gladstone [11] examined the two parallel approaches to lower blepharoplasty. An unpublished review of 4,460 transcutaneous blepharoplasty cases and 3,438 transconjunctival blepharoplasties was discussed. Malposition of the lid was the most frequently reported complication associated with the transcutaneous approach, occurring in 1.4% of patients vs. 0.7% with the transconjunctival technique. Patients who underwent transconjunctival blepharoplasty experienced considerably more edema, 18.4 vs. 0.2% for the contrasting method (VI/C).

A review of 1,340 transconjunctival lower eyelid laser blepharoplasty cases in Asian patients by Kim et al. [20] also reported edema as the most common complication. Approximately, 90% of patients between the ages of 20–30 reported good to excellent results with this technique, while only 74% of those over the age of 40 gave the same rating (V/B) [20].

Baylis et al. [21] reviewed 122 patients who underwent transconjunctival blepharoplasty. The main complication was under-excision of fat (7.4%). The authors had no cases of lower lid retraction, the most common complication of the transcutaneous technique. A more recent review of the literature by Baylis et al. [22] also reports inadequate removal of fat as the most common complication after transconjunctival blepharoplasty, occurring in as many as 20% of cases. The author advises patients that the goal of lower blepharoplasty is to remove 90% of the excess fat (VI/C).

Griffin et al. [23] performed a randomized control trial of 36 patients to compare transcutaneous blepharoplasty without resurfacing to transconjunctival blepharoplasty with resurfacing. The study found no statistically significant difference in lower lid bulging and wrinkles between the two groups. Lateral lid rounding with scleral show and ectropion developed in 3.2% of the transcutaneous patients. The authors point out that the main advantages of the transconjunctival technique, namely lack of eyelid malposition and visible scar formation, can become a concern when transconjunctival surgery is combined with adjuvant $CO_2$ laser resurfacing or chemical peels (II/A).

Rizk and Matarasso [5] reported that the transconjunctival approach for lower eyelid blepharoplasty avoids damage to the orbital septum as compared to the transcutaneous approach. In addition to trauma to the septum, the transcutaneous technique may lead to denervation with consequent retraction, scarring, and rounding of the eye and scleral show, even with conservative technique. However, the transconjunctival approach limits the surgeon's ability to address redundant skin (V/B). Castro [24] conducted a similar prospective study of 100 lower eyelid blepharoplasty cases. The transcutaneous approach (with and without canthopexy) was compared to the transconjunctival approach (with and without fat removal and canthopexy). The author found that each patient's treatment must be individually tailored (V/B).

A modified transconjunctival approach was introduced in a review of 300 patients by Perkins et al. [25]. The authors advocate an initial incision through the conjunctiva, followed by separation of the orbicularis muscle from the orbital septum in an anterior approach (V/B).

Kim and Bucky [26] published a retrospective review of 71 patients who underwent pinch blepharoplasty of the lower lid, a technique which does not involve skin undermining. The authors believe the avoidance of undermining leads to less potential for contraction and, therefore, less postoperative lower lid malposition. As the incidence of lower lid malposition after conventional transcutaneous blepharoplasty is reported to be 15–20%, this method offers an alternative to the standard technique. Their study also found that the pinch method allows resection of more skin and allows the addition of simultaneous laser resurfacing (V/B).

A randomized control trial by Greene et al. [27] assessed the efficacy of octyl-2-cyanoacrylate tissue glue in blepharoplasty against traditional running suture closure. Twenty upper blepharoplasty patients were studied. One surgical site was closed with tissue glue; the opposite incision was closed with running suture. Five blinded observers did not find any statistically significant difference in wound quality using a visual analog scale and modified Hollander scale. No significant difference was found in duration of healing, inflammation, and wound complications. The authors conclude that octyl-2-cyanoacrylate glue is an excellent alternative to suture closure. Tissue glue did not result in any inflammatory complications and withstood the forces of closure (II/A).

Scaccia et al. [28] conducted a prospective study of 30 patients to compare subcuticular closure using 5-0 polypropylene suture with running 6-0 fast-absorbing catgut suture for approximation after blepharoplasty. Both materials resulted in comparable morbidity and postoperative discomfort levels (V/B).

Blepharoplasty of the Asian eyelid requires an understanding of the particular anatomy of the Asian eyelid and the use of modified techniques. A review by Kim and Bhatki [29] summarized the unique features of blepharoplasty in the Asian eyelid as the following: the Asian lid contains an increased amount of preseptal fat, the characteristics of the superior palpebral fold vary considerably in Asian patients and many Asian patients have a medial epicanthal fold (VI/C).

## Complications

Morax and Touitou [30], Glavas [31] and Fulton [32] have published reviews on the complications of blepharoplasty. Although complications are rare, surgeons should be aware of expected inherent tissue reactions and true complications. Table 24.2 is a comprehensive list of the known complications. Ocular complications include diplopia, keratoconjunctivitis sicca, chemosis, blurred vision, changes in visual acuity, epiphora, and dry-eye syndrome. Structural complications include ptosis, lagophthalmos, ectropion, enophthalmia, scleral show, round eye, asymmetry, lacrimal gland prolapse, eyelid fold abnormalities, and superior sulcus syndrome. Hematoma, retrobulbar hemorrhage, ecchymosis, wound dehiscence, abnormal scarring/webbing, infection, and undercorrections can also occur (VI/C).

The most dreaded complication of blepharoplasty is retrobulbar hemorrhage with blindness. DeMere et al. reported the incidence of this complication as 0.04% [33]. More recently, Hass et al. [34] conducted an analysis of 237 questionnaires completed by members of the ASOPRS. They found the incidence of orbital hemorrhage after cosmetic eyelid surgery is 0.055% (1:2,000). The incidence of hemorrhage with permanent visual loss is 0.0045% (1:22,000). The authors

**Table 24.2** Complications of blepharoplasty

| Ocular | Structural | Vascular | Wound healing | Infection | Other |
|---|---|---|---|---|---|
| Blindness | Eyelid ptosis | Retrobulbar hematoma | Wound dehiscence | Cellulitis | Inadequate fat removal |
| Blurred vision | Lagophthalmos | Hemorrhage | Abnormal scarring | Abscess | Allergic reaction |
| Change in visual acuity | Lower lid retraction | Ecchymosis | Epicanthus | Necrotizing fasciitis | Pyogenic granuloma |
| Chemosis/conjunctivitis | Ectropion | Edema | Hypertrophic scar | | Lipogranuloma |
| Diplopia | Enophthalmia | Optic nerve infarction | Altered pigmentation | | Cysts |
| Dry-eye syndrome | Scleral show | | | | |
| Glaucoma | Round eye | | | | |
| Epiphora | Asymmetry | | | | |
| Myopic changes | Lacrimal gland prolapse | | | | |
| Grave's orbitopathy | Eyefold abnormalities | | | | |
| Ophthalmoplegia | Superior sulcus syndrome | | | | |
| Keratopathy | | | | | |

recommend that physicians remain available for at least 24 h after surgery as the majority of cases occur in the immediate postoperative period (VI/C).

Delayed cases have been reported and surgeons should be cognizant of this complication even 2 weeks after initial surgery. Cruz et al. [35] published a case of hematoma and vision loss 7 days after surgery (V/B). Teng et al. [36] reported a case of retrobulbar hemorrhage resulting in permanent visual field loss 9 days after upper blepharoplasty (V/B). Yachouh et al. [37] recommend testing visual acuity prior to surgery and specifically stating blindness as a complication in the informed consent (V/B).

A suspicion of orbital hemorrhage and/or vision loss should not be taken lightly. Total vascular insufficiency of 60–120 min can produce permanent visual loss. Presenting signs include eye pain, pressure, loss of vision, diplopia, nausea, vomiting, proptosis, dilated or unresponsive pupils, limited extraocular movement, and lid ecchymosis [34, 38, 39]. A review of retrobulbar hematoma and blepharoplasty by Wolfort et al. [40] also includes scintillating scotomas, chemosis, hemianopsia, amaurosis fugax, loss of light perception, retinal or optic disc pallor, increased intraocular pressure, and scleral hematoma as alarming signs

**Table 24.3** Retrobulbar hematoma: signs and symptoms

| Signs and symptoms | |
|---|---|
| Blindness | Increased intraocular pressure |
| Change in visual acuity | Dilated/unresponsive pupils |
| Loss of light perception | Limited extraocular movement |
| Ocular pain | Scintillating scotoma |
| Ocular pressure | Amaurosis fugax |
| Diplopia | Scleral hematoma |
| Proptosis | Retinal/optic disc pallor |
| Lid ecchymosis | Hemianopsia |
| Chemosis | Nausea/vomiting |

(VI/C). A summary of the signs and symptoms of a retrobulbar hematoma is provided in Table 24.3.

Comorbidities associated with orbital hemorrhage include hypertension, postoperative vomiting or coughing, aspirin use, increased physical activity, history of vascular disease, bleeding disorders, and glaucoma.

The exact mechanism of retrobulbar hemorrhage is unknown. The most accepted theory is that the posterior orbital vessels are damaged from excessive traction during anterior fat excision. Gentle handling to avoid traction injury is therefore advised [34, 40]. Other possible mechanisms of hemorrhage include: failure to cauterize excised

**Table 24.4** Management of retrobulbar hematoma

| Medical | Surgical | Adjuvant |
|---|---|---|
| Mannitol | Hemostasis | Remove dressing |
| Acetazolamide | Hematoma drainage | Remove sutures |
| IV steroids | Lateral canthotomy | Ophthalmology consult |
| Steroid eyedrops | Lateral orbitotomy | Elevate head |
| Beta-blocking eyedrops | Bony orbital decompression | Irrigate eyes |
| 95% $O_2$/5% $CO_2$ | Anterior chamber paracentesis[a] | |

[a]Controversial

fat pads, rebound vasodilation after epinephrine is metabolized, oozing from incised orbicularis muscle, increased vascular pressure with Valsalva maneuver, damage to neovascularization from previous orbital surgery, and delayed fibrinolysis of a clot.

The mechanism of blindness following retrobulbar hemorrhage is also poorly understood. Potential mechanisms of visual loss include retinal ischemia caused by central retinal artery occlusion or compression from hemorrhage, optic nerve ischemia caused by compression of nutrient vessels or direct pressure from hemorrhage, and vasospasm of vessels from local anesthetic and optic nerve damage from blood waste products [31, 34, 39–43]. Increased intraocular pressure can also precipitate acute angle-closure glaucoma in susceptible individuals.

Many believe damage to the optic nerve plays a greater role in visual loss than damage from central retinal artery occlusion [40, 41]. Anderson and Edwards [41] performed electrophysiologic studies which support this idea. The data reveal the nutrient vessels to the optic nerve are more easily compromised than the central retinal artery and are therefore more likely to be responsible for visual loss (V/B). Goldberg et al. [42] also confirmed optic nerve damage on electrophysiologic studies in two cases of visual loss after blepharoplasty. Central retinal artery occlusion was not found (V/B). Good et al. [43] demonstrated infarction of the posterior intraorbital optic nerve on MRI (V/B).

Brancato et al. [44] reported a sudden drop in visual acuity after central retinal artery occlusion presumably secondary to injection of lidocaine without epinephrine in the surrounding vascular

arcade (V/B). Kelly and May [38] published an analogous case of central retinal artery occlusion after blepharoplasty. The authors advise surgeons to perform meticulous dissection and achieve complete hemostasis intraoperatively (V/B). The authors also warn against postoperative dressings, stating dressings can raise intraorbital pressure and can obstruct postoperative observation, which can lead to a delay in detecting vision loss.

In addition to blindness associated with retrobulbar hemorrhage, the ASOPRS questionnaire analysis found visual loss in the absence of orbital hemorrhage in 0.003% of cases [34]. Kordic et al. [45] presented such a case of visual deterioration after blepharoplasty in which no hemorrhage was found on MRI. The authors attribute the visual changes to perioperative ischemic posterior optic neuropathy (V/B).

Treatment of intraorbital hemorrhage requires immediate intervention. Table 24.4 summarizes the medical, surgical, and adjuvant treatment options in the management of a retrobulbar hematoma. Initial measures include obtaining an ophthalmology consult, removing dressings/sutures, and keeping the head elevated. Medical therapy includes medications aimed at lowering intraocular pressure such as mannitol, acetazolamide, steroids, and beta-blocking eye drops. The wound should be explored, any hematoma should be evacuated, and meticulous hemostasis of active bleeding sites must be achieved. Lateral canthotomy, bony orbital decompression, anterior chamber paracentesis, and lateral orbitotomy may be necessary (VI/C) [30–32, 42].

Lagophthalmos can occur as a consequence of unintentional removal of an excessive amount of upper eyelid skin. This condition can lead to

**Table 24.5** Management of chemosis

| Medical | Surgical | Adjuvant |
|---|---|---|
| Moisturizing eyedrops | Conjunctivotomy | Cool compress |
| Lubricating ointment | Tarsorrhaphy | Ice packs |
| Decongestant eyedrops | | Massage |
| Steroid eyedrops | | Head elevation |
| Oral steroids | | Eye pressure |
| | | Eye patching |

keratopathy, corneal infection, and loss of vision. Shorr et al. [46] published a retrospective analysis of 20 patients after upper eyelid skin grafting for the treatment of lagophthalmos. Skin grafts were placed in the supraciliary position. A mean improvement of 2 mm of lagophthalmos was observed. Keratopathy improved in 71% of patients. Evaluating surgeons found the grafts to have excellent color match (84%) and overall appearance (81%). Grafts from the posterior auricular skin gave the best cosmetic result. The authors recommend placing the graft over the pretarsal orbicularis, immobilizing the graft with a bolster dressing, thinning the tissue as necessary, sizing the graft exactly to the recipient site, and approximating wound edges with care (V/B).

Temporary paresis or permanent paralysis of the extraocular muscles may occur after blepharoplasty. Diplopia is the presenting symptom. Proposed mechanisms include dysfunction due to intramuscular hemorrhage or edema, structural damage from cautery or excision of the muscle, scar tissue development, aggressive removal of fat, entrapment of the muscle, and pressure injury from extramuscular hematoma. Kushner and Jethani [47] published a case series focusing on superior oblique injury from blepharoplasty. They note the superior oblique muscle tendon may be damaged from surgery in the medial aspect of the upper eyelid (V/B). Ghabrial et al. [48] published a series of six patients presenting with diplopia. The inferior rectus, inferior oblique, and lateral rectus were involved (V/B). Mazow et al. [49] presented a case of scar and fat surrounding the medial rectus (V/B). Jameson et al. [50] published a similar case of fat adherence on the inferior rectus simulating inferior oblique palsy (V/B). Alfonso et al. [51] presented a case of inferior rectus paresis after secondary

blepharoplasty (V/B). A related case report by Schlenker and Slavin [52] involved acute postoperative proptosis due to intramuscular inferior rectus hematoma (V/B). These cases illustrate that surgeons must consider the anatomy of the globe and understand which muscles are vulnerable when using different techniques.

Weinfield et al. [53] conducted a retrospective review of 312 bilateral lower transcutaneous blepharoplasties to study postoperative chemosis. The incidence of chemosis after lower lid blepharoplasty was 11.5%. The majority of cases presented intraoperatively or up to 1 week following the procedure. Associated factors included conjunctival exposure intraoperatively, lagophthalmos from upper lid surgery or brow lift, periorbital or facial edema, and lymphatic dysfunction. Although most cases resolved spontaneously, a treatment protocol was defined in the following progressive manner: ophthalmic lubricating ointment, ocular decongestants, ophthalmic steroid drops/ointment, eye patch, eye patch with bandage, conjunctivotomy and/or tarsorrhaphy, and oral steroids (V/B). Table 24.5 reviews the treatment options for blepharoplasty-induced chemosis. Enzer and Shorr [54] described three cases of persistent conjunctival prolapse after both transconjunctival and transcutaneous blepharoplasty, challenging the notion that chemosis only occurs with extensive manipulation of the tissue. The authors urge surgeons to ask about prior episodes of chemosis in the preoperative assessment (V/B).

Acute angle-closure glaucoma is a serious complication of blepharoplasty. Bleyen et al. [55] reported two cases of painful eyes, decreased visual acuity, and increased intraocular pressure after surgery (V/B). Wride and Sanders [56] described a case of acute angle-closure glaucoma that progressed to blindness. Risk factors include glaucoma-prone anatomy, prolonged pupillary dilation, and epinephrine exposure. Plain lidocaine, anticholinergic medications, anxiety, and dilation of the eye under postoperative bandaging can also cause mydriasis and potential glaucoma (V/B).

Other ocular complications have been described. Temporary myopic changes after $CO_2$ transconjunctival blepharoplasty were reported in a case by Ogata et al. [57]. The authors believe the laser caused inadvertent thermal injury to the adjacent globe, resulting in mild deformity of the eyeball (V/B). Rosenthal and Baker [58] described activation of previously undiagnosed Graves orbitopathy after four-lid blepharoplasty (V/B). Perlman and Conn [59] presented a series of three patients with transient ophthalmoplegia during blepharoplasty. All three had dilated pupils not reactive to light or accommodative stimulus. The authors attribute the mydriasis and lack of accommodation to local anesthesia diffusing into the orbit (V/B).

Infection rarely occurs after blepharoplasty due to the extensive vascularization of the region. Moorthy and Rao [60] discussed a case of atypical mycobacterial infection after bilateral blepharoplasty. *Mycobacterium chelonae* was identified despite strict sterile technique employed during the procedure. The infection was treated with antituberculosis medications, including clarithromycin (V/B). Yang and Kim [61] published a similar case in which *Mycobacterium tuberculosis* infection occurred after eyelid surgery (V/B). Rao et al. [62] reported a parallel case of *Mycobacterium fortuitum* infection after blepharoplasty and full-face resurfacing with the $CO_2$ laser. The infection developed 2 months after blepharoplasty, making the authors believe the bacteria originated from the patient's own skin or saliva after laser ablation. The authors state it was unlikely that the bacteria was introduced exogenously during blepharoplasty (V/B). Case reports of postoperative infection with *Group A Beta-hemolytic Streptococcus* have been described. Suner et al. [63] presented a case of necrotizing fasciitis after bilateral upper blepharoplasty in a patient with diabetes mellitus (V/B). Jordan et al. [64] reported the same after four-lid blepharoplasty. In this case,

the patient's son was found to have had impetigo before the procedure (V/B). Goldberg and Li [65] described a comparable case which presented 30 h postoperatively. The authors emphasize necrotizing fasciitis is initially indistinguishable from cellulitis (V/B). A case of orbital abscess diagnosed with ultrasonography has been described by Rees et al. [66]. Early postoperative pain and edema should not be taken lightly. Immediate treatment with intravenous antibiotics, debridement, drainage, and possible hyperbaric oxygen is recommended (V/B).

Other uncommon complications have been reported. Nonsutured transconjunctival blepharoplasty incisions have been associated with the formation of pyogenic granuloma [67] (V/B), progressive multinodular eyelid lipogranuloma [68] (V/B), and cyst formation in the lower eyelid fat compartment [69]. The latter two cases were believed to be caused by direct introduction of lubricating ointment into the open wound. Kavouni recommends placing a silk suture in the center of the incision if an eye shield is being positioned for an adjunctive laser procedure. This should prevent inoculation of ointment. The suture should be removed after the eye shields are removed (V/B). Baylis et al. closed their transconjunctival incisions in their review on the technique (VI/C) [21].

## Conclusion

Blepharoplasty is a commonly performed surgery to correct dermatochalasis. Many different cutting devices can be used, including $CO_2$ laser, radiofrequency, cold steel scalpel, and electrocautery. Each offers its own advantage. Similarly, various techniques can be employed depending on the surgeon's preference and the desired outcome. Although complications are rare, they can be serious. Retrobulbar hemorrhage and blindness require immediate medical and surgical intervention. A detailed preoperative evaluation, thorough understanding of the anatomy and an anticipation of uncommon complications should lead to a pleasant experience for both the patient and surgeon.

## Evidence-Based Summary

| Findings | Evidence level |
|---|---|
| Patients undergoing blepharoplasty should have a thorough periorbital and ophthalmologic examination. They should be asked about specific medical conditions which could affect the procedure and postoperative healing | VI/C |
| Blepharoplasty may be performed post-LASIK after an interval of time | III/B |
| Patients should be told that consistent use of eye drops and lubricating ointment is necessary to prevent corneal abrasions during the initial postoperative period | VI/C |
| Compared to cold steel surgery, the $CO_2$ laser leads to improved hemostasis, reduced operative time, less bleeding, greater intraoperative visibility, and decreased ecchymosis and edema | II/A; VI/C |
| No statistically significant difference in wound healing has been found when comparing the $CO_2$ laser with cold steel scalpel, diamond laser scalpel, or the Colorado needle | II/A; VI/C |
| No statically significant difference in wound healing has been found when comparing radiosurgery with the $CO_2$ laser or conventional scalpel | II/A; V/B |
| The laser diamond scalpel and Colorado needle offer the surgeon tactile feedback | II/A |
| Malposition of the lid is the most frequently reported complication associated with transcutaneous blepharoplasty | VI/C |
| Inadequate removal of fat is the most common complication after transconjunctival blepharoplasty | VI/C |
| Patients who undergo transconjunctival blepharoplasty may experience more edema than with the transcutaneous approach | V/B |
| Eyelid malposition and visible scar formation can become a concern when transconjunctival surgery is combined with adjuvant $CO_2$ laser resurfacing or chemical peels | II/A |
| The transconjunctival approach limits the surgeon's ability to address redundant skin | V/B |
| No significant difference was found in duration of healing, inflammation, and wound complications when tissue glue was compared to running suture closure | II/A |
| Asian eyelid surgery requires modified techniques because of the unique anatomy of the Asian eyelid | VI/C |
| Patients with a predisposition to acute angle-closure glaucoma and dry-eye syndrome should be carefully considered before surgery | V/B |
| Surgeons must consider the extraocular muscles when performing blepharoplasty | V/B |
| Patients should be informed complications can occur. These complications can be ocular, structural, involve bleeding, abnormal healing, infection, and loss of vision | VI/C |
| Over-excision of upper eyelid skin can be corrected with a posterior auricular graft | V/B |
| Surgeons should be aware of delayed cases of retrobulbar hematoma and blindness | V/B |
| Surgeons should be aware of the medical and surgical treatment of retrobulbar hematoma | VI/C |
| Surgeons should achieve meticulous hemostasis to prevent postoperative hematoma | V/B |
| Damage to the optic nerve likely plays a greater role in visual loss from retrobulbar hemorrhage than damage caused by central retinal artery occlusion | V/B |

# References

1. American Academy of Facial Plastic and Reconstructive Surgery. 2006 membership survey: trends in facial plastic surgery; 2007. http://www.aafprs.org/media/stats_polls/aafprsMedia2006.pdf. Accessed 13 Jan 2009.
2. Rohrich RJ, Coberly DM, Fagien S, Stuzin JM. Current concepts in aesthetic upper blepharoplasty. Plast Reconstr Surg. 2004;113(3):32e–42.
3. American Society of Plastic Surgeons. Practice parameter for blepharoplasty; 2007. http://www.plasticsurgery.org/Medical_Professionals/Health_Policy_and_Advocacy/Health_Policy_Resources/Evidence-based_GuidelinesPractice_Parameters.html. Accessed 13 Jan 2009.
4. American Academy of Ophthalmology. Functional indications for upper and lower eyelid blepharoplasty: a report by the American academy of ophthalmology ophthalmic technology assessment committee; 1995. http://one.aao.org/CE/PracticeGuidelines/Ophthalmic_Content.aspx?cid=352adf24-e6aa-4454-839b-a10033727dbc&popup=. Accessed 13 Jan 2009.
5. Rizk SS, Matarasso A. Lower eyelid blepharoplasty: analysis of indications and the treatment of 100 patients. Plast Reconstr Surg. 2003;111(3):1299–306.
6. Trussler AP, Rohrich RJ. MOC-PSSM CME article: blepharoplasty. Plast Reconstr Surg. 2008;121 (1 Suppl): 1–10.
7. Griffin RY, Sarici A, Ayyildizbayraktar A, Ozkan S. Upper eyelid blepharoplasty in patients with LASIK. Orbit. 2006;25(2):103–6.
8. Rees TD, LaTrenta GS. The role of the Schirmer's test and orbital morphology in predicting dry-eye syndrome after blepharoplasty. Plast Reconstr Surg. 1988;82(4):618–25.
9. Fincher EF, Moy RL. Cosmetic blepharoplasty. Dermatol Clin. 2005;23(3):431–42.
10. Coleman III WP. Cold steel for blepharoplasty. Dermatol Surg. 2000;26(9):886–7.
11. Gladstone HB. Blepharoplasty: indications, outcomes, and patient counseling. Skin Therapy Lett. 2005;10(7): 4–7.
12. David LM, Sanders G. $CO_2$ laser blepharoplasty: a comparison to cold steel and electrocautery. J Dermatol Surg Oncol. 1987;13(2):110–4.
13. Morrow DM, Morrow LB. $CO_2$ laser blepharoplasty. A comparison with cold-steel surgery. J Dermatol Surg Oncol. 1992;18(4):307–13.
14. Biesman BS. Blepharoplasty: laser or cold steel? Skin Therapy Lett. 2003;8(7):5–7.
15. Baker SS, Hunnewell JM, Muenzler WS, Hunter GJ. Laser blepharoplasty: diamond laser scalpel compared to the free beam $CO_2$ laser. Dermatol Surg. 2002;28(2):127–31.
16. Rokhsar CK, Ciocon DH, Detweiler S, Fitzpatrick RE. The short pulse carbon dioxide laser versus the Colorado needle tip with electrocautery for upper and lower eyelid blepharoplasty. Lasers Surg Med. 2008; 40(2):159–64.
17. Lessner AM, Fagien S. Laser blepharoplasty. Semin Ophthalmol. 1998;13(3):90–102.
18. Niamtu III J. Radiowave surgery versus CO laser for upper blepharoplasty incision: which modality produces the most aesthetic incision? Dermatol Surg. 2008;34(7):912–21.
19. Ritland JS, Torkzad K, Juul R, Lydersen S. Radiosurgery versus conventional surgery for dermatochalasis. Ophthal Plast Reconstr Surg. 2004;20(6):423–5.
20. Kim SW, Kim WS, Cho MK, Whang KU. Transconjunctival laser blepharoplasty of lower eyelids: Asian experience with 1,340 cases. Dermatol Surg. 2003;29(1):74–9.
21. Baylis HI, Long JA, Groth MJ. Transconjunctival lower eyelid blepharoplasty. Technique and complications. Ophthalmology. 1989;96:1027–32.
22. Baylis HI, Goldberg RA, Kerivan KM, Jacobs JL. Blepharoplasty and periorbital surgery. Dermatol Clin. 1997;15(4):635–47.
23. Griffin RY, Sarici A, Ozkan S. Treatment of the lower eyelid with the $CO_2$ laser: transconjunctival or transcutaneous approach? Orbit. 2007;26(1):23–8.
24. De Castro CC. A critical analysis of the current surgical concepts for lower blepharoplasty. Plast Reconstr Surg. 2004;114(3):785–93.
25. Perkins SW, Dyer II WK, Simo F. Transconjunctival approach to lower eyelid blepharoplasty. Experience, indications, and technique in 300 patients. Arch Otolaryngol Head Neck Surg. 1994;120(2):172–7.
26. Kim EM, Bucky LP. Power of the pinch: pinch lower lid blepharoplasty. Ann Plast Surg. 2008;60(5):532–7.
27. Greene D, Koch RJ, Goode RL. Efficacy of octyl-2-cyanoacrylate tissue glue in blepharoplasty. A prospective controlled study of wound-healing characteristics. Arch Facial Plast Surg. 1999;1(4): 292–6.
28. Scaccia FJ, Hoffman JA, Stepnick DW. Upper eyelid blepharoplasty. A technical comparative analysis. Arch Otolaryngol Head Neck Surg. 1994;120(3): 827–30.
29. Kim DW, Bhatki AM. Upper blepharoplasty in the Asian eyelid. Facial Plast Surg Clin North Am. 2007;15(3):327–35.
30. Morax S, Touitou V. Complications of blepharoplasty. Orbit. 2006;25(4):303–18.
31. Glavas IP. The diagnosis and management of blepharoplasty complications. Otolaryngol Clin North Am. 2005;38(5):1009–21.
32. Fulton JE. The complications of blepharoplasty: their identification and management. Dermatol Surg. 1999;25(7):549–58.
33. DeMere M, Wood T, Austin W. Eye complications with blepharoplasty or other eyelid surgery. Plast Reconstr Surg. 1974;53:634–7.
34. Hass AN, Penne RB, Stefanyszyn MA, Flanagan JC. Incidence of postblepharoplasty orbital hemorrhage and associated visual loss. Ophthal Plast Reconstr Surg. 2004;20(6):426–32.
35. Cruz AA, Ando A, Monteiro CA, Elias Jr J. Delayed retrobulbar hematoma after blepharoplasty. Ophthal Plast Reconstr Surg. 2001;17(2):126–30.

36. Teng CC, Reddy S, Wong JJ, Lisman RD. Retrobulbar hemorrhage nine days after cosmetic blepharoplasty resulting in permanent visual loss. Ophthal Plast Reconstr Surg. 2006;22(5):388–9.
37. Yachouh J, Arnaud D, Psomas C, Arnaud S, Goudot P. Amaurosis after lower eyelid laser blepharoplasty. Ophthal Plast Reconstr Surg. 2006;22(3):214–5.
38. Kelly PW, May DR. Central retinal artery occlusion following cosmetic blepharoplasty. Br J Ophthalmol. 1980;62(12):918–22.
39. Medina FM, Pierre-Filho P, Freitas HB, Rodrigues FK, Caldato R. Blindness after cosmetic blepharoplasty: case report. Arq Bras Oftalmol. 2005;68(5):697–9.
40. Wolfort FG, Vaughan TE, Wolfort SF, Nevarre DR. Retrobulbar hematoma and blepharoplasty. Plast Reconstr Surg. 1999;104(7):2154–62.
41. Anderson RL, Edwards JJ. Bilateral visual loss after blepharoplasty. Ann Plast Surg. 1980;5(4):288–92.
42. Goldberg RA, Marmor MF, Shorr N, Chirstenbury JD. Blindness following blepharoplasty: two case reports, and a discussion of management. Ophthalmic Surg. 1990;21(2):85–9.
43. Good CD, Cassidy LM, Moseley IF, Sanders MD. Posterior optic nerve infarction after lower lid blepharoplasty. J Neuroophthalmol. 1999;19(3):176–9.
44. Brancato R, Pece A, Carassa R. Central retinal artery occlusion after local anesthesia for blepharoplasty. Graefes Arch Clin Exp Ophthalmol. 1991;229(6):593–4.
45. Kordic H, Flammer J, Mironow A, Killer HE. Perioperative posterior ischemic optic neuropathy as a rare complication of blepharoplasty. Ophthalmologica. 2005;219(3):185–8.
46. Shorr N, Goldberg RA, McCann JD, Hoenig JA, Li TG. Upper eyelid skin grafting: an effective treatment for lagophthalmos following blepharoplasty. Plast Reconstr Surg. 2003;112(5):1444–8.
47. Kushner BJ, Jethani JN. Superior oblique tendon damage resulting from eyelid surgery. Am J Ophthalmol. 2007;144(6):943–8.
48. Ghabrial R, Lisman RD, Kane MA, Milite J, Richards R. Diplopia following transconjunctival blepharoplasty. Plast Reconstr Surg. 1998;102(4):1219–25.
49. Mazow ML, Avilla CW, Morales HJ. Restrictive horizontal strabismus following blepharoplasty. Am J Ophthalmol. 2006;141(4):773–4.
50. Jameson NA, Good WV, Hoyt CS. Fat adherence simulating inferior oblique palsy following blepharoplasty. Arch Ophthalmol. 1992;110(10):1369.
51. Alfonso E, Levada AJ, Flynn JT. Inferior rectus paresis after secondary blepharoplasty. Br J Ophthalmol. 1984;68(8):535–7.
52. Schlenker JD, Slavin SA. Proptosis immediately following blepharoplasty due to an inferior rectus intramuscular hematoma. Ann Plast Surg. 2006;56(4):437–8.
53. Weinfeld AB, Burke R, Codner MA. The comprehensive management of chemosis following cosmetic lower blepharoplasty. Plast Reconstr Surg. 2008;122(2):579–86.
54. Enzer YR, Shorr N. Medical and surgical management of chemosis after blepharoplasty. Ophthal Plast Reconstr Surg. 1994;10(1):57–63.
55. Bleyen T, Rademaker R, Wolfs RC, van Rij G. Acute angle closure glaucoma after oculoplastic surgery. Orbit. 2008;27(1):49–50.
56. Wride NK, Sanders R. Blindness from acute angle-closure glaucoma after blepharoplasty. Ophthal Plast Reconstr Surg. 2004;20(6):476–8.
57. Ogata H, Kurosaka D, Nakajima T, Sasaki K, Oshiro T. Myopic change after transconjunctival blepharoplasty during carbon dioxide laser: case report. Aesthetic Plast Surg. 2005;29(4):313–6.
58. Rosenthal EL, Baker SR. Development of Graves orbitopathy after blepharoplasty. A rare complication. Arch Facial Plast Surg. 1999;1(2):127–9.
59. Perlman JP, Conn H. Transient internal ophthalmoplegia during blepharoplasty. A report of three cases. Ophthal Plast Reconstr Surg. 1991;7(2):141–3.
60. Moorthy RS, Rao NA. Atypical mycobacterial wound infection after blepharoplasty. Br J Ophthalmol. 1995;79(1):93.
61. Yang JW, Kim YD. A case of primary lid tuberculosis after upper lid blepharoplasty. Korean J Ophthalmol. 2004;18(2):190–5.
62. Rao J, Golden TA, Fitzpatrick RE. Atypical mycobacterial infection following blepharoplasty and full-face resurfacing with $CO_2$ laser. Dermatol Surg. 2002;28(8):768–71.
63. Suner IJ, Meldrum ML, Johnson TE, Tse DT. Necrotizing fasciitis after cosmetic blepharoplasty. Am J Ophthalmol. 1999;128(3):367–8.
64. Jordan DR, Mawn L, Marshall DH. Necrotizing fasciitis caused by group A streptococcus infection after laser blepharoplasty. Am J Ophthalmol. 1998;125(2):265–6.
65. Goldberg RA, Li TG. Postoperative infection with group A beta-hemolytic Streptococcus after blepharoplasty. Am J Ophthalmol. 2002;134(6):908–10.
66. Rees TD, Craig SM, Fisher Y. Orbital abscess following blepharoplasty. Plast Reconstr Surg. 1984;73(1):126–7.
67. Soll SM, Lisman RD, Charles NC, Palu RN. Pyogenic granuloma after transconjunctival blepharoplasty: a case report. Ophthal Plast Reconstr Surg. 1993;9(4):298–301.
68. Heltzer JM, Ellis DS, Stewart WB, Spencer WH. Diffuse nodular eyelid lipogranuloma following sutureless transconjunctival blepharoplasty dressing with topical ointment. Ophthal Plast Reconstr Surg. 1999;15(6):438–41.
69. Kavouni A, Stanek JJ. Lower eyelid cysts following transconjunctival blepharoplasty. Plast Reconstr Surg. 2002;109(1):400–1.

## Self-Assessment

1. Patient often seek elective eyelid surgery because they believe their eyelids make them appear:
   (a) Beautiful and charming
   (b) Fatigued and sad
   (c) Cheerful and vibrant
   (d) Intelligent and confident
   (e) Younger than their age

2. Prior to surgery, patients should be screened for all of the following *except*:
   (a) Bleeding disorders
   (b) Thyroid disease
   (c) Glaucoma risk
   (d) Ulcerative colitis
   (e) Prior refractive surgery

3. Blepharoplasty of the lower lid is commonly performed using which approach:
   (a) Transconjunctival
   (b) Transcutaneous
   (c) Transpupillary
   (d) a and b
   (e) a and c

4. True or False: Compared to the transcutaneous approach to blepharoplasty, the transconjunctival approach leads to more lower lid retraction and a more visible scar.
   (a) True
   (b) False

5. Which statement is true?
   (a) The $CO_2$ laser cannot coagulate vessels
   (b) The Colorado needle cannot provide tactile feedback
   (c) The cold steel scalpel allows coagulation
   (d) The $CO_2$ laser, Colorado needle, and radiofrequency device allow simultaneous cutting and coagulation
   (e) The $CO_2$ laser and cold steel scalpel provide tactile feedback

6. Reported complications of blepharoplasty include all of the following *except*:
   (a) Chemosis
   (b) Lagophthalmos
   (c) Decreased appetite
   (d) Eyelid cysts
   (e) Inferior rectus dysfunction

7. Proposed mechanisms of blindness following retrobulbar hemorrhage include all of the following *except*:
   (a) Retinal ischemic changes from central retinal artery occlusion
   (b) Retinal ischemic changes from compression from hemorrhage
   (c) Optic nerve ischemia caused by compression of nutrient vessels
   (d) Optic nerve damage from direct pressure from hemorrhage
   (e) Retinal detachment after metabolism of lidocaine

8. Comorbidities associated with retrobulbar hemorrhage include all of the following *except*:
   (a) Hypertension
   (b) Obesity
   (c) Increased physical activity
   (d) Postoperative vomiting
   (e) Aspirin use

9. A patient presents with proptosis, increasing eye pain and increased intraocular pressure 3 h after blepharoplasty. You suspect retrobulbar hemorrhage. You tell the patient:
   (a) This is common. Do not worry about it.
   (b) Apply ice packs overnight. Call me in the morning.
   (c) Apply ice packs overnight. Return for your scheduled suture removal appointment.
   (d) Take some acetaminophen for the pain. Elevate your head to reduce the swelling.
   (e) This is an emergency. I need to see you immediately.

10. True or False: *Streptococcus* infection of a blepharoplasty wound has never been reported in the literature.
    (a) True
    (b) False

## Answers

1. b: Fatigued and sad
2. d: Ulcerative colitis
3. d: a and b
4. b: False
5. d: The $CO_2$ laser, Colorado needle, and radiofrequency device allow simultaneous cutting and coagulation
6. c: Decreased appetite
7. e: Retinal detachment after metabolism of lidocaine
8. b: Obesity
9. e: This is an emergency. I need to see you immediately
10. b: False

# Cellulite

**25**

Jennifer L. MacGregor, Brenda LaTowsky,
Kenneth A. Arndt, and Jeffrey S. Dover

## Introduction

The term cellulite is derived from the French word *cellule*, literally meaning "small cell." It describes the dimpled appearance of skin created by pebbly subcutaneous fat that occurs in nearly all postpubertal women, most commonly on the buttocks, hips, and thighs (Fig. 25.1). Although, cellulite can appear on any area of the body with subcutaneous adipose tissue. It is not specifically associated with obesity, or any other pathologic condition, and is considered a normal variant in healthy individuals [1]. Archaic synonyms such as edematous fibrosclerotic panniculopathy, protrusis cutis, adiposis edematosa, dermopanniculosis deformans, and gynoid lipodystrophy have fallen out of favor. The designation "cellulite" has become universal in the medical literature, industry, with lay individuals, and the media. Its appearance is upsetting to many and it is a frequent complaint of those seeking cosmetic treatment in the offices of dermatologists and plastic surgeons. With progress over the past decades, we have therapies to improve many cosmetic cutaneous concerns including brown and red facial discoloration, excessive hair, rhytids, localized adiposity, and a multitude of other conditions with relatively less invasive procedures than in the past; however, the same is not true for cellulite. Patients are looking for simple, safe effective solution – and many are even willing to undergo multiple, costly procedures to improve cellulite. There has been a recent explosion in the number of devices and treatments claiming to erase, improve, or diminish cellulite, but evidence is lacking that any of these therapies can effect a long lasting change in its appearance (See Evidence-Based Summary). Some novel noninvasive modalities to shape and smooth the appearance of subcutaneous fat have transient beneficial effects and may hold promise for the future.

J.L. MacGregor (✉)
SkinCare Physicians, 1244 Boylston Street, Suite 103,
Chestnut Hill, MA 02467, USA

Division of Dermatology, Georgetown University
Hospital, Washington, DC, USA
e-mail: jmacgregor@skincarephysicians.net

B. LaTowsky
Skin Care Physicians, 1244 Boylston Street, Suite 103,
Chestnut Hill, MA 02467, USA

Paradise Valley Dermatology, Phoenix, AZ, USA

K.A. Arndt • J.S. Dover
SkinCare Physicians, 1244 Boylston Street, Suite 103,
Chestnut Hill, MA 02467, USA

Section of Dermatologic Surgery and Cutaneous
Oncology, Yale University School of Medicine,
New Haven, CT, USA

Dartmouth Medical School, Hanover, NH, USA

M. Alam (ed.), *Evidence-Based Procedural Dermatology*,
DOI 10.1007/978-0-387-09424-3_25, © Springer Science+Business Media, LLC 2012

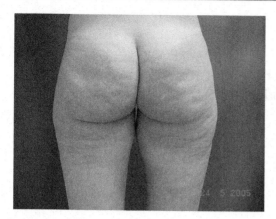

**Fig. 25.1** Dimpled appearance of cellulite on the buttocks and posterior thigh of a 24 year-old female. From Goldman et al. [49]

## The Structure and Etiology of Cellulite

The etiology and pathogenesis of cellulite is incompletely understood. It is not entirely weight related as patients who are at or near ideal body weight, who eat a well balanced diet, and exercise regularly develop cellulite. Its development is likely multifactorial and related to hormonal, genetic, anatomic, vascular, and inflammatory factors. Gender differences are well-known, with nearly all post pubertal females having some degree of cellulite. Cellulite is aggravated by pregnancy, nursing, and estrogen therapy in women, and is also seen in men with androgen deficiency, such as those with hypogonadism, Klienfelters, postcastration, those receiving estrogen for prostate cancer [2, 3]. It is almost never seen in healthy males. All races are affected, but Caucasian women seem to have more severe cellulite than Asians [4]. Lifestyle factors such as alcohol (increases lipogenesis), sedentary lifestyle, chronic stress (catecholamines stimulate lipogenesis), and smoking (alters microcirculation) may theoretically exacerbate cellulite [3]. Microcirculatory insufficiency has also been reported [3].

Anatomic differences include those that are body site specific (i.e., abdomen vs. thigh) and those related to the structure of the dermis and subcutis that are gender specific. There are differences in blood flow and lipolytic responsiveness that may explain why certain body regions are predisposed to the development of cellulite. In the gluteo-femoral region of women, as compared to abdominal fat deposits, there is weaker blood flow and an abundance of $\alpha$-2 adrenergic receptors leading to relative decrease of $\beta$-adrenergic responsiveness to catecholamines, resistance to lipolysis, and sluggish fat turnover [5, 6]. Structurally, the subcutaneous compartment is different in patients with and without cellulite. Based on analysis of adipose tissue, Nurnberger and Muller reported indentations into the deep adipose tissue through the dermis and perpendicular fibrous septae in women [1]. In contrast, the fibrous septae run in a crisscross pattern in men. Thus, the horizontal, crisscross pattern of connective tissue at the dermal-subcutaneous junction and thicker dermis prevents bulging or dimpling of fat in men (Fig. 25.2). Subcutaneous adipose tissue is thicker with larger adipocyte lobules in skin with cellulite compared with unaffected skin [7]. This principle has been confirmed by analysis of wedge biopsy specimens from affected female and unaffected male patients [8], examination of autopsy specimens [9], and by ultrasound and MRI imaging modalities [7, 8, 10, 11]. Patients with cellulite also tend toward having increased skin laxity and elastic deformation than those without [12].

## Standardizing Our Evaluation of Treatment Modalities for Cellulite

The treatment of cellulite is challenged by a lack of standardized clinical and photographic evaluation among existing studies. At the initial visit, a uniform visual assessment should be used to define clinical severity. Different clinical grading systems have been used to assess severity based on clinical appearance. Some scales for grading cellulite rely on changes in skin appearance when positioning patient from standing to laying down [1] or with and without muscular contraction or tissue compression [13]. More recently proposed clinical scales can be used without manipulating

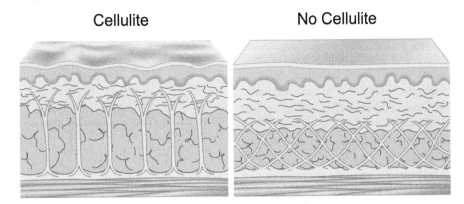

Cellulite                    No Cellulite

**Fig. 25.2** The structure of cellulite

**Table 25.1** Visual grading scale for cellulite [7]

| Grading scale | Clinical appearance |
|---|---|
| 0 | Smooth skin with no visible dimpling |
| 1 | Few number of small, shallow, sparse dimples |
| 2 | Moderate number of dimples (some large) |
| 3 | Large number of visible dimples (many large) |
| 4 | Diffuse "cottage-cheese" appearance of skin with no intervening smooth skin |

**Table 25.2** Comprehensive cellulite grading scale [14]

| Grading scale | Contour | Dimple density | Dimple distribution | Dimple depth |
|---|---|---|---|---|
| 0 | Smooth | 0 | 0 | 0 |
| 1 | 1 indent | 1–2/site | 1 site | Shallow (1–2 mm) |
| 2 | 2 indents | 3–5/site | 2 sites | Moderate (3–4 mm) |
| 3 | 3 indents | 6–8/site | 3 sites | Advanced (5–6 mm) |
| 4 | >3 indents | >9/site | 4 sites | Deep (>7 mm) |

patient position and are much more practical for blinded-rater assessments of photographs in clinical trials (Tables 25.1 and 25.2) [7, 14]. Alster and Tehrani also suggest the following practical considerations when studying new devices for cellulite: select treatment candidates with moderate, photographable skin contour irregularities of the buttock and posterior thigh, confirm patient adherence to regular diet and exercise, and lack of weight fluctuations exceeding 10 lb in the month preceding treatment [15]. Weight and body measurements should be documented and photographs should be taken as described by Gherardini et al. [16]. Standardized photography in black bikini underwear with overhead light without flash, or a single lateral light in the foreground from 75 to 90° angle to highlight skin contour irregularities is recommended [16]. Patient position for evaluation must also be consistent throughout the study as the skin and subcutaneous structures change orientation and appearance with pressure and weight bearing. Imaging modalities have improved our ability to visualize cellulite and may advance our ability to correlate clinical with radiographic improvement following treatment. Although ultrasound has been used most commonly, newer high-resolution imaging with MRI and ultrasound can clearly confirm the structure of cellulite – with superficial fat herniations through connective tissue bands into the thinned dermis in patients affected [7, 11]. Visual grades of cellulite images by both patients and physicians can also be highly correlated with quantitative three-dimensional surface roughness as measured by laser surface scanning [10]. Baseline and long-term follow-up of at least 1 year will be essential to imply sustained value for any treatment modality. With varying clinical grading scales and subjective endpoints used in most existing studies, results should be interpreted with caution.

## Treatment of Cellulite

There are no policy papers, multicenter consensus documents, or guidelines regarding the treatment of cellulite published in peer-reviewed scientific journals. There are, however, critical and detailed reviews regarding treatments, their proposed mechanism of action, and evidence for their clinical efficacy [17–19].

Recent research efforts have focused on two main goals for treating cellulite: (1) Tighten and strengthen lax connective tissue and bolster underlying subcutaneous fat; (2) Target and reduce the actual subcutaneous fat that contributes to the "lumpy" surface appearance of cellulitic skin. Traditional carbon dioxide resurfacing with ablation of the superficial layers produces a deeper zone of residual thermal damage that stimulates wound healing and collagen contracture, and tightens skin [20]. Nonablative modalities that selectively focus thermal injury into the dermis while sparing the epidermis, such as radiofrequency devices, are being explored to tighten facial skin, but may also produce similar effects in patients with cellulite [14]. Targeted reduction of subcutaneous fat with nonablative laser devices and focused ultrasound is also the subject of investigation. Anderson et al. [21] recently showed that the 1,210 and 1,720-nm wavelengths, where the absorption coefficient of human fat is greater than that of water, may allow selective heating of adipose tissue with minimal damage to surrounding structures (Fig. 25.3). There are no commercially available devices utilizing these wavelengths.

Numerous therapies including topical preparations, mechanical massage, surgical correction, and injectables have been used and popularized for the treatment of cellulite. Laser and light based technology has also been combined with massage and/or radiofrequency with transient improvement in a limited number of patients. We will focus this review on controlled trials and quality case studies of existing modalities for cellulite treatment published in peer-reviewed medical journals.

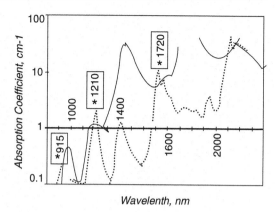

**Fig. 25.3** Infrared absorption spectra of water (*solid line*) and human fat (*dotted line*), noting approximate wavelengths where fat absorption exceeds that of water. From Anderson et al. [21]

## Randomized Controlled Trials and Meta-Analyses

### Endermologie

Endermologie (LPG, France), is a handheld massage device that was the first FDA-approved treatment for cellulite. A body stocking is worn to prevent friction between the device and the skin as it suctions the tissue between rollers to provide deep mechanical massage and can produce up to 500 mbar of low pressure [22]. It purports to increase lymphatic drainage, stimulate circulation, and disorganize the adipose tissue and smooth dimpled skin over several treatments. There are no controlled clinical studies to support this claim. In a porcine model, however, similar mechanical massage was shown to increase longitudinal collagen bundles in the deep subcutis and histologically shrink adipocytes following sequential treatments [23]. Though the Yucatan minipigs studied have a dermis and subcutis similar to that of humans, they do not suffer from cellulite and thus a clinical benefit was not assessed. Another interesting finding is that 12 sessions of Endermologie over a month induced an increase in the lipid-mobilizing effect of isoproterenol as measured by microdialysis in nine patients [24]. This may indicate an enhanced responsiveness to lipolysis, but again did not correlate clinically with a significant result.

Clinical studies with Endermologie have been disappointing to date. In a randomized, single blinded study with internal control, only 5/17 treated patients thought the Endermologie treated leg improved (V/C). The blinded investigator was only able to detect a difference in two patients [25]. Other studies claiming improvement in body circumference, and weight loss with Endermologie fail to demonstrate actual improvement in the condition of cellulite [22, 26]. The Cellu M6 (LPG, France) is a newer, roller device with suction and massage that recently received FDA approval for the treatment of lymphedema.

## Laser, Light, and Radiofrequency Devices

Table 25.3 outlines a summary of recent studies utilizing noninvasive light and radiofrequency based devices in the treatment of cellulite.

The Triactive System (Cynosure, Westford, MA) combines a low-fluence 810-nm diode laser with cooling and suction massage. It received FDA approval for the treatment of cellulite in 2004. Its limited, reported efficacy appears to depend on the presence of the 810-nm component, rather than the cooling and suction alone [27–29]. Reports of efficacy using this device vary widely and appear in uncontrolled, observational, and comparative studies with limited follow-up (IV/B) [30]. SmoothShapes 100 (SmoothShapes, Merrimack, NH) combines dual wavelength $650 \pm 20$ and $915 \pm 10$-nm light with massage. After a mean of 14 treatments delivered over 4–6 weeks, 65 patients had reduced fat thickness of 1.19 cm and improvement in appearance of cellulite in the treated leg as quantified by MRI scan measurements of fat pad dimensions [31]. The difference in fat thickness was significant as compared to massage alone at 2 weeks, but no definite improvement in cellulite contour was determined or quantified as an end point in this study (VI/C). The Synergie Aesthetic Massage

System (Dynatronics, Salt Lake City, UT) has not been studied with data published in peer-reviewed medical journals.

The VelaSmooth (Syneron Medical, Ontario, Canada and Israel) device features a combination of bipolar radiofrequency and infrared light (700–2,000 nm) emitted at up to 20 W (or J/s). It also includes mechanical rollers with 200 mbar (or 750 mmHg negative pressure) vacuum. Though treatment parameters, duration, and area size differ slightly between treatment sessions, several well-designed studies (Table 25.3) have demonstrated significant (up to 50% clinically) improvement with at least biweekly treatments over a 4-week period, though the benefits diminish in some patients over a period of 2–6 month follow-up (III/B) (Fig. 25.4a, b) [32–36]. Limited temporary improvement is a clear disadvantage to the treatment. Further studies are needed to determine if monthly treatments may maintain clinical results [32]. Reported side effects are mild and included transient erythema, bruising, and two reports of blister/burns that resolved without scarring [34, 37]. Wanitphakdeeca and Manuskiatti also report improvement in six patients treated with the VelaSmooth device using similar treatment parameters, though the data reported primarily indicates improvement in circumferential reduction and not a maintained benefit in the appearance of cellulite [37]. Though Sadick reported no histological change following treatment with VelaSmooth [35], a recent evaluation found adipocyte contraction and membrane disruption occurred within 2 h following treatment [38]. Syneron recently refined the VelaSmooth device, featuring increase in the bipolar radiofrequency component, with up to 5 mm depth of optical and 5–15 mm radiofrequency heating. The newer device is, termed VelaShape, is FDA-approved for cellulite and circumferential reduction, though studies are needed to evaluate clinical efficacy.

The Alma Accent RF System® (Alma Lasers, Israel) and ThermaCool® (Thermage, Hayward, CA) represent radiofrequency devices that were initially employed to induce tissue tightening by controlled volumetric heating of the dermis,

**Table 25.3** Devices to treat cellulite with laser, light, radiofrequency, and ultrasound: an evidence-based summary of recent studies

| Study | Device | Pts. | Design | Results |
|---|---|---|---|---|
| Controlled | | | | |
| Alster and Tanzi [32] | VelaSmooth | 20 | Controlled, split-leg, blinded-rater study of moderate thigh cellulite 8 treatments over 4 weeks (biweekly) | 90% patients improved. Rating of improvement was 50% at 1 month and diminished to approximately 25% by 6 month follow-up |
| Sadick and Magro [35] | VelaSmooth | 16 | Controlled, split-leg, blinded-rater study of thigh cellulite 12 treatments over 6 weeks (biweekly) | All patients improved. Rating of improvement was greater than 25% for more than half of patients at 2 month follow-up. No histological changes or changes in blood tests were noted |
| Romero et al. [33] | VelaSmooth | 10 | Controlled, split-leg, blinded-rater, and patient-rated study of buttock cellulite 12 treatments over 6 weeks (biweekly) | All patient and blinded-raters reported improvement at final treatment. Patients maintained satisfaction by 2 months. Not statistically significant |
| Alexiades-Armenakas et al. [14] | Accent RF system – unipolar | 10 | Controlled, split-leg, blinded-rater study of thigh cellulite – mean of 4 unilateral treatments (range 3–6) at 2 week intervals | All patients improved. At 3 month follow-up 11% grading improvement in dimple density and distribution, but only 2.5% for dimple depth. Not statistically significant |
| Lach [31] | SmoothShapes | 74 | Controlled (massage alone), randomized, split-leg study of thigh cellulite – mean of 14.3 treatments over 4–6 weeks | Fat thickness reduction was significant, but no quantification of cellulite improvement. No long-term follow-up |
| Teitelbaum et al. [41] | Contour 1 Ultrashape | 164 | Controlled, prospective study of localized adiposity over 12-week period following a single treatment to either the abdomen, thighs, or flanks (137 treated, 27 untreated) | Fat thickness reduction was significant, but no quantification of cellulite improvement. Effect achieved within 2 weeks and sustained at 12 weeks |
| Comparative | | | | |
| Nootheti et al. [30] | Triactive vs. VelaSmooth | 20 | Split-leg, blinded-rater, comparative, prospective study of grade 3 thigh cellulite 12 treatments over 6 weeks (biweekly) | 25% patients improved for both devices at 6 weeks. Rating of cellulite grade and smoothness showed no significant difference between devices. No long-term follow-up |
| Uncontrolled | | | | |
| Frew and Katz [27] | Triactive | 10 | Split leg observational study of triactive with and without diode laser component 16 treatments over | 83 vs. 17% in the laser on vs. laser off treatment sides, respectively at 1 month post treatment |
| Boyce et al. [29] | Triactive | 16 | Observational series of 12 treatments over 6 weeks (biweekly) | 21% improvement that diminished by 1 month follow-up |

(continued)

**Table 25.3** (Continued)

| Study | Device | Pts. | Design | Results |
|---|---|---|---|---|
| Sadick and Mulholland [36] | VelaSmooth | 35 | Uncontrolled**, blinded-rater, prospective study in thigh cellulite 8 treatments over 4 weeks or 16 treatments over 8 weeks (biweekly) **no comparison to untreated sites | All patients improved, with an average of 40% improvement noted 1 month after final treatment. No long-term follow-up. No histological changes observed on hemotoxylin and eosin, Masson, or van Gieson staining of biopsy specimens |
| Kulick [34] | VelaSmooth | 16 | Uncontrolled, physician-rated, prospective study in thigh cellulite 8 treatments over 4 weeks (biweekly) | All patients improved, with an average of 62% improvement at 3 and 50% at 6 months |
| Del Pino [11] | Accent RF system – unipolar | 26 | Uncontrolled, observational study in thigh and buttock cellulite 2 treatments spaced 15 days apart | 20% volumetric reduction in the subcutaneous space measured by ultrasound at 1 month (15 days after last treatment). No follow-up |
| Goldberg et al. [40] | Accent RF system – unipolar | 27 | Uncontrolled, blinded-rater, prospective study of grade 3 or 4 thigh cellulite 6 treatments at 2-week intervals | 90% patients improved an average of 2.9 points on a 4 point scale at 6 month follow-up. Histological evidence of dermal fibrosis occurred without any subcutaneous changes |
| Foster et al. [43] | Medsculpt | 5 | Uncontrolled, observational study of 12 treatments at 2 week intervals | All patients with "mild" improvement in skin tone, texture, and cellulite appearance |
| Goldman et al. [49] | Subdermal 1,064-nm Nd:YAG plus fat transplantation and triactive | 52 | Uncontrolled, observational study of combined therapy on severe thigh and buttock cellulite | 84.6% patients rated improvement as good or excellent |

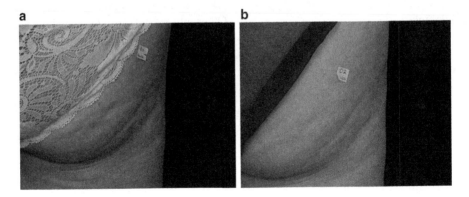

**Fig. 25.4** Posterior thigh and buttock before (**a**) and 3 months after a series of 8 twice weekly VelaSmooth treatments (**b**). From Alster and Tehrani [15]

contracture of collagen, and neocollagenesis [14, 39, 40]. Unlike optical devices that target a chromophore, radiofrequency produces heat based on the electrical resistance of tissue and specifically produces subtle damage to collagen that is then remodeled. Radiofrequency devices range from 3 to 300 kHz on the electromagnetic spectrum and deliver energy as monopolar (energy between tip and grounding plate), bipolar (energy between two points on the treatment tip), and unipolar (electromagnetic radiation delivery without the use of grounding plate). The energy travels to an approximate depth of only 2–6 mm in the bipolar mode but to 20 mm depth of penetration in the unipolar mode [11]. At this depth, the unipolar RF handpiece of the Alma Accent RF device delivers energy into the subcutaneous adipose tissue, which may account for the contraction of the subcutaneous space, collagen remodeling and neocollagenesis at the dermal-subcutaneous junction, and improvements in the appearance of cellulite observed in some studies (III/B) [11, 14, 40]. Though, no blinded controlled trials demonstrate statistically significant results, well-designed trials trend toward cellulite improvement. Alexiades-Armenakas et al. demonstrated clear clinical improvement in a controlled, split-leg, blinded-rater study of ten patients following treatment with this device [14]. These results did not reach significance based on the comprehensive cellulite grading scale (Table 25.2), but clinical evaluation was more rigorous and scientific than most other clinical cellulite studies. The side-effect profile is similar to that of other devices, but fewer treatments spaced over 2 week intervals may signify a logistical advantage over other modalities. There are no published studies evaluating the ThermaCool system for the treatment of cellulite, however, it is FDA-approved for use on the abdomen, buttocks, and thighs.

## Ultrasound

There are currently no ultrasound devices approved by the FDA for the treatment of cellulite. There has been success with noninvasive reduction of localized adiposity using focused ultrasound devices. The Contour 1 (UltraShape Ltd., Israel) emits focused ultrasound waves to induce mechanical, nonthermal acoustic energy penetration to the adipose tissue, with selective disruption of fat cells. The higher energy levels are focused to correspond with the depth of the subcutaneous fat in order to protect the epidermis and dermis from damage. A recent, controlled, pivotal phase II clinical trial of 137 patients and 27 controls evaluated patients for a 12-week

period following a single treatment to either the abdomen, thighs, or flanks [41]. There was a mean reduction of approximately 2 cm in treatment area circumference and approximately 2.9 mm in skin fat thickness as measured by ultrasound. These results were statistically significant when compared to controls at all time points, with the majority of the effect achieved within 2 weeks and sustained at 12 weeks (VI/C). There were no severe or sustained adverse events associated with treatment [41]. These results confirm the results of a smaller, uncontrolled study that found a mean 2.28 cm reduction in fat thickness at 1 month following the last of 3 monthly treatments [42]. No study has evaluated this device specifically for the treatment of cellulite appearance. The MedSculpt (Alderm, Irvine, CA) combines 850 mbar vacuum-assisted massage, with continuous sinusoidal pulsed ultrasound energy delivered at a frequency range between 2.7 and 3.3 MHz. Reductions in circumference and "mild" improvements in cellulite appearance were noted in a small observational study of 12 treatments delivered at 2-week intervals (V/C) [43]. Taken together, studies indicate that ultrasound may be useful for noninvasive body shaping, but studies to specifically address improvements in cellulite, if any, are needed. Other ultrasound devices such as SonoSculpt (LipoSonix, Bothell, WA) and Dermasonic (Symedex, Minneapolis, MN) are not yet FDA-approved and have no studies published in the peer-reviewed medical literature.

## Case Series and Cohort Studies

### Weight Reduction

Weight loss is not definitively associated with improvement in cellulite. Twenyt-eight subjects with cellulite who lost weight in a medically supervised program and eight subjects with stable weight (controls) completed a 6 month study observation period for cellulite severity and skin quality [44]. Methods of weight loss included liquid diet, medication management, bariatric surgery, liquid diet, and low-fat meals. On average, those with greater weight loss and more severe cellulite at baseline experienced some improvement in their cellulite with reduction in body mass index. The effects were highly variable and 9/28 patients (32%) experienced worsening (V/C). Those who developed more severe cellulite trended toward having smaller reductions in weight and body mass index, as well as significant increase in skin compliance (i.e., their skin became looser) as measured by elastic deformation stiffness, energy absorption, and elasticity percentage using the BTC-2000 (SRLI Technologies, Nashville, TN) [10]. While obesity may accentuate the appearance of cellulite, weight loss does not definitively improve its appearance if increases in skin laxity develop.

## Liposuction

Liposuction is a safe and effective procedure to reduce localized adiposity in the subcutaneous planes. Superficial or "subdermal" liposuction has been suggested as a method of improving cellulite [45, 46], though we know from clinical experience that it is not effective for cellulite (VI/C). Further, a complication of oversuctioning or superficial suctioning is exaggerated, sometimes linear, indentations in the skin. Internal ultrasonic assistance has been employed, with no additional benefit in the appearance of cellulite [47].

## Laser-Assisted Liposuction

Laser-assisted lipolysis is an emerging field where subdermal energy is delivered by one or several wavelengths to create photothermal energy and subsequent adipocyte lysis [48]. Diode and Nd:YAG systems have been studied to enhance adipocyte membrane disruption and facilitate fat removal. There is theoretical potential for collagen remodeling and tissue tightening with these devices, though there are no controlled or well-designed studies demonstrating clinical improvements in cellulite with the use of subdermal laser treatment alone.

## Combined Subdermal Nd:YAG Laser Lipolysis, Autologous Fat Transplantation, and Triactive (Cynosure, Westford, MA)

Subdermal Nd:YAG pulsed 1,064-nm laser (Smartlipo DEKA, Calenzano, Italy and Cynosure Westford, MA) treatment of thigh and buttock cellulite was combined with autologous fat transplantation to dimpled areas in a recent observational study of 52 female patients with severe cellulite [49]. The areas were infiltrated using tumescent technique, treated with subdermal Nd:YAG laser application (total energies ranged from 2,000 to 12,000 J), followed by microlipoinjection to the most atrophic areas, and finally treatment with the Triactive System (Cynosure, Westford, MA) during the post operative period. 84.6% of patients rated their outcome as good or excellent and follow-up ranged from 12 to 30 months during which time results were maintained (V/C). Multiple modalities were used in this study and there was no control group. Controlled, split-leg, blinded-rater studies are necessary to determine what effect, if any, could be attributed to the use of subdermal Nd:YAG 1,064-nm laser component.

## Subcision

The term subcision, described by Orentreich and Orentreich [50], is a technique whereby vertical bands of connective tissue are physically disrupted with an 18-gauge needle. Although it is more invasive than newer modalities, requires local anesthesia, and results in transient bruising and pain for up to 4 months, there was a very high patient satisfaction rate (79%) in a large observational study of 232 patients treated with subcision (IV/B) [51]. However, all patients (100%) in this study developed hemosiderin pigmentation at the site of resolving bruises that lasted up to 10 months. Despite the evidence that this may be a useful therapy for cellulite, less invasive therapies with more benign side-effect profiles are more attractive options.

## Intense Pulsed Light

Intense pulsed light (IPL) is known to induce new collagen formation in the superficial papillary dermis [52], which could theoretically strengthen dermal connective tissue and prevent the dermal fat herniations characteristic of cellulite. The Quadra Q4® IPL (DermaMedUSA, Media, PA) is a 510–1,200-nm broad band light emitting device with peak energy delivery at 585 nm. Fink et al. used IPL alone between 8 and 14 J/cm² for a total of 12 weekly treatments, or in combination with retinyl-based cream in an uncontrolled pilot study (V/C) [53]. 4/6 patients in the IPL group assessed themselves as having significant improvement, though expert evaluation or blinded photographs were not studied. Two patients did not present for their follow-up and 3/4 felt they maintained a benefit after 8 months.

## LED Plus Topical Phosphatidylcholine-Based Gel

Sasaki et al. conducted a randomized, blinded study of a phosphatidylcholine-based gel for the treatment of cellulite in nine healthy females. They included a red 660-nm and near-infrared 950-nm light (LED) device in their treatment protocol, but treated both thighs with the LED and only one with the active topical agent [54]. Thus, the thigh treated with the LED alone served as a control and any effect produced by the LED alone was not evaluated (V/C). Though 8/9 patients reported greater improvement in the thigh with the active topical at 3 months, these effects diminished in the majority of patients by the 18 month follow-up.

## Extracorporeal Pulse Activation Therapy

Extracorporeal acoustic pulses transmit energy from the point of generation a target region and have been used to stimulate circulation and improve cell permeability [55]. The effects on connective tissue were studied by Christ et al. in a pilot observational study in 59 female patients with severe thigh and buttock cellulite (IV/B). Following either 6 or 8 biweekly treatments with the C-Actor handpiece of the Cellactor SC1 device (Storz Medical AG, Tagerwilen, Switzerland) and ultrasound gel coupling, increased density in the network of collagen/elastic fibers in the dermis and subcutis was measured by ultrasound in the majority of patients at both 3 and 6 month follow-up time points [55]. Clinical improvements correlated with measured improvements, but controlled trials are needed to critically evaluate these results.

## Mesotherapy

Mesotherapy involves the injection of compounds into the subcutaneous space for the treatment of local and medical conditions [56]. The term "mesotherapy" does not denote any particular compound or medical treatment, but rather a method of drug delivery. Lipolytic activities of various compounds including: melilotus, aminophylline, yohimbine, and isoproterenol have been confirmed by in vitro analysis in a human fat cell assay, but have not been studied clinically [57]. Local anesthetics such as lidocaine have been found to inhibit lipolysis and could potentially counteract a lipolytic effect if added to a mesotherapy solution. At present, there are no FDA-approved compounds for cellulite or localized adiposity. As reviewed by Rotunda and Kolodney, phosphatidylcholine injections, including the clinically active deoxycholate component, have been shown to induce clinical and histological evidence of adipocyte lysis and fat loss in lipomas, lipodystrophy associated with HIV, infraorbital fat, trunk, chin, neck, and extremity adiposities [56]. Controlled studies using phosphatidylcholine and deoxycholate are underway to determine just how safe and effective these treatments are. At present, a clinical application for cellulite has not been established.

## Carbon Dioxide Therapy

There are reports that injecting carbon dioxide into subcutaneous tissue may reduce localized adiposities and improve circulation when used alone [58] or as a complement to liposuction [59]. Though neither study proves a specific benefit for cellulite, a significant increase in skin elasticity of 55% was reported as measured by Cuteometer skin elastic measurement (SEM) 474 before and after treatment [59].

## Pharmacotherapy

There are multiple oral and topical preparations being marketed for the treatment of cellulite, including a great number of herbal products that have never been tested. There are no reliable, consistent studies that demonstrate efficacy for any of these agents and countless products have never been evaluated for safety. Only methylxanthines (aminophylline, caffeine, and theophylline) and topical retinoids have been critically evaluated and reported to have some mild benefit, though these results are not consistent between studies [17–19]. Iontophoresis is not established as a treatment for cellulite, but is known to cause cutaneous vasodilatation [60] and has been suggested as a method to enhance the delivery and efficacy of topical anti-cellulite drugs. At present, there is no reliable data in the peer-reviewed medical literature to support the use of oral or topical agents for cellulite.

## Conclusions

Cellulite treatment is a great frontier for clinical and technological research. With recent progress, new laser, light, radiofrequency, ultrasound, and combination devices are able to temporarily improve this common cosmetic concern. However, there is a clear demand for solutions that permanently alter subcutaneous architecture and provide significant and lasting results. With new devices that combine of dermal tightening and reduction in subcutaneous adiposity, it is likely that we will be able to shape and smooth the appearance of cellulite in the very near future. Exciting research and clinical trials are underway to evaluate new therapies for cellulite.

**Evidence-Based Summary**

| Treatment | FDA approval | Mechanism of action | Evidence for efficacy |
|---|---|---|---|
| Weight reduction[a] | N/A | Decreasing fat globule protrusion into the dermis | V/C |
| Endermologie (LPG, France) | Cellulite | Handheld roller device provides deep massage in an effort to alter structure | V/C |
| Cellu M6 (LPG, France) | For lymphedema | Handheld roller device with suction and deep massage | VI/C |
| Intense pulsed light | Pigmentary and vascular lesions, textural changes and hair reduction | Light stimulation of new collagen formation and increased dermal thickness | V/C |
| Synergie Aesthetic Massage System | Cellulite | Vacuum massage ±660–880 nm probe or 880 nm pad | VI/C |
| SmoothShapes (Eleme Medical Merrimack, NH) | Cellulite | Suction and massage with 650 nm light and 915 nm laser | VI/C[b] |
| TriActive (Cynosure, Westford, MA) | Cellulite | Low-fluence 810 nm diode laser with cooling and massage | IV/B |
| VelaSmooth (Syneron Medical, Ontario, Canada and Israel) | Cellulite | Infrared light, bipolar radiofrequency, and massage | III/B |
| VelaShape (Syneron Medical, Ontario, Canada and Israel) | Cellulite and circumferential reduction | Infrared light, bipolar radiofrequency, and massage | VI/C |
| Alma Accent RF System (Alma Lasers, Israel) | Cellulite (unipolar handpiece) and tightening/rhytides on and off the face (unipolar and bipolar) | Unipolar and bipolar radiofrequency, with only the unipolar handpiece studied for cellulite | III/B |
| ThermaCool (Thermage, Hayward, CA) | For tightening/rhytides on and off the face | Monopolar radiofrequency | VI/C |
| MedSculpt (Alderm, Irvine, CA) | For cellulite | Continuous ultrasound combined with vacuum suction and massage | V/C |
| Contour I (UltraShape Ltd., Israel) | Awaiting FDA approval | Focused ultrasound | VI/C[b] |
| SonoSculpt (LipoSonix, Bothell, WA), | Awaiting FDA approval | Ultrasound, vacuum suction, and massage | VI/C |
| Dermasonic (Symedex, Minneapolis, MN) | Awaiting FDA approval | Ultrasound, vacuum suction, and massage | VI/C |
| Subcision | N/A | Disruption of vertical subcutaneous fibrous bands with 18-gauge needle | IV/B |
| Phosphatidyl choline injections | Awaiting FDA approval | Causes adipocyte lysis, cell death, fat necrosis, and reduction in size | VI/C[b] |
| Nd:YAG laser-assisted lipolysis | Multiple devices approved for laser-assisted lipolysis and surgical incision, excision, vaporization, ablation, and coagulation of soft tissues | Enhance adipocyte membrane disruption and theoretical potential for collagen remodeling and tissue tightening | VI/C |
| Cellactor SC1 device (Storz Medical AG, Tägerwilen, Switzerland) | For muscle pain and local circulation | Acoustic wave therapy applies energy to subcutaneous target and alters connective tissue | IV/B |

*N/A* not applicable

[a]Weight reduction may worsen cellulite in some patients

[b]Evidence for reduction in fat thickness but no data regarding cellulite appearance

# References

1. Nurnberger F, Muller G. So-called cellulite: an invented disease. J Dermatol Surg Oncol. 1978;4: 221–9.
2. Avram MM. Cellulite: a review of its physiology and treatment. J Cosmet Laser Ther. 2004;6:181–5.
3. Rossi ABR, Vergnanini AL. Cellulite: a review. J Eur Acad Dermatol Venereol. 2000;14:251–62.
4. Draelos ZD. In search of answers regarding cellulite. Cosmet Dermatol. 2001;14:55–8.
5. Lafontan M, Berlan M. Do regional differences in adipocyte biology provide new pathophysiological insights? Trends Pharmacol Sci. 2003;24:276–83.
6. Bjorntorp P. The regulation of adipose tissue distribution in humans. Int J Obes Relat Metab Disord. 1996;20:291–302.
7. Mirrashed F, Sharp JC, Krause V, Morgan J, Tomanek B. Pilot study of dermal and subcutaneous fat structures by MRI in individuals who differ in gender, BMI, and cellulite grading. Skin Res Technol. 2004;10:161–8.
8. Rosenbaum M, Prieto V, Hellmer J, Boschmann M, Krueger J, Leibel RL, et al. An exploratory investigation of the morphology and biochemistry of cellulite. Plast Reconstr Surg. 1998;101(7):1934–9.
9. Pierard GE, Nizet JL, Perard-Franchimont C. Cellulite: from standing fat herniation to hypodermal stretch marks. Am J Dermatopathol. 2000;22:34–7.
10. Smalls LK, Whitestone J, Kitzmiller WJ, Wicket RR, Visscher MO. Quantitative model of cellulite: three dimensional skin surface topography, biophysical characterization and relationship to human perception. J Cosmet Sci. 2005;56:105.
11. Del Pino E, Rosado R, Azuela A, Guzman G. Effect of controlled volumetric tissue heating with radiofrequency on cellulite and subcutaneous tissue of the buttocks and thighs. J Drugs Dermatol. 2006;5(8): 714–22.
12. Dobke MK, DiBernardo B, Thompson C. Assessment of biochemical skin properties: is cellulite skin different? Aesthet Surg J. 2002;22:260–6.
13. Curri SB. Las paniculopatias de estasis venosa: Diagnostico clinico e instrumental. Barcelona: Hausmann; 1991.
14. Alexiades-Armenakas M, Dover JS, Arndt KA. Unipolar radiofrequency treatment to improve the appearance of cellulite. J Cosmet Laser Ther. 2008;10: 148–53.
15. Alster TS, Tehrani M. Treatment of cellulite with optical devices: an overview with practical considerations. Lasers Surg Med. 2006;38:727–30.
16. Gherardini G, Matarasso A, Serure AS, Toledo LS, DiBernardo BE. Standardization in photography for body contour surgery and suction-assisted lipectomy. Plast Reconstr Surg. 1997;100:227–37.
17. Wanner M, Avram M. An evidence-based assessment of treatments for cellulite. J Drugs Dermatol. 2008; 7(4):341–5.
18. Rawlings AV. Cellulite and its treatment. Int J Cosmet Sci. 2006;28:175–90.
19. Van Vliet M, Ortiz A, Avram MM, Yamauchi PS. An assessment of traditional and novel therapies for cellulite. J Cosmet Laser Ther. 2005;7:7–10.
20. Ross EV, McKinlay JR, Anderson RR. Why does carbon dioxide resurfacing work? Arch Dermatol. 1999;135:444–54.
21. Anderson RR, Farinelli W, Laubach H, Manstein D, Yaroslavsky AN, Gubeli J, et al. Selective photothermolysis of lipid-rich tissues: a free electron laser study. Lasers Surg Med. 2006;38:913–9.
22. Chang P, Wiseman J, Jacoby T, Salisbury AV, Ersek RA. Noninvasive mechanical body contouring: (endermologie) a one-year clinical outcome study update. Aesthetic Plast Surg. 1998;22:145–53.
23. Adcock D, Paulsen S, Jabour K, Davis S, Nanney LB, Shack BR. Analysis of the effects of deep mechanical massage in the porcine model. Plast Reconstr Surg. 2001;108(1):223–40.
24. Monteux C, Lafontan M. Use of the microdialysis technique to assess lipolytic responsiveness of femoral adipose tissue after 12 sessions of mechanical massage technique. J Eur Acad Dermatol Venereol. 2008;22:1465–70.
25. Collins NB, Elliot LA, Sharpe C, Sharpe DT. Cellulite treatment: a myth or reality: a prospective randomized, controlled trial of two therapies, endermologie and aminophylline cream. Plast Reconstr Surg. 1999;104:1110–7.
26. Ersek RA, Mann GE, Salisbury S, Salisbury AV. Noninvasive mechanical body contouring: a preliminary clinical outcome study. Aesthetic Plast Surg. 1997;21(2):61–7.
27. Frew K, Katz B. The efficacy of a diode laser with contact cooling and suction (Triactive System®) in the treatment of cellulite. In: Presented at the 13th congress of the European Academy of Dermatology and Venerology; 2004.
28. Boyce SM. A comparison study: tri-active with and without the 800 nm diode laser component. Am J Cosmetic Surg. 2003;4.
29. Boyce S, Pabby A, Chuchaltkaren P, Brazzini B, Goldman MP. Clinical evaluation of a device for the treatment of cellulite: Triactive. Am J Cosmetic Surg. 2005;22:233–7.
30. Nootheti PK, Magpantay A, Yosowitz G, Calderon S, Goldman MP. A single center, randomized, comparative, prospective clinical study to determine the efficacy of the VelaSmooth system versus the TriActive system for the treatment of cellulite. Lasers Surg Med. 2006;38:908–12.
31. Lach E. Reduction of subcutaneous fat and improvement in cellulite appearance by dual-wavelength, low-level laser energy combined with vacuum massage. J Cosmet Laser Ther. 2008;10(4):2002–9.
32. Alster TS, Tanzi EL. Cellulite treatment using a novel combination radiofrequency, infrared light, and mechanical tissue manipulation device. J Cosmet Laser Ther. 2005;7:81–5.

33. Romero C, Caballero N, Herrero M, Ruiz R, Sadick NS, Trelles MA. Effects of cellulite treatment with RF, IR light, mechanical massage and suction treating one buttock with the contralateral as a control. J Cosmet Laser Ther. 2008;10(4):193–201.

34. Kulick M. Evaluation of the combination of radiofrequency, infrared energy and mechanical rollers with suction to improve skin surface irregularities (cellulite) in a limited treatment area. J Cosmet Laser Ther. 2006;8:185–90.

35. Sadick NS, Magro C. A study evaluating the safety and efficacy of the VelaSmooth system in the treatment of cellulite. J Cosmet Laser Ther. 2007;9:15–20.

36. Sadick NS, Mulholland RS. A prospective clinical study to evaluate the efficacy and safety of cellulite treatment using the combination of optical and RF energies for subcutaneous tissue heating. J Cosmet Laser Ther. 2004;6:187–90.

37. Wanitphakdeedecha R, Manuskiatti W. Treatment of cellulite with a bipolar radiofrequency, infrared heat and pulsatile suction device: a pilot study. J Cosmet Dermatol. 2006;5:284–8.

38. Mordon SR, Trelles MA. Adipocyte membrane lysis observed after cellulite treatment is performed with radiofrequency. Aesthetic Plast Surg. 2009;33:125–8.

39. Sukal SA, Geronemus RG. Thermage: the nonablative radiofrequency for rejuvenation. Clin Dermatol. 2008;26:602–7.

40. Goldberg DJ, Fazeli A, Berlin AL. Clinical, laboratory, and MRI analysis of cellulite treatment with a unipolar radiofrequency device. Dermatol Surg. 2008;34(2):204–9.

41. Teitelbaum SA, Burns JL, Junichiro K, Hidenori M, Otto MJ, Shirakabe Y, et al. Noninvasive body contouring by focused ultrasound: safety and efficacy of the contour I device in a multicenter, controlled, clinical study. Plast Reconstr Surg. 2007;120(3):779–89.

42. Moreno-Mraga J, Valero-Altes T, Riquelme AM, Isarria-Marcosy MI, de la Torre JR. Body contouring by non-invasive transdermal focused ultrasound. Lasers Surg Med. 2007;39:315–23.

43. Foster KW, Douba DJ, Hayes J, Freeman V, Moy RL. Reductions in thigh and infraumbilical circumference following treatment with a novel device combining ultrasound, suction, and massage. J Drugs Dermatol. 2008;7(2):113–5.

44. Smalls LK, Hicks M, Passeretti D, Gersin K, Kitzmiller JW, Bakhsh A, et al. Effect of weight loss on cellulite: gynoid lypodystrophy. Plast Reconstr Surg. 2006;118(2):510–6.

45. Gasperoni C, Gasperoni P. Subdermal liposuction: long-term experience. Clin Plast Surg. 2006;33:63–73.

46. Gasparotti M. Superficial liposuction: a new application of the technique for aged and flaccid skin. Aesthetic Plast Surg. 1992;16:141–53.

47. Igra H, Satur N. Tumescent liposuction versus internal ultrasonic-assisted lipoplasty. Dermatol Surg. 1997;23:1213–8.

48. Parlette EC, Kaminer MS. Laser-assisted liposuction: here's the skinny. Semin Cutan Med Surg. 2008;27(4):259–63.

49. Goldman A, Gotkin RH, Sarnoff DS, Prati C, Rossato F. Cellulite: a new treatment approach combining subdermal Nd:Yag laser lipolysis and autologous fat transplantation. Aesthet Surg J. 2008;28(6):619–26.

50. Orentreich DS, Orentreich NA. Subcutaneous incisionless (subcision) surgery for the correction of depressed scars and wrinkles. Dermatol Surg. 1995;21:543–9.

51. Hexsel DM, Mazzuco R. Subcision: a treatment for cellulite. Int J Dermatol. 2000;39:539–44.

52. Goldberg DJ. New collagen formation after dermal remodeling with an intense pulsed light source. J Cutan Laser Ther. 2000;2:59–61.

53. Fink JS, Mermelstein H, Thomas A, Trow R. Use of intense pulsed light and a retinyl-based cream as a potential treatment for cellulite: a pilot study. J Cosmet Dermatol. 2006;5:254–62.

54. Sasaki GH, Oberg K, Tucker B, Gaston M. The effectiveness and safety of topical PhotoActif phosphatidylcholine based anti-cellulite gel and LED (red and near-infrared) light on Grade II–III thigh cellulite: a randomized, double-blinded study. J Cosmet Laser Ther. 2007;9:87–96.

55. Christ C, Brenke R, Sattler G, Siems W, Novak P, Daser A. Improvement in skin elasticity in the treatment of cellulite and connective tissue weakness by means of extracorporeal pulse activation therapy. Aesthet Surg J. 2008;28(5):538–44.

56. Rotunda AM, Kolodney MS. Mesotherapy and phosphatidylcholine injections: historical clarification and review. Dermatol Surg. 2006;32:465–80.

57. Caruso MK, Roberts AT, Bissoon L, Self S, Guillot TS, Greenway FL. An evaluation of mesotherapy solutions for inducing lipolysis and treating cellulite. J Plast Reconstr Aesthet Surg. 2008;61:1321–4.

58. Brandi C, D'Aniello C, Grimaldi L, Bosi B, Dei I, Lattarulo P, et al. Carbon dioxide therapy in the treatment of localized adiposities: clinical study and histopathological correlations. Aesthetic Plast Surg. 2001;25(3):170–4.

59. Brandi C, D'Aniello C, Grimaldi L, Caiazzo E, Stanghellini E. Carbon dioxide therapy: effects on skin irregularity and its use as a complement to liposuction. Aesthetic Plast Surg. 2004;28(4):222–5.

60. Asberg A, Holm T, Vassborn T, Andreassen AK, Hartmann A. Nonspecific vasodilation during iontohoresis is attenuated by application of hyperosmolar saline. Microvasc Res. 1999;58:41–58.

# Non-Invasive Body Contouring

## 26

### Misbah H. Khan, Neil S. Sadick, and Babar K. Rao

## Introduction

Body contouring or soi-disant Liposculpting is an effective method for surgically improving localized subcutaneous areas of adiposity. The idea of removing excess fat from skin is not new [1]. In 1921 Charles Dujarrier, in France, attempted to remove subcutaneous fat using a uterine curette on a dancer's calves and knees. A tragic result occurred due to injury of the femoral artery leading to amputation of one of the dancer's legs. Today, liposculpting can be safely performed in an office setting. Conservative techniques ensure fewer complications. Substantial amounts of subcutaneous fat can be contoured with acceptable esthetic outcomes using minimally invasive methods.

Tumescent liposuction using suction cannulas is among the most common cosmetic procedures in the United States [2] (V/B). A conservative estimate is that there are 300,000–400,000 procedures performed in the US annually. Despite its overwhelming popularity, the risk of serious complications due to its invasive nature remains of significant concern. Complications ranging in spectrum from prolonged swelling, areas of numbness, bruising, persistent erythema to abdominal perforation [3], thrombophlebitis, and pulmonary embolism have been reported [4] (V/B).

Greater demand in body esthetic medicine for noninvasive procedures has motivated researchers to develop new techniques to replace traditional treatments for body contouring. Transdermally focused ultrasound, radiofrequency (RF), laser-assisted lipolysis, and selective cryolipolysis are the leading technologies for improving the appearance of body silhouette noninvasively. Focusing (ultrasound), greater intensity in subcutaneous fat (laser, RF), and/or concurrent application of cooling are used to generate maximum effects of emitted energy below the surface at the level of fatty tissue. The selectivity of such modalities is achieved by the physical interaction between the tissue and emitted energy.

We discuss herein some of the commonly employed noninvasive procedures used for body contouring.

## Intradermally Focused Ultrasound

Although postliposuction ultrasound has been recommended for many years in an attempt to facilitate healing, interest in using therapeutic ultrasound in liposuction preoperatively for fat dissolution is relatively recent. Moy published

M.H. Khan (✉)
Department of Dermatology, Weill Cornell
Medical College, New York, NY, 10075, USA
e-mail: mkhan@sadickdermatology.com

N.S. Sadick
Weil Medical College,
Cornell University, New York, NY, USA
e-mail: nssderm@sadickdermatology.com

B.K. Rao
Department of Dermatology, Robert-Wood Johnson
University Hospital, University of Medicine
and Dentistry New Jersey, New Brunswick, NJ, USA

M. Alam (ed.), *Evidence-Based Procedural Dermatology*,
DOI 10.1007/978-0-387-09424-3_26, © Springer Science+Business Media, LLC 2012

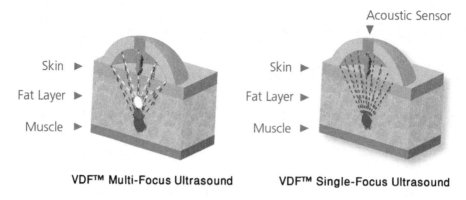

**Fig. 26.1** Cross-section of the contour I transducer, courtesy of UltraShape Ltd., TelAviv, Israel

the first report of this [5] and Cook published a second favorable report in December 1997 [6].

## Mechanism of Action of Ultrasound Assisted Liposculpting (UAL)

In a conducive setting, ultrasonic energy affects tissue destruction through three mechanisms: cavitation, micromechanical disruption, and thermal damage. It is thought that cavitation is predominantly responsible for tissue destruction in internal ultrasound assisted liposculpting (UAL). It is postulated that external ultrasound prior to liposuction works either through thermal or micromechanical effects [7].

A nonablative thermal treatment would not be expected to have a significant or durable effect on fat. In fact, external nonfocused therapeutic ultrasound has been applied to body contouring but was found to be effective only as an adjunct to tumescent liposuction, improving tissue hydration and distribution of the tumescent solution [8]. In the context of benefits and drawbacks of previously available therapeutic ultrasound technology, Contour I UltraShape™ system was designed to be noninvasive and focused, but well-tolerated for office based use without the need for any sedation or anesthesia, downtime or recovery period.

Transdermally focused Contour I UltraShape™ (Tel Aviv, Israel) uses focused ultrasound to deliver a finite amount of acoustic energy at a controlled distance from the ultrasound transducer to achieve noninvasive body contouring.

Ultrasound energy is emitted from a hemispherical transducer (Fig. 26.1). In this geometry, the energy is low near the transducer surface and is concentrated in an additive manner at a distant focus. The transducer is placed directly on the skin and focuses the energy at the depth of the subcutaneous fat. As a result, the energy can be delivered through the skin, with low energy density at the epidermis and dermis, and with a high energy density in the subcutaneous fat. The ultrasound energy is delivered in pulses, using parameters that provide a nonthermal effect. High levels of ultrasound energy within the subcutaneous fat can disrupt adipose tissue safely and effectively, as has been demonstrated in ultrasound-assisted liposuction. A unique central tracking and guidance system provides a crucial element of safety and quality control. A real-time video image of the treatment area is displayed on the LCD monitor. The tracking component captures the region of interest and generates a treatment algorithm, such that each spot is treated once and only once. The tracking system does not allow a pulse of energy to be delivered outside the region that the physician marked before initiating the treatment, obviating the potential for accidental treatment in undesired areas.

## Therapeutic Utility of UAL

A method of delivering ultrasound to the fat without depositing significant ultrasound energy in the skin provides the benefits of ultrasound disruption of fat with greater safety. Furthermore, noninvasive method of delivering energy reduces periprocedural morbidity such as infection, scarring, anesthesia-related complications, and other risks associated with surgical procedures.

One of the largest studies conducted by Teitelbaum et al. [9] (III/B) was the pivotal clinical trial that demonstrates the safety and efficacy of the Contour I (UltraShape Ltd., Tel Aviv, Israel), a noninvasive device for body contouring. One hundred and sixty-four healthy volunteers were enrolled in this prospective, comparative study conducted at five centers (two in the United States, one in the United Kingdom, and two in Japan) between August of 2004 and June of 2005, designed to assess the safety and efficacy of a single treatment with the Contour I system at different body areas (abdomen, thighs, or flanks). One hundred and thirty-seven study subjects were treated while 27 served as controls. The results of their multicenter study revealed that a single treatment resulted in a mean circumference reduction of 1.9 cm at 12 weeks, with a response rate of 82%. In the experimental (treated) group, the mean circumference reduction from baseline was significant at all time points except day 1 ($p<0.001$ on days 14, 28, and 84; $p=0.223$ on day 1). Approximately 77% of the observed circumference reduction occurred within 14 days of treatment. The response of the abdomen, thighs, and flanks was comparable. They also found no statistically significant difference in the mean circumference reduction at any of these treatment areas [abdomen, $-2.3\pm 0.32$ cm, flanks, $-1.8\pm0.31$ cm, thighs, $-1.6\pm0.39$ cm; differences among sites, not significant ($p= 0.366$)]. The response of men and women was similar, with a mean circumference reduction of 1.8 cm in women and 2.2 cm in men on day 84 ($p=0.368$).

Safety assessments including various laboratory testing such as complete blood count, serum chemistry (sodium, potassium, creatinine, urea, calcium), fasting lipids (total cholesterol, high-density lipoprotein, low-density lipoprotein, and triglycerides), liver markers (alanine aminotransferase, aspartate aminotransferase, lactate dehydrogenase, alkaline phosphatase, total bilirubin, albumin), and complete urinalysis were performed at each visit. No clinically significant treatment-associated changes in laboratory values were observed. Notably, no treatment-induced elevations in serum lipids or lipoprotein levels were detected in any of the study participants. Approximately, 85% of the reduction in fat thickness occurred within 14 days of treatment shows a representative sonogram, demonstrating a 4-mm reduction in fat thickness at day 14.

A prospective study conducted by Moreno-Moraga et al. [10] (II/A) on 30 adult healthy volunteers using Contour I UltraShape™ however showed significant reduction in the subcutaneous fat within the treated areas after three treatments, performed at 1-month intervals. The mean reduction in fat thickness as measured by ultrasound was found to be approximately 3.0 cm with a mean circumferential reduction on the treated areas of $3.95\pm1.99$ cm. They also reported no adverse effects or significant changes in laboratory values of lipids and liver enzymes. The authors of this particular study recommended multiple treatments combined with appropriate patient selection in order to achieve significant results.

Although Contour I UltraShape™ is widely used for noninvasive body contouring, data regarding the long-term efficacy and persistence of satisfactory results is still lacking. Whether the treated patients will require regular treatments for maintenance of achieved results indefinitely, is still a query.

## Laser-Assisted Lipolysis (LAL)

Laser lipoplasty with pulsed neodymium, yttrium, aluminum, garnet (Nd:YAG) laser, also called interstitial laser lipolysis was first described in 1994 [11] (III/A). This technique is widely used in Europe and Latin America, and has recently been introduced in Japan and the United States. Less trauma, bleeding, and pain have been the main advantages of this technique.

The Nd: YAG laser was proposed first for use in laser lipolysis because of the penetration depth of its wavelength (1,064 nm). However, diode lasers, which can typically emit at 810, 940, and

980 nm, offer an alternative. Their wavelengths are in the same spectral region, and they offer the advantages of higher efficiency (usually 30%) and higher power (25 W or more). The absorption spectrum of mammalian fat obtained by van Veen et al. [12] using three independent methods show that the absorption coefficient obtained with a wavelength of 980 nm is very similar to that obtained with a wavelength of 1,064 nm. Similarly, coefficients of human fatty tissue reported by Altshuler et al. [13] were found to be very similar. Nowadays pulsed Nd:YAG (1,064 nm, SmartLipo, Deka Italy) and continuous wave (CW) diode (980 nm, Pharaon, Osyris, France) are both employed for laser-assisted lipolysis (LAL).

## Mechanism of Action of Laser Lipolysis

The mechanisms leading to laser lipolysis are temperature dependent. A histologic analysis performed by Zulmira et al. [14] compared traditional liposuction with LAL on the same patient. Their analysis showed areas of reversible cellular damage (tumefaction), irreversible cellular damage (lysis), and a reduced intensity of bleeding, as compared with the tissue products of conventional liposuction. The degree of tumefaction and lysis varied proportionally with the intensity of energy accumulated to the target.

Another study on the effects of laser lipolysis was done by Ichikawa et al. [15] (III/B), done on freshly excised human subcutaneous fat exposed to pulsed Nd:YAG laser at 150 mJ and 100 μs. Scanning electron microscopy after irradiation showed greater destruction of human adipocytes than in the control. Degenerated cell membrane, vaporization, liquefaction, carbonization, and heat-coagulated collagen fibers were observed.

The effects of human adipocytes to pulsed Nd:YAG laser vs. CW 980 nm diode were compared histologically by Mordon et al. [16]. Their work showed that at low-energy settings, tumescent adipocytes were observed. At higher energy settings, cytoplasmic retraction, disruption of membranes, and heat-coagulated collagen fibers were noted; coagulated blood cells were also present.

For the highest energy settings, carbonization of fat tissue involving fibers and membranes was clearly seen. For given energy settings, 1,064 and 980-nm wavelengths gave similar histologic results.

## Therapeutic Utility of Laser Lipolysis

Laser lipolysis is a new technique still under development. The use of 1,064 nm-Nd:YAG and the 980-nm diode laser as an auxiliary tool has refined the traditional liposuction technique. Under local tumescent anesthesia, a small puncture is made in the skin and laser light is conveyed through the insertion of a micro-cannula of 1 mm diameter into which an optical fiber has been inserted. Red aiming beam at the tip guides the surgeon. The subcutaneous fat is then liquefied by back and forth movement of the cannula. Due to small size of cannulas used for LAL, the procedure is considered minimally invasive. Delicate areas of fat such as face, arms, medial thighs, knees, and upper abdomen are preferred areas of treatment.

A randomized and prospectively analyzed double blinded clinical trial was performed by Prado et al. [17] (II/B), which compared LAL with traditional liposuction side by side.

Laser-assisted lipoplasty and suction-assisted lipoplasty sides of 25 patients were compared with preoperative and postoperative photographs at 3–5 days, 12–15 days, and 6–11 months. Statistical analysis considered surgeon and patient satisfaction, time used in the procedures, learning curves, lipocrits, operative technique, postoperative pain, edema, ecchymosis, time of recovery, body mass index, DNA proteins, free fatty acids, and cytologic patterns of post–laser-assisted lipoplasty and suction-assisted lipoplasty adipocyte architecture. Photographs were sent to the patients (blinded to the operated sides) and two plastic surgeons unfamiliar with the cases for evaluation of results.

No complications were observed among the study participants. Less pain, higher triglycerides, and DNA cellular membrane traces were detected in the laser-assisted lipoplasty sides. Cytologic studies showed more damage of the adipocytes in the laser-assisted lipoplasty sides. All other considerations studied showed no differences with either technique in the three periods of the follow-up controls. Their study clearly revealed no significant differences in the sites treated with LAL vs. traditional liposuction. However, the elevated triglycerides observed in their study participants treated with LAL warn caution if chosen as a preferred treatment method.

A recently published retrospective study done by Katz and McBean [18] evaluated 537 patients treated with LAL with tumescent anesthesia between January 2006 and November 2007 at a single center, to determine the number of adverse events associated with the procedure and number of touch-up procedures performed (V/B). Their analysis reported a complication rate of 0.93%. These included one local infection and four skin burns. The rate of touch-up procedures was 3.5%.

The authors recommend LAL as a safe and useful adjunct to tumescent liposuction. Smaller size of cannulas limits the ability of this technology to be used on areas other than face, medial arms, knees, peri-umbilical and perhaps medial thighs as a sole treatment.

## Selective Cryolipolysis

Cooling is commonly employed to protect the epidermis during laser or intense pulsed light treatments without any therapeutic effects per se. In contrast, cryosurgery is widely used for nonselective destruction of actinic keratosis, warts, lentigines, superficial benign and malignant tumors, etc. Cell death occurs due to a rapid decrease in intracellular water below the freezing point of tissue water [19].

There is evidence that adipose tissue is selectively sensitive to cold injury. A rare entity of cold-induced fat necrosis of the newborns and infants called "popsicle panniculitis" has been described in the literature [20]. The most likely mechanism hypothesized when popsicle panniculitis was first described, is that crystallization of cytoplasmic lipids in adipocytes occurs at temperatures well above the freezing point of tissue water.

## Proposed Mechanisms of Selective Cryolipolysis

Cryolysis of fatty tissue is possible due to biological selectivity. Biologic selectivity is referred to a specific response (e.g., inflammation) that is confined to a certain tissue (e.g., fat).

The potential for tissue-specific cold injury was first investigated and recently reported by Anderson and coworkers [21] in an animal model. Black Yucatan pigs were exposed to temperatures of 20, −1, −3, −5, and −7°C for 10 min using the Zeltiq prototype device (Zeltiq, Pleasonton CA). At 3.5 month follow-up, some treated areas showed grossly obvious loss of several millimeters of subcutaneous fat. The investigators did not find any significant change in serum lipid values.

The investigators of this study clearly concluded that a delayed, cold-induced lobular panniculitis is involved; presumably in response to direct cold-induced injury of adipocytes, In this study, inflammation and adipose tissue loss were well correlated. Both proceeded for many weeks following a single, local exposure to cold, reaching an apparent maximum at 4 weeks after and resolving about 3 months after cold exposure. In its early inflammatory phase, panniculitis may further damage adipocytes. In its later phase however, phagocytosis appears to account for removal of adipocytes and loss of fat tissue.

Temperature and time of application are both important to induce selective cryolysis of fatty tissue. A skin surface temperature as high as −1°C induced within the various tested anatomical locations in average a mild superficial panniculitis, and the anatomic depth of panniculitis and of fat loss was increased when lower temperatures are applied.

Several factors seem to play a significant role in the "lipid ice" formation further leading to cryolysis. Of interest is the fact that pig fat solidifies and crystallizes at 10°C, as well as the triglycerides;

depending upon the chain length, cooling rate and degree of saturation [22]. Crystallization requires energy, which is expressed as latent heat of freezing.

In the aforementioned study by Anderson and coworkers [21], the investigators found that the rate of temperature decrease in superficial fat during treatment with a flat applicator, changes at around 10°C. This deflection is consistent with a latent heat exchange due to crystallization of adipocyte lipids. It appears that heat must be extracted from the fat, not only to cool it, but also to crystallize it. Taken together, these observations suggest but do not prove that lipid crystallization is responsible for selective injury to adipose tissue.

## Therapeutic Challenges of Selective Cryolysis

Many important details about selective cryolysis remain to be studied. Most importantly, there is not enough information available in published literature regarding the mechanisms of adipocyte injury in adult humans when sub-zero temperatures are applied to a fold of skin suctioned in between two cold applicators, for varying times.

Certain dermatoses such as sclerema neonatorum, subcutaneous necrosis of the newborn popsicle panniculitis and steroid panniculitis, all characterized by needle shaped crystal formation within adipocytes, are by far most commonly seen in infants. Subcutaneous fat of the infants is more prone to developing crystals due to higher concentration of saturated fatty acids such as palmitic and stearic acids, as compared to unsaturated fatty acids such as oleic acid, seen in adults [23]. The increased saturated to unsaturated fatty acid ratio results in a higher melting point for stored fat and promotes crystallization under certain conditions. Microsized crystals (type A) are too small to elicit an inflammatory reaction. However, larger crystals (type B) are arranged in rosettes and are capable of inducing an inflammatory response characterized by lobular panniculitis. Spontaneous resolution of these lesions is the rule, sometimes in association with lipoatrophy.

Work done by Anderson and coworkers [21] suggests that lipid crystallization is perhaps responsible for lipoatrophy seen in their Yucatan pig models. This mechanism will pose challenges to the development of selective cryolysis for clinical use, as pigs have a higher content of saturated compared to unsaturated fatty acids. Additionally, it is not apparent that the intracellular crystals seen in adipocytes were large enough to elicit the inflammatory panniculitis, largely responsible for producing the effects.

At this point, we know little or nothing about the longevity of the fat lost as a result of selective cryolysis. The possibility of fat regenerating itself after a certain period of time still remains. Additional mechanisms, such as oxidative stress or reperfusion injury [24] (V/B) responsible for adipocyte death, might also play a role in loss of subcutaneous volume.

Finally there is a question of the "fate of fat." Although in the study done by Anderson and coworkers [21] no significant rise in serum lipids was seen, the possibility of fatty infiltration of liver cannot be excluded. Histologic analysis revealed shrunken adipocytes and lipid laden macrophages suggesting that perhaps apoptosis and phagocytosis of adipocytes is responsible for their localized loss. This process is likely to follow usual pathways for adipocyte tissue turnover, which accounts for 10% of body fat recycling each year.

The authors of this chapter believe that potentially, selective cryolysis, might develop into a clinical alternative treatment for fat removal. Selective cryolysis warrants further human studies as a local treatment for subcutaneous adiposities.

## Bipolar and Unipolar Radiofrequency Devices

Recently, noninvasive devices employing RF technology have gained acceptance and supremacy in the treatment of cellulite and localized adiposities. These include the TriActive (Cynosure,

USA) and Velasmooth (Syneron Medical Ltd., Israel). Of the available devices with RF only, VelaSmooth has been approved by the FDA specifically for cellulite treatment. The TriActive laser combines low-energy diode laser, contact cooling, suction, and massage. This system has been shown to reduce cellulite [25]. The VelaSmooth combines infrared light (700–2,000 nm) bipolar RF and suction, and mechanical massage.

## Mechanisms of Action of Radiofrequency Devices for Fat Removal

The precise mechanism by which the two systems work is yet to be elucidated. Bipolar RF devices are based on the principle of heat generation as a result of poor electrical conductance, according to the Ohms Law:

$$H = J2\rho \text{ (heat generation is directly correlated with tissue resistance).}$$

Generated heat is strong enough to cause thermal damage to the surrounding adipose tissue and connective tissue septae.

Bipolar RF devices have a penetration depth of >3 mm and allow for better control and localized adipose tissue alteration.

Unipolar devices utilize high frequency electromagnetic radiation (EMR). High frequency EMR induces high frequency rotational oscillations in water molecules which in turn produce heat, i.e., greater the presence of water, greater is the tissue heat generation. The depth and breadth of thermal damage is greater and in a rather diffuse pattern with little control than bipolar RF devices. End result is the creation of dermal fibrosis or so-called "appearance-enhancing scarring" that leads to long-term improvement after fewer treatments.

Unipolar and bipolar RF technologies also exist as combination Accent/ Alma device (Alma lasers, Buffalo Groove, IL).

## Therapeutic Applications of Radiofrequency Devices

In the largest study of VelaSmooth, Sadick evaluated 35 patients who completed either 8 or 16 treatments with VelaSmooth [26] (III/B). A blinded dermatologist evaluated the photographs and found 40% improvement on average.

A more recent study of VelaSmooth found a statistically significant decrease in thigh circumference at 4 weeks, but no immediate change or a persistent decrease at 8 weeks [27] (V/B). Visual improvement of less than 50% was noted in the majority of subjects. 31% of the subjects experienced bruising.

Work done by Goldman and coworkers [28] (V/B) compared the efficacy of treatment of cellulite using two novel modalities, TriActive vs. VelaSmooth. Patients were treated twice weekly for 6 weeks with either VelaSmooth or TriActive. They calculated a 28 vs. a 30% improvement rate, respectively, in the upper thigh circumference measurements, while a 56 vs. a 37% improvement rate was observed, respectively, in lower thigh circumference measurements. Statistical significance of these results was $p > 0.05$. Incidence and extent of bruising was higher in VelaSmooth than in TriActive system which may be attributed to mechanical manipulation.

Like the VelaSmooth, the Alma Accent RF system (Alma lasers, Buffalo Groove, IL) and ThermaCool (Thermage, Hayward, CA) utilize RF and maybe useful in the treatment of cellulite. Both the Accent and ThermaCool are FDA approved for the treatment of wrinkles and rhytides. The ThermaCool is a unipolar RF, while the Accent system is a unipolar and bipolar RF device. Of the two devices, only Accent system has been evaluated for the treatment of localized adiposities. Study done by Goldberg et al. [29] (V/B) used Accent unipolar RF device for cellulite treatment. Their study included subjects with higher grade cellulite of upper thighs. They were treated every other week for a total of six treatments. Results obtained 6 months after the last treatment showed an average 2.45 cm reduction in thigh circumference with minimal side effects, and no changes in serum lipid abnormalities and MRI were seen. They attribute their longer lasting effects to the formation of dermal fibrosis in the upper dermis and increased contraction between the dermis and camper's fascia, which has been previously reported in ultrasound imaging studies [30]. The presence of thickened dermal fibrous band or so-called "scarring" is concerning regarding long-term effects. As it is known that postmenopausal women tend to lose more weight in the femoral area as compared to premenopausal women, who tend to gain more. For women who would undergo unipolar RF treatment in their reproductive years might lose weight later on. Since scarring induced by unipolar RF devices is permanent, long-term improvement is questionable and concerning.

# Conclusions

Noninvasive body contouring techniques such as transdermally focused ultrasound, LAL, and RF devices can be a safe, effective, and well-tolerated alternative to conventional invasive tumescent liposuction for body contouring. These techniques can be a safer choice for patients who decline or are not suitable candidates for surgical approaches to body contouring. Selective cryolipolysis is a new and emerging technology on the horizon; several aspects of which need to be studied in greater depth. The concept of cryolipolysis has a potential to be one of the most exciting techniques that can be utilized for noninvasive lipolysis with minimal down time. However, to this date, there is limited data available to support this theory in a clinical setting.

Based on the published literature, noninvasive body contouring is rather more effective for individuals at or near their ideal body weight; who desire treatment of localized adiposities. It is not a treatment for obesity. We recommend all patients to adopt and maintain a healthy lifestyle in order to retain the effects of treatment.

### Evidence-Based Summary

| Findings | Evidence level |
| --- | --- |
| Even though traditional tumescent liposuction is one of the most commonly performed cosmetic procedures, serious adverse events such as abdominal perforation, thrombophlebitis, and pulmonary embolism have been reported | (V/B) |
| Noninvasive body contouring is an acceptable alternative for patients who are at or near their ideal body weight and desire treatment for localized adiposities. It is not a treatment for obesity | (III/B) |
| Transdermally focused ultrasound technology can be used for body contouring with acceptable outcomes. However, the number of treatments required to achieve and maintain the desired effects is still under investigation | (III/B) |
| Laser-assisted lipolysis is a safe and useful adjunct to tumescent liposuction for larger body surface areas | (II/B) |
| Although selective cryolysis is a new and emerging technology for noninvasive lipolysis, the precise mechanism of action and its utility as a useful clinical tool is still under investigation | (IV) |
| Unipolar and bipolar Radiofrequency devices are used for noninvasive contouring of cellulite prone areas with grossly visible results. The long-term efficacy of this technology and maintenance of achieved results is still being investigated | (V/B) |

# References

1. Flynn T, Coleman WP, Filed LM, Klein JA, Hanke W. History of liposuction. Dermatol Surg. 2000;26: 515–20.
2. Coleman III WP, Hanke CW, Glogau RG. Does the speciality of the physician affect fatality rates in liposuction? A comparison of specialty specific data. Dermatol Surg. 2000;26:611–5.
3. Talmor M, Hoffman LA, Lieberman M. Intestinal perforation after suction lipoplasty; a case report and review of literature. Ann Plast Surg. 1997;38: 169–72.
4. Bernstein G, Hanke CW. Safety of liposuction; a review of 9478 cases performed by dermatologists. J Dermatol Surg Oncol. 1988;14:1112–4.
5. Havoonjian HH, Luftman DB, Menaker GM, et al. External ultrasonic tumescent liposuction: a preliminary study. J Dermatol Surg. 1997;23:1201–6.
6. Cook Jr WR. Utilizing external ultrasonic energy to improve the results of tumescent liposculpture. J Dermatol Surg. 1997;23:1207–12.
7. Lawrence N, Coleman III WP. Ultrasonic-assisted liposuction, internal and external. Dermatol Clin. 1999;17(4):761.
8. Silberg BN. The technique of external ultrasound-assisted lipoplasty. Plast Reconstr Surg. 1998;101(2): 552.
9. Teitelbaum SA, Burns JL, Kubota J, et al. Noninvasive body contouring by focused ultrasound: safety and efficacy of the Contour I device in a multicenter controlled clinical study. Plast Reconstr Surg. 2007;120(3): 779–89.
10. Moreno-Moraga J, Valero-Altes T, Riquelme MA, Issarria-Marcosy MI, Royo de la Torre J. Body contouring by non-invasive transdermal focused ultrasound. Lasers Surg Med. 2007;39:315–23.
11. Apfelberg DB, Rosenthal S, Hunstad JP, Achauer B, Fodor PB. Progress report on multicenter study of laser-assisted liposuction. Aesthetic Plast Surg. 1994;18(3):259–64.
12. van Veen RL, Sterenborg HJ, Pifferi A, Torricelli A, Chikoidze E, Cubeddu R. Determination of visible near-IR absorption coefficients of mammalian fat using time-and spatially resolved diffuse reflectance and transmission spectroscopy. J Biomed Opt. 2005;10:054004.
13. Altshuler GB, Anderson RR, Manstein D. Method and apparatus for the selective targeting of lipid-rich tissues. Boston: Massachusetts General Hospital Corporation; 2003.
14. Zulmira A, Badin ED, Luciana BE, Gondek M, Choppa L, Fabiane BZ, et al. Analysis of laser lipolysis effects on human tissue samples obtained from liposuction. Aesthetic Plast Surg. 2005;29(4):281–6.
15. Ichikawa K, Miyasaka M, Tanaka R, Tanino R, Mizukami K, Wakaki M. histologic evaluation of the pulsed Nd:YAG laser for laser lipolysis. Lasers Surg Med. 2005;36(1):43–6.
16. Mordon S, Eymard-Maurin AF, Wassmer B, Ringot J. Histologic evaluation of laser lipolysis: pulsed 1064 nm laser versus CW 980 nm diode laser. Aesthet Surg J. 2007;27(3):263–8.
17. Prado A, Andrades P, Danilla S, Leniz P, Castillo P, Gaete F. A prospective randomized controlled double blinded clinical trial comparing laser-assisted lipoplasty with suction assisted lipoplasty. Plast Reconstr Surg. 2006;118(4):1032–45.
18. Katz B, McBean J. Laser-assisted lipolysis: a report on complications. J Cosmet Laser Ther. 2008;17:1–3.
19. Karow Jr AM, Webb WR. Tissue freezing. A theory for injury and survival. Cryobiology. 1965;2(3): 99–108.
20. Epstein Jr EH, Oren ME. Popsicle panniculitis. New Engl J Med. 1970;282(17):966–7.
21. Manstein D, Laubach H, Watanabe K, Farinelli W, Zurakowski D, Anderson RR. Selective cryolysis: a novel method of non-invasive fat removal. Lasers Surg Med. 2008;40:595–604.
22. Sventrup G, Bruggemann DB, Kristensen L, Risbo J. The influence of pretreatment on pork fat crystallization. Eur J Lipid Sci Technol. 2005;107(9):607–15.
23. Fretzin DF, Arias AM. Sclerema neonatorum and subcutaneous fat necrosis of the newborn. Pediatr Dermatol. 1987;4:112–22.
24. Nishikawa H, Gower JD, Fryer PR, Charlett A, Manek S, Green CJ. Ultrastructural changes and lipid peroxidation in rat adipomusculocutaneous flap isotransplants after normothermic storage and reperfusion. Transplantation. 1992;54(5):795–801.
25. Boyce S, Pabby A, Brazzini B, Goldman MP. Clinical evaluation of a device for the treatment of cellulite: TriActive. Am J Cosmetic Surg. 2005;22:233–7.
26. Sadick NS, Mulholland RS. A prospective clinical study to evaluate the efficacy and safety of cellulite treatment using the combination of optical and RF energies for subcutaneous tissue heating. J Cosmet Laser Ther. 2004;6:187–90.
27. Sadick NS, Margo C. A study evaluating the safety and efficacy of the Velasmooth system in the treatment of cellulite. J Cosmet Laser Ther. 2007;9:15–20.
28. Nootheti PK, Magpantay A, Yosowitz G, Calderon S, Goldman MP. A single center, randomized comparative, prospective clinical study to determine the efficacy of the VelaSmooth system versus the Triactive system for the treatment of cellulite. Lasers Surg Med. 2003;38:908–12.
29. Goldberg D, Fazeli A, Berlin A. Clinical, laboratory and MRI analysis of cellulite treatment with a unipolar radiofrequency device. J Dermatol Surg. 2008; 34(2):204–9.
30. del Pino M, Rosado RH, Azuela A, et al. Effects of controlled volumetric tissue heating with radiofrequency on cellulite and the subcutis of the buttocks and thighs. J Drugs Dermatol. 2006;5:714–22.

## Self-Assessment

1. Which of the following is the most mechanism(s) of action of ultrasound assisted liposculpting?
   (a) Cavitation
   (b) Micromechanical disruption
   (c) Thermal damage
   (d) a and b
   (e) a, b, and c

2. Laser lipolysis can be preferably used as the sole technique for the treatment of which of the following areas?
   (a) Lateral thighs
   (b) Large pendulous abdomen
   (c) Calves
   (d) Localized areas such as neck, face, and knees
   (e) Essentially any area can be treated with lasers

3. Mechanism of laser-assisted lipolysis is:
   (a) Evaporation of adipocytes
   (b) Thermal necrosis of adipocytes
   (c) Cytoplasmic retraction, disruption of membranes, and heat-coagulated collagen fibers
   (d) a and b
   (e) None of the above

4. Panniculitis characterized by needle shaped crystals within the adipocytes include which of the following?
   (a) Sclerema neonatorium
   (b) Steroid panniculitis
   (c) Popsicle panniculitis
   (d) Subacute fat necrosis of the newborn
   (e) All of the above

5. Selective cryolysis is a new and evolving technology that causes adipocyte damage by virtue of:
   (a) Causing adipocyte rupture
   (b) Creating cold-induced skin necrosis
   (c) Causing intense vasospasm leading to ischemia
   (d) Selective adipocyte necrosis by causing intracellular crystallization followed by an inflammatory response
   (e) Mechanism of action of selective cryolysis is unclear

## Answers

1. e: a, b and c
2. d: Localized areas such as neck, face, and knees
3. c: Cytoplasmic retraction, disruption of membranes, and heat-coagulated collagen fibers
4. e: All of the above
5. d: Selective adipocyte necrosis by causing intracellular crystallization followed by an inflammatory response

# Index

M. Alam (ed.), *Evidence-Based Procedural Dermatology*,
DOI 10.1007/978-0-387-09424-3, © Springer Science+Business Media, LLC 2012

prophylactic systemic antibiotics
administration, 180
case series and cohort studies, 183–185
consensus documents, 181–182
herpes simplex virus (HSV) reactivation, 181
randomized controlled trials and meta-analyses, 185–186
wound treatment
case series and cohort studies, 196
CDC guidelines, 195
dermatologic procedures, 195
dermatologic surgery, 194, 195
evidence-based summary, 196–197
Gram's stain and culture, 194
infection risk, 196
meta-analyses, 196
MRSA, 194
NICE stress, 194
postoperative monitoring, 194
substantial edema, 194
Prolopenko, I., 297
Prophylactic systemic antibiotics
administration, 180
case series and cohort studies, 183–185
consensus documents, 181–182
herpes simplex virus (HSV) reactivation, 181
randomized controlled trials and meta-analyses, 185–186
Prophylaxis
antibiotic, 183
antimicrobialv, 183
dermatologic surgery, 181
dosage, 184
high-risk cardiac conditions, 181
infected tissue, 182
Provan, A., 143
Provost, N., 45
Psomas, C., 409
Pulsed dye laser (PDL)
and $CO_2$, 151
copper based technologies, 215–216
ice pick scars, 163
KTP, 226
585 nm, 219
585-nm and 595-nm, 162
photodynamic therapy, 216
scar texture, 161
second-generation, 216
settings, 226
treatment, 225
Pulzi, P., 150
Punjabi, S., 50

**Q**

Q-switched laser
Becker's nevus, 236
melanin-containing epidermis, 236
pigmented lesions, 236
scar-free elimination, 237
Quaedvlieg, P.J.F., 66, 67

**R**

Rabinovitz, H., 12
Rachel, J.D., 186
Radakovic-Fijan, S., 106, 107
Rademaker, R., 411
Radiation
microscopic nodal disease, 92–93
monotherapy, 92
Radiofrequency (RF)
Accent, 293
dermal heating, 291
ThermaCool
Asian skin, 292
eyelid rejuvenation, 293
Fitzpatrick Wrinkle Classification Scale (FWCS), 291–292
Leal Laxity Classification System, 292
tissue tightening
Accent system, 289
appropriate candidate, 289
company-supplied grid, 289
cryogen cooling system, 288
devices, 288
electrocautery, 287
energy output, 288
ThermaCool TC™ system, 288
Rahimi, A.D., 396
Rahman, Z., 169
Randall, P.E., 188
Randle, H.W., 19
Randolph, M.A., 303
Rand, R., 338
Rao, B.K., 433
Rao, J., 412
Rao, N.A., 412
Rassman, W.R., 377, 380
Rassner, G., 63
Ratner, D., 11, 18, 19, 33
Ratz, J.L., 19
Rau, K.A., 260, 261
Rawnsley, J.D., 379
Rayatt, S.S., 18
Rebrin, I., 325
Recovery, 271
Recurrence
BCC
low *vs.* high risk factors, 36
and metastasis, 36
cryosurgery ranges, 81
decription, 91
disease progression, 62
local, 65
margins, 92
Mohs surgical technique, 81
rates, 78
SCC, risk factors, 59
Reddy, S., 409
Red light, 104
Reed, J.T., 261
Rees, T.D., 405, 412
Reifenberger, J., 47

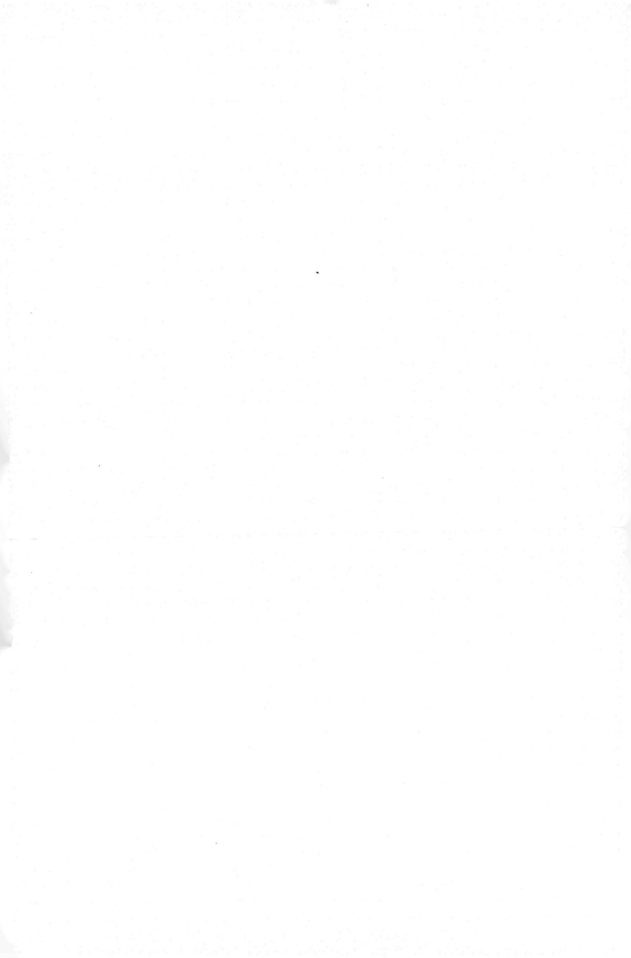

CPSIA information can be obtained
at www.ICGtesting.com
Printed in the USA
LVOW02*2329120516

488030LV00004B/5/P

9 780387 094236